# Neuroscience for Addiction Medicine: From Prevention to Rehabilitation

# Neuroscience for Addiction Medicine: From Prevention to Rehabilitation

Editor: Lois Rivera

FOSTER ACADEMICS

www.fosteracademics.com

www.fosteracademics.com

FOSTER ACADEMICS

**Cataloging-in-Publication Data**

Neuroscience for addiction medicine : from prevention to rehabilitation / edited by Lois Rivera.
p. cm.
Includes bibliographical references and index.
ISBN 978-1-64646-577-4
1. Substance abuse--Treatment. 2. Neurosciences--Therapeutic use. 3. Addicts--Medical care.
4. Addicts--Rehabilitation. 5. Substance abuse--Physiological aspects.
6. Compulsive behavior--Treatment. I. Rivera, Lois.
RC564 .N48 2023
362.29--dc23



Foster Academics,
118-35 Queens Blvd., Suite 400,
Forest Hills, NY 11375, USA

ISBN 978-1-64646-577-4 (Hardback)

# Contents

# Preface

Addiction refers to a complex and chronic brain illness influenced by the environment and genes. It is characterized by substance abuse or compulsive behaviors that persist despite negative consequences. Commonly abused substances include intoxicants like heroin and alcohol, and milder stimulants like nicotine and caffeine. Addiction is recognized as a mental illness and it causes significant economic, health, and social difficulties. Addiction medicine is a subspecialty of medicine that involves the diagnosis, evaluation, prevention, and treatment of addiction. Neuroscience can be used to study the brain mechanisms behind behaviors related to addiction, in order to further the understanding of the addictive processes. It also studies the actions of drug abuse. This book aims to understand the role of neuroscience in the field of addiction medicine. It covers in detail some existent theories and innovative concepts revolving around the prevention and rehabilitation of addictive behaviors. The readers would gain knowledge that would broaden their perspective with respect to this area of medicine.

This book has been the outcome of endless efforts put in by authors and researchers on various issues and topics within the field. The book is a comprehensive collection of significant researches that are addressed in a variety of chapters. It will surely enhance the knowledge of the field among readers across the globe.

It gives us an immense pleasure to thank our researchers and authors for their efforts to submit their piece of writing before the deadlines. Finally in the end, I would like to thank my family and colleagues who have been a great source of inspiration and support.

**Editor**

# 1

# Increased Neural Activity in Hazardous Drinkers during High Workload in a Visual Working Memory Task: A Preliminary Assessment through Event-Related Potentials

*Elisa Schroder†, Clémence Dousset†, Xavier Noel, Charles Kornreich and Salvatore Campanella**

*Laboratoire de Psychologie Médicale et d'Addictologie, ULB Neuroscience Institute (UNI), CHU Brugmann-Université Libre de Bruxelles (U.L.B.), Brussels, Belgium*

***Correspondence:**
*Salvatore Campanella*
*salvatore.campanella@chu-brugmann.be or salvatore.campanella@ulb.ac.be*

*†These authors have contributed equally to this work.*

Despite equated behavioral performance levels, hazardous drinkers generally exhibited increased neural activity while performing simple cognitive tasks compared to light drinkers. Here, 49 participants (25 hazardous and 24 light drinkers) participated in an event-related potentials (ERPs) study while performing an *n*-back working memory task. In the control zero-back (N0) condition, the subjects were required to press a button when the number "2" or "6" was displayed. In the two-back and three-back (N2; N3) conditions, the subjects had to press a button when the displayed number was identical to the number shown two/three trials earlier. To assess for the impact of alcohol consumption on the updating of working memory processes under various cognitive loads, difference waveforms of "N2 minus N0" and "N3 minus N0" were computed by subtracting waveforms in the N0 condition from waveforms in the N2 and N3 conditions, for the light and the hazardous drinkers. Three main ERP components were noted for both groups: a P200/N200 complex, a P300 component, and an N400/P600 activity. The results show that, to perform the task at the same level as the light drinkers, the hazardous drinkers exhibited larger amplitude differences, mainly around the P300 and P600 components. These data may be considered, at the preventive level, as vulnerability factors for developing adult substance use disorders, and they stress the importance, at a clinical level, to consider such working memory processes in the management of alcohol dependence.

**Keywords: heavy social drinking, alcohol, working memory, cognitive workload, *n*-back task, event-related potentials**

## INTRODUCTION

Working memory (WM), the capacity to store information in short-term registers and simultaneously manipulate it online, is required for most key daily living activities such as planning, engaging in active conversation, or solving complex problems (1). At the functional level, three categories covering most of the functions indexing WM have been well-described: storage and processing, executive processes, and coordination (2). Indeed, one of the main characteristics of WM refers to a capacity limited mental workspace used to store and process information for use in ongoing cognition (3). This WM load is, therefore, a reasonable measure of the cognitive effort dedicated to holding information in mind for short periods of time while performing a cognitive task (4). It was traditionally proposed by Miller (5) as the "magical number seven plus or minus two" items that can be remembered. Neuroimaging studies have shown that when the WM load exceeds the individual short-term memory capacity, the dorsal prefrontal cortex (PFC)—in addition to ventral PFC regions—may be recruited to mediate strategic processes necessary for the maintenance of a high WM load [e.g., Ref. (6)]. In recent years, there has been considerable debate regarding the notion of a capacity limitation in WM as well as on whether mechanisms of interference, rather than capacity limits, might explain performance limitations [e.g., see Ref. (7)]. Also, WM executive processes refer to three main functions identified as mental set shifting (e.g., the ability to shift from one task to another one), inhibition of prepotent responses (e.g., the ability to suppress a dominant motor response), and information updating (e.g., the ability to update relevant information compared to nonrelevant ones in WM) (8). A third important role of WM is to coordinate elements and build new relations to integrate them into structures (e.g., representing different visual objects in a three-dimensional space). These three different functional facets can be isolated and described on their own. Nevertheless, WM functions as a whole, and all these different facets interact for higher level processes (2). The main point we will focus on here is that *individual differences in WM load* correspond to fundamental differences in *executive control skills* [e.g., Ref. (9)] that might impact some dysfunctional behaviors such as impulsive decision-making typically observed in addictive behaviors [e.g., Ref. (10)].

In dual-process neurocognitive models, the persistence of heavy alcohol consumption results from a) an abnormal bottom-up system generating craving and automatic alcohol-approach tendencies; paired with b) an abnormal top-down system generating reduced cognitive control upon long-term prospects [e.g., Ref. (11)]. The underlying neural mechanisms of these phenomena are defined by increased dopamine release in the cortico-striatal reward circuit triggered by drug stimuli [e.g., Ref. (12)], which draws the subject's attention to the drug-related stimulus [e.g., Ref. (13)], while hypoactivation of frontal regions indicates that alcoholics lack the executive resources needed to inhibit the salient and dominant response [e.g., Ref. (14)]. In this view, a lot of empirical research has been devoted to the role of neurocognitive processes such as cue reactivity [e.g., see Ref. (15) for a meta-analysis] or inhibitory skills [e.g., see Ref. (16) for a review] in the onset, development, and persistence of heavy alcohol consumption. Indeed, both of these processes appear to be promising targets for interventions aimed at treating patients with alcohol disorder [e.g., Refs. (17, 18)].

However, WM capacity has also been shown to impact cognitive control of impulsivity by way of keeping future goals in mind when making decisions when faced with rewarding/arousing distractions (19). This fits perfectly with the dual-process model of cognitive control, whereby executive functions are used to regulate bottom-up implicit arousal responses (14, 20). Indeed, a threshold of PFC activation is needed for effective modulation of bottom-up processes, and is associated with WM [e.g., Ref. (21)]. In such a view, low WM capacity can exacerbate the worse impulse control that results from excessive consumption of alcohol [e.g., Ref. (22)], by triggering poor inhibition of immediate behavior as well as poor longer-term planning of future options (10). Chronic heavy users of alcohol often exhibit lower levels of WM capacity [e.g., Refs. (23, 24)]. However, although some of these deficits appear to result from heavy alcohol use [e.g., Ref. (25)], there is also evidence suggesting that low capacity WM problems contribute to the development of alcohol abuse [e.g., Ref. (26)]. WM deficits are then considered to contribute to the core pathology of addiction [e.g., Ref. (14)]. Indeed, Brooks and colleagues conducted a review yielding 93 studies that examined WM and cognitive control, between 2010 and 2017, in patients with substance use disorders (SUD; including stimulants such as nicotine, opioids, and marijuana, and alcohol use). The majority of the studies (72%) reported worse WM performances compared to healthy drug-naive controls or nondrug-taking control groups. From these insights, training WM has been shown to be highly relevant for reducing stimulant (27) as well as alcohol use [e.g., Ref. (28)] by increasing control over automatic impulses, even though different training techniques appear to produce differential impacts on the broader landscape of cognitive abilities (3). Indeed, there is some evidence that suggests that nonsequential and nonadaptive training paradigms should not be effective (29), while "core training programs" using tasks that commonly involve sequential processing and frequent memory updating appear to produce more far-reaching transfer effects, most likely because they target domain-general mechanisms of WM (3). A good illustration of such a training program relates to *the n-back task*, which requires continuous upgrades of the memory store (i.e., a memory updating process) and which is particularly suited for the study of varying levels of WM load (30).

This *n*-back task requires online monitoring, updating, and manipulation of remembered information, and it is, therefore, assumed to place great demands on a number of key processes within WM subtended by widespread neural areas (31). Indeed, frontal regions have been implicated in numerous cognitive functions that are relevant to the *n*-back task, including monitoring and manipulation within WM (32); the parietal cortex is thought to be involved in the implementation of stimulus-response mapping (33) and in the storage of WM contents (34) as a kind of "buffer for perceptual attributes" (35); while activation of the precuneus during the visual WM task is consistent with a recollection process aided by visual imagery (36), and insula activation is considered to be a part of the inferior frontoparietal network, which responds to behaviorally relevant rather than to expected stimuli (37).

This task has been extensively tested in heavy alcohol users to outline WM disturbances linked with high workloads, but it yielded heterogeneous results. Indeed, decreased PFC activation and worse WM were observed, for instance, in adolescent alcohol users [e.g., Ref. (38)] and in youths with a family history of alcoholism (FHA) (39). However, while many functional magnetic resonance imaging (fMRI) studies have reported insignificant differences in behavioral performances between healthy control groups and heavy alcohol users, significant neural differences can be discerned by including brain imaging measures [e.g., Refs. (40–42)], indexing compensatory neural processing during variation in cognitive load (43). The bulk of the reported data consisted of *reduced* activation of the PFC network (including insula, cerebellar, anterior cingulate, and/or parietal regions) in alcoholic patients [e.g., Refs. (40, 44)] or (conversely) *increased* PFC network activation in heavy social drinkers (i.e., people characterized by excessive alcohol consumption, without a clinical state of dependence) (42, 45, 46). According to a "functional compensation view," decreases or absences in activation reflect deficits in brain function, and the concomitant increases in activation reflect "attempted" or "successful" compensation for these deficits (47). Aside from fMRI studies, differences in electrophysiological [electroencephalogram (EEG)] components are considered to be sensitive indicators of workload (48, 49). Indeed, a decrease in alpha power is associated with an increase in arousal, resource allocation, or workload [e.g., Ref. (50)], and an increase in theta power (most profound over frontal electrodes) has been observed as task requirements increase [e.g., Ref. (51)]. Event-related potentials (ERPs), derived from EEGs, also convey relevant information about an individual's workload. Throughout the information processing stream, ERP components such as the P100 [e.g., Ref. (52)], the N100 [e.g., Ref. (53)], the N200 (54), a positive/negative component between 140 and 280 ms (55), and the P300 [e.g., Ref. (56)] have been shown to be modulated by the WM workload and task difficulty. By using a visual task with a high WM load (57, 44) or through a spatial 2-back task (58), several ERP studies have determined that memory load capacity is affected in heavy users of alcohol.

However, to our knowledge, there has not been a study to date that specifically investigated the impact of *increasing visual memory load* on neural activity in healthy vs. heavy alcohol users based on ERPs. In light of its high temporal resolution, we sought to define whether increasing WM visual load specifically impacts hazardous vs. light drinkers at specific time intervals throughout the information processing stream. To address this, we chose 1) to use a visual WM *n*-back task (N = 0; 2; or 3), forcing subjects to continuously remember the last two or three rapidly changing items, to induce different levels of visual workload; and 2) to compare light versus heavy social drinkers, as done previously in an fMRI experiment (only comparing N2 vs. N0 conditions) suggesting increased pre-supplementary motor area, PFC, and cerebellar activations in heavy drinkers despite similar behavioral performances (42). In the present ERP study, increasing memory load was applied to participants through N2 and N3-back tasks, and this parametric manipulation of the task variable (visual memory workload) was compared in light vs. heavy alcohol drinkers by use of a subtraction method (N2 minus N0; N3 minus N0) that is well-known to index specific WM processes such as storage and manipulation (updating) (34). Light and hazardous drinkers were enrolled in the study as our aim was to show the potential differences induced by different alcohol consumption patterns (rather than between drinkers and nondrinkers). This strategy appears to be congruent with most earlier studies on heavy social drinking (e.g., cited in this paper) (57, 59), where the control group was composed of light drinkers. Moreover, recent studies have shown that control teetotalers appear to represent a specific population that results in unexpected results (e.g., worse executive performance) (60), which constitutes an additional reason to avoid including nondrinkers in the present study. Our main hypotheses are that 1) light and heavy alcohol drinkers will exhibit similar behavioral performances [see Ref. (61) for a review]; and 2) compared to light drinkers, the higher the memory load, the more that heavy drinkers will recruit neural resources. Moreover, as a result of the optimal temporal resolution of ERPs compared to fMRI (62), a precise temporal window can be defined for this enhanced neural activity recruitment. Such results could have the highest relevance at a prevention level, as these under-investigated WM load processes (compared to executive or cue-reactivity ones) in alcohol disorders could index "biological vulnerability factors" that may trigger further onset of alcohol dependence.

## MATERIALS AND METHODS

### Participants

First, we conducted a general screening of 120 students from the Faculty of Psychology of the University of Brussels (Belgium) in order to ascertain sociodemographic variables (age, gender, education level, and native language) and patterns of alcohol consumption. On the basis of these self-reported data, groups of participants were defined as detailed below. Exclusion criteria for participants included major medical issues, conditions relating to impairment of the central nervous system (including epilepsy and a prior history of brain injury), visual impairments, and past or current drug consumption (other than alcohol and tobacco use). Our main objective was to select two groups of participants who only exhibited differences in terms of their alcohol-drinking patterns (see **Table 1** for the complete descriptive data). Therefore, subjects concurrently consuming cannabis (defined as at least once in the month prior to the study) were not included. Also, a similar number of participants with a family history of alcoholism (FHA) (63) were included in the final groups (only one by group). In line with earlier studies [e.g., Refs. (42, 59, 64, 65)], three variables (self-reported by participants through the use of a timeline follow-back method questionnaire assessing alcohol–drug consumption characteristics) were used to determine control and heavy alcohol user groups: the mean number of drinking occasions per week (DOW: "how many times do you typically consume alcohol in a week?"), the mean number of alcohol doses per drinking occasion (ADO: "how many drinks do you generally consume during one drinking occasion?"), and the mean number of alcohol doses per week (ADW: "how many drinks do you generally consume in a week?"; one dose corresponding to 10 g of pure ethanol). According to the definition of binge drinking used in European countries, participants who drank six or more standard alcoholic drinks (10 g of alcohol) on the same occasion at a rate of at least two drinks per hour and at most two or three times per week were classified as hazardous drinkers. Those who drank 1 to 30 days a month, but never more than five standard alcoholic drinks on the same occasion and at a maximum rate of two drinks per hour, were classified as controls. This classification was confirmed utilizing the AUDIT-C consumption subscore, which is defined by three items of the complete 10-item AUDIT instrument (66), and which can help identify people who are hazardous drinkers (67). The AUDIT-C is scored on a scale 0–12. A score of 3 for women and 4 for men is considered optimal for identifying hazardous drinkers; the higher the score, the more likely the drinking pattern affects the participants' safety (68). Hazardous drinking, which can significantly impact public health despite the absence of any *bona fide* disorder in the individual users, is defined as a level of alcohol consumption that is likely to result in harm to the user or other individuals (69).

In order to ensure that any potential difference in the ERP data would be due to alcohol consumption and not to other variables, the groups were balanced for age, gender, and level of education (i.e., the number of years of education completed since starting primary school). The participants were also asked to fill out questionnaires assessing psychological measures. These were the State-Trait Anxiety Inventory (STAI A and B) to assess state and trait anxiety (70); the Beck Depression Inventory (BDI-II) (71) to assess depression; and the Urgency Premeditation Perseverance and Sensation Seeking Impulsive Behavior Scale (UPPS) (72), which is a measure of impulsivity as a personality trait. Control of all of these variables is important, as drinkers with depression, anxiety, as well as high impulsivity symptoms have been shown to be at increased risk of developing alcohol dependence (73–75). Therefore, it can be seen that the participants of both groups did not exhibit any difference in terms of these variables (see **Table 1**). Indeed, based on these criteria, 60 undergraduate students were selected for the ERP study and classified as light ($n$ = 30) or heavy (hazardous) drinkers ($n$ = 30). Among these, 11 participants exhibiting EEG artifact contamination were removed. Therefore, the final groups were represented by 24 light and 25 hazardous drinkers. We obtained informed written consent from the participants after they were fully informed about the study. The local ethics committee of the Brugmann Hospital approved the study ("Comité d'Ethique Hospitalier CE 2010/156"). The participants were instructed to abstain from consuming alcohol in the 24 h before the ERP recording.

## Working Memory *n*-Back Task

WM performance and the underlying neural activity were measured using a visual $n$-back task under three different conditions. The stimuli were white numbers (Arial font, size 74) displayed on a black background on the center of the screen, presented successively in a pseudo-random order. In the vigilant/control zero-back (N0) condition, the subjects were asked to press a button with their right hand whenever the number "2" was displayed (block 1) or "6" (block 2). In the WM two-back (N2) and three-back (N3) conditions, the subjects had to press the button when the displayed number was identical to the number displayed two or three trials earlier (see **Figure 1** for an illustration). The subjects were successively administered two blocks in the N0 condition, then two blocks in the N2 and two blocks in the N3 conditions. This order was kept constant across the participants in order to ensure that all of the groups were exposed to exactly the same manipulation of tasks with increasing complexity (from N0 to N2 and then N3). Each N0 block consisted of a sequence of 80 trials (including 20 targets), while the N2 and N3 conditions consisted of a sequence of 86 (104) trials, respectively, also including 20 targets each. Each stimulus was displayed for 1,750 ms with an interstimulus interval of 250 ms. This way, 40 targets were available for each condition across the participants. The pseudo-random order ascertained that, in N0, two targets were not successively presented; and, in N2 and N3, that the same number was not repeatedly used as a target (but instead varied randomly from 1 to 9). All of the participants performed one practice block for each condition (N0, N2, and N3).

## EEG Recordings

During the ERP recordings, each participant sat alone in a darkened room, on a chair placed 1 m from the screen. EEG activity was recorded with 32 electrodes mounted on a Quick-Cap and placed in standard (based on the 10–20 system) and intermediate positions (Fpz, Fp1, Fp2, Fz, F3, F7, F4, F8, FC1, FC5, FC2, FC6, Cz, C3, C4, T7, CP5, CP1, CP2, CP6, T8, P7, P3, Pz, P4, P8, POz, O1, Oz, and O2). Recordings were made with a linked mastoid physical reference. The EEG was amplified

**TABLE 1** | The light and the hazardous drinkers were equivalent in terms of age, gender, depression [Beck Depression Inventory (BDI)-II scores], anxiety [State-Trait Anxiety Inventory (STAI)-trait and STAI-state scores], and impulsivity [Urgency Premeditation Perseverance and Sensation Seeking Impulsive Behavior Scale (UPPS) total score] (all $p$'s > 0.05). The two groups differed solely on alcohol variables: the Alcohol Use Disorders Identification Test - Alcohol Consumption questions (AUDIT-C) subscore [$t(47) = -10.836$; $p < 0.001$], the mean number of alcohol doses per drinking occasion (ADO), the mean number of drinking occasions per week (DOW), and the mean number of alcohol doses per week (ADW).

| | Light drinkers ($n$ = 24) | Hazardous drinkers ($n$ = 25) | *T* value | *P* value |
|---|---|---|---|---|
| Age | 26.79 ± 9.3 | 23.96 ± 2.4 | 1.442 | 0.161 |
| Gender (M/F) | 11/13 | 13/12 | $\chi^2 = 0.186$ | 0.666 |
| AUDIT-C | 2.92 ± 1.2 | 6.76 ± 1.2 | −10.836 | <0.001 |
| ADO | 0.95 ± 0.6 | 2.12 ± 1.3 | −3.977 | <0.001 |
| DOW | 1.71 ± 1.2 | 5.16 ± 2.4 | −6.236 | <0.001 |
| ADW | 1.8 ± 1.5 | 7.3 ± 4.9 | −5.255 | <0.001 |
| BDI-II | 6.92 ± 4.9 | 5.36 ± 4.3 | 1.171 | 0.248 |
| STAI-trait | 46.54 ± 8.8 | 44.72 ± 9.1 | 0.712 | 0.48 |
| STAI-state | 46.67 ± 9.6 | 43.92 ± 6.4 | 1.177 | 0.245 |
| UPPS | 101.67 ± 12.1 | 105.36 ± 11.195 | −1.108 | 0.273 |

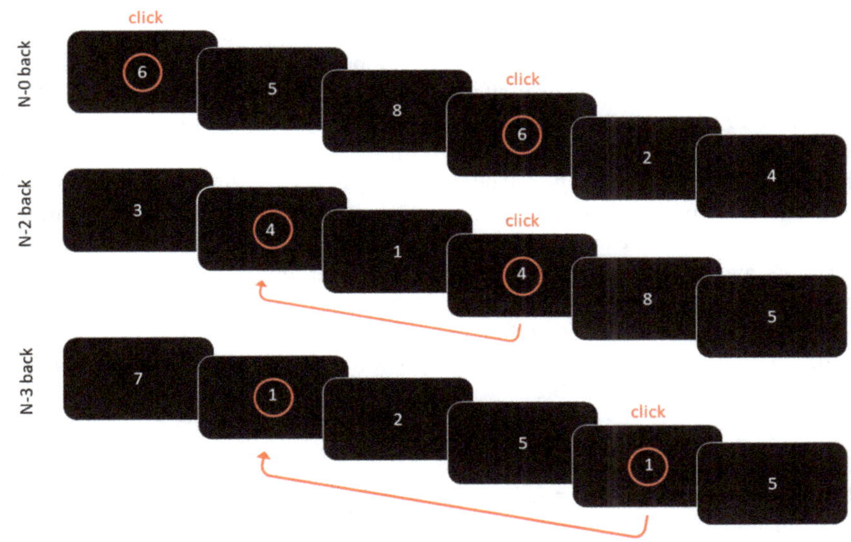


**FIGURE 1 |** Visual N-back working memory task. In the N0 condition, the participants had to as quickly as possible detect the number 6. In the N2/N3 conditions, the participants had to press the button when the displayed number was identical to the number displayed two/three trials earlier.

with battery-operated ANT® amplifiers with a gain of 30,000 and a bandpass of 0.01–100 Hz. The ground electrode (AFz) was positioned between Fpz and Fz along the midline. The impedance of all of the electrodes was maintained below 10 kΩ during all the experiments. EEG was recorded continuously at a sampling rate of 500 Hz with ANT Eeprobe software. Approximately 20% of the trials were contaminated (a cutoff of 30 mV was used to define trials that were contaminated either by eye movements or muscular artifacts), and they were eliminated offline in order to only analyze the artifact-free trials. Epochs starting 200 ms before the onset of the stimulus and lasting for 800 ms were created. The data were filtered with a 30-Hz low-pass filter. A baseline correction (from −200 to 0 ms) was computed. Only trials that were correctly performed were included in these averages [i.e., correct hits for targets, while hits for nontargets (false alarms) were eliminated]. Two parameters were coded for each stimulus: i) the condition (N0; N2; N3) and ii) the type of response (key press for targets, no key press for the other stimuli). This coding allowed us to compute different averages of ERP target stimuli. The averages were computed for each subject individually. Grand-averages were then computed for the three conditions (N0, N2, and N3) for each group (light vs. hazardous drinkers).

## Statistical Analyses

For the behavioral data, three ANOVAs were computed on the correct hits, the reaction times, and the false alarms with level (N0, N2, and N3) as within-subject variables, and group (light vs. hazardous drinkers) as a between-subject variable. The Greenhouse–Geisser correction was applied to all of the ANOVAs when necessary. For the ERP data, we first analyzed the two classical ERP components associated with the control N0 condition: 1) the P100 component, measured as a mean amplitude value over O1, Oz, and O2 electrodes in the latency range [80–140 ms] (55); and 2) the P300 component, measured as a mean amplitude value over P3, Pz, and P4 electrodes in the latency range [280–450 ms] (55). Then, as no group difference emerged on this baseline condition, the main analyses of this study consisted of subtracting it from the WM conditions (N2, N3) in order to isolate specific WM processes such as storage and manipulation (updating) (34, 42, 55). Subtractions "N2 minus N0" as well as "N3 minus N0" were then computed for each participant of each group and were subsequently grand-averaged. Significant effects were calculated at four selected electrode clusters [i.e., Frontal (mean of electrodes F3, F4, and Fz), Central (mean of Cz, C3, and C4), Parietal (mean of P3, Pz, and P4), and Occipital (mean of O1, Oz, and O2)] through Student's *t*-tests (amplitude of the difference wave compared to zero from 0 to 800 ms) (76, 77). These *t*-values were significant at the level $p < .01$ if they were above 2.79/below −2.79 for the hazardous drinkers (significance threshold computed on the basis of a sample size of $n = 25$) or above 2.81/below −2.81 for the light drinkers [$n = 24$; see the critical values (percentiles) for the *t* distribution at https://faculty.washington.edu/heagerty/Books/Biostatistics/TABLES/t-Tables/]. Only spatiotemporal patterns whose *t*-values were significant *for at least 20 ms* were considered as relevant (76–78). All of the analyses were conducted with SPSS 20 software.

# RESULTS

## Behavioral Data

The light and the hazardous drinkers were equivalent in terms of age, gender, depression (BDI-II scores), anxiety (STAI-trait and STAI-state scores), and impulsivity (UPPS total score; all *p*'s > 0.05). The two groups differed solely on "alcohol" variables, i.e., on the AUDIT-C subscore [$t(47) = -10.836$; $p < 0.001$], and on the DOW [$t(47) = -6.236$; $p < 0.001$], ADO [$t(47) = -3.977$; $p < 0.001$], as well as ADW [$t(47) = -5.255$; $p < 0.001$] variables. The complete demographic characteristics of the cohort are reported in **Table 1**. The ANOVAs revealed a significant principal effect of level on correct hits [F(2,94) = 197.549; $p < 0.001$; observed power = 1], reaction times [F(2,94) = 171.15; $p < 0.001$; observed power = 1], and false alarms [F(2,94) = 89.012; $p < 0.001$; observed power = 1]. This suggests a "complexity effect," as the more difficult the task (N3 > N2 > N0), the more the participants made errors (fewer correct hits and more false alarms) and had longer response latencies. However, no significant effects of group or significant level × group interactions were found (all *p*'s > 0.05), suggesting that both groups performed the task similarly. Detailed analysis results are presented in **Table 2**.

## Event-Related Potential Data

At a technical level, we first ensured that the same number of trials was included in ERP analyses for both groups across conditions. An ANOVA 2 × 3 with group (light vs. hazardous drinkers) as a between-subject variable and condition (N0, N2, N3) as a within-subject variable was computed. As only correct hits for targets were entered in ERP analyses, we were able to show a main condition effect [F(2,94) = 60.582; $p < 0.001$; observed power = 1], indexing an increased number of errors as a function of task complexity [mean number of trials ± SD: N0 Light: 29 (7.6), Hazardous: 32 (6.8); N2: Light: 22 (6.9), Hazardous: 25 (7.9); N3: Light: 18 (7), and Hazardous: 20 (7)]. However, this complexity effect was not modulated by the group [no group effect: F(1,47) = 2.575; $p = 0.115$; no interaction condition × group: F(2,94) = 0.231; $p = 0.779$], suggesting that a similar signal-to-noise ratio was ensured for each condition between groups. Waveforms recorded on target and nontarget trials in each condition (N0, N2, and N3) are shown in **Figure 2**. As expected, the targets involved widespread higher amplitudes than the nontargets [e.g., Ref. (55)].

We then compared P100 and P300 amplitudes on the baseline N0 condition between the light and the hazardous drinkers. We used two ANOVAs with group (light vs. hazardous drinkers) as a between-subject variable. No significant difference emerged (all *p*'s > 0.05). Therefore, as expected [e.g., Ref. (42)], we were able to compute "N2 minus N0" as well as "N3 minus N0" subtractions.

The subtraction "N2 minus N0" revealed three main components in both groups: 1) a widespread positivity (with maximal amplitudes visible at occipital sites) associated with a negativity maximally recorded at occipital sites around 150–250 ms: such a pattern exhibited high similarity with the P200/N200 recorded by Missonnier and colleagues (55); 2) a positive activity around 280–400 ms, mainly visible at frontal sites, that can refer to the well-known P300 component, as in Johnson and colleagues' (79) study; and 3) a large negativity around 300–500 ms associated with a long-lasting positivity starting around 500 ms on all of the electrodes (Fz, Cz, Pz, and Oz) that can be linked to the "old/new" N400/P600 memory effect (80). In the same way, the subtraction "N3 minus N0" also revealed these three main components. This is illustrated in **Figure 3** and **Table 3**.

In order to compare these "subtracted waveforms" (N2 minus N0; N3 minus N0), between groups, we submitted these data to Student's *t*-tests (amplitude of the difference wave compared to zero from 0 to 800 ms) (76, 77) in order to isolate specific spatiotemporal electrophysiological patterns devoted to the WM processes involved in our task (such as storage and updating) (34, 42, 55). To achieve this, and to deal with the multiple comparisons that we computed, we considered that patterns for which the *t*-values were above 2.79/below −2.79 ($p < .01$) for the hazardous drinkers ($n = 24$) or above 2.81/below −2.81 ($p < .01$) for the light drinkers ($n = 25$) were significant *only if they lasted for at least 20 ms* (76–78).

For "N2 minus N0," the light drinkers exhibited 1) at frontal sites, no significant difference while the hazardous drinkers exhibited three patterns of significant "difference" activities at ms [306-361], [533–564], and [581–819]; 2) at central sites, a small late difference at ms [751–819], while this difference was more sustained in the hazardous drinkers at ms [532–819]; 3) at parietal sites, a similar pattern to the one described at central sites, i.e., a significant activity around [747–819] ms for the light drinkers and a more sustained one in the hazardous participants around [527–819] ms; and 4) at occipital sites, two significant differences, at [143–180] ms and [379–421] ms intervals, that were not observable in the hazardous drinkers, who always exhibited a sustained later activity around ms [545–819]. The results are shown in **Figure 4A** and **Table 4A**.

For "N3 minus N0," one can observe 1) at frontal sites, no significant difference for the light drinkers while the hazardous drinkers exhibited three patterns of significant "difference" activities at ms [182–211], [544–659], and [676–736]; 2) at central sites, no significant difference for the light drinkers while the hazardous drinkers exhibited three significant intervals at ms [415-467], [632–659], and [668–819]; 3) at parietal sites, a significant activity around [356–475] ms for the light drinkers and two for the hazardous participants around [346–476] and [597–819] ms; and 4) at occipital sites, two significant differences, at [146–178] and [337–443] ms intervals, that emerged for the light drinkers while the hazardous drinkers exhibited four significant patterns of activities at ms [211–231], [300–435], [585–702], and [730–769]. The results are illustrated in **Figure 4B** and **Table 4B**.

**TABLE 2 |** The ANOVAs revealed a significant principal effect of level on correct hits [F(2,94) = 197.549; $p < 0.001$; observed power = 1], reaction times [F(2,94) = 171.15; $p < 0.001$; observed power = 1], and false alarms [F(2,94) = 89.012; $p < 0.001$; observed power = 1]. No significant effects of groups or significant level × group interactions were found (all *p*'s > 0.05), suggesting that both groups performed the task similarly.

| | Level | Light drinkers | Hazardous drinkers |
|---|---|---|---|
| Correct hits (/40) | N0 | 40 ± 0 | 39.88 ± 0.3 |
| | N2 | 33.79 ± 2.6 | 35.2 ± 2.08 |
| | N3 | 28.25 ± 5.2 | 28.04 ± 4.8 |
| Reaction times | N0 | 422 ± 54.4 | 423 ± 71.4 |
| | N2 | 586 ± 110.2 | 549 ± 98.6 |
| | N3 | 741 ± 148.3 | 777 ± 141.4 |
| False alarm | N0 | 0.13 ± 0.3 | 0.2 ± 0.5 |
| | N2 | 3.12 ± 2.3 | 2.96 ± 1.5 |
| | N3 | 7.79 ± 4.5 | 8.28 ± 5.5 |

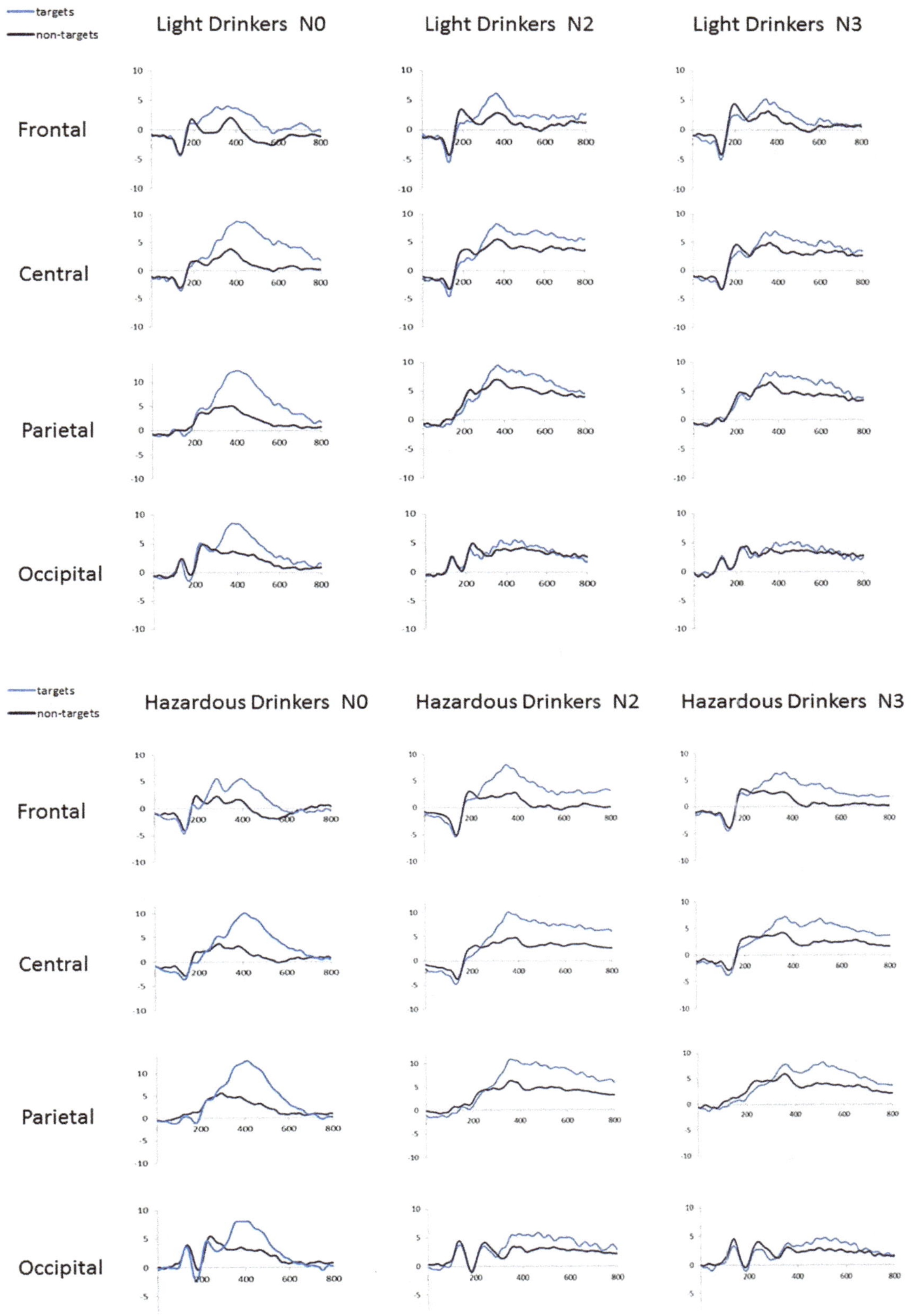


**FIGURE 2 |** Waveforms recorded at frontal (mean amplitudes for F3, Fz, F4), central (C3, Cz, C4), parietal (P3, Pz, P4), and occipital (O1, Oz, O2) sites for the light ($n$ = 24) and the hazardous ($n$ = 25) drinkers on each condition (N0, N2, N3) for target and nontarget trials.

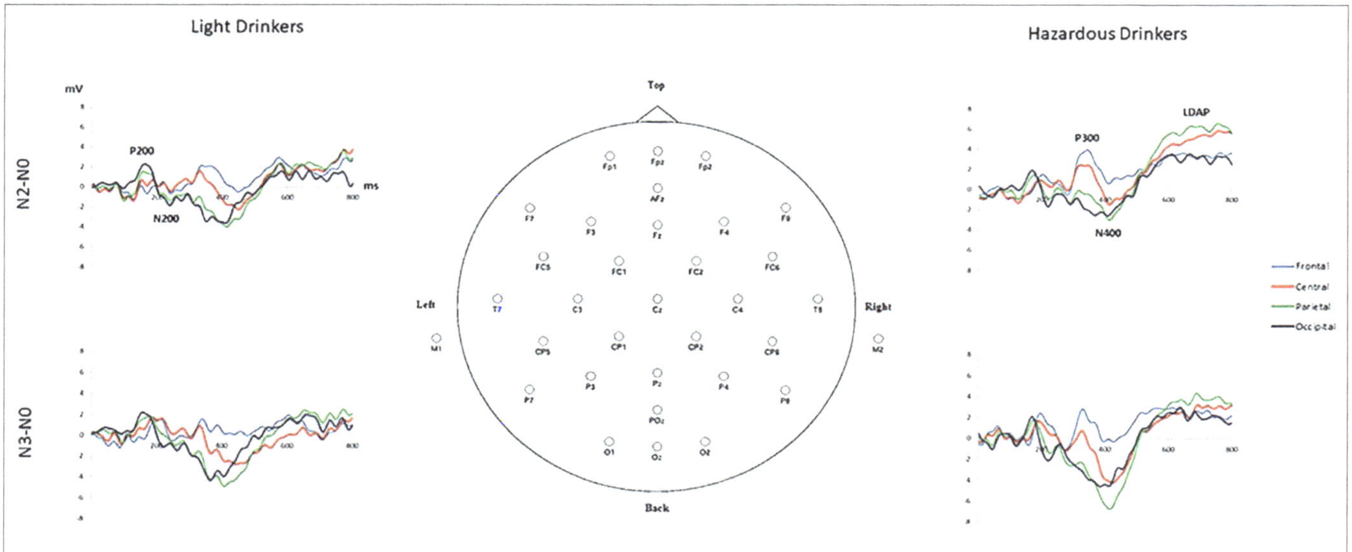


**FIGURE 3 |** Subtracted grand-average waveforms "N2 minus N0" and "N3 minus N0" at frontal (mean amplitudes for F3, Fz, F4), central (C3, Cz, C4), parietal (P3, Pz, P4), and occipital (O1, Oz, O2) sites for the light ($n$ = 24) and the hazardous ($n$ = 25) drinkers.

Overall, the hazardous drinkers exhibited enhanced amplitude activities compared to the light drinkers, to perform N2 and N3-back conditions. More precisely, the hazardous drinkers exhibited higher amplitude differences, mainly at frontal P300 and widespread P600 components, whereas the light drinkers exhibited enhanced amplitudes around the P200 and N400 components. It should also be noted that, even though the hazardous drinkers exhibited a higher number of significant activities in the N3-back condition compared to the N2-back condition (suggesting incremental activity with task complexity), group differences between the light and the hazardous drinkers were of higher amplitudes for the N2 minus N0 condition than for the N3 minus N0 one. This suggests that the hazardous drinkers exhibited higher processing intensity throughout the information-processing stream, notably around the P300 and the late directing attention positivity (LDAP) components, while the light drinkers can just increase early visual attention (P200) in order to obtain a better memory trace (N400) to deal with the $n$-back task implying different cognitive loads.

## DISCUSSION

Although many $n$-back studies have not reported any significant difference between healthy participants and excessive alcohol drinkers, significant neural differences have been found indexing compensatory neural processing during variation in the cognitive load (40–44, 46). Moreover, these neural differences appear to be observable throughout the information processing stream when electrophysiological measures (characterized by a better temporal resolution) are used (52–56). In the present ERP study, and for the first time to our knowledge, increasing memory load (N2 and N3-back tasks) has been placed on light and hazardous drinkers.

The main result of the present study is that, even though the performances were equal between the groups, the hazardous drinkers exhibited more intense and widespread activities than the light drinkers. These data are in total agreement with previous data obtained in our lab through an fMRI study (42), in which hazardous drinkers exhibited higher bilateral activity in the pre-supplementary motor area as well as specific positive correlations between the number of alcohol doses consumed per occasion and higher activity in the dorsomedial PFC, and between the number of drinking occasions per week and higher activity in cerebellum, thalamus, and insula while performing the N2 memory task. The present study extended these results, as it showed that 1) these enhanced activities are also present in the N3-back task; and 2) as a result of the optimal resolution of ERPs, it specified the *temporal dynamic* of these increased activities.

At the behavioral level, our results confirmed that the N3 condition was considerably more difficult than the N2-back task,

**TABLE 3 |** Mean amplitude values (± SD) for the main ERP components resulting from "N2 minus N0" and "N3 minus N0" subtractions on time intervals and on sites of maximally recorded amplitudes for the light and the hazardous drinkers.

| | | | Light (N2–N0) | Hazardous (N2–N0) |
|---|---|---|---|---|
| **P200** | 100–200 ms | Occipital | 1.15 (± 0.82) | 0.77 (± 0.68) |
| **N200** | 200–300 ms | Occipital | −1.16 (± 0.35) | −0.96 (± 0.47) |
| **P300** | 300–400 ms | Frontal | 1.57 (± 0.62) | 2.80 (± 0.90) |
| **N400** | 300–500 ms | Parietal | −2.45 (± 0.97) | −1.19 (± 0.96) |
| **LDAP** | 500–800 ms | Parietal | 1.89 (± 1.03) | 5.14 (± 1.52) |
| | | | **Light (N3–N0)** | **Hazardous (N3–N0)** |
| **P200** | 100–200 ms | Occipital | 1.16 (± 0.74) | 0.40 (± 0.96) |
| **N200** | 200–300 ms | Occipital | −1.03 (± 0.30) | −1.57 (± 0.60) |
| **P300** | 300–400 ms | Frontal | 0.76 (± 0.49) | 1.36 (± 0.85) |
| **N400** | 300–500 ms | Parietal | −3.34 (± 1.14) | −4.17 (± 1.62) |
| **LDAP** | 500–800 ms | Parietal | 1.25 (± 1.08) | 2.98 (± 1.22) |

*LDAP, Late Directing Attention Positivity.*

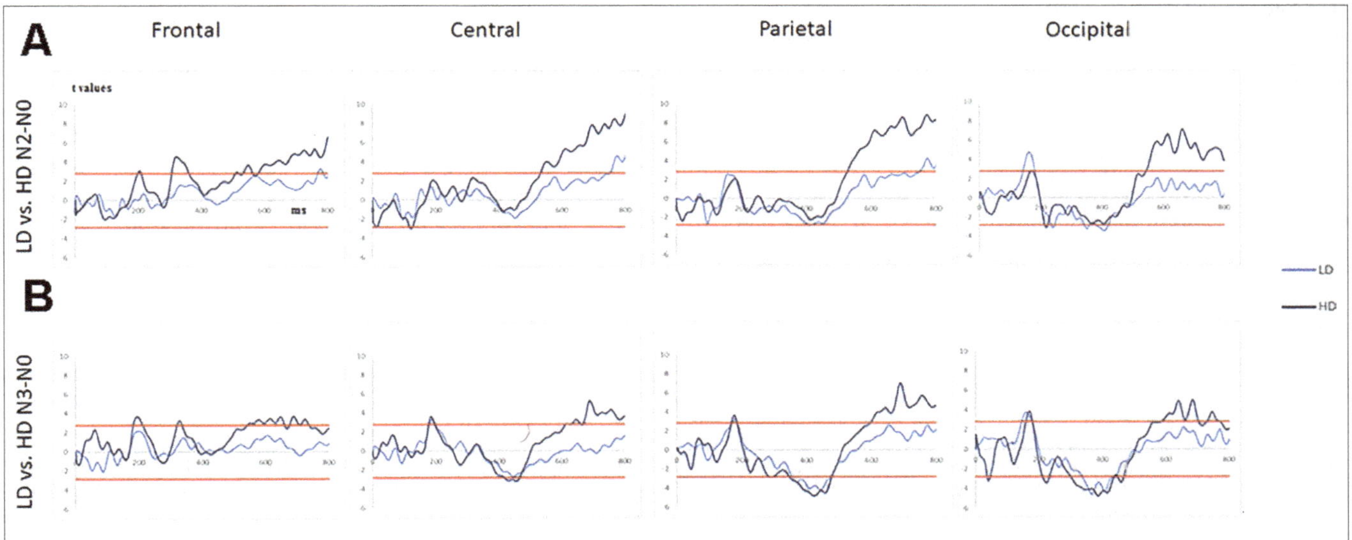


**FIGURE 4 | (A)** T-values obtained for the subtraction "N2 minus N0" (significance levels are represented by red lines) for the light and the hazardous drinkers at frontal, central, parietal, and occipital sites. **(B)** *T*-values obtained for the subtraction "N3 minus N0" (significance levels are represented as red lines) for the light and the hazardous drinkers at frontal, central, parietal, and occipital sites.

but also that no difference was observable between the groups (as expected) (42). At the ERP level, as the baseline N0 condition was similar across the groups, we computed subtraction "N2 minus N0" and "N3 minus N0" to isolate WM processes (34). By visual inspection, three patterns of activities could be discerned: one around 150 to 250 ms with a maximal activity at posterior sites (P200/N200 complex), one around 300 to 400 ms at frontal sites (P300), and one around 400 to 800 ms as a late positive potential (N400/P600 complex). Therefore, Student's *t*-tests (amplitude of the difference wave compared to zero from 0 to 800 ms) (76, 77) were applied in order to assess statistically significant differences among these three spatiotemporal patterns of activities between the light and the hazardous drinkers.

According to a "functional compensation view," increases in activation reflect "attempted" or "successful" compensation for these deficits during more complex cognitive tasks (47). These changes in cerebral responses may be considered, at the preventive level (particularly for young drinkers), as vulnerability factors for the development of adult SUD (42), but also stressed the importance, at a more clinical level, to consider such WM processes (such as the ability to deal with a high cognitive load) in the management of alcohol dependence. Some studies aiming to train WM efficiency in excessive alcohol users have already been published, disclosing encouraging results (27, 28). Moreover, it has also been shown that prior WM training with a high memory load interferes with the reconsolidation of alcohol-related memories in a sample of nontreatment-seeking heavy drinkers (81). However, more studies tagged dual-process mechanisms [cue reactivity/inhibition; for instance, Refs. (17, 18)]. As WM capacity has been shown to impact cognitive control of impulsivity by way of keeping future goals in mind when making decisions when faced with rewarding/arousing distractions (19), a point that perfectly fits with the dual-process model of cognitive control, further studies aiming to develop cognitive training procedure for alcohol-dependent patients should include the WM process.

Also, it is worth noting that the ERP data we obtained are in line with several previous ERP studies. First, the P200/N200 component has already been described by Missonnier and colleagues (55), by subtracting ERP waveforms from memory-free control tasks (detection) from memory tasks (1-back and 2-back tasks), its amplitude increasing significantly in healthy subjects with higher memory load (2-back vs. 1-back). At the functional level, this complex was interpreted as an *intermediate* phase, as short-term storage should directly follow

**TABLE 4A |** Statistically significant time intervals (in ms) for the subtracted waveforms exhibited at frontal, central, parietal, and occipital sites for the subtraction "N2 minus N0." A significant interval was considered as relevant (in green) when it lasted for at least 20 ms (76–78). Other intervals (in red) were neither considered nor discussed. P for positive activity; N for negative activity.

| | Light drinkers (*n* = 24) | Hazardous drinkers (*n* = 25) |
|---|---|---|
| Frontal | P [769; 786]<br>P [806; 819] | P [198; 209]<br>P [306; 361]<br>P [508; 520]<br>P [533; 564]<br>P [581; 819] |
| Central | P [751; 819] | P [11; 15]<br>P [117; 127]<br>P [532; 819] |
| Parietal | P [406; 419]<br>P [747; 819] | P [527; 819] |
| Occipital | P [143; 180]<br>N [234; 245]<br>N [343; 361]<br>P [379; 421] | P [167; 174]<br>P [213; 223]<br>P [545; 819] |

**TABLE 4B** | Statistically significant time intervals (in ms) for the subtracted waveforms exhibited at frontal, central, parietal, and occipital sites for the subtraction "N3 minus N0." A significant interval was considered as relevant (in green) when it lasted for at least 20 ms (76–78). Other intervals (in red) were neither considered nor discussed. P for positive activity; N for negative activity.

| | Light drinkers (*n* = 24) | Hazardous drinkers (*n* = 25) |
|---|---|---|
| Frontal | Ø | P [182; 211]<br>P [320; 335]<br>P [544; 659]<br>P [676; 736] |
| Central | P [180; 196] | P [177; 196]<br>N [415; 467]<br>P [613; 622]<br>P [632; 659]<br>P [668; 819] |
| Parietal | P [169; 186]<br>N [356; 475]<br>P [808; 819] | P [168; 187]<br>N [283; 295]<br>P [346; 476]<br>P [597; 819] |
| Occipital | P [146; 178]<br>N [337; 443] | N [36; 45]<br>P [159; 178]<br>N [211; 231]<br>N [300; 435]<br>N [447; 466]<br>P [585; 702]<br>P [730; 769] |

pure sensory-driven processes (such as the P100) and precede execution-related processes (300 ms or later). Therefore, the P200/N200 complex could refer to the visual encoding of the stimulus, translated into its corresponding phonological representations (1), which is created and stored in the posterior parietal cortex, remains active for a few seconds, and constitutes *the storage function of verbal working memory* (82). It needs to be emphasized that the light drinkers exhibited higher responses (for the P200 in the N2-back task) than the hazardous ones. Usually, when task-relevant images are displayed, the early/sustained attention increases, thereby increasing the impact of the stimuli [e.g., Ref. (83)]. This could suggest that the light drinkers generally exhibited an *enhanced early visual attentional process* to ease task performance compared to the hazardous drinkers (consistent with a recollection process aided by visual imagery) (36). Secondly, similarities were also found with a study by Johnson et al. (79), which focused on the *refreshing* process. Refreshing is thought to be a key process for selecting, maintaining, and manipulating information within WM (84), and is, therefore, a critical component in tasks that require manipulation such as updating (e.g., *n*-back) (85). In that study, ERP analyses showed that a typical refresh task does have a distinct electrophysiological response compared to a control condition, and it includes at least two main temporal components: an earlier (~400 ms) positive peak reminiscent of a P3a/P3b response and a later (~800–1,400 ms) sustained positivity over several sites reminiscent of the late directing attention positivity (P600 or LDAP) (79). In our study, we found a positive component around 280 to 400 ms, and one around 500 to 800 ms as a late positive potential. These two distinct component cognitive processes are consistent with a two-phase model predicted from fMRI: the first phase referring to the initiation of an appropriate nonautomatic cognitive or motor action based on the interpretation of a cue, and the second reflecting top-down modulation carrying meaningful information about currently active mental representation (79). In this view, it seems reasonable to draw some connections between these two components and the P3 family of responses (typically occurring around 280–500 ms) (86) and the P600 or LDAP (typically arising around 500 ms post-cue) (87). On the one hand, our component around 280 to 400 ms could be related to both the P3a, which is related to the initial orientation to and evaluation of a stimulus, driven primarily by prefrontal regions (88), and the P3b, which appears to be related more to the resolution of uncertainty about stimuli and the concomitant updating of expectancies or context, potentially engaging additional attentional or memory processes, and driven primarily by temporoparietal activity (86, 88). On the other hand, our late positive component from 500 to 800 ms may be seen as similar to a P600 or LDAP, a late positive potential associated with perceptual attention, lasting up to several hundred milliseconds. It has been interpreted as arising from the anticipatory top-down modulation of visual regions in response to the refreshing of a visual representation [e.g., Ref. (89)]. Such WM processes required more intense and sustained activities in the hazardous drinkers compared to the light ones, therefore suggesting a type of vulnerability of these cognitive processes. Thirdly, it is also worth noting that such an LDAP has also been previously linked to an N400 component. Indeed, Finnigan and colleagues (80) recorded ERPs while subjects made old/new recognition judgments on new unstudied words and old words that had been presented in the study either once ("weak") or three times ("strong"). They showed that the N400 component was found to be modulated in a graded manner by the memory trace strength (i.e., an "N400 strength effect") while the amplitude of the LDAP was sensitive to confidence in the decision accuracy. In the present study, the light drinkers exhibited higher amplitudes for this N400 component compared to the hazardous drinkers, suggesting a more intense memory trace.

Overall, one of the main strengths of ERPs is to be able to provide *a dynamic temporal view* of a cognitive process. Using visual *n*-back WM with different cognitive loads (N2-back, N3-back) appears to reveal such an information-processing stream, impacted by alcohol consumption: aside from physical processing of visual stimuli, participants have 1) to translate, encode, and store visual stimuli in short-term verbal memory (i.e., the P200/N200 complex); 2) to orient attention to stimuli (P3a), update short-term memory, and make decisions (P3b); and 3) this decision being impacted by the memory trace strength (N400) and confidence in the decision accuracy (LDAP). *To perform the task at the same level as the light drinkers, the hazardous drinkers exhibited a higher processing intensity throughout the information-processing stream, notably around the P300 and the LDAP components, while the light drinkers could merely increase early visual attention (P200) in order to obtain a better memory trace (N400).* This increment in the neural resources needed to accomplish a more and more complex task can be seen as a compensation strategy. According to a "functional compensation view," concomitant increases in activation reflect "successful" compensation for these deficits (47). Indeed, due to neuronal loss induced by the neurotoxic effect of alcohol, excessive drinkers need more resources to successfully perform a task. This could imply that 1) once the threshold of available resources is reached (for instance, by making the task more and more complex), a behavioral deficit will appear; and 2) with a less efficient WM load process, excessive drinkers may have fewer resources to plan long-term goals (e.g., be healthy), increasing propensity (i.e., decreasing cognitive control) towards an immediate reward (e.g., a drink). Therefore, it is important to highlight such data for at least two main reasons. First, at a preventive level, it seems important to stress that, *at a stage at which behavioral manifestations are not yet observable*, social heavy drinking is not just trivial social fun, as it induces substantial neural modifications subtending cognitive functions such as WM processes that may impact continuation of excessive alcohol consumption (for instance, by minimizing the impact of long-term consequences). And second, at a clinical level, training WM load capacity may reduce future alcohol consumption by increasing attention toward long-term goals, by increasing control toward immediate rewards that are not relevant to long-term prospects, and by facilitating reconsolidation of alcohol-related memories [e.g., Refs. (27, 28, Kaag et al., 2017)].

Clearly, we are fully aware that our present findings do not allow us to map ERP phenomena directly onto specific cortical areas, and that the relationships that we present above (even though theoretically grounded) are speculative. Such clear associations can, for instance, be obtained through combined ERP-fMRI studies [e.g., Ref. (90)]. We are also aware that it is not possible, from the present study, to completely discount the possibility that the differential effects observed for the hazardous drinkers are pre-morbid in nature, i.e., they existed prior to any alcohol consumption. In this view, further longitudinal studies should be designed in order to verify whether the emergence of brain differences in heavy drinkers did or did not follow the onset of drinking habits. Also, even though the N3-back tasks were more difficult than the N2-back tasks at the behavioral level, electrophysiological group differences between N2 and N0 conditions revealed *higher amplitude differences* than those between N3 and N0 conditions. This could be due to an "order effect," as the participants were always exposed to N2-back tasks *before* N3 ones. This ensured that all of the participants were exposed to conditions that were entirely similar. However, the participants could also develop a strategy to perform the N2-back condition and then apply it in the N3-back tasks so that the latter could require fewer neural resources than if they had been performed first (i.e., when the participants were still "naive" and have to adapt to the task). A fatigability effect cannot be excluded either. Therefore, further studies should alter the order of the presentation of these different conditions in order to be able to directly compare N3-back and N2-back tasks. Indeed, such a comparison would be biased in the present study as neural activities recorded in the N3-back condition appear to be decreased compared to the N2-back ones due to a type of "habituation" effect. This way, one could investigate whether differences between light and hazardous drinkers increase as a function of the cognitive load.

## AUTHOR CONTRIBUTIONS

ES and CD contributed equally to the paper (coauthors). They acquired and processed the data and wrote the paper. XN and CK participated to writing the paper. SC participated to task design and paper writing.

## ACKNOWLEDGMENTS

ES is a research fellow at the Fond pour la Recherche en Sciences Humaines (FRESH) from the Belgian Fund for Scientific Research (FRS-FNRS, Belgium). SC is a senior research associate (FRS-FNRS).

## REFERENCES

1. Baddeley A. The episodic buffer: a new component of working memory? *Trends Cogn Sci* (2000) 4(11):417–23. doi: 10.1016/S1364-6613(00)01538-2
2. Oberauer K, Süß HM, Wilhelm O, Wittman WW. The multiple faces of working memory: storage, processing, supervision, and coordination. *Intelligence* (2003) 31(2):167–93. doi: 10.1016/S0160-2896(02)00115-0
3. Morrison AB, Chein JM. Does working memory training work? The promise and challenges of enhancing cognition by training working memory. *Psychon Bull Rev* (2011) 18(1):46–60. doi: 10.3758/s13423-010-0034-0
4. Baddeley A, Hitch G. Working memory. In: Bower GH *The psychology of learning and motivation: advances in research and theory*. vol. 8 New York: Academic Press (1974). p. 47–89. doi: 10.1016/S0079-7421(08)60452-1
5. Miller GA. The magical number seven, plus or minus two: some limits on our capacity for processing information. *Psychol Rev* (1956) 63:81–97. doi: 10.1037/h0043158
6. Rypma B, D'Esposito M. The roles of prefrontal brain regions in components of working memory: effects of memory load and individual differences. *Proc Natl Acad Sci* (1999) 96(11):6558–63. doi: 10.1073/pnas.96.11.6558
7. Cowan N. The magical number 4 in short-term memory: a reconsideration of mental storage capacity. *Behav Brain Sci* (2001) 24(1):87–114. doi: 10.1017/S0140525X01003922
8. Miyake A, Friedman NP, Emerson MJ, Witzki AH, Howerter A, Wager T. The unity and diversity of executive functions and their contributions to complex "frontal lobe" tasks: a latent variable analysis. *Cog Psychol* (2000) 41:49–100. doi: 10.1006/cogp.1999.0734
9. Kane MJ, Bleckley MK, Conway AR, Engle RW. A controlled-attention view of working-memory capacity. *J Exp Psychol: Gen* (2001) 130(2):169. doi: 10.1037/0096-3445.130.2.169
10. Hinson JM, Jameson TL, Whitney P. Impulsive decision making and working memory. *J Exp Psychol: Learn, Mem, Cogn* (2003) 29(2):298. doi: 10.1037/0278-7393.29.2.298
11. Evans JSB. In two minds: dual-process accounts of reasoning. *Trends Cog Sci* (2003) 7(10):454–9. doi: 10.1016/j.tics.2003.08.012
12. Robinson TE, Berridge KC. The neural basis of drug craving: an incentive-sensitization theory of addiction. *Brain Res Rev* (1993) 18(3):247–91. doi: 10.1016/0165-0173(93)90013-P
13. Vollstädt-Klein S, Loeber S, Richter A, Kirsch M, Bach P, von der Goltz C, et al. Validating incentive salience with functional magnetic resonance imaging: association between mesolimbic cue reactivity and attentional bias in alcohol-dependent patients. *Addict Biol* (2012) 17(4):807–16. doi: 10.1111/j.1369-1600.2011.00352.x
14. Bechara A. Decision making, impulse control and loss of willpower to resist drugs: a neurocognitive perspective. *Nat Neurosci* (2005) 8(11):1458. doi: 10.1038/nn1584

15. Littel M, Euser AS, Munafò MR, Franken IH. Electrophysiological indices of biased cognitive processing of substance-related cues: a meta-analysis. *Neurosci Biobehav Rev* (2012) 36(8):1803–16. doi: 10.1016/j.neubiorev.2012.05.001
16. Luijten M, Machielsen MW, Veltman DJ, Hester R, de Haan L, Franken IH. Systematic review of ERP and fMRI studies investigating inhibitory control and error processing in people with substance dependence and behavioural addictions. *J Psychiatry Neurosci* (2014) 39(3):149. doi: 10.1503/jpn.130052
17. Fadardi JS, Cox WM. Reversing the sequence: reducing alcohol consumption by overcoming alcohol attentional bias. *Drug Alcohol Depend* (2009) 101(3): 137–45. doi: 10.1016/j.drugalcdep.2008.11.015
18. Houben K, Havermans RC, Nederkoorn C, Jansen A. Beer à No-Go: learning to stop responding to alcohol cues reduces alcohol intake *via* reduced affective associations rather than increased response inhibition. *Addiction* (2012) 107(7):1280–87. doi: 10.1111/j.1360-0443.2012.03827.x
19. Brooks SJ, Funk SG, Young SY, Schiöth HB. The role of working memory for cognitive control in anorexia nervosa versus substance use disorder. *Front Psychol* (2017) 8(1651):1–28. doi: 10.3389/fpsyg.2017.01651
20. Sofuoglu M, DeVito EE, Waters AJ, Carroll KM. Cognitive function as a transdiagnostic treatment target in stimulant use disorders. *J Dual Diagn* (2016) 12(1):90–106. doi: 10.1080/15504263.2016.1146383
21. Goldman-Rakic PS. Cellular basis of working memory. *Neuron* (1995) 14(3):477–85. doi: 10.1016/0896-6273(95)90304-6
22. Finn PR, Justus A, Mazas C, Steinmetz JE. Working memory, executive processes and the effects of alcohol on Go/No-Go learning: testing a model of behavioral regulation and impulsivity. *Psychopharmacol* (1999) 146(4): 465–72. doi: 10.1007/PL00005492
23. Bechara A, Martin EM. Impaired decision making related to working memory deficits in individuals with substance addictions. *Neuropsychol* (2004) 18(1):152. doi: 10.1037/0894-4105.18.1.152
24. Goudriaan AE, Oosterlaan J, de Beurs E, van den Brink W. Decision making in pathological gambling: a comparison between pathological gamblers, alcohol dependents, persons with Tourette syndrome, and normal controls. *Cogn Brain Res* (2005) 23(1):137–51. doi: 10.1016/j.cogbrainres.2005.01.017
25. Fillmore MT, Vogel-Sprott M. Acute effects of alcohol and other drugs on automatic and intentional control. *Handbook of implicit cognition and addiction* (2006) 293–306. doi: 10.4135/9781412976237.n20
26. Finn PR, Hall J. Cognitive ability and risk for alcoholism: short-term memory capacity and intelligence moderate personality risk for alcohol problems. *J Abn Psychol* (2004) 113(4):569. doi: 10.1037/0021-843X.113.4.569
27. Bickel WK, Yi R, Landes RD, Hill PF, Baxter C. Remember the future: working memory training decreases delay discounting among stimulant addicts. *Biol Psychiatry* (2011) 69:260–5. doi: 10.1016/j.biopsych.2010.08.017
28. Houben K, Nederkoorn C, Wiers RW, Janses A. Resisting temptation: decreasing alcohol-related affects and drinking behavior by training response inhibition. *Drug Alcohol Depend.* (2011) 116:132–6. doi: 10.1016/j.drugalcdep.2010.12.011
29. Olson IR, Jiang Y. Visual short-term memory is not improved by training. *Mem Cog* (2004) 32(8):1326–32. doi: 10.3758/BF03206323
9. Kane MJ, Bleckley MK, Conway AR, Engle RW. A controlled-attention view of working-memory capacity. *J Exp Psychol: Gen* (2001) 130(2):169. doi: 10.1037/0096-3445.130.2.169
10. Hinson JM, Jameson TL, Whitney P. Impulsive decision making and working memory. *J Exp Psychol: Learn, Mem, Cogn* (2003) 29(2):298. doi: 10.1037/0278-7393.29.2.298
11. Evans JSB. In two minds: dual-process accounts of reasoning. *Trends Cog Sci* (2003) 7(10):454–9. doi: 10.1016/j.tics.2003.08.012
12. Robinson TE, Berridge KC. The neural basis of drug craving: an incentive-sensitization theory of addiction. *Brain Res Rev* (1993) 18(3):247–91. doi: 10.1016/0165-0173(93)90013-P
13. Vollstädt-Klein S, Loeber S, Richter A, Kirsch M, Bach P, von der Goltz C, et al. Validating incentive salience with functional magnetic resonance imaging: association between mesolimbic cue reactivity and attentional bias in alcohol-dependent patients. *Addict Biol* (2012) 17(4):807–16. doi: 10.1111/j.1369-1600.2011.00352.x
14. Bechara A. Decision making, impulse control and loss of willpower to resist drugs: a neurocognitive perspective. *Nat Neurosci* (2005) 8(11):1458. doi: 10.1038/nn1584
36. Ishai A, Haxby JV, Ungerleider LG. Visual imagery of famous faces: effects of memory and attention revealed by fMRI. *NeuroImage* (2002) 17:1729–41. doi: 10.1006/nimg.2002.1330
37. Corbetta M, Patel G, Shulman GL. The reorienting system of the human brain: from environment to theory of mind. *Neuron* (2008) 58:306–24. doi: 10.1016/j.neuron.2008.04.017
38. Bava S, Jacobus J, Mahmood O, Yang TT, Tapert SF. Neurocognitive correlates of white matter quality in adolescent substance users. *Brain Cogn* (2010) 72:347–54. doi: 10.1016/j.bandc.2009.10.012
39. Cservenka A, Herting MM, Nagel BJ. Atypical frontal lobe activity during verbal working memory in youth with a family history of alcoholism. *Drug Alcohol Depend* (2012) 123:98–104. doi: 10.1016/j.drugalcdep.2011.10.021
40. Pfefferbaum A, Desmond JE, Galloway C, Menon V, Glover GH, Sullivan EV. Reorganization of frontal systems used by alcoholics for spatial working memory: an fMRI study. *NeuroImage* (2001) 14:7–20. doi: 10.1006/nimg.2001.0785
41. Crews FT, Buckley T, Dodd PR, Ende G, Foley H, Harpey C, et al. Alcoholic neurobiology: changes in dependence and recovery. *Alcohol Clin Exp Res* (2005) 29:1504–13. doi: 10.1097/01.alc.0000175013.50644.61
42. Campanella S, Peigneux P, Petit G, Lallemand F, Saeremans M, Noël X, et al. Increased cortical activity in binge drinkers during working memory task: a preliminary assessment through a functional magnetic resonance imaging study. *PLOS ONE* (2013a) 8:e62260. doi: 10.1371/journal.pone.0062260
43. Clark CM, Lawlor-Savage L, Goghari VM. Functional brain activation associated with working memory training and transfer. *Behav Brain Res* (2017) 15:34–49. doi: 10.1016/j.bbr.2017.07.030
44. Crego A, Rodriguez-Holguín S, Parada M, Mota N, Corral M, Cadaveira F. Reduced anterior prefrontal cortex activation in young binge drinkers during a visual working memory task. *Drug Alcohol Depend* (2010) 109:45–56. doi: 10.1016/j.drugalcdep.2009.11.020
45. Vollstädt-Klein S, Hermann D, Rabinstein J, Wichert S, Klein O, Ende G, et al. Increased activation of the ACC during a spatial working memory task in alcohol-dependence versus heavy social drinking. *Alcohol Clin Exp Res* (2010) 34:771–6. doi: 10.1111/j.1530-0277.2010.01149.x
46. Squeglia LM, Schweinsburg AD, Pulido C, Tapert SF. Adolescent binge drinking linked to abnormal spatial working memory brain activation: differential gender effects. *Alcohol Clin Exp Res* (2011) 35:1831–41. doi: 10.1111/j.1530-0277.2011.01527.x
47. Cabeza R. Hemispheric asymmetry reduction in older adults: the HAROLD model. *Psychol Aging* (2002) 17:85–100. doi: 10.1037/0882-7974.17.1.85
48. Grimes D, Tan DS, Hudson SE, Shenoy P, Rao RP. Feasibility and pragmatics of classifying working memory load with an electroencephalograph. In *Proceedings of the SIGCHI Conference on Human Factors in Computing Systems*. ACM (2008). p. 835–44.
49. Brouwer AM, Hogervorst MA, Van Erp JB, Heffelaar T, Zimmerman PH, Oostenveld R. Estimating workload using EEG spectral power and ERPs in the n-back task. *J Neural Engin* (2012) 9(4):045008. doi: 10.1088/1741-2560/9/4/045008
50. Fink A, Grabner RH, Neuper C, Neubauer AC. EEG alpha band dissociation with increasing task demands. *Cogn Brain Res* (2005) 24:252–9. doi: 10.1016/j.cogbrainres.2005.02.002
51. Esposito F, Aragri A, Piccoli T, Tedeschi G, Goebel R, Di Salle F. Distributed analysis of simultaneous EEG-fMRI time-series: modeling and interpretation issues. *Magn Reson Imaging* (2009) 27:1120–30. doi: 10.1016/j.mri.2009.01.007
52. Pratt N, Willoughby A, Swick D. Effects of working memory load on visual selective attention: behavioral and electrophysiological evidence. *Front Hum Neurosci* (2011) 5:57. doi: 10.3389/fnhum.2011.00057
53. Allison BZ, Polich J. Workload assessment of computer gaming using a single-stimulus event-related potential paradigm. *Biol Psychol* (2008) 77(3): 277–83. doi: 10.1016/j.biopsycho.2007.10.014
54. Kramer AF, Trejo LJ, Humphrey D. Assessment of mental workload with task-irrelevant auditory probes. *Biol Psychol* (1995) 40(1–2):83–100. doi: 10.1016/0301-0511(95)05108-2
55. Missonnier P, Leonards U, Gold G, Palix J, Ibáñez V, Giannakopoulos P. A new electrophysiological index for working memory load in humans. *Neuroreport* (2003) 14(11):1451–5. doi: 10.1097/00001756-200308060-00009

56. Evans JL, Selinger C, Pollak SD. P300 as a measure of processing capacity in auditory and visual domains in specific language impairment. *Brain Res.* (2011) 1389: 93–102. doi: 10.1016/j.brainres.2011.02.010
57. Crego A, Rodriguez-HolguõÂn S, Parada M, Mota N, Corral M, Cadaveira F. Binge drinking affects attentional and visual working memory processing in young university students. *Alcohol Clin Exp Res* (2009) 33(11):1870–9. doi: 10.1111/j.1530-0277.2009.01025.x
58. Park S, Kim MS. An event-related potential study of spatial working memory in binge drinking college students. *PloS one* (2018) 13(9):e0203696. doi: 10. 1371/journal.pone.0203696
59. Petit G, Kornreich C, Noël X, Verbanck P, Campanella S. Alcohol-related context modulates performance of social drinkers in a visual Go/No-Go task: a preliminary assessment of event-related potentials. *PLoS One* (2012) 7(5):e37466. doi: 10.1371/journal.pone.0037466
60. Gil-Hernandez S, Garcia-Moreno LM. Executive performance and dysexecutive symptoms in binge drinking adolescents. *Alcohol* (2016) 51:79–87. doi: 10.1016/j.alcohol.2016.01.003
61. Petit G, Maurage P, Kornreich C, Verbanck P, Campanella S. Binge drinking in adolescents: a review of neurophysiological and neuroimaging research. *Alcohol Alcoholism* (2013) 49(2):198–206. doi: 10.1093/alcalc/agt172
62. Rugg MD, Coles MGH. *Electrophysiology of mind. Event-related brain potentials and cognition.* Oxford: Oxford University Press, Oxford Psychology Series (1995).
63. McGue M. Genes, environment, and the etiology of alcoholism. In: Zucker R, Boyd G, Howard J, editor. *The development of alcohol problems: exploring the biopsychosocial matrix of risk.*Washington, DC: US Government Printing Office (1994). p. 1–40. (NIAAA Research Monograph No. 26).
64. Campanella S, Absil J, Carbia Sinde C, Schroder E, Peigneux P, Bourguignon M, et al. Neural correlates of correct and failed response inhibition in heavy versus light social drinkers: an fMRI study during a go/no-go task by healthy participants. *Brain Imaging Behav* (2016) 11(6):1796–811. doi: 10.1007/ s11682-016-9654-y
65. Petit G, Kornreich C, Dan B, Verbanck P, Campanella S. Electrophysiological correlates of alcohol-and non-alcohol-related stimuli processing in binge drinkers: a follow-up study. *J Psychopharmacol* (2014) 28(11):1041–52. doi: 10.1177/0269881114545663
66. Saunders JB, Aasland OG, Babor TF, de la Fuente JR, Grant M. Development of the Alcohol Use Disorders Identification Test (AUDIT): WHO collaborative project on early detection of persons with harmful alcohol consumption—II. *Addiction* (1993) 88:791–804. doi: 10.1111/j.1360-0443.1993.tb02093.x
67. Bush K, Kivlahan DR, McDonell MB, Fihn SD, Bradley KA. The AUDIT alcohol consumption questions (AUDIT-C): an effective brief screening test for problem drinking. *Arch Int Med* (1998) 158(16):1789–95. doi: 10.1001/ archinte.158.16.1789
68. Bradley KA, Bush KR, Epler AJ, Dobie DJ, Davis TM, Sporlede JL, et al. Two brief alcohol-screening tests from the Alcohol Use Disorders Identification Test (AUDIT): validation in a female Veterans Affairs patient population. *Arch Int Med* (2003) 163(7):821–29. doi: 10.1001/archinte.163.7.821
69. Babor T, Campbell R, Room R, Saunders J. *Lexicon of alcohol and drug terms.* Geneva: World Health Organization (1994).
70. Spielberger CD. *Manual for the State-Trait Anxiety Inventory (STAI).* Palo Alto, CA: Consulting Psychologists Press (1983).
71. Beck AT, Steer RA, Brown GK. Beck depression inventory-II. *San Antonio* (1996) 78(2):490–8.
72. Whiteside SP, Lynam DR. Understanding the role of impulsivity and externalizing psychopathology in alcohol abuse: application of the UPPS impulsive behavior scale. *Exp Clin Psychopharmacol* (2003) 11:210–17. doi: 10.1037/1064-1297.11.3.210
73. McKenzie M, Jorm AF, Romaniuk H, Olsson CA, Patton GC. Association of adolescent symptoms of depression and anxiety with alcohol use disorders in young adulthood: findings from the Victorian Adolescent Health Cohort Study. *Med J Aust* (2011) 195:27–30. doi: 10.5694/j.1326-5377.2011. tb03262.x
74. Norberg MN, Oliver J, Alperstein DM, Zvolensky MJ, Norton AR. Adverse consequences of student drinking: the role of sex, social anxiety, drinking motives. *Addict Behav* (2011) 36:821–8. doi: 10.1016/j. addbeh.2011.03.010
75. Henges AL, Marczinski CA. Impulsivity and alcohol consumption in young social drinkers. *Addict Behav* (2012) 37(2):217–20. doi: 10.1016/j.addbeh. 2011.09.013
76. Joassin F, Maurage P, Bruyer R, Crommelinck M, Campanella S. When audition alters vision: an event-related potential study of the crossmodal interactions between faces and voices. *Neurosci Lett* (2004) 369:132–7. doi: 10.1016/j.neulet.2004.07.067
77. Joassin F, Meert G, Campanella S, Bruyer R. The associative processes involved in faces-proper names versus animals-common names binding: a comparative ERP study. *Biol Psychol* (2007) 75(3):286–99. doi: 10.1016/j. biopsycho.2007.04.002
78. Rugg MD, Doyle MC, Wells T. Word and non-word repetition within- and across-modality: an event-related potential study. *J Cogn Neurosci* (1995) 7:209–27. doi: 10.1162/jocn.1995.7.2.209
79. Johnson MR, McCarthy G, Muller KA, Brudner SN, Johnson MK. Electrophysiological correlates of refreshing: event-related potentials associated with directing reflective attention to face, scene, or word representations. *J Cogn Neurosci* (2015) 27(9):1823–39. doi: 10.1162/jocn_a_00823
80. Finnigan S, Humphreys MS, Dennis S, Geffen G. ERP 'old/new' effects: memory strength and decisional factor (s). *Neuropsychologia* (2002) 40(13): 2288–304. doi: 10.1016/S0028-3932(02)00113-6
81. Kaag AM, Goudriaan AE, De Vries TJ, Pattij T, Wiers RW. A high working memory load prior to memory retrieval reduces craving in non-treatment seeking problem drinkers. *Psychopharmacology* (2018) 235(3):695–708. doi: 10.1007/s00213-017-4785-4
82. Smith EE, Jonides J. Neuroimaging analyses of human working memory. *Proc Natl Acad Sci* (1998) 95(20):12061–8. doi: 10.1073/pnas.95.20.12061
83. Delle-Vigne D, Kornreich C, Verbanck P, Campanella S. Subclinical alexithymia modulates early audio-visual perceptive and attentional event-related potentials. *Front Hum Neurosci* (2014) 8:106. doi: 10.3389/ fnhum.2014.00106
84. Chun MM, Johnson MK. Memory: enduring traces of perceptual and reflective attention. *Neuron* (2011) 72:520–35. doi: 10.1016/j. neuron.2011.10.026
85. Cohen JD, Perlstein WM, Braver TS, Nystrom LE, Noll DC, Jonides J, et al. Temporal dynamics of brain activation during a working memory task. *Nature* (1997) 386:604–08. doi: 10.1038/386604a0
86. Polich J. Updating P300: an integrative theory of P3a and P3b. *Clin Neurophysiol* (2007) 118:2128–48. doi: 10.1016/j.clinph.2007.04.019
87. Johnson MR, Mitchell KJ, Raye CL, D'Esposito M, Johnson MK. A brief thought can modulate activity in extrastriate visual areas: top–down effects of refreshing just-seen visual stimuli. *Neuroimage* (2007) 37:290–9. doi: 10. 1016/j.neuroimage.2007.05.017
88. Bledowski C, Prvulovic D, Hoechstetter K, Scherg M, Wibral M, Goebel R, et al. Localizing P300 generators in visual target and distractor processing: a combined event-related potential and functional magnetic resonance imaging study. *J Neurosci* (2004) 24:9353–60. doi: 10.1523/JNEUROSCI. 1897-04.2004
89. Johnson MR, Johnson MK. Top–down enhancement and suppression of activity in category selective extrastriate cortex from an act of reflective attention. *J Cog Neurosci* (2009) 21:2320–7. doi: 10.1162/jocn. 2008.21183
90. Campanella S, Bourguignon M, Peigneux P, Metens T, Nouali M, Goldman S, et al. BOLD response to deviant face detection informed by P300 event-related potential parameters: a simultaneous ERP–fMRI study. *NeuroImage* (2013b) 71:92–103. doi: 10.1016/j.neuroimage.2012.12.077

2

# Learning from Loss after Risk: Dissociating Reward Pursuit and Reward Valuation in a Naturalistic Foraging Task

*Samantha V. Abram[1,2], A. David Redish[3] and Angus W. MacDonald III[1,4]**

*[1] Department of Psychology, University of Minnesota Twin Cities, Minneapolis, MN, United States, [2] Sierra Pacific Mental Illness Research Education and Clinical Centers, San Francisco VA Medical Center, and the University of California, San Francisco, San Francisco, CA, United States, [3] Department of Neuroscience, University of Minnesota Twin Cities, Minneapolis, MN, United States, [4] Department of Psychiatry, University of Minnesota Twin Cities, Minneapolis, MN, United States*

***Correspondence:***
*Angus W. MacDonald III*
*angus@umn.edu*

A fundamental feature of addiction is continued use despite high-cost losses. One possible driver of this feature is a dissociation between reward pursuit and reward valuation. To test for this dissociation, we employed a foraging paradigm with real-time delays and video rewards. Subjects made stay/skip choices on risky and non-risky offers; risky losses were operationalized as receipt of the longer delay after accepting a risky deal. We found that reward likability following risky losses predicted reward pursuit (i.e., subsequent choices), while there was no effect on reward valuation or reward pursuit in the absence of such losses. Individuals with high trait externalizing, who may be vulnerable to addiction, showed a dissociation between these phenomena: they liked videos more after risky losses but showed no decrease in choosing to stay on subsequent risky offers. This suggests that the inability to learn from mistakes is a potential component of risk for addiction.

**Keywords: risk, regret, foraging, decision-making, externalizing**

## INTRODUCTION

Many choices, like starting a new relationship or accepting a job out of state, involve some level of risk that can be expressed as a win or loss relative to baseline (1). Such decisions can lead to negative affective experiences, particularly if an individual chooses to take a risk and then receives an unfavorable outcome (2). While some individuals learn to make choices that minimize future negative outcomes (3, 4), the inability to learn from such losses may be integral to certain externalizing psychopathologies like addiction (5, 6). In this study, we examined relations between risky losses and externalizing tendencies by modifying a newly established human foraging paradigm (the *Web-Surf Task*) (7).

An earlier version of the Web-Surf Task was based on a rodent neuroeconomic task (*Restaurant Row*) (8). These parallel tasks entailed serial stay/skip choices regarding offers of real-time delays and primary rewards (food from four feeder sites in Restaurant Row, video clips from four galleries in the Web-Surf Task). On each encounter in the Web-Surf Task, the subject was informed of a required delay before the reward would be delivered, indicated by a download bar and numeric text instruction. The subject could either accept the deal and *stay* through the delay for the reward, or *skip* the deal and try his or her luck at the next reward site (video gallery). Reward kind (genre of video) remained constant at each gallery. Subjects had a limited time to spend on the task, thus creating delay-related trade-offs between galleries. Delay was random (selected uniformly from 1 to 30 s) on each offer encounter.

In our earlier work, we observed comparable decision valuation processes across species using these analogous tasks (9). Each subject revealed different, but reliable, delay-dependent preferences (i.e., thresholds) for each restaurant/gallery, taking delays below that threshold and skipping delays above. We also observed a high correspondence between choices and consummatory responses among humans (delay thresholds related to video enjoyment ratings), and between choices and stated preferences (delay thresholds related to rankings of video galleries assessed at the end of the task) (7).

Our initial work using the original Web-Surf Task bridged cross-species models of decision-making while also demonstrating the task's capacity to parse different valuation processes (7). A critical next step is to understand whether foraging task parameters predict meaningful individual differences, like those observed on the externalizing psychopathology spectrum (including addiction). We were motivated to use the Web-Surf Task to assess externalizing tendencies for two reasons: 1) the rodent analogue (Restaurant Row) has been used to assess the effects of different substances (i.e., cocaine and morphine) on deliberation and post-decisional commitment (6), highlighting the value of this paradigm for understanding substance use disorders. 2) Recent theories suggest that foraging models of decision-making are a promising approach for studying addiction, as these tasks measure how a subject allocates scarce resources (e.g., time) when searching for valuable goods (e.g., food, drug) (10). For instance, drug users can be conceptualized as foraging for resources in a patchy environment, e.g., smokers looking for the cheapest cigarettes (11).

To better assess for behavioral markers of addiction vulnerabilities using the Web-Surf Task, we added a risk component to the task, given accumulating evidence that risky decisions represent a vulnerability for substance use disorder (12). We then characterized risky outcomes according to prospect theory (13), which raises the possibility that subjects might reframe their enjoyment with regard to post-decisional outcomes. That is, they might reframe the outcome of an incurred risk (e.g., a win or loss) relative to the mid-point of the option, independent of whether the choice was the right option to take given the information at the time. For instance, the act of losing on a risky decision may impact video enjoyment regardless of whether their choice to stay and wait for that video was consistent with the offer's value.

Our overarching goal for the current study was to test whether an experiential foraging task can measure addiction-relevant behaviors, following from theories that conceptualize risky substance use within foraging models (14). More specifically, we aimed to determine 1) whether subjects showed differential responses to risky losses with respect to their enjoyment of reward and acceptance of subsequent risky deals, and 2) whether individual differences in response to risky losses predicted variation in trait-level externalizing, a risk factor for substance use disorders (15–17). We expected bad outcomes to reduce one's likelihood of accepting subsequent risky offers and for this pattern to be reversed among high-externalizing subjects (suggesting continued risk-taking despite negative outcomes).

# METHODS

## Subjects

One hundred five undergraduate students (81% female, average age 20.2 years) from the University of Minnesota completed the current study and received compensation in the form of extra credit towards psychology courses. We targeted a sample size of around 100 subjects for our individual differences analyses (i.e., relations with externalizing scores), given an *a priori* power analysis indicating the need for 84 subjects to have 80% power for detecting a moderate effect size of $r = 0.3$ when employing a 0.05 criteria for statistical significance (based on a meta-analysis indicating small to moderate effect sizes for risk-taking and externalizing trait correlations) (18). The racial/ethnic breakdown of the sample was as follows: 63% Caucasian, 26% Asian, 4% Black/African American, 3% Hispanic, 1% American Indian/Alaskan Native, 1% Native Hawaiian/Pacific Islander, 2% other. The University of Minnesota Institutional Review Board approved the study procedures, and all subjects provided written informed consent.

## Experimental Design

In the risk variant of the Web-Surf Task (**Figure 1A**), subjects had 40 min to travel between galleries that provided video rewards from the four galleries described in Abram et al. (7): kittens, dance, landscapes, and bike accidents. As in the original Web-Surf and Restaurant Row tasks, subjects had a fixed amount of time to forage; this means that subjects should have made economically maximizing decisions and stayed when the subjective value of an offer exceeded its cost.

Subjects encountered serial offers that presented a set of possible delays (**Figure 1B, C**): on entry into a gallery, the subject was shown a gallery icon, a textual representation of the offer, a pair of web-page like delay bars showing the maximum and minimum delays that could be received on that trial (possible delays ranged from 3 to 30 s), and the option to wait through the delay for a video from that gallery or move on. If the subject chose to wait, the actual delay was revealed, the delay counted down, and a 4 s video was shown; the subject then rated the video from 1 to 4 as an indicator of how much he or she liked it (4 = highest). Enjoyment ratings were made with key presses, and the task did not proceed until subjects input a rating (thus, there were no missing ratings). Importantly, in this version of the task, punishment was inescapable: subjects were locked in after making a stay choice (after which the delay began to count down). After each trial (regardless of the choice to stay or skip), the subject had to perform a short "travel" task, which entailed clicking the numbers 1 to 4 (presented in a darker shade of gray) as they randomly appeared around the screen (shown in a lighter gray). This travel task produced a cost to leaving an offer before getting to the next offer and was analogous to the travel time required as rats move between feeders during Restaurant Row.

Risky and non-risky trials were intermixed. Risk level was reflected by the variance of an offer and was either 0 (non-risky) or greater than 0 (risky, see **Figure 1**). *Risky trials* consisted of an offer with a range of delays (e.g., 5, 10, or 15 s), and each offer varied according to the set of possible delays and spread between

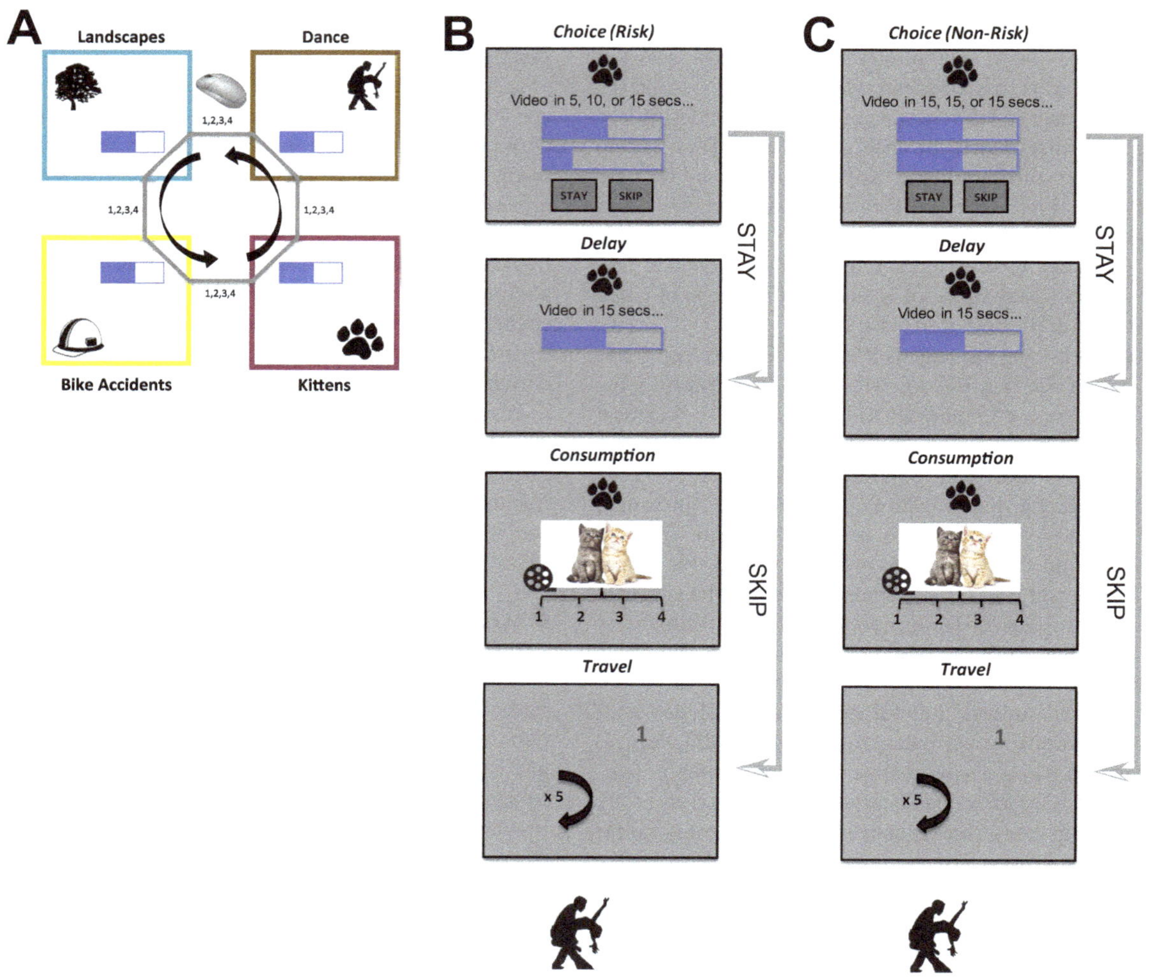


**FIGURE 1** | Overview of task layout. **(A)** Schematic representation of the Web-Surf Task. Subjects cycled between four video galleries (kittens, dance, landscapes, bike accidents) in a constant order. **(B, C)** Flow diagram illustrates sequencing between risky **(B)** and non-risky **(C)** trials. For a risky trial, the true delay was only revealed if the subject stayed. If they instead skipped, they advanced directly to the travel task before encountering the next offer. The travel task entailed clicking the numbers 1–4 as they appeared around the screen (traveling required five random number selections).

the shortest and longest delay. (We did not allow for non-integer mid values in the risky trials, e.g., "Video in 5, 5.5, or 6 secs..." could not occur.) Critically, for risky trials, the true delay was only revealed if the subject elected to stay. Subjects were not informed of the probabilities associated with receipt of the different delays on risky trials. In comparison, *non-risky trials* presented offers with three identical delays, e.g., "Video in 7, 7, or 7 secs..."

We further classified risky trials as good or bad based on their outcome: receipt of the low delay on a risky trial was a "good" outcome, while receipt of the high delay was a "bad" outcome. (Following the framing effects from prospect theory, our definitions derive from an offer's outcome *type* but not *value*, meaning that a bad outcome could have a delay below one's threshold.) We were particularly interested in situations where the subject accepted a risky offer and received the bad outcome, i.e., the subject took a risk and "lost." We contrasted these trials with a control condition, in which the subject accepted a non-risky offer of equivalent value, and with situations characterized by relief, where the subject received the good outcome on a risk trial, i.e., the subject took a risk and "won". Importantly, the decision to *stay* or *skip* the offer on a non-risky trial, in which the true offer delay is known, can be assumed to be economically valid (i.e., correctly judged, not a mistake).

All subjects first underwent a training phase that entailed eight practice trials (two cycles through all four galleries, presented in the same order as the main task). After completion of the training phase, the subject had the opportunity to ask questions of the examiner before advancing to the main test phase.

## Trait-Level Externalizing Measure

Subjects completed the 100-item version of the Externalizing Spectrum Inventory (ESI; 19), which has been employed in several studies of undergraduate students (20–23). This inventory captures a range of traits and behaviors associated with the externalizing spectrum of psychopathology, including general disinhibition processes (e.g., theft, irresponsibility), substance use/abuse, and callous aggression.[1] Total ESI scores were acquired by summing across all items in the inventory (20) and then applying a log-transformation to improve normality.

To assess whether behavior on the risk variant of the Web-Surf Task was related specifically to substance abuse tendencies versus externalizing behavior more broadly, we computed the three ESI subfactors: *general disinhibition* (which captures impulsivity and irresponsibility), *substance abuse* (which captures recreational and problematic substance use), and *callous aggression* (which captures physical/relational aggression and lack of empathy) (21, 24). Lastly, we computed three subscales from the substance abuse subfactor that measure problems associated with substance use: *alcohol problems*, *marijuana problems*, and *drug problems*; here, our aim was to further explore whether task behaviors predicted substance-related consequences or harms. Examples of questions in these subscales are: "My drinking led to problems at home," "I've broken the law to get money for drugs," and "At times, marijuana has been more important to me than work, friends, or school." Because many subjects were non-responders on the problem scales, we encountered a zero-inflation problem. We thus isolated subjects who endorsed at least one item on the subscale, as individuals already experiencing negative consequences (evidence of behavioral disinhibition) are at greater risk for developing an alcohol or substance use disorder (25); 22 subjects (21%) were retained for the alcohol problem subscale analyses, versus 18 subjects (17%) for the marijuana problem subscale analyses, and 19 subjects (18%) for the drug problem subscale analyses.

## Analyses

### Specialized Procedures

**Heaviside step function:** a piecewise function denoted H($x$), where H($x$) = 0 for $x < 0$, H($x$) = ½ when $x = 0$, and H($x$) = 1 for $x > 0$. This function captures the point at which a signal switches from 0 to 1. We used this function to identify the point at which subjects reliably began to skip offers (which we refer to as *delay thresholds*; see below for details). We used a Heaviside step function as an alternative to the logistic fit function described in Abram et al. (7), as the Heaviside approach is better equipped to handle extreme cases (i.e., when a subject stayed or skipped all offers in a gallery). In such instances, the Heaviside step function produces a reasonable value (e.g., the minimal or maximal delay offered), whereas the logistic function can produce values approaching infinity.

**Subject-specific delay thresholds** were computed separately for each trial using a leave-one-out approach; this yielded four thresholds, one per gallery. Thresholds were indicative of revealed preferences, reflecting the delay time at which a subject reliably began to skip offers for a particular gallery. To obtain the threshold for trial *i*, we fit a Heaviside step function to all trials in gallery *x* excluding trial *i*. This produced a vector of thresholds with length equal to the number of trials in gallery *x*. Importantly, thresholds were computed using the mid value of each offer for risky trials only. Non-risky trials were then assigned a threshold equal to the mean of the threshold vector for the respective gallery.

**Expected value for non-risky trials (with a given delay):** defined as the difference between the gallery-specific threshold and the offered delay. **Expected value for risky trials:** calculated as the average expected value of the three delays, assuming an equal likelihood for each delay (low, mid, high; see **Figure 1C**). For simplicity, we assumed a linear difference. Values ranged from −27 to 27, with a value of 0 meaning that the delay offer was equivalent to the revealed threshold.

**Mixed-effects models:** We used linear mixed-effects models to assess for group-level effects; all reported models include original p-values as well as false discovery rate (FDR)—adjusted p-values using Benjamini and Hochberg's FDR control algorithm (26). We fit models using the MCMCglmm package in R (27), which uses Markov chain Monte Carlo techniques (see below), and lmer and lsmeans, which provided nearly identical estimates, for plotting (28, 29). The tilde (~) in all regression models can be read as "is modeled as a function of" (30).

**Markov chain Monte Carlo (MCMC) techniques:** an approach that uses random sampling to approximate the posterior distribution of a variable of interest within a probabilistic space.

### Validity Analyses

We evaluated the *external and face validity* of the risk variant of the Web-Surf Task using methods described in Abram et al. (7). For each subject, for each gallery, we averaged the vector of delay thresholds produced using the leave-one-out method described above; this yielded four thresholds per subject. We measured external validity by correlating delay thresholds with stated preferences (i.e., average gallery ratings and post-test gallery rankings) and obtained two validity correlations per subject.

### Group-Level Choice, Rating, and Reaction Time Models

Our *primary choice/rating models* evaluated the impact of framing (i.e., good/bad outcome) on risk seeking (i.e., subsequent choices) and reward valuation (i.e., immediate video enjoyment ratings).

The *primary choice model* evaluated whether the type of outcome on the previous trial influenced subsequent risk seeking or aversion. This model included choice at the current trial as the dependent variable, actual value received and outcome type at the previous trial as fixed-effect independent variables, and subject as a random effect: [$Choice_t \sim actual\ value_{t-1} + outcome\ type_{t-1} + (1|subject)$]. This model included risky trials where the subject stayed and also received a risky offer at the next trial.

The *primary rating model* assessed the impact of framing effects on immediate reward valuation and included mean-centered rating as the dependent variable (i.e., centered to the average of the respective gallery), actual value and outcome type at the previous trial as fixed-effect independent variables, and subject as a random effect: [$Rating_t \sim actual\ value_t + outcome\ type_t + (1|subject)$]. This model included risky trials for which the subject stayed.

[1] Missing self-report data for 1 subject.

Lastly, we computed a *secondary group-level model* to examine direct relations between risk seeking/aversion and reward valuation, while considering the effects of framing and risk. In particular, we were interested in whether affective responses interacted with actual value or offer type when predicting subsequent decisions (building off the prior choice model detailed above). This model included choice at the current trial as the dependent variable; actual value, mean-centered rating, and outcome type of the previous trial, and two interaction terms as fixed-effect independent variables; and subject as a random effect: [$Choice_t \sim actual\ value_{t-1} + rating_{t-1} + outcome\ type_{t-1} + actual\ value_{t-1}{:}rating_{t-1} + actual\ value_{t-1}{:}outcome\ type_{t-1} + (1|subject)$]. In this model, outcome type coded good outcomes, bad outcomes, and non-risky offers; this metric then reflected the framing and risk manipulations.

To assess whether bad outcomes influenced the speed at which subjects made subsequent decisions, we tested a *supplemental reaction time model* that included logged reaction times as the dependent variable, actual value received and outcome type at the previous trial as fixed-effect independent variables, and subject as a random effect: [$logRT_t \sim actual\ value_{t-1} + outcome\ type_{t-1} + (1|subject)$].

## Global Risk-Aversion Trend and Control Models

We also constructed a set of models to investigate global trends in risk seeking/aversion and reward valuation, i.e., address the possibility that any trial-by-trial effects were better explained by cross-session effects. The *global risk-aversion model* included choice as the dependent variable; number of videos viewed (i.e., consumed up to trial *t*), expected value, a risky/non-risky categorical indicator, and a video consumption × risky/non-risky interaction term as the fixed-effect independent variables; and subject as a random effect: [$Choice_t \sim number\ videos\ consumed_t + expected\ value_t + risky/non\text{-}risky_t + number\ consumed\ videos_t{:}risky/non\text{-}risky_t + (1|subject)$]. All trials were included in the choice model.

The global risk-aversion rating model was structurally equivalent to the first but included mean-centered ratings as the dependent variable: [$Rating_t \sim number\ videos\ consumed_t + expected\ value_t + risky/non\text{-}risky_t + number\ consumed\ videos_t{:}risky/non\text{-}risky_t + (1|subject)$]. Only stay trials were included in the rating model, as subjects only rated videos during stay trials.

Based on the results of the global trend models above, we constructed a *control model* to assess whether any trial-by-trial effects were better explained by other risk-aversion patterns. Within this model, we controlled for global risk-aversion trends (number of videos consumed), as well as categorical (high, low, mid) and continuous (0–30 s) risk dimensions. Our intention was to determine if cross-session declines in accepting risky deals and/or the general tendency to prefer offers with lower risk, i.e., a more narrow offer window, could better account for the sequential choice effects seen. The control model was structured as follows: [$Choice_t \sim actual\ value_{t-1} + outcome\ type_{t-1} + number\ videos\ consumed_t + risk_t + (1|subject)$].

## Subject-Specific Choice and Rating Models

To examine individual differences, we fit subject-specific models based on the main choice and rating group-level models. For the *subject-specific choice models*, we included choice at the current trial as the dependent variable and actual value and outcome type of the prior trial as the independent variables: [$Choice_t \sim actual\ value_{t-1} + outcome\ type_{t-1}$]. We extracted the unstandardized outcome-type coefficient that reflected the subject's likelihood to stay following receipt of the good versus bad outcome, with higher values indicating an increased tendency to stay after receiving the bad outcome.

For the *subject-specific rating models*, we included mean-centered ratings as the dependent variable and actual value and outcome type of the prior trial as independent variables: [$Rating_t \sim actual\ value_{t-1} + outcome\ type_{t-1}$]. We again extracted the unstandardized outcome-type coefficient for good versus bad outcomes, with higher coefficients reflecting better ratings for the bad versus good outcome.

We correlated the subject-specific coefficients with trait-level externalizing, using robust partial correlation methods to reduce the influence of outliers and control for age, sex, and ethnicity. We included the age and sex demographic covariates based on prior research linking these variables with self-report and behavioral impulsivity measures (31), and more broadly with externalizing tendencies (32–34). We also included race/ethnicity, as substance use trajectories through young adulthood may differ by this factor (35). Our *primary partial correlations* related the two subject-specific coefficients with total ESI scores (distributions shown in **Figure 7**), and *follow-up partial correlations* assessed for associations with the substance abuse subfactor and subscales.

## Delay-Discounting Comparison Models

Given the extensive literature using traditional binary choice tasks to evaluate externalizing and impulsivity (36–38), we tested whether metrics from a computerized monetary delay- and probability-discounting paradigm better explained individual differences in externalizing.[2] This entailed subjects making a series of binary choices between hypothetical monetary rewards of different reward magnitudes associated with different temporal delays (e.g., "Would you prefer $5 now or $10 in two weeks?") or probabilities (e.g., "Would you prefer $5 for sure or $10 with a 75% chance?"). Offers ranged from 50 cents to $10. The task lasted approximately 10 min.

A discounting rate (or k-value) was computed for the delay and probability trials separately using a hyperbolic function (39), yielding two k-values per subject. Higher k-values reflect more rapid discounting of delayed rewards and have been linked with impulsivity and addiction (40). For each subject, we checked for nonsystematic data using criteria outlined by Johnson and Bickel (41), and an $R^2$ value was calculated to determine how well the data points fit the hyperbolic function.[3] The median $R^2$ was 0.86 and 0.91 for the delay- and probability-discounting rates

[2] Missing delay- and probability-discounting data for three subjects.

[3] We excluded nine subjects with invalid k-values (discounting rates of 0), one subject with a k-value more than 4 standard deviations above the mean, and one subject with nonsystematic data.

(i.e., logged k-values), respectively. Logged parameter distributions of k from the delay-discounting experiment showed median = −5.26 days$^{-1}$, SD = 2.05, and from the probability experiment showed median = 0.28% chance$^{-1}$, SD = 0.84. These results are comparable to those reported in a large sample of healthy adults (31) and suggest that, for our sample, a $10 reward would be generally worth $9.52 after a 10-day delay or $8.75 when equated with a 90% chance.

## RESULTS

### Subjects Were Willing to Wait for Videos and Showed Individual Preferences

Subjects performed similarly on this task to what was seen in the original Web-Surf Task (7). As shown in **Figure 2D** and **E**, subjects showed reliable thresholds that were generally correlated with ratings (median $r = 0.66$) and with rankings (median $r = 0.60$). The decision curves of both risky and non-risky decisions depict the expected sigmoid shape, where subjects typically skipped low-valued offers (i.e., expected value < 0) and stayed for high-valued offers (i.e., expected value > 0).

### Loss After Risk Influences Choice and Reward Valuation

To address questions of how subjects responded to loss after risk, we examined how risky outcomes impacted decision behaviors and video ratings. Here, a given delay was framed as good, bad, or in-between (mid) depending on its placement within an offer on a risky trial. Note that the true delay was known at the outset of the non-risky trials but was only revealed after the decision to stay on risky trials. Our *primary choice model* shows that, when controlling for actual value, subjects were less likely to accept a successive risky offer if they previously received a bad outcome than if they had previously received a good outcome ($p$-adj = 0.01; **Figure 3A**; **Table 1a**). Subjects were also slower to make decisions following receipt of the bad outcome (**Figure 4**; **Table 2**), suggestive of post-error slowing in response to risky losses.

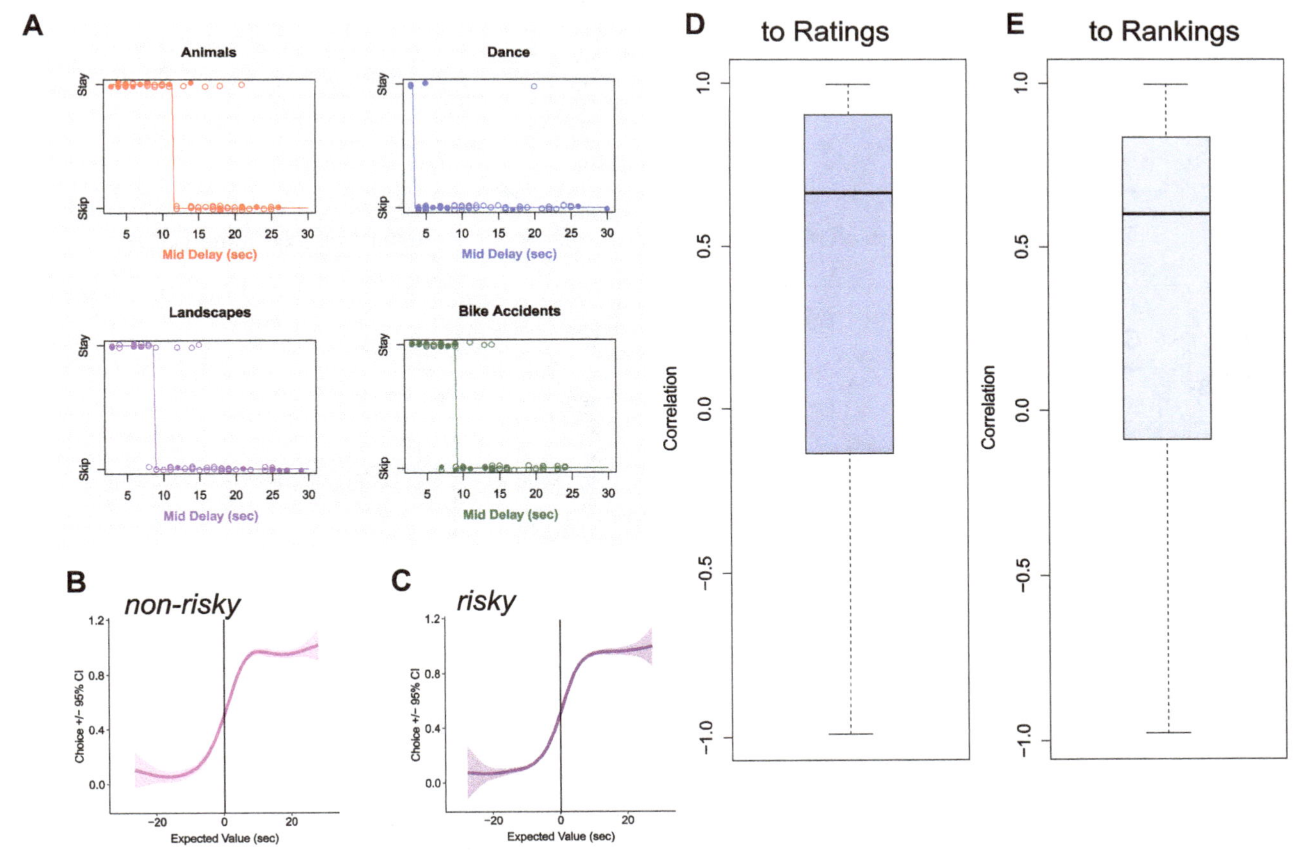


**FIGURE 2 |** Thresholds reveal valuations. **(A)** Example thresholds identified for a typical subject. Open circles show risky trials; closed circles show non-risky trials. Threshold marked with solid line. **(B)** Average psychophysics curve for non-risky decisions, aligned to threshold for each video gallery for each subject. **(C)** Average psychophysics curve for risky decisions, aligned to threshold for each video gallery for each subject. Panels **(B)** and **(C)** are aligned to the same threshold, calculated for each gallery for each subject. **(D)** Distribution of observed correlations between revealed thresholds and video ratings. **(E)** Distribution of observed correlations between revealed thresholds and post-task stated rankings.

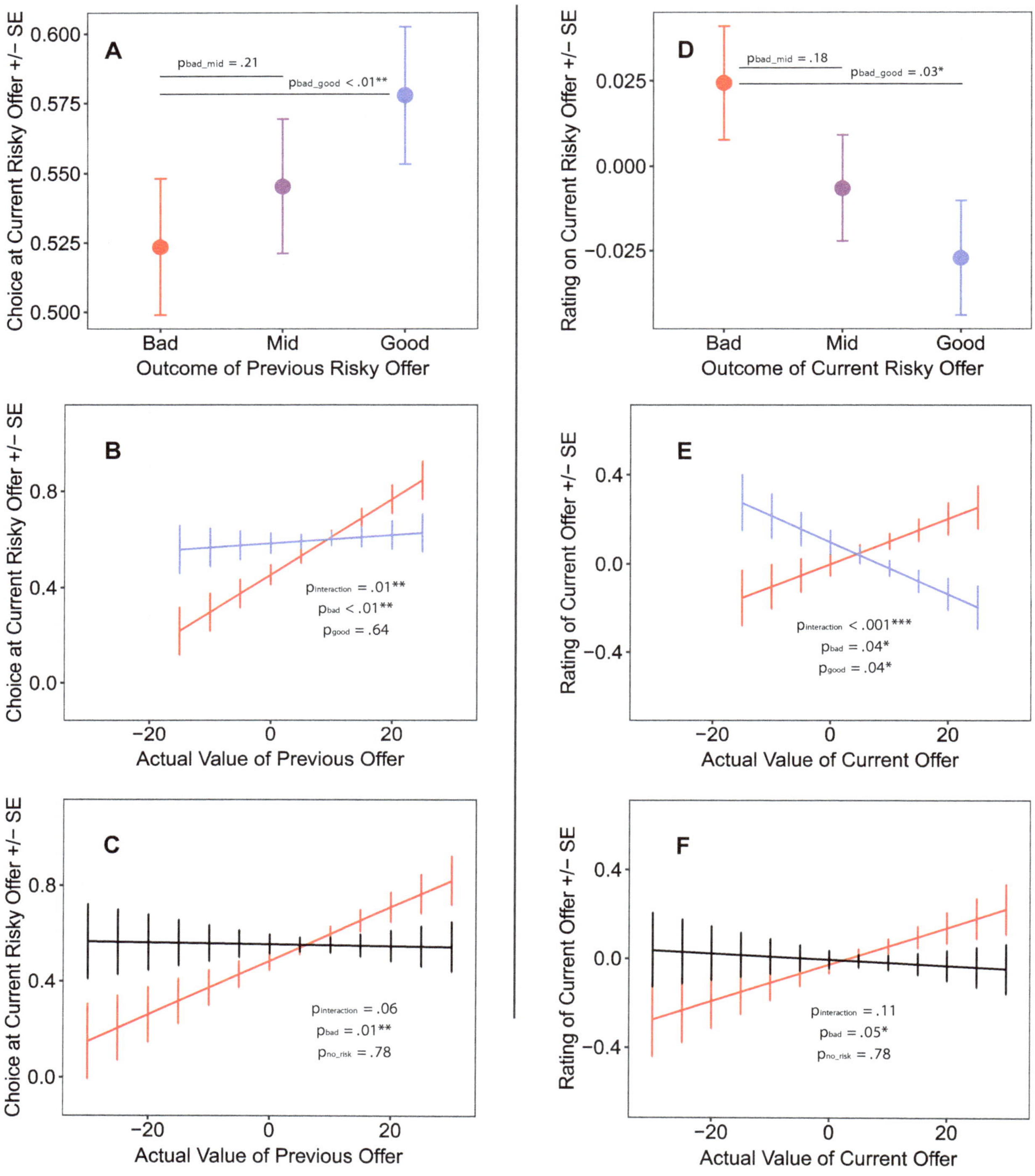


**FIGURE 3 |** Group- and individual-level effects of risky losses on deliberation and reward likability. **(A)** Proportion of stay choices on current risky offers following receipt of the good, bad, or mid outcome on the previous risk trial. Red represents a bad outcome after accepting a risky offer; blue indicates a relief-inducing situation (good outcome after accepting a risky offer), with higher values indicating an increased likelihood of staying. Subjects were more risk-averse after risky losses. **(B, C)** Interactions between previous outcome type and actual value when predicting choices on subsequent risky offers. Black represents the control condition (equivalently valued non-risk offers). Subjects became risk-averse following risky losses of low value, versus risk seeking after risky losses of high value (whereas no associations between value and choice were detected for the relief and control conditions). **(D)** Mean-centered likability ratings following the receipt of the good, bad, and mid outcomes on the current risk trial. Subjects rated videos that followed bad outcomes more highly than those that followed good outcomes. **(E, F)** Interactions between previous outcome type and actual value when predicting immediate likability ratings (mean-centered). After a risky loss, subjects tended to rate videos that followed a low-value offer worse than those that followed a high-value offer; the inverse pattern was found for videos linked to good outcomes. A similar pattern emerged when comparing bad outcomes and control trials. Error bars indicate within-subject standard errors. *$p < 0.05$; **$p < 0.01$; ***$p < 0.001$.

**TABLE 1** | Choice/rating by framing models.

| Predictor variable | B | CI | *P*-value | *P*-adj |
|---|---|---|---|---|
| (a) Choice by framing (main) | | | | |
| Actual value | −.006 | [−.008, −.004] | **.001** | **.002** |
| Outcome type (bad vs. good) | −.055 | [−.098, −.020] | **.008** | **.01** |
| Outcome type (mid vs. good) | −.033 | [−066, .005] | .10 | .10 |
| (b) Choice bad vs. good framing (follow-up) | | | | |
| Actual value | .013 | [.004, .023] | **.004** | **.008** |
| Outcome type (bad vs. good) | .134 | [.010, .236] | **.02** | **.02** |
| Actual value × outcome type | −.014 | [−026, −.002] | **.01** | **.02** |
| (c) Choice by bad vs. non-risk framing (follow-up) | | | | |
| Actual value | .011 | [.002, .019] | **.02** | **.03** |
| Outcome type (bad vs. non-risk) | .056 | [−.048, .144] | .24 | .24 |
| Actual value × outcome type | −.010 | [−.020, .000] | .06 | .08 |
| (d) Rating by framing (main) | | | | |
| Actual value | .002 | [.000, .004] | **.04** | **.05** |
| Outcome type (bad vs. good) | .051 | [.005, .100] | **.03** | **.05** |
| Outcome type (mid vs. good) | .020 | [−.022, .065] | .38 | .38 |
| (e) Rating by bad vs. good framing (follow-up) | | | | |
| Actual value | .010 | [.000, .020] | **.04** | .08 |
| Outcome type (bad vs. good) | .100 | [−.046, .244] | .17 | .23 |
| Actual value × outcome type | −.022 | [−.038, −.009] | **<.001** | **.004** |
| (f) Rating by bad vs. non-risk framing (follow-up) | | | | |
| Actual value | .008 | [.000, .016] | **.04** | .37 |
| Outcome type (bad vs. non-risk) | .021 | [−.087, .128] | .68 | 1.00 |
| Actual value × outcome type | −.010 | [−.021, .004] | .11 | .48 |

*B, unstandardized coefficient; CI, confidence interval; P-adj, FDR-adjusted p-values. Bolded text indicates p-values that are below 0.05.*

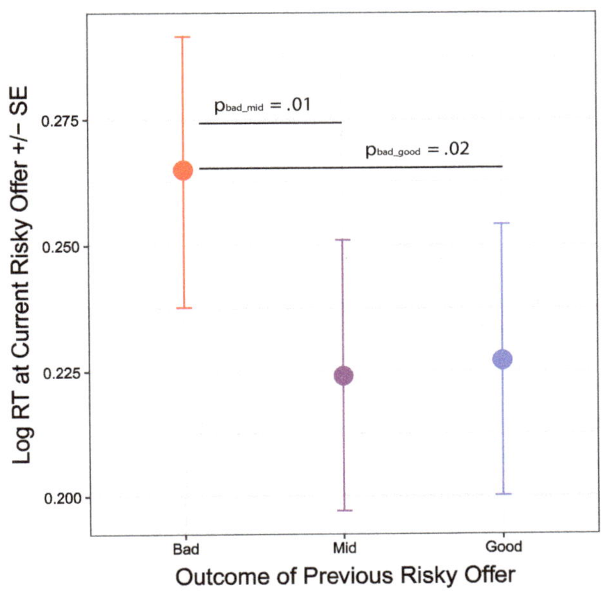


**FIGURE 4** | Loss after risk influences reaction times. Receipt of the bad (long-delay) outcome (red) resulted in slower reaction times (log RT) on subsequent trials, as compared to other risky conditions. Error bars represent within-subject standard errors.

*Follow-up models* clarified these sequential choice effects using subsets of trials matched by the actual value of the previous trial. The first subset included trials for which subjects stayed and received the good or bad outcome on a risky trial and encountered risk on the following trial. The second subset included trials for which subjects stayed and received the bad outcome or stayed on a non-risky trial and encountered risk on the subsequent trial. Trials were matched on a subject-by-subject basis and then combined for the group analysis. Because each subject's contributing trials only included a portion of the possible values, we included actual value as a nested variable in the following model: [$Choice_t \sim actual\ value_{t\text{-}1} + outcome\ type_{t\text{-}1} + actual\ value_{t\text{-}1}{:}outcome\ type_{t\text{-}1} + (actual\ value_{t\text{-}1}|subject)$]. We included the interaction term to test whether framing effects differentially shaped value-by-choice sequencing effects.

**TABLE 2** | Logged choice reaction time by framing model.

| Predictor variable | B | CI | *P*-value | *P*-adj |
|---|---|---|---|---|
| Actual value | .001 | [−.001, .003] | .33 | .44 |
| Outcome type (bad vs. good) | .041 | [.008, .071] | **.02** | **.04** |
| Outcome type (mid vs. good) | .001 | [−.028, .032] | .95 | .95 |

*B, unstandardized coefficient; CI, confidence interval; P-adj, FDR-adjusted p-values. Bolded text indicates p-values that are below 0.05.*

For the subset that matched bad- with good-outcome trials, we observed a significant outcome-by-value interaction ($p$-adj = 0.02; **Table 1b**); further analyses revealed that the negative framing of the previous outcome impacted relations between value of the previous trial and choice on the current trial ($\beta = 0.014$, CI = [0.004, 0.023], $p = 0.004$; **Figure 3B**). That is, subjects became risk-averse after receiving a bad offer of lower value and risk seeking after a bad offer of higher value. In contrast, we did not detect an association between the previous trial's value and successive choice after receipt of a good outcome ($\beta = 0.002$, CI = [−0.007, 0.011], $p = 0.64$). We identified a similar (but trend-level) effect for the subset that matched bad outcome with equivalent non-risk offers (outcome-by-value interaction, $p$-adj = 0.08; **Table 1c**); follow-up analyses indicated a positive association between value and choice following receipt of a bad outcome ($\beta = 0.012$, CI = [0.004, 0.020], $p = 0.012$; **Figure 3C**), versus no association for non-risky decisions ($\beta = 0.001$, CI = [−0.007, 0.009], p = 0.78). Together, these results suggest that receipt of negatively framed outcomes (or losses), in particular, changed subsequent reward pursuit and decision-making.

But to what extent do losses after risk impact the liking of a reward? Experiments have suggested that subjects take expended costs into account when making valuations (42, 43). To address this question, we tested the impact of framing on ratings. We observed an opposite pattern in the *primary rating model* as compared to the *primary choice model*: where subjects rated videos that followed a *bad* outcome more highly than those that followed a good outcome ($p$-adj = 0.05; **Figure 3D–F**; **Table 1d**). We clarified these rating effects using *follow-up* matched-trial *models* that compared ratings that followed good versus bad outcomes and ratings that followed bad outcomes versus non-risky offers. We then fit the following model: [$Rating_t \sim actual\ value_{t-1} + outcome\ type_{t-1} + actual\ value_{t-1}{:}outcome\ type_{t-1} + (actual\ value_{t-1}|subject)$].

These follow-up analyses revealed an interaction between actual value and rating for bad versus good outcomes ($p$-adj = 0.004; **Figure 3E**; **Table 1e**), with bad outcomes yielding a positive association between value and rating ($\beta = 0.010$, CI = [0.000, 0.020], $p = 0.04$) and good outcomes a negative association ($\beta = -0.012$, CI = [−0.022, −0.001], $p = 0.04$). Although not significant (interaction term in **Table 1f**), we saw a similar pattern for the interaction between risky and non-risky trials, with risky trials having a more substantial impact on the relationship between bad outcomes and ratings than non-risky trials (bad outcomes: $\beta = 0.008$, CI = [0.000, 0.017], $p = 0.05$; non-risky: $\beta = -0.001$, CI = [−0.010, 0.007], $p = 0.78$; **Figure 3F**).

## Global Trends Impacted Choices But Not Ratings

We found that subjects were less likely to accept a risky offer versus a non-risky offer as they consumed more videos (significant number of consumed videos × risk interaction, $p$-adj = 0.004; **Figure 5A**; **Table 3a**); that is, subjects became more risk-averse across the session. This interaction remained significant if the consumption variable was replaced with the number of good outcomes or bad outcomes, suggesting that this effect was not solely driven by accumulated negative experiences (but rather, risky rewards became progressively less effective in eliciting reward seeking with ongoing exposure). In comparison, we did not observe a consumption history x risk interaction ($p$-adj = 0.67) for the rating model (**Figure 5B**; **Table 3b**), suggesting that ratings were less impacted by these factors.

## Sequential Choice Effects Remained When Accounting for Global Trends

Based on the evidence that subjects grew risk-averse across the session, we built a *control model* to test whether the global risk-aversion trends (noted above) confounded trial-by-trial framing effects. The control model indicated that trial-by-trial choice effects were not better explained by consumption history (i.e., number of videos consumed) or risk level (i.e., spread of delays on a risky offer; **Table 4**).

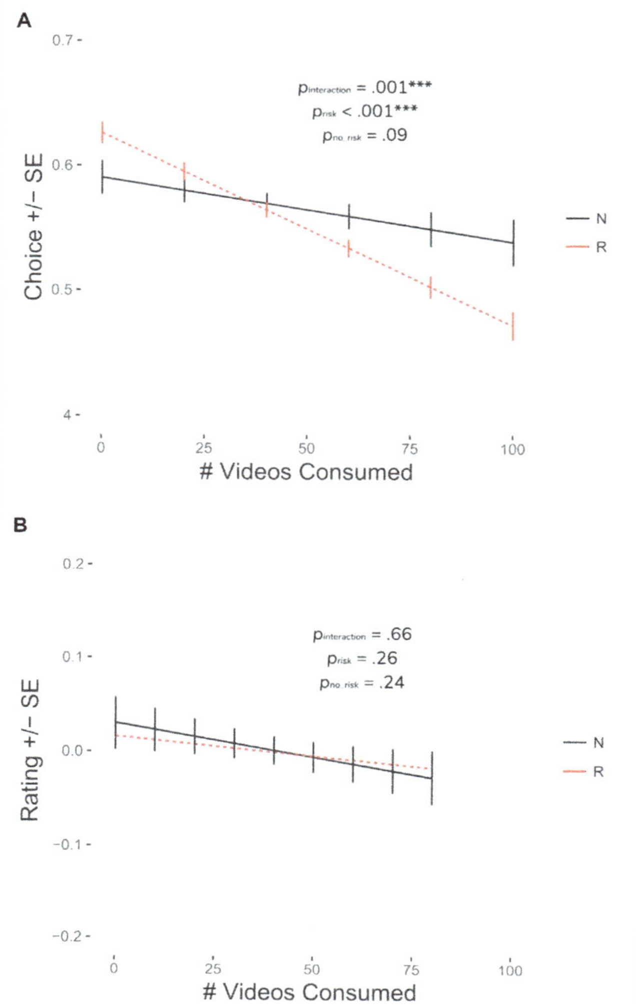


**FIGURE 5 |** Global risk trends. **(A)** Subjects became more risk-averse as the task progressed. **(B)** Subjects' likability ratings decreased over time but did not differ between risky and non-risky offers. Error bars represent within-subject standard errors. ***$p < 0.001$.

## Is the Effect Simply Due to Seeking Gains and Avoiding Losses?

The analyses above showed that the effect of risky trials on subsequent choices depended on the unexpected costs of the trial: a bad outcome meant spending more time than expected and was therefore a loss (worse than expected), while a good outcome meant spending less time than expected and was therefore a gain (better than expected). To test whether this was a general property of unexpected gains and losses, we turned to variability in the ratings within each gallery. While all the videos within a gallery were similar (e.g., cute videos of kittens), each individual video was different. Thus, subjects had an expectation of video quality based on their gallery preferences, but observed a specific video on completion of the delay that might have been better or worse than the average. This produced variability in the post-video ratings: for example, seeing a video rated worse

**TABLE 3 |** Choice/rating by consumption models.

| Predictor variable | B | CI | P-value | P-adj |
|---|---|---|---|---|
| (a) Choice | | | | |
| # videos consumed | −.001 | [−.001, .000] | **.07** | .17 |
| Expected value | .032 | [.031, .033] | **.001** | **.004** |
| Risk/non-risk | .036 | [.007, .061] | **.006** | **.02** |
| # videos consumed x risk/ non-risk | −001 | [−.002, .000] | **.001** | **.004** |
| (b) Rating | | | | |
| # videos consumed | −.001 | [−.002, .001] | .25 | .62 |
| Expected value | .002 | [.000, .004] | **.02** | .11 |
| Risk/non-risk | −014 | [−.086, .048] | .67 | .67 |
| # videos consumed x risk/ non-risk | .000 | [−.001, .002] | .66 | .67 |

*B, unstandardized coefficient; CI, confidence interval; P-adj, FDR-adjusted p-values. Bolded text indicates p-values that are below 0.05.*

**TABLE 4 |** Choice by consumption and risk confound model.

| Predictor variable | B | CI | P-value | P-adj |
|---|---|---|---|---|
| Actual value | −.007 | [−.008, −.005] | **<.001** | **.002** |
| Outcome type (bad vs. good) | −.055 | [−.092, −.017] | **.006** | **.01** |
| Outcome type (mid vs. good) | −.036 | [−.068, −.001] | **.04** | **.05** |
| # videos consumed | −.001 | [−.002, −.001] | **<.001** | **.002** |
| Risk | −.002 | [−005, .000] | .07 | .07 |

*B, unstandardized coefficient; CI, confidence interval; P-adj, FDR-adjusted p-values. Bolded text indicates p-values that are below 0.05.*

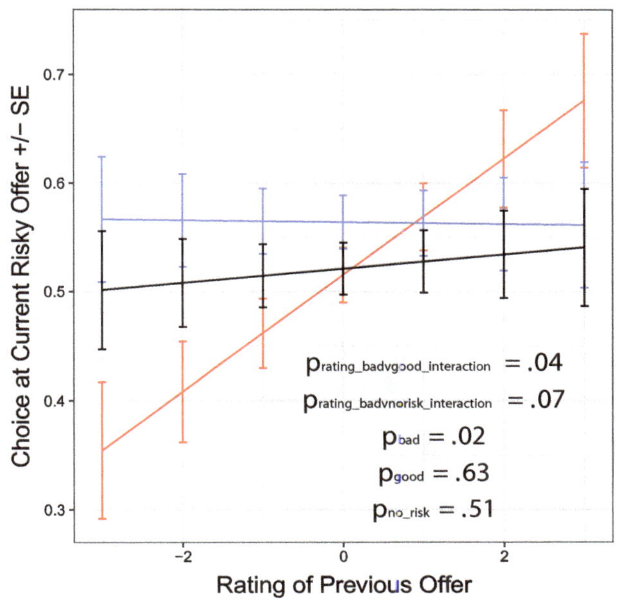


**FIGURE 6 |** Interaction between previous outcome type and rating when predicting choices on subsequent risky offers. Following receipt of the bad outcome, subjects were more risk-averse after lower-rated videos and more risk seeking after higher-rated videos; no association was detected for the other conditions; ratings are mean-centered. Error bars represent within-subject standard errors.

than average was effectively a loss, while a video rated better than average was effectively a gain. In general, we can consider video ratings themselves as a measure of gain/loss.

We used a *secondary model* to test whether video ratings directly guided future choices under the different conditions of interest (**Figure 6**; **Table 5**). We found trend-level interactions between outcome and rating ($p$-adj = 0.06, $p$-adj = 0.09): following risky losses, relatively lower ratings predicted risk aversion, whereas relatively higher ratings yielded risk-seeking behaviors ($\beta$ = 0.040, CI = [0.005, 0.071], $p$ = 0.02). We did not detect associations between video ratings and subsequent choice following good outcomes ($\beta$ = 0.009, CI = [-0.028, 0.039], $p$ = 0.63) or non-risky trials ($\beta$ = 0.011, CI = [-0.017, 0.043], $p$ = 0.51). Thus, ratings only produced changes in risk seeking if in the context of bad outcomes on risky trials (akin to a win–stay/lose–shift strategy) (44). This implies that there was something different about risky losses that went beyond the mere experience of a less enjoyable reward (since a good outcome of the risky trial leading to a poorly rated video was still a loss but did not impact subsequent reward pursuit). We note that these effects remained when accounting for the number of prior videos consumed.

**TABLE 5 |** Choice by rating integrated model.

| Predictor variable | B | CI | P-value | P-adj |
|---|---|---|---|---|
| Actual value | −.006 | [−.008, −.004] | **<.001** | **.004** |
| Rating | .040 | [.005, .073] | **.03** | .06 |
| Outcome type (good vs. bad) | .049 | [.015, .090] | **.01** | **.03** |
| Outcome type (non-risk vs. bad) | .006 | [−.028, .039] | .74 | .74 |
| Actual value × rating | .002 | [.000, .004] | .12 | **.14** |
| Rating × outcome type (good vs. bad) | −.055 | [−.110, −.004] | .04 | .06 |
| Rating × outcome type (non-risk vs. bad) | −.047 | [−.102, .001] | .07 | .09 |

*B, unstandardized coefficient; CI, confidence interval; P-adj, FDR-adjusted p-values. Bolded text indicates p-values that are below 0.05.*

## Failure to Learn from Loss After Risk Correlated With Externalizing Traits

To explore the importance of personality traits to risky decision-making, we investigated whether individuals scoring high on the Externalizing Spectrum Inventory (ESI, 19, which measures a range of impulsive, substance use, and aggressive behaviors) were less influenced by risk when making choices. **Figure 7A** and **B** shows the distribution of observed ESI values. Many subjects who typically score high on externalizing inventories, such as chronic smokers and individuals at risk for addiction, have been seen to be less influenced by risk when making choices (45, 46). We examined whether such individuals exhibited similar risk-induced effects on reward valuation (i.e., video ratings).

Informed by the group-level model, we computed a parameter that compared a subject's likelihood of accepting a risky offer after receipt of a good versus bad outcome on the prior trial. Individuals scoring high on the ESI showed an inverse pattern to that observed

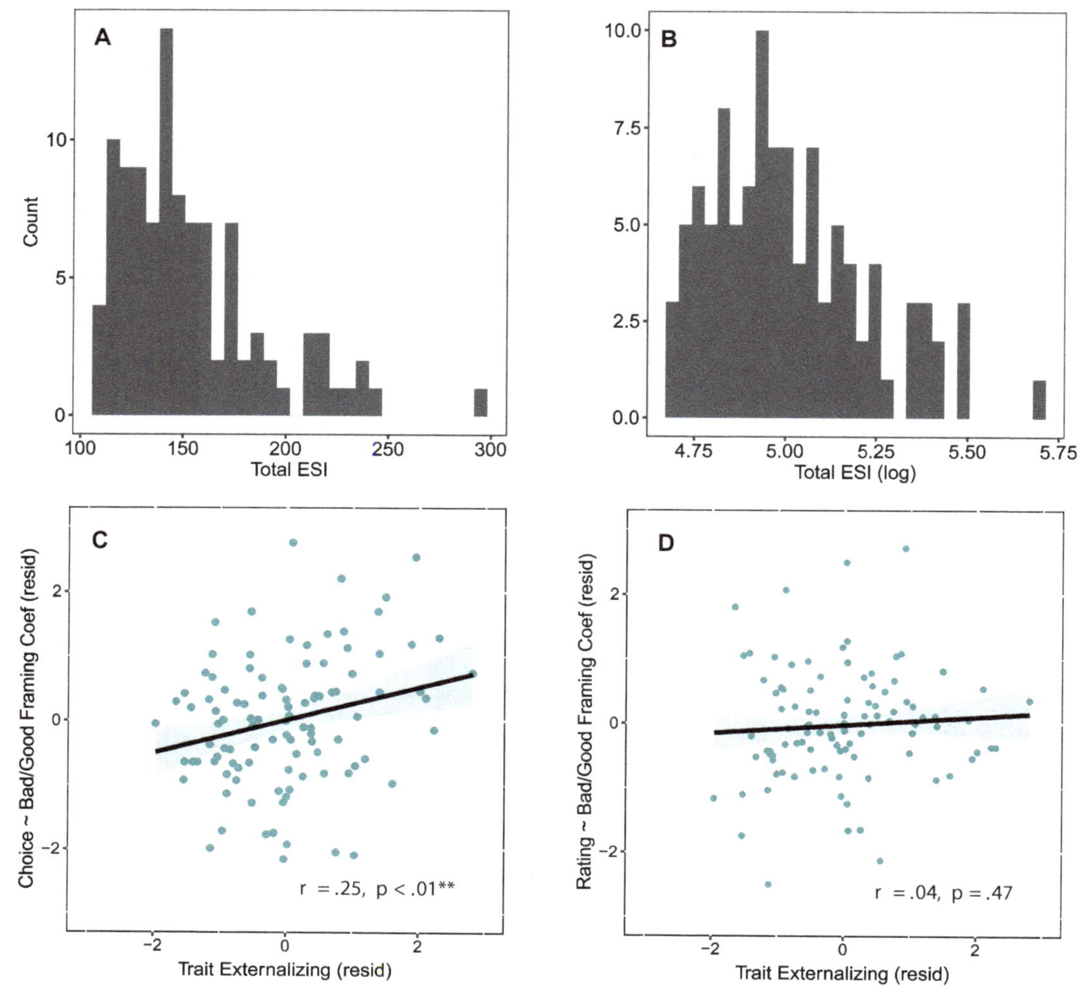


**FIGURE 7 |** Externalizing Spectrum Inventory distributions and risky loss associations. Distribution of scores from the Externalizing Spectrum Inventory (ESI), shown as raw values **(A)** and logged values **(B)**. **(C)** Relationship between trait-level externalizing and the likelihood of accepting a risk offer after previously receiving the bad outcome. Impulsive subjects showed less risk aversion in response to bad outcomes. **(D)** Relations between trait-level externalizing and immediate likability ratings (mean-centered). Impulsive subjects did not differ in their ratings following bad outcomes. $^{**}p < 0.01$.

at the group level (partial $r = 0.25$, $p = 0.008$; **Figure 7C**); these individuals were more likely to accept a risky offer after having just received a bad outcome, signifying a potential deficiency in learning from risky losses. In contrast, the association between outcome type and ratings was unrelated to ESI scores (partial $r = 0.04$, $p = 0.47$; **Figure 7D**).[4] Together, these results indicate that these externalizing traits affected individual differences in reward pursuit but not reward valuation.

Based on the group-level results above, we used *follow-up partial correlations* to probe whether reward pursuit was related to the broader *substance abuse* subfactor (versus *general disinhibition* and *callous aggression*), as well as its underlying problem subscales (i.e., *alcohol problems, marijuana problems, drug problems*. We computed one-tailed robust correlations (i.e., assuming more risk seeking after bad outcomes) and report original and FDR-adjusted p-values that account for the six follow-up correlations.

Our results revealed that two of the three ESI subcomponents were correlated with reward pursuit when accounting for multiple comparisons (general disinhibition partial $r = 0.16$, $p = 0.05$, $p$-adj = 0.08; substance abuse partial $r = 0.24$, $p = 0.005$, $p$-adj = 0.01; callous aggression partial $r = 0.20$, $p = 0.02$, $p$-adj = 0.05; **Figure 8A–C**); however, only substance abuse remained a significant predictor when accounting for the other two subcomponents (partial $r = 0.18$, $p = 0.03$). Further, for individuals endorsing alcohol problems, we found a positive association between reward pursuit after risk and the alcohol problem subscale ($r = 0.59$, $p = 0.004$, $p$-adj = 0.01; **Figure 8D**), versus no association with the marijuana ($r = -.22$, $p = 0.14$, $p$-adj = 0.17; **Figure 8E**) and drug problem ($r = 0.19$, $p = 0.75$, $p$-adj = 0.75; **Figure 8F**) subscales.

[4] We excluded one subject with a coefficient less than 4 standard deviations below the mean.

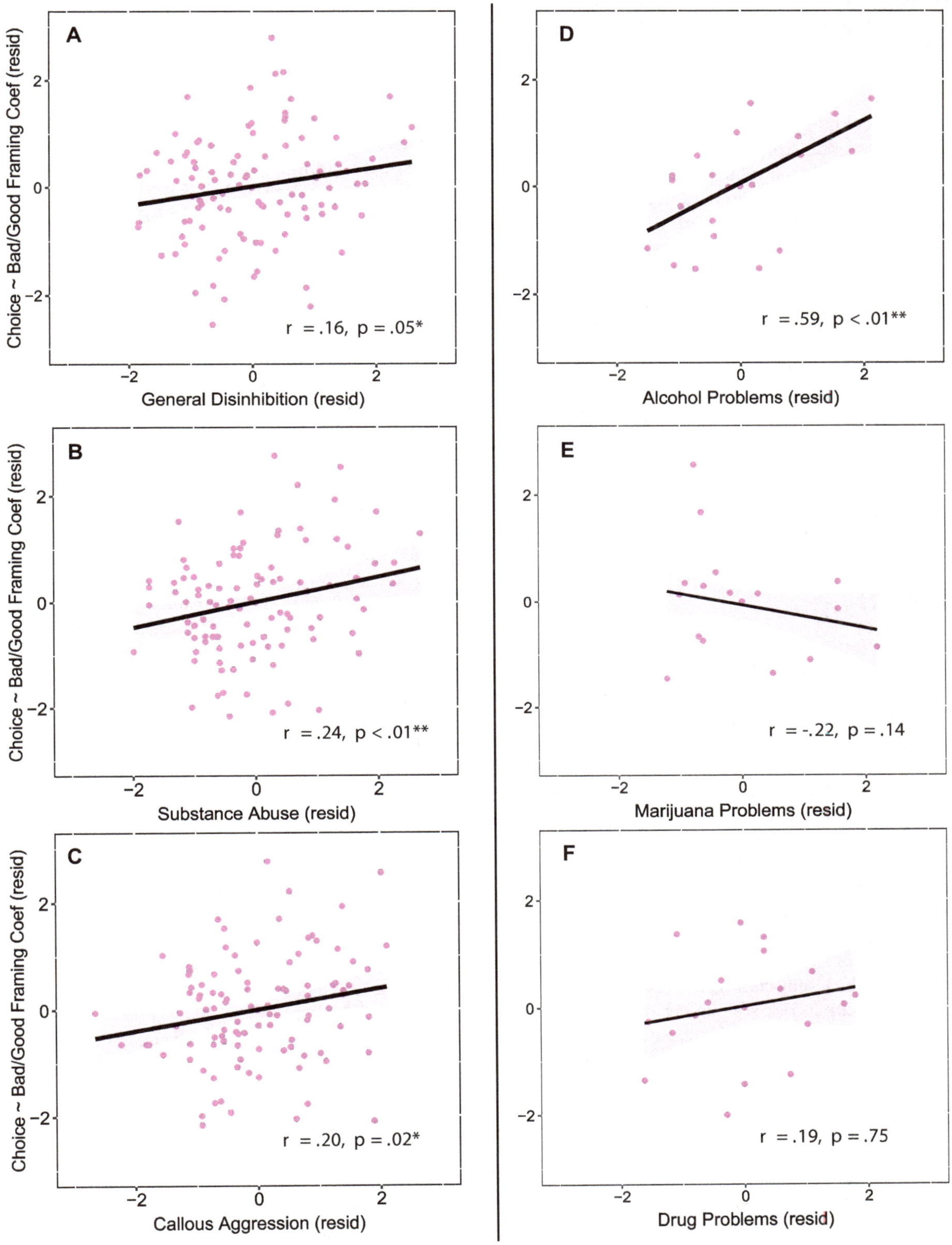


**FIGURE 8 |** Risky losses influence each ESI subfactor and alcohol problems. The left trio of panels **(A, B, C)** shows the correlation between each ESI subfactor and the likelihood of accepting a risk offer after previously receiving a bad outcome. More externalizing subjects showed less risk aversion in response to bad outcomes for each subfactor. The right trio of panels **(D, E, F)** shows correlations with the three problem subscales of the substance abuse subfactor; more problematic alcohol use was associated with less risk aversion after a bad outcome. $^{*}p < 0.05$; $^{**}p < 0.01$.

### Discounting Rates Did Not Explain the Effects of Externalizing Traits on Reward Pursuit

We computed a series of follow-up robust partial correlations to compare Web-Surf Task–derived metrics with those from a traditional discounting task. The first two correlations predicted total ESI scores from the log-transformed delay and probability k-values, while controlling for age, sex, and ethnicity. Here we found that discounting rates did not significantly predict externalizing (delay k-value: partial $r = 0.08$, $p = 0.46$; probability k-value: partial $r = 0.02$, $p = 0.88$). We then checked whether k-values were related specifically to the substance abuse subfactor, given null associations with the total score and our interest in addiction liability. Similarly, k-values were unrelated to substance abuse (delay k-value: partial $r = 0.05$, $p = 0.68$; probability k-value: partial $r = -.07$, $p = 0.57$). Lastly, we tested whether the subject-level coefficient from the Web-Surf Task that indicated sequencing responses following receipt of a good versus bad outcome still predicted ESI scores, after controlling for the two k-values and additional covariates. Importantly, the Web-Surf Task parameter capturing reward pursuit following risk still predicted ESI scores, even when accounting for the two k-values (partial $r = 0.25$, $p = 0.03$).

## DISCUSSION

We assessed the effects of wins and losses on reward valuation and reward pursuit in a new risk variant of the Web-Surf Task. We found that receipt of the bad outcome on a risky gamble influenced both reward valuation and reward pursuit, but in opposite directions; that is, bad outcomes after risk led to reduced reward pursuit and higher reward valuation. Follow-up analyses showed that offer value impacted these effects, whereby low-value risky losses led to risk aversion and lower-than-normal reward valuations, while high-value losses led to risk seeking and higher-than-normal reward valuations. Subjects were also slower to make decisions after bad outcomes, which points to a post-error slowing effect. There was no impact on willingness to take risks following wins after risk situations (better than expected) or after non-risky control trials. Thus, there was something unique about situations in which subjects lost after deciding to take a risk that increased plasticity in risk-seeking behaviors. Importantly, we also found that trait-level externalizing, particularly substance use tendencies, tracked whether these situations influenced future decisions. Externalizing behaviors were not better explained by performance on a traditional discounting task, highlighting the value of foraging behaviors in capturing substance use disorder vulnerabilities.

In line with our hypotheses and prospect theory (13), the *framing* of an offer relative to the mid-point (versus its absolute value) impacted subsequent reward pursuit and reward valuation. That is, whether an outcome was good or bad relative to the mid-point influenced a subject's performance regardless of whether he or she took the correct action, as determined by comparing risky and non-risky offers of equivalent value, where non-risky outcomes did not influence performance. Framing effects were also not better explained by global trends in risk aversion. Global trend analyses showed that subjects accepted fewer risky deals as the session progressed, which could suggest that subjects become more sensitive to punishment over time and/or that they experienced reward satiety from ongoing reward exposure. Regardless, the tendency to turn down risky deals following bad outcomes remained when accounting for global risk-aversion trends, highlighting the impact of framing effects on risky choices above and beyond other influences.

Choosing to accept a risky deal and finding oneself in the bad outcome, i.e., with a longer delay than expected, may also be seen as a regret-inducing situation. Constructs of regret suggest that regret occurs at the intersection of agency and mistake (47, 48), where a subject recognizes that an alternate choice (counterfactual) would have led to a better outcome (49). Counterfactually, the subject could have "just skipped it" if only they had known they were going to get the bad deal. A similar phenomenon has been found in mice running the Restaurant Row task, in which mice show regret-related behaviors after accepting a deal and then quitting out of it, but not after spending the same amount of time deliberating over the offer before skipping it (50).

The finding for slowed reaction times after risky losses is consistent with observations in humans of post-error slowing (51–53) but contrasts with findings that rats and mice respond more quickly to the next trial after making a mistake of their own agency (8, 50). There remain several differences between these tasks: 1) the human task presented here included chance and risk, while the rodent tasks were deterministic; 2) humans had brief pre-training, while rodents had months of training; and 3) humans were working for luxury items (videos), while rodents were working for their basic necessities (food intake for the day). And because rodents had a fixed amount of time to consume their meal, there was potentially more impetus to move quickly and consume more food before time ran out. Of course, it is also possible that there could be a species difference in how humans and rodents respond to these tasks, e.g., cross-species divergences in self-evaluation processes following loss could contribute to the observed reaction time differences, although given the similarities recently seen in their response to deliberation and sunk costs (9), this may be less likely. Whether this post-error response inconsistency arises from cross-species differences in response to regret or unique task attributes remains unknown and will have to be left for future study. One possibility is that "regret" is more complicated and that there are differences between realizing that you made a mistake in a situation in which you had all the necessary information to make a better decision versus taking a risk only to find that the answer is not what you hoped for.

Our analyses also revealed that risky losses had an opposite impact on reward valuation, whereby subjects liked videos that followed a bad (long-delay) outcome more than those following a good (short-delay) outcome on risky trials, though we note that the effects of reward valuation were less robust than those for reward pursuit and should be interpreted with caution. These reward valuation results are consistent with economic observations that humans rate outcomes higher when they have spent more on them (54). This suggests that subjects have a backwards-looking view when rating videos that is consistent with explanations of sunk-cost effects seen in human and non-human subjects (9, 55, 56) and with economic explanations for the effect of anticipation on subsequent reward valuation (57). A desire to reduce cognitive dissonance, an aversive mental state that occurs when there is a discrepancy between behavior and attitude (58), could also explain higher ratings following bad outcomes. That is, subjects may have been trying to alter their attitude as a means to reduce psychological discomfort (59).

A key result from this study is that individuals exhibiting greater externalizing disorder vulnerability were more likely to accept a risky offer after receipt of a bad outcome. Critically, our findings were strongest for the substance abuse subfactor, and largely, the alcohol problem subscale, which could reflect the nature of an undergraduate sample. This risky decision–externalizing association is consistent with notions that addiction involves continued reward pursuit despite negative outcomes (60), and could reflect an inability to learn from mistakes (61). These results also speak to dimensional models of psychopathology, given that behavior is correlated with externalizing problems even in the absence of clinical diagnoses.

Compared to reward pursuit, we saw no relation between externalizing and reward evaluation following regret, suggesting that externalizing may have different associations with different facets of the decision process. One hypothesis is that high externalizers do not show differentiation in reward valuation because of a tendency to respond in a socially conforming manner. For instance, prior research suggests that striatal dopamine availability is a common link between the tendency to "fake good," i.e., respond in a socially desirable way (62, 63), and impulsivity (64). It is then possible that high-externalizing subjects may conform to the socially expected pattern when evaluating rewards. Similarly, externalizing problem behavior is highly related to cognitive distortions, which is an umbrella term that includes the rationalization (or neutralization) of deviant behavior (65). Here, high-externalizing subjects may rationalize their bad decisions with positive ratings. Future research could directly test these theories by including scales that measure socially desirable responding (e.g., the Marlowe–Crowne Social Desirability Scale; 66) or pre-conscious rationalization (65).

Our data could be explained in part by differences in temporal attention, whereby reward valuation is done by looking backwards, while changes in reward pursuit are done by looking forwards. This leads to a key question of whether these two processes are linked. We found them linked in typical subjects, but our individual-differences analyses revealed that these effects occur through separable processes: more externalizing individuals showed comparable effects of risk on reward valuation but did not subsequently modulate their reward pursuit following regret. In fact, **Figure 4** suggests that people scoring high on the ESI may even show the opposite effect, becoming risk seeking after regret-inducing instances. These results are consistent with application of the temporal attention hypothesis to delay discounting, in which a preference for immediate rewards among individuals with addiction is due to a narrowing of temporal attention (67); perhaps high-externalizing subjects have a narrowed attention window that leaves valuation of recent consummatory experiences intact but reduces their capacity to evaluate distal outcomes.

As noted above, externalizing tendencies were not associated with performance on a traditional discounting task. This result diverges from established links between substance abuse and discounting (68, 69). One possible explanation is that steeper discounting is more strongly tied to *current* substance abuse versus a *liability* towards substance abuse. For instance, while steeper discounting rates are observed in chronic nicotine users, discounting rates have been shown to normalize among ex-smokers (70, 71). Gowin et al. (69) observed similar results, where individuals with current alcohol use disorder (AUD) had steeper discounting rates than healthy controls, but individuals with past AUD showed no difference from controls. The fact that our sample includes both individuals with a substance use/abuse history and individuals who are prone to substance use may have reduced our likelihood of capturing such a link. This explanation is in line with Isen et al. (72), who found that hypothetical delay-discounting behaviors did not predict latent trait-externalizing tendencies as similarly measured with the ESI. This again suggests that there may be weaker relationships between discounting behaviors and externalizing liability.

## Limitations

A recognized limitation of the current study is the use of an undergraduate sample that was not specifically recruited based on substance use history. However, the fact that we still detected foraging–substance use relations suggests that the task is sensitive to behaviors that are likely present even at the lower end of the externalizing spectrum; this study also provides a set of foundational findings that can be tested in a confirmatory manner to clarify whether reward pursuit during foraging similarly tracks recreational and problematic substance use in the broader community and among individuals with varying levels of usage. Another limitation is the lack of consumption or craving measurements, as these factors could moderate the observed effects. We also acknowledge that the consequences of a risky loss on the Web-Surf Task is small relative to real-life consequences like filing for bankruptcy, losing transportation options following a DUI, or being imprisoned; but if we find substance use associations when the stakes are low, we might expect greater effects as substance use becomes more chronic and/or problematic.

## Conclusions

Our results suggest a dissociation among individuals with greater substance use disorder vulnerability: costly experiences serve to enhance reward value but did not impact subsequent reward pursuit following regret. Taken together, a blunted sense of regret may result in an overvaluation of risky losses that in turn drives the continued pursuit of risky endeavors. Future work will assess the impact of risky losses while foraging in clinical samples.

## AUTHOR CONTRIBUTIONS

SA, AR, and AM designed the experiment. AR and AM supervised the project. SA carried out the experiments and analyzed the data. SA, AR, and AM wrote the manuscript.

## ACKNOWLEDGMENTS

We thank the members of the TRiCAM lab for assistance with data collection. We also thank both the TRiCAM and Redish labs for providing helpful discussion. Some of the content included in the current manuscript first appeared in a doctoral thesis (73), which is available online at: https://conservancy.umn.edu/handle/11299/200236.

## REFERENCES

1. Tom SM, Fox CR, Trepel C, Poldrack RA. The neural basis of loss aversion in decision-making under risk. *Science* (2007) 315:515–8. doi: 10.1126/science.1134239
2. Connolly T, Zeelenberg M. Regret in decision making. *Curr Dir Psychol Sci* (2002) 11:212–6. doi: 10.1111/1467-8721.00203
3. Coricelli G, Dolan RJ, Sirigu A. Brain, emotion and decision making: the paradigmatic example of regret. *Trends Cogn Sci* (2007) 11(6);258–65. doi: 10.1016/j.tics.2007.04.003
4. Loomes G, Sugden R. Regret theory: an alternative theory of rational choice under uncertainty. *Econ J* (1982) 92:805. doi: 10.2307/2232669
5. Chiu PH, Lohrenz TM, Montague PR. Smokers' brains compute, but ignore, a fictive error signal in a sequential investment task. *Nat Neurosci* (2008) 11:514–20. doi: 10.1038/nn2067
6. Sweis BM, Redish AD, Thomas MJ. Prolonged abstinence from cocaine or morphine disrupts separable valuations during decision conflict. *Nat Commun* (2018) 1–9. doi: 10.1038/s41467-018-04967-2
7. Abram SV, Breton Y-A, Schmidt B, Redish AD, MacDonald AW. The Web-Surf Task: a translational model of human decision-making. *Cogn Affect Behav Neurosci* (2016) 16(1):37–50. doi: 10.3758/s13415-015-0379-y
8. Steiner AP, Redish AD. Behavioral and neurophysiological correlates of regret in rat decision-making on a neuroeconomic task. *Nat Neurosci* (2014) 17(7):995–1002. doi: 10.1038/nn.3740
9. Sweis BM, Abram SV, Schmidt BJ, Seeland KD, MacDonald AW, Thomas MJ, et al. Sensitivity to "sunk costs" in mice, rats, and humans. *Science* (2018) 361:178–81. doi: 10.1126/science.aar8644
10. Stephens DW. Decision ecology: foraging and the ecology of animal decision making. *Cogn Affect Behav Neurosci* (2008) 8(4):475–84. doi: 10.3758/CABN.8.4.475
11. Feighery EC, Schleicher NC, Boley Cruz T, Unger JB. An examination of trends in amount and type of cigarette advertising and sales promotions in California stores, 2002–2005. *Tob Control* (2008) 17:93–8. doi: 10.1136/tc.2007.022046
12. De Wit H. Impulsivity as a determinant and consequence of drug use: a review of underlying processes. *Addict Biol* (2009) 14(1):22–31. doi: 10.1111/j.1369-1600.2008.00129.x
13. Kahneman D, Tversky A. Prospect theory: an analysis of decision under risk. *Econometrica* (1979) 47:263–92. doi: 10.1111/j.1536-7150.2011.00774.x
14. Phillips JG, Currie J, Ogeil RP. Consumption and foraging behaviors for common stimulants (nicotine, caffeine). *J Addict Dis* (2016) 35:15–21. doi: 10.1080/10550887.2015.1094721
15. Kendler KS, Prescott C, Myers J, Neale MC. The structure of genetic and environmental risk factors for common psychiatric and substance use disorders in men and women. *Arch Gen Psychiatry* (2003) 60(9):929–37. doi: 10.1001/archpsyc.60.9.929
16. Krueger RF, Hicks BM, Patrick CJ, Carlson SR, Iacono WG, McGue M. Etiologic connections among substance dependence, antisocial behavior and personality: modeling the externalizing spectrum. *J Abnorm Psychol* (2002) 111(3):411–24. doi: 10.1037//0021-843X.111.3.411
17. Krueger RF, Markon KE, Patrick CJ, Iacono WG. Externalizing psychopathology in adulthood: a dimensional-spectrum conceptualization and its implications for DSM-V. *J Abnorm Psychol* (2005) 114:537–50. doi: 10.1037/0021-843X.114.4.537
18. Lauriola M, Panno A, Levin IP, Lejuez CW. Individual differences in risky decision making: a meta-analysis of sensation seeking and impulsivity with the Balloon Analogue Risk Task. *J Behav Decis Mak* (2014) 27(1):20–36. doi: 10.1002/bdm.1784
19. Krueger RF, Markon KE, Patrick CJ, Benning SD, Kramer MD. Linking antisocial behavior, substance use, and personality: an integrative quantitative model of the adult externalizing spectrum. *J Abnorm Psychol* (2007) 116(4):645–66. doi: 10.1037/0021-843X.116.4.645
20. Blonigen DM, Patrick CJ, Gasperi M, Steffen B, Ones DS, Arvey RD, et al. Delineating the construct network of the personnel reaction blank: associations with externalizing tendencies and normal personality. *Psychol Assess* (2011) 23:18–30. doi: 10.1037/a0021048
21. Brislin SJ, Yancey JR, Perkins ER, Palumbo IM, Drislane LE, Salekin RT, et al. Callousness and affective face processing in adults: behavioral and brain-potential indicators. *Personal Disord* (2018) 9:122–32. doi: 10.1037/per0000235
22. Hall JR, Bernat EM, Patrick CJ. Externalizing psychopathology and the error-related negativity. *Psychol Sci* (2007) 18:326–33. doi: 10.1111/j.1467-9280.2007.01899.x
23. Meehan KB, De Panfilis C, Cain NM, Clarkin JF. Effortful control and externalizing problems in young adults. *Pers Individ Dif* (2013) 55:553–8. doi: 10.1016/j.paid.2013.04.019
24. Patrick CJ, Kramer MD, Krueger RF, Markon KE. Optimizing efficiency of psychopathology assessment through quantitative modeling: development of a brief form of the Externalizing Spectrum Inventory. *Psychol Assess* (2013) 25(4):1332–48. doi: 10.1037/a0034864
25. Zucker RA. Anticipating problem alcohol use developmentally from childhood into middle adulthood: what have we learned? *Addiction* (2008) 103:100–8. doi: 10.1111/j.1360-0443.2008.02179.x
26. Benjamini Y, Hochberg Y. Controlling the false discovery rate: a practical and powerful approach to multiple testing. *J Royal Stat Soc B* (1995) 57(1):289–300. doi: 10.1111/j.2517-6161.1995.tb02031.x
27. Hadfield JD. MCMC methods for multi-response generalized linear models. *J Stat Softw* (2010) 33:1–22. doi: 10.1002/ana.22635
28. Bates D, Maechler M, Walker S. Package "lme4": linear mixed-effects models using "Eigen" and S4. *CRAN Repository* (2016) 1–113. doi: 10.18637/jss.v067.i01
29. Lenth RV. Least-squares means: the R package lsmeans. *J Stat Softw* (2016) 69(1):1–33. doi: 10.18637/jss.v069.i01
30. Hahn PR (n.d). Statistical formula notation in R. Retrieved from https://faculty.chicagobooth.edu/richard.hahn/teaching/formulanotation.pdf.
31. de Wit H, Flory JD, Acheson A, McCloskey M, Manuck SB. IQ and nonplanning impulsivity are independently associated with delay discounting in middle-aged adults. *Pers Individ Dif* (2007) 42(1):111–21. doi: 10.1016/j.paid.2006.06.026
32. Eaton NR, Keyes KM, Krueger RF, Balsis S, Skodol AE, Markon KE, et al. An invariant dimensional liability model of gender differences in mental disorder prevalence: evidence from a national sample. *J Abnorm Psychol* (2012) 121(1):282–8. doi: 10.1037/a0024780
33. Kramer MD, Krueger RF, Hicks BM. The role of internalizing and externalizing liability factors in accounting for gender differences in the prevalence of common psychopathological syndromes. *Psychol Med* (2008) 38:51–61. doi: 10.1017/S0033291707001572
34. Romer D, Hennessy M. A biosocial-affect model of adolescent sensation seeking: the role of affect evaluation and peer-group influence in adolescent drug use. *Prev Sci* (2007) 8:89–101. doi: 10.1007/s11121-007-0064-7
35. Chen P, Jacobson KC. Developmental trajectories of substance use

from early adolescence to young adulthood: gender and racial/ethnic differences. *J Adolesc Health* (2012) 50:154–63. doi: 10.1016/j.jadohealth.2011.05.013

36. Anokhin AP, Golosheykin S, Grant JD, Heath AC. Heritability of delay discounting in adolescence: a longitudinal twin study. *Behav Genet* (2011) 41(2):175–83. doi: 10.1007/s10519-010-9384-7
37. Olson EA, Hooper CJ, Collins P, Luciana M. Adolescents' performance on delay and probability discounting tasks: contributions of age, intelligence, executive functioning, and self-reported externalizing behavior. *Pers Individ Dif* (2007) 43(7):1886–97. doi: 10.1016/j.paid.2007.06.016
38. Reynolds B. A review of delay-discounting research with humans: relations to drug use and gambling. *Behav Pharmacol* (2006) 17(8):651–67. doi: 10.1097/FBP.0b013e3280115f99
39. Ainslie G, Haslam N. Hyperbolic discounting. In Loewenstein G, Elster J (Eds.), *Choice over Time*. New York: Russell Sage Foundation. p. 57–92.
40. Bickel WK, Jarmolowicz DP, Mueller ET, Koffarnus MN, Gatchalian KM. Excessive discounting of delayed reinforcers as a trans-disease process contributing to addiction and other disease-related vulnerabilities: emerging evidence. *Pharmacol Ther* (2012) 134(3):287–97. doi: 10.1016/j.pharmthera.2012.02.004
41. Johnson MW, Bickel WK. An algorithm for identifying nonsystematic delay-discounting data. *Exp Clin Psychopharmacol* (2008) 16:264–74. doi: 10.1037/1064-1297.16.3.264
42. Plassmann H, O'Doherty J, Shiv B, Rangel A. Marketing actions can modulate neural representations of experienced pleasantness. *Proc Natl Acad Sci U S A* (2008) 105(3):1050–54. doi: 10.1073/pnas.0706929105
43. Sweis BM, Abram SV, Schmidt BJ, Seeland KD, MacDonald AW, Thomas MJ, Redish AD. Sensitivity to "sunk costs" in mice, rats, and humans. *Science* (2018b) 361:178–81. doi: 10.1126/science.aar8644
44. Worthy DA, Hawthorne MJ, Otto AR. Heterogeneity of strategy use in the Iowa gambling task: a comparison of win–stay/lose–shift and reinforcement learning models. *Psychon Bull Rev* (2013) 20(2):364–71. doi: 10.3758/s13423-012-0324-9
45. Benegal V, Antony G, Venkatasubramanian G, Jayakumar PN. Gray matter volume abnormalities and externalizing symptoms in subjects at high risk for alcohol dependence. *Addict Biol* (2007) 12:122–32. doi: 10.1111/j.1369-1600.2006.00043.x
46. Carroll AJ, Sutherland MT, Salmeron BJ, Ross TJ, Stein EA. Greater externalizing personality traits predict less error-related insula and anterior cingulate cortex activity in acutely abstinent cigarette smokers. *Addict Biol* (2015) 20:377–89. doi: 10.1111/adb.12118
47. Van Dijk WW, Zeelenberg M. Investigating the appraisal patterns of regret and disappointment. *Motiv Emot* (2002) 26:321–31. doi: 10.1023/A:1022823221146
48. Zeelenberg M, Van Dijk WW, Manstead ASR, Van Der Pligt J. The experience of regret and disappointment. *Cogn Emot* (1998) 12:221–30. doi: 10.1080/026999398379727
49. Bell DE. Regret in decision making under uncertainty. *Oper Res* (1982) 30:961–81. doi: 10.1287/opre.30.5.961
50. Sweis BM, Thomas MJ, Redish AD. Mice learn to avoid regret. *PLoS Biol* (2018) 16(6) 1–21. doi: 10.1371/journal.pbio.2005853
51. Dutilh G, Vandekerckhove J, Forstmann BU, Keuleers E, Brysbaert M, Wagenmakers EJ. Testing theories of post-error slowing. *Atten Percept Psychophys* (2012) 74(2):454–65. doi: 10.3758/s13414-011-0243-2
52. Laming D. Choice reaction performance following an error. *Acta Psychol* (1979) 43(3):199–224. doi: 10.1016/0001-6918(79)90026-X
53. Rabbitt P, Rodgers B. What does a man do after he makes an error? an analysis of response programming. *Q J Exp Psychol* (1977) 29(4):727–43. doi: 10.1080/14640747708400645
54. Cunha M, Caldieraro F. Sunk-cost effects on purely behavioral investments. *Cogn Sci* (2009) 33:105–13. doi: 10.1111/j.1551-6709.2008.01005.x
55. Aronson E. The effect of effort on the attractiveness of rewarded and unrewarded stimuli. *J Abnorm Psychol* (1961) 63:375–80. doi: 10.1037/h0046890
56. Wikenheiser AM, Stephens DW, Redish AD. Subjective costs drive overly patient foraging strategies in rats on an intertemporal foraging task. *Proc Natl Acad Sci* (2013) 110(20):8308–13. doi: 10.1073/pnas.1220738110
57. Loewenstein G. Anticipation and the valuation of delayed consumption. *Econ J* (1987) 97(387):666. doi: 10.2307/2232929
58. Festinger L. *An introduction to the theory of dissonance. a theory of cognitive dissonance*. Stanford, CA: Stanford University Press (1957). doi: 10.1037/10318-001
59. Elliot AJ, Devine PG. On the motivational nature of cognitive dissonance: dissonance as psychological discomfort. *J Pers Soc Psychol* (1994) 67(3):382–94. doi: 10.1037/0022-3514.67.3.382
60. Hyman SE. Addiction: a disease of learning and memory. *Am J Psychiatry* (2005) 162(8):1414–22. doi: 10.1176/appi.ajp.162.8.1414
61. Bechara A. Risky business: emotion, decision-making, and addiction. *J Gambl Stud* (2003) 19:23–51. doi: 10.1023/A:1021223113233
62. Egerton A, Rees E, Bose SK, Lappin JM, Stokes PRA, Turkheimer FE, et al. Truth, lies or self-deception? Striatal D2/3 receptor availability predicts individual differences in social conformity. *NeuroImage* (2010) 53:777–81. doi: 10.1016/j.neuroimage.2010.06.031
63. Reeves SJ, Mehta MA, Montgomery AJ, Amiras D, Egerton A, Howard RJ, et al. Striatal dopamine (D2) receptor availability predicts socially desirable responding. *NeuroImage* (2007) 34:1782–9. doi: 10.1016/j.neuroimage.2006.10.042
64. Anderson BA, Kuwabara H, Wong DF, Courtney SM. Density of available striatal dopamine receptors predicts trait impulsiveness during performance of an attention-demanding task. *J Neurophysiol* (2017) 117(1):64–8. doi: 10.1152/jn.00125.2017
65. Helmond P, Overbeek G, Brugman D, Gibbs JC. A meta-analysis on cognitive distortions and externalizing problem behavior: associations, moderators, and treatment effectiveness. *Crim Justice Behav* (2015) 42(3):245–62. doi: 10.1177/0093854814552842
66. Crowne DP, Marlowe D. A new scale of social desirability independent of psychopathology. *J Consult Psychol* (1960) 24:349–54. doi: 10.1037/h0047358
67. McClure SM, Bickel WK. A dual-systems perspective on addiction: contributions from neuroimaging and cognitive training. *Ann N Y Acad Sci* (2014) 1327:62–78. doi: 10.1111/nyas.12561
68. Bickel WK, Marsch LA. Toward a behavioral economic understanding of drug dependence: delay discounting processes. *Addiction* (2001) 96:73–86. doi: 10.1046/j.1360-0443.2001.961736.x
69. Gowin J, Sloan ME, Swan JE, Momenan R, Ramchandani VA. The relationship between delay discounting and alcohol dependence in individuals with and without comorbid psychopathology. *Psychopharmacology* (2019) 236(2):775–85. doi: 10.1007/s00213-018-5113-3
70. Bickel WK, Odum AL, Madden GJ. Impulsivity and cigarette smoking: delay discounting in current, never, and ex-smokers. *Psychopharmacology* (1999) 146:447–54. doi: 10.1007/PL00005490
71. Secades-Villa R, Weidberg S, García-Rodríguez O, Fernández-Hermida JR, Yoon JH. Decreased delay discounting in former cigarette smokers at one year after treatment. *Addict Behav* (2014) 39(6):1087–93. doi: 10.1016/j.addbeh.2014.03.015
72. Isen JD, Sparks JC, Iacono WG. Predictive validity of delay discounting behavior in adolescence: a longitudinal twin study. *Exp Clin Psychopharmacol* (2014) 22(5):434–43 doi: 10.1037/a0037340
73. Abram SV. *Towards a translational model of decision-making: findings from the Web-Surf Task*. University of Minnesota (2017).

# 3

# Rewiring the Addicted Brain through a Psychobiological Model of Physical Exercise

*Kell Grandjean Costa*[1], *Daniel Aranha Cabral*[1], *Rodrigo Hohl*[2] *and Eduardo Bodnariuc Fontes*[1*]

[1] *NEUROex: Research Group in Physical Activity, Cognition and Behavior, Center of Health Sciences, Federal University of Rio Grande do Norte, Natal, Brazil,* [2] *Department of Physiology, Federal University of Juiz de Fora, Juiz de Fora, Brazil*

***Correspondence:***
*Eduardo Bodnariuc Fontes*
*eduardobfontes@gmail.com*

Drug addiction is a worldwide public health problem, resulting from multiple phenomena, including those both social and biological. Chronic use of psychoactive substances has been shown to induce structural and functional changes in the brain that impair cognitive control and favor compulsive seeking behavior. Physical exercise has been proven to improve brain function and cognition in both healthy and clinical populations. While some studies have demonstrated the potential benefits of physical exercise in treating and preventing addictive behaviors, few studies have investigated its cognitive and neurobiological contributions to drug-addicted brains. Here, we review studies in humans using cognitive behavioral responses and neuroimaging techniques, which reveal that exercise can be an effective auxiliary treatment for drug addictive disorders. Moreover, we describe the neurobiological mechanisms by which exercise-induced neuroplasticity in the prefrontal cortex improves executive functions and may decrease compulsive behaviors in individuals prone to substance use disorders. Finally, we propose an integrative cognitive-psychobiological model of exercise for use in future research in drug addiction and practical guidance in clinical settings.

**Keywords: aerobic exercise, neuralplasticity, substance use disorder, addiction, alcohol abuse**

## INTRODUCTION

Addiction to psychoactive substances (e.g., nicotine, cocaine, marijuana, alcohol, heroin, inhalants, LSD, and ecstasy) is a public health problem of the modern world (1). The Diagnostic and Statistical Manual of Mental Disorders of the American Psychiatric Association (DSM-V 2013) classifies drug addiction as a substance use disorder (SUD) when an individual meets two or more of the following criteria regarding the use of psychoactive substances: tolerance, craving, repeated attempts to stop use, or social, personal, physical, or psychological problems related to drug use (2). In addition to the influences of biological, cultural, social, economic, and psychological factors on individuals with SUD (3), studies in animal models and humans have shown that psychoactive substance use induces epigenetic, molecular, structural, and functional changes to the brain (4). Thus, the neurobiological model of drug addiction has proposed a complex interaction between biological and environmental factors and created new integrative perspectives for prevention, treatment, and pharmacological targets (5).

SUD is traditionally related to abnormal dopamine release and sensitivity in the brain reward system. This neural network is composed of several interconnected brain areas, including the ventral tegmental area, nucleus accumbens, amygdala, striatum, hippocampus, and prefrontal cortex (PFC) (6). The PFC is an integrated neural system in humans required for normal executive functioning, including decision-making and inhibitory control, and beneficial socio-emotional functioning (7). Studies using positron emission tomography (PET) and functional magnetic resonance imaging (fMRI) have demonstrated that individuals with SUD present decreased activityin the PFC (8). This condition seems to be related to a reduced number of dopamine receptors and an abnormal firing rate of dopaminergic neurons (9). These changes in the dopamine system and PFC activity may favor compulsive substance intake and seeking behaviors, as well as loss of control over drug consumption (8). Similarly, incomplete prefrontal cortex development and the resulting decrease in ability to control impulsive decisions has been suggested as an explanation for adolescents' particular vulnerability to drug abuse (10), highlighting the importance of preventing the use of addictive psychoactive drugs during this period of brain development. Hence, contemporary rehabilitation programs have emphasized the importance of interdisciplinary treatment approaches that target the reestablishment of normal PFC functioning while combining the use of medication, social care, and behavioral therapy supported by psychiatrists, psychologists, social workers, and family (5).

Physical exercise has been proposed as a complementary therapy for individuals with SUD undergoing treatment at different stages of addiction rehabilitation (11–13). Preclinical animal research has shown evidence of neurobiological mechanisms induced by physical exercise that support its potential use as a therapeutic strategy to treat drug addiction. Examples are the following: normalizing dopaminergic and glutaminergic transmissions, promoting epigenetic interactions mediated by BDNF (brain-derived neurotrophic factor), and modifying dopaminergic signaling in the basal ganglia (11, 14). However, identifying similar molecular interactions between exercise and the human brain presents significant methodological challenges that need to be overcome in order totranslate these findings from animal models to humans.

The benefits of physical exercise for cognitive functioning and brain structure in humans are, on the other hand, well documented in literature (15). For instance, aerobic exercise is linked to improvements in executive functions and increased gray matter volume and activity in PFC regions (16, 17). Furthermore, children and adults with higher cardiorespiratory fitness (i.e., $VO_2$ max) show improved cognitive performance and neuronal activity in the PFC and anterior cingulate cortex (ACC) (18). The results of preclinical animal studies show that these brain adaptations seem to be related to the release of exercise-induced molecules, such as BDNF (19) and IGF-1 (insulin-like growth factor 1) (20). Both molecules act as neurotrophic factors and create new synapses, neurons, and neural networks (18). These adaptations are facilitated by an increase in cerebral blood flow during exercise (21) and a release of a vascular endothelial growth factor (VEGF) (22), which promotes mitotic activity in vascular endothelial cells, thereby promoting angiogenesis and enhancing the oxygen and nutrient supply to neurons (18). Additionally, exercise is also related to the integrity of the brain-blood barrier (23). However, despite the wide range of benefits of the exercising brain, its effects on individuals with SUD who have impaired PFCs and cognitive functions need to be further investigated.

In this mini review, we present the results of a review of the current literature on exercise and SUD. We limited our search to studies that investigated the effect of acute or chronic aerobic exercise on cognitive and/or neurobiological markers in humans with SUD. The search terms used to select the articles were "tobacco cigarettes," "nicotine," "alcohol," "methamphetamine," "crack," "cocaine and marijuana," "physical activity," "endurance exercise," "aerobic exercise," "addiction,":substance use disorder," "executive functions," "prefrontal cortex," "cognition," and "brain." Two authors selected the published and peer-reviewed articles identified on electronic databases (Pubmed Central, Medline, Scopus, and Web of Science) in February 2019, while a third author resolved differences in opinion. Only articles published in English were considered. Finally, we propose an integrative cognitive-psychobiological model of exercise to support future research on the subject and provide methodological guidance for its application in clinical settings as a therapeutic tool for the treatment of SUD.

## The Effect of Aerobic Exercise on Brain and Cognitive Function in Individuals With SUD

Aerobic exercise is typically performed at submaximal intensity for a long duration with most of the energy consumption coming from mitochondrial oxygen-dependent production of ATP. Organic adaptations of the cardiorespiratory system as a result of aerobic training are mainly reflected by higher values of $VO_2$ max, which has been associated with improvements in several health parameters, as well as brain and cognitive functioning (18, 24). Examples of aerobic exercise include running, swimming, and cycling among summer sports and cross-country skiing or speed skating among winter sports (25). **Table 1** describes studies that investigated the effect of aerobic exercise on the brain and cognitive functions in individuals with SUD. Acute effects of aerobic exercise (i.e., immediately after exercise cessation) have been shown to include increases in PFC oxygenation associated with greater inhibitory control (26) and improved memory, attention, and speed processing in polysubstance users (27). Similarly, methamphetamine users who exercised on a stationary cycling ergometer exhibited improvements afterward, such as better drug-specific inhibitory control, reduced craving levels, and enhanced brain activity in the ACC, the area involved in conflict monitoring and inhibition (28). Wang et al. (29) and Wang, Zhou, and Chang (30) also studied methamphetamine users and showed that exercise performed at moderate intensity (i.e., 65–75% of maximum heart rate) elicits a decrease in craving levels, improves performance on a go/no-go task, and increases N2 amplitude during no-go conditions when the individuals have to inhibit the impulse to press the bottom of the computer screen after a visual cue. Notably, the N2 is an event-related potential, monitored using non-invasive electroencephalography (EEG), that originates from the fronto-parietal cortex and is directly associated with inhibitory control (31).

**TABLE 1** | Studies investigating the effects of physical exercise on the brain and cognitive functions in individuals with substance use disorders.

**Results from acute exercise studies**

| Reference | Study procedures | Drug type | Exercise (type; intensity; time) | Neurobiological marker and cognitive test | Outcomes |
|---|---|---|---|---|---|
| Janse Van Rensburg and Taylor, (2008) (32) | Smokers (N=23) underwent to conditions (Exercise and passive resting). They performed a cognitive test before and after the conditions. | Nicotine | Aerobic exercise on a treadmill; Light self-paced intensity; 2min warm-up and 15min exercise | Stroop test | Following the exercise session, smokers did not improve on the cognitive test performance compared to the control session. |
| Janse Van Rensburg et al., (2009) (33) | Smokers (N=10) underwent to conditions (Exercise and passive resting) followed by fMRI scanning while watching smoking and neutral images. | Nicotine | Aerobic exercise on cycleergometer; Moderate-intensity (RPE 11-13); 2min warm-up, 10min exercise. | fMRI | Smokers presented reduced brain activity in areas related to reward, motivation and visuo-spatial attention following exercise, compared to the control condition. |
| Rensburg et al., (2012) ( 34) | Smokers (N=20) underwent to conditions (Exercise and passive resting) followed by fMRI scanning while watching smoking and neutral images. | Nicotine | Aerobic exercise on cycleergometer; Moderate-intensity (RPE 11-13); 2min warm-up, 10min exercise) | fMRI | Smokers presented decreased activity in visual processing (i.e., occipital cortex) areas during smoking images after the exercise session |
| Wang, Zhou and Chang., 2015 (30) | Participants (N=24) performed two conditions: exercise and reading control sessions The cognitive tests and the brain electroactivity were measured following each condition. | Methamphetamine | Aerobic exercise on cycle-ergometer; 65-75% of estimated maximum HR, 30min (5min warm-up, 20min of exercise and 5min cool-down) | Electroencephalogram (EEG), GoNoGo | Both general and methamphetamine specific inhibitory control were improved after the exercise session compared to the control session. Greater N2 amplitude was observed during the cognitive tests on the Nogo conditions of both inhibitory control tests compared to the control session. |
| Wang et al., 2016 (29) | Participants (N=92) were randomly assigned to 4 groups: light exercise, moderate exercise, vigorous exercise and reading control group. Cognitive test and brain electroactivity were measure before and 20min after the exercise or reading session. | Methamphetamine | Aerobic exercise on a cycle-ergometer; each group had its own intensity based on estimated maximum HR (40-50%, 65-75% and 85-95%, corresponding to light, moderate and high intensities, respectively); 30min of exercise (5min warm-up, 20min of exercise and 5min cool-down) | Electroencephalogram (EEG) a while performing a general GoNogo task and a methamphetamine specific GoNogo task. | Moderate intensity group showed better reaction time and lower number of errors. The same group showed greater N2 amplitude during Nogo conditions of both general and meth-specific inhibitory control. |
| Da Costa et al., 2017 (35) | Individuals with substance use disorder (N=15) were compared with 15 healthy individuals during a maximum effort exercise session. During the session, all volunteers had their prefrontal cortex oxygenation measured while performing a cognitive test. | Multiple drug users (35.5% were addicted to one substance, 43% to two substances and 21.1% to three substances). 8 reported to be crack/cocaine user, 6 were alcohol users and 3 were marijuana users. | Aerobic exercise until voluntary exhaustion [20 on Borg Scale (6-20)]. The cycloergometer was kept in 60-70 rpm. The initial load was 25w and in every two minutes, 25w increment occurred. | Near infrared spectroscopy (NIRS) and Stroop test | Individuals with substance use disorder increased prefrontal cortex oxygenation during exercise associated to better reaction time on the Stroop test. Also, lower cravings was reported after the exercise session. |

(Continued)

**TABLE 1** | Continued

| Results from chronic exercise studies | | | | | |
|---|---|---|---|---|---|
| **Reference** | **Study design** | **Drug type** | **Exercise (type; intensity; frequency; time)** | **Neurobiological marker and cognitive test** | **Outcomes** |
| Da Costa et al., (2016) (36) | Individuals with substance abuse (N=9) performed 3 months of exercise intervention. They performed a cognitive test before and after the exercise protocol. | Crack and cocaine | Aerobic exercise (free running), self-selected intensity; 3 sessions/ week; 36-60min/session. The protocol lasted for 3 months. | Stroop test | It was found that the participants decreased the reaction time associated with improvements on cardiorespiratory fitness. The number of errors on the Stroop test kept the same comparing pre and post intervention. |
| Cabral et al., (2017) (37)(a) | Case report. The subject performed prefrontal cortex oxygenation during incremental exercise before, 45 days after and 90 days after the beginning of the running protocol. | Alcohol and nicotine | Aerobic exercise (free running); self-selected intensity; 3 sessions/ week; the running time was increased along the weeks (first week: 3-6min, last week: 40-50min). The protocol lasted for 12 weeks. | Near infrared spectroscopy (NIRS). Stroop test | After 90 days of running, the subject improved prefrontal cortex oxygenation in 921% at ventilatory threshold, 604.2% at respiratory compensation point and 76.1% at maximum effort. Moreover, the individual increased number of correct answers during inhibitory control test by 266.6% and reaction time by 23%. |
| Wang et al., (2017) (38) | Randomized controlled trial study. Participants were divided in two groups: exercise (N=25) and control group (N=25). Cognitive tests and electroencephalogram were measured in both groups before and after 12 weeks. | Methamphetamine | Aerobic exercise (cycling, jogging, jump rope); 65-75% of estimated maximum HR; 3 sessions/ week; 40min/session (5min warm-up, 30min of aerobic exercise and 5min cool-down). The protocol was conducted for 12 weeks. | Electroencephalogram (EEG), Go/NoGo | Both general and methamphetamine specific inhibitory control were improved after the exercise session compared to the control group. Greater N2 amplitude was observed during the cognitive tests on the Nogo conditions of both inhibitory tests compared to the control group. |
| Cabral et al., (2018) (39) (b) | Case report. The participant had its brain activity measured before and after the exercise protocol during rest, while doing a cognitive test. Moreover, prefrontal cortex oxygenation was measured during incremental treadmill exercise. | Crack/cocaine and alcohol | High intensity aerobic exercise; all out for 30s and resting for 4:30min 3 sessions a week. The protocol lasted for 4 weeks. | Electroencephalogram (EEG) and Near infrared spectroscopy (NIRS), Stroop test | Prefrontal cortex oxyhemoglobin increased 228.2% at the beginning of the treadmill test, 305.4% at the middle and 359.4% at the end of the test. Prefrontal cortex activity during the Stroop test was enhanced. The Stroop effect was decreased by 327%. |

In nicotine users, a meta-analysis (40) and a systematic review (41) show little or no effect of exercise in smoking cessation. However, those reviews did not include studies using cognitive or neurobiological markers as outcomes. On the other hand, Rensburg et al. (32–34) conducted a series of important experiments that suggest potential benefits of aerobic exercise to the brain and cognitive functions of nicotine users. The first study showed that 15 min of light-intensity treadmill exercise reduced craving levels compared to a control condition (passive resting) but did not find improvements in inhibitory control. However, performance on the inhibitory control task was only measured by reaction time and not by the number of errors, which might limit our interpretation of the results (32). In the second experiment, 10 min of moderate-intensity cycling exercise elicited decreases in craving levels compared to a control condition (passive sitting for 10 min). After each condition, participants underwent fMRI scanning while viewing neutral pictures and pictures related to smoking. While viewing smoking images participants demonstrated reduced activation in brain areas related to reward (i.e., caudate nucleus), motivation (i.e., orbitofrontal cortex), and visuo-spatial attention (i.e., parietal lobe and parahippocampal gyrus) after exercise (33). Another study replicated the same experimental design with a larger sample of smokers. The results showed that 10 min of moderate-intensity exercise also reduced craving levels, and the fMRI analyses revealed decreased activity in visual processing (i.e., occipital cortex) areas during smoking images for the exercise condition but not for the control condition (passive sitting) (34). Thus, these results show the potential effects of aerobic exercise in modulating craving and correlated brain areas in nicotine users.

Therefore, despite the limited amount of studies available in the literature so far, it is apparent that acute sessions of aerobic exercise decrease craving levels and seem to benefit cognitive and brain functions in these individuals. However, it could also be important to understand if regularly performed exercise (i.e., chronic effects) may potentialize the acute benefits to the brain and cognition of individuals with SUD throughout weeks and months of exercise training. To date, only two studies have investigated the chronic effects of aerobic exercise in individuals with SUD using neurobiological and cognitive markers (**Table 1**). In one study, methamphetamine users showed improved inhibitory control and greater activation of the ACC during an inhibition task after performing 3 months of moderate-intensity exercise for 30 min three times a week (38). Curiously, this pioneering work by Wang et al. (38) did not report changes in cardiorespiratory fitness, which limited the association between the cardiorespiratory adaptations induced by exercise and improvements in brain and cognitive functioning. However, the results of a different pilot longitudinal study with polysubstance users showed that 3 months of aerobic exercise improved inhibitory control and was correlated with cardiorespiratory fitness improvements (36).

Because of the lack of longitudinal studies in the literature, we have conducted two case reports, in which we tested two different exercise interventions. The first one was a 3-month running program (three times a week), based on self-selected moderate-intensity exercise. The study was conducted with a chronic alcohol user receiving treatment in a public psychiatric hospital. Measures of PFC oxygenation, inhibitory control, and the need for medical intervention were assessed before and after the exercise program. At the end of the 3-month period, the participant demonstrated improved PFC oxygenation, decreased reaction time in the inhibitory control task, and reduced need for medical intervention (37). The second case report involved a crack/cocaine and alcohol user receiving treatment. They engaged in 4 weeks of high-intensity exercise (three times a week), and we measured PFC oxygenation, brain activity through electroencephalography, and inhibitory control before and after the intervention. The participant showed increased PFC activity during the inhibitory control test and increased PFC oxygenation during exercise (39). Taken together, the relationship between cognitive abilities and brain function and regular exercise suggests a promising role of physical exercise in promoting greater executive control on the compulsive behavior of individuals with SUD.

## PSYCHOBIOLOGY OF SELF-SELECTED EXERCISE INTENSITY: PRACTICAL TOOL FOR CLINICAL SETTINGS AND RESEARCH

From an evolutionary perspective, humans have adapted to withstanding prolonged aerobic exercise through the search for food and persistence hunting of prey (supposedly pursued until physical exhaustion) (42). Aerobic self-selected exercise along with the cognitive appraisal of environmental cues for the acquisition of food and survival have been postulated to be key features in the development of the human brain (43). However, modern society has removed the need for humans to run/walk for food or shelter. As a result there is an increasing rate of hypokinetic behavior and related diseases such as diabetes, obesity, and hypertension (44, 45). Rational declarative decision-making concerning the volume, intensity, and frequency of exercise has not been sufficient to change sedentary behavior. Therefore, methods are being proposed to promote greater adherence to physical activity regiments, and a psychobiological integrative perspective appears to be a promising approach to achieve this goal (46, 47).

Cognitive and affective regulation of exercise intensity have been suggested to play a key role in both tolerance and adherence to exercise programs. For instance, homeostatic disturbances caused by high-intensity exercise have been associated with negative affective states and lower pleasure during exercise in sedentary individuals (45), leading to lower rates of adherence (48). Conversely, self-selected exercise intensity has been associated with positive affective states and higher levels of pleasure during exercise (45). Self-selected exercise intensity emphasizes the brain as the central governor of exercise intensity fluctuations (46), whereas the decision-making to increase and decrease velocity or tolerate or terminate the exercise session is controlled by the PFC through a bi-directional mind/body integration (49). Within this framework, top-down mechanisms are those initiated *via* declarative or non-declarative mental processing at the PFC level, which regulates muscle recruitment and alters physiological and behavioral responses. On the other hand, bottom-up mechanisms are initiated by sensitizing the ubiquitous somato-, viscero-, chemo-, and mechanical sensory receptors that influence central neural processing from the periphery to the brainstem, limbic system, and cerebral cortex (50). While performing any physical activity with self-selected intensity, the cognitive interpretation of the physiological state may be constantly working to preserve body homeostasis in order to reach the established goal (46, 51). In other words, fluctuations in pace while running are a behavioral outcome monitored by the brain (52). This behavioral modification results from integrating the task cognitive appraisal with afferent information related to biochemical and biophysical changes, such as temperature, heart and respiratory rate, blood pressure, blood concentrations of metabolites (e.g., $PO_2$, $PCO_2$, $H^+$, $HCO_3^-$, and lactate), intramuscular $H^+$, and energy substrate availability during the exercise (53).

Furthermore, feelings of fatigue and self-defeating thoughts demand inhibitory control mediated by the PFC in order to maintain physical activity (54). In this context, decision-making might be based on feelings such as perceived exertion (i.e., how hard the exercise is), affect (i.e., generic valence for good and bad feelings), and internal conversations such as "I cannot do it," "I will give up," or "it is very difficult" (53, 55). Therefore, self-selected exercise intensity emphasizes cognitive control (top-down) under the physiological changes (bottom-up) during physical effort (**Figure 1**), and it can be used as a strategy to develop self-monitoring and self-control abilities during the treatment of individuals with SUD. For instance, when setting a goal during an exercise session, such as running for a specific time or distance (i.e., time trial exercise), individuals need to regulate their pace to successfully complete that task. Thus, during the exercise, the decision to regulate the pace (running velocity) will be influenced by several environmental stimuli (i.e. weather, terrain, competitors, verbal instructions, and time or distance feedbacks) combined with the physiological state.

Several therapies focusing on this mind-body interaction through the top-down and bottom-up bi-directional mechanism have been suggested as promising rehabilitation tools in regulating stress and the immune system (56, 57). Therefore, we hypothesize

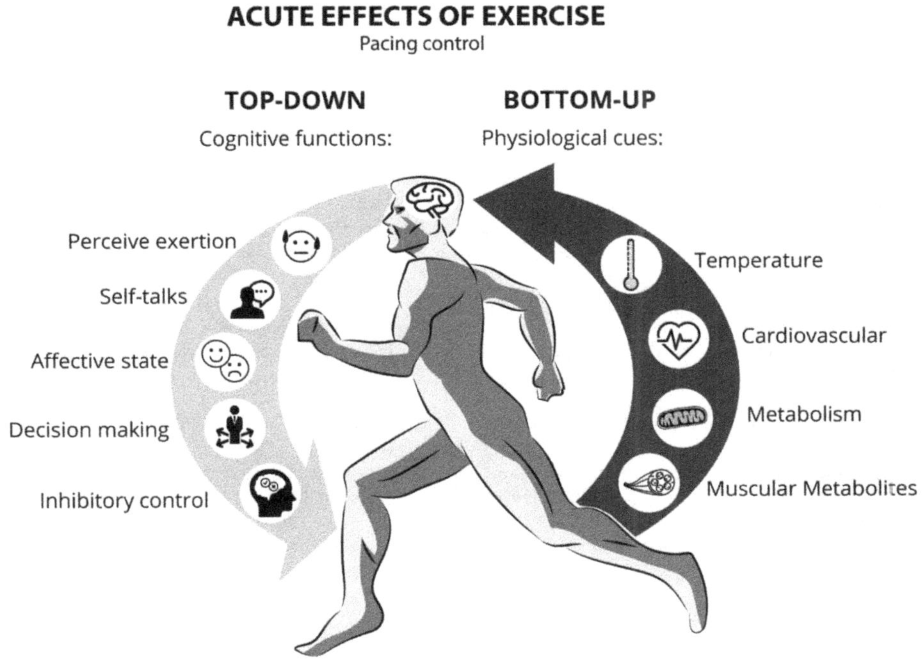


**FIGURE 1** | Pace control during continuous exercise while integrating top-down (cognitive functions) and bottom-up processing factors (physiological responses).

that self-selected exercise intensity employs the bi-directional mechanism enabling improvements in self-control abilities associated with brain exercise-induced neuroplasticity. This cognitive regulation can be tested in humans while investigating perceptual responses, exercise-induced effects, and PFC function using neuroimaging methods (e.g., fMRI, PET scan, and fNIRS) and/or electroencephalogram. In addition, the brain responses can be associated with tests that evaluate the executive constructs of SUD-specific decision-making and inhibitory control, such as cue-reactivity go/no-go tests in which individuals have to inhibit their responses to salient stimuli relating to drug-related cues (e.g., drug behavior pictures). This cue-reactivity response has been shown to activate areas of the PFCand to predict relapses in different substances disorders (58, 59). Thus, we suggest that randomized clinical trials could follow the neuroscience paradigm and cognitive methodologies to test this hypothesis. In addition, the implementation of a control group would play a key role in these experimental designs in order to compare the self-selected intensity of exercise with other types of exercise intensity regulation to demonstrate its efficacy.

## CONCLUSION

Despite the need for further prospective studies and clinical trials to test the efficacy of the psychobiological model of exercise as an intervention and treatment for SUD, physical exercise has been shown to be an effective and promising additional therapeutic tool for individuals with SUD. Here, we have described the brain areas affected by chronic substance use in patients with SUD as well as those improved by aerobic exercise. Some of these areas are primarily related to executive functions, which refer to a set of self-regulatory processes associated with the control of thoughts and behavior, including inhibitory control and decision-making. Therefore, in the same way that physical exercise is advised for treating other diseases, the neuroplasticity promoted by aerobic exercise may indicate its usefulness as a potential additional treatment for individuals with SUD. Specifically, these benefits may be seen in brain areas related to executive control, such as those areas involved in inhibition of drug-seeking behavior and impulsivity, as well as in decision-making regarding drug consumption. Furthermore, individuals with SUD who improve their fitness levels may enhance PFC function and cognition. These benefits should improve an individual's ability to inhibit drug consumption behavior when exposed to environmental cues and, consequently, their ability to maintain abstinence. However, this is still a hypothesis, and further studies are necessary to provide evidence of the effectiveness of exercise on maintaining drug abstinence, specifically exercise of self-regulated intensity. Thus, we propose an integrative cognitive-psychobiological model of exercise for future research and provide practical guidance to optimize its potential benefits during rehabilitation programs.

## AUTHOR CONTRIBUTIONS

KC and EF conceived the idea, draft, figure and final revision. DC reviewed literature for table, described the results and final revision. RH reviewed manuscript and added theoretical framework, practical application and final revision.

## REFERENCES


1. Ali SF, Onaivi ES, Dodd PR, Cadet JL, Schenk S, Kuhar MJ, et al. Understanding the global problem of drug addiction is a challenge for IDARS scientists. *Curr Neuropharmacol* (2011) 9(1):2–7. doi: 10.2174/157015911795017245
2. Hasin DS, O'Brien CP, Auriacombe M, Borges G, Bucholz K, Budney A, et al. DSM-5 criteria for substance use disorders: recommendations and rationale. *Am J Psychiatry* (2013) 170(8):834–51. doi: 10.1176/appi.ajp.2013.12060782
3. Farisco M, Evers K, Changeux J-P. Drug addiction: from neuroscience to ethics. *Front Psychiatry* (2018) 9:595. doi: 10.3389/fpsyt.2018.00595
4. Volkow Nora D, Koob GF, McLellan AT. Neurobiologic advances from the brain disease model of addiction. *N Eng J Med* (2016) 374(4):363–71. doi: 10.1056/NEJMra1511480
5. Volkow Nora D, Boyle M. Neuroscience of addiction: relevance to prevention and treatment. *Am J Psychiatry* (2018) 175(8):729–40. doi: 10.1176/appi.ajp.2018.17101174
6. Leshner AI. Addiction is a brain disease, and it matters. *Science* (1997) 278(5335):45–7. doi: 10.1126/science.278.5335.45
7. Damasio AR. The somatic marker hypothesis and the possible functions of the prefrontal cortex. *Philos Trans R Soc Lond B Biol Sci* (1996) 351(1346):1413–20. doi: 10.1098/rstb.1996.0125
8. Goldstein RZ, Volkow ND. Dysfunction of the prefrontal cortex in addiction: neuroimaging findings and clinical implications. *Nat Rev Neurosci* (2011) 12(11):652–69. doi: 10.1038/nrn3119
9. Volkow ND, Fowler JS, Wang GJ, Baler R, Telang F. Imaging dopamine's role in drug abuse and addiction. *Neuropharmacology* (2009) 56 Suppl 1:3–8. doi: 10.1016/j.neuropharm.2008.05.022
10. Winters KC, Arria A. Adolescent brain development and drugs. *Prev Res* (2011) 18(2):21–4. doi: 10.1037/e552592011-006
11. Lynch WJ, Peterson AB, Sanchez V, Abel J, Smith MA. Exercise as a novel treatment for drug addiction: a neurobiological and stage-dependent hypothesis. *Neurosci Biobehav Rev* (2013) 37(8):1622–44. doi: 10.1016/j.neubiorev.2013.06.011
12. Smith MA, Lynch WJ. Exercise as a potential treatment for drug abuse: evidence from preclinical studies. *Front Psychiatry* (2011) 2 82. doi: 10.3389/fpsyt.2011.00082
13. Wang D, Wang Y, Wang Y, Li R, Zhou C. Impact of physical exercise on substance use disorders: a meta-analysis. *PLoS ONE* (2014) 9(10):e110728. doi: 10.1371/journal.pone.0110728
14. Robison LS, Swenson S, Hamilton J, Thanos PK. Exercise reduces dopamine D1R and increases D2R in rats: implications for addiction. *Med Sci Sports Exerc* (2018) 50(8):1596–602. doi: 10.1249/MSS.0000000000001627
15. Baek S-S. Role of exercise on the brain. *J Exerc Rehabil* (2016) 12(5):380–5. doi: 10.12965/jer.1632808.404
16. Colcombe S, Kramer AF. Fitness effects on the cognitive function of older adults: a meta-analytic study. *Psychol Sci* (2003) 14(2):125–30. doi: 10.1111/1467-9280.t01-1-01430
17. Erickson KI, Kramer AF. Aerobic exercise effects on cognitive and neural plasticity in older adults. *Br J Sports Med* (2009) 43(1):22–4. doi: 10.1136/bjsm.2008.052498
18. Hillman CH, Erickson KI, Kramer AF. Be smart, exercise your heart: exercise effects on brain and cognition. *Nat Rev Neurosci* (2008) 9(1):58–65. doi: 10.1038/nrn2298
19. Griffin ÉW, Mullally S, Foley C, Warmington SA, O'Mara SM, Kelly AM. Aerobic exercise improves hippocampal function and increases BDNF in the serum of young adult males. *Physiol Behav* (2011) 104(5):934–41. doi: 10.1016/j.physbeh.2011.06.005
20. Trejo JL, Llorens-Martín MV, Torres-Alemán I. The effects of exercise on spatial learning and anxiety-like behavior are mediated by an IGF-I-dependent mechanism related to hippocampal neurogenesis. *Mol Cell Neurosci* (2008) 37(2):402–11. doi: 10.1016/j.mcn.2007.10.016
21. Ogoh S, Ainslie PN. Cerebral blood flow during exercise: mechanisms of regulation. *J Appl Physiol (1985)* (2009) 107(5):1370–80. doi: 10.1152/japplphysiol.00573.2009
22. During MJ, Cao L. VEGF, a mediator of the effect of experience on hippocampal neurogenesis. *Curr Alzheimer Res* (2006) 3(1):29–33. doi: 10.2174/156720506775697133
23. Buttler L, Jordão MT, Fragas MG, Ruggeri A, Ceroni A, Michelini LC. Maintenance of blood-brain barrier integrity in hypertension: a novel benefit of exercise training for autonomic control. *Front Physiol* (2017) 8:1048. doi: 10.3389/fphys.2017.01048
24. Ruegsegger GN, Booth FW. Health benefits of exercise. *Cold Spring Harb Perspect Med* (2018) 8(7). doi: 10.1101/cshperspect.a029694
25. Morici G, Gruttad'Auria CI, Baiamonte P, Mazzuca E, Castrogiovanni A, Bonsignore MR. Endurance training: is it bad for you? *Breathe* (2016) 12(2):140–7. doi: 10.1183/20734735.007016
26. Grandjean da Costa K, Soares Rachetti V, Quirino Alves da Silva W, Aranha Rego Cabral D, Gomes da Silva Machado D, Caldas Costa E, et al. Drug abusers have impaired cerebral oxygenation and cognition during exercise. *PLoS ONE* (2017) 12(11):e0188030. doi: 10.1371/journal.pone.0188030
27. Ferreira SE, dos Santos AK, de M, Okano AH, Gonçalves B, da SB, et al. Efeitos agudos do exercício físico no tratamento da dependência química. *Revista Bras Ciênc Do Esporte* (2017) 39(2):123–31. doi: 10.1016/j.rbce.2016.01.016
28. Leland DS, Arce E, Miller DA, Paulus MP. Anterior cingulate cortex and benefit of predictive cueing on response inhibition in stimulant dependent individuals. *Biol Psychiatry* (2008) 63(2):184–90. doi: 10.1016/j.biopsych.2007.04.031
29. Wang D, Zhou C, Zhao, M, Wu X, Chang, YK. Dose-response relationships between exercise intensity, cravings, and inhibitory control in methamphetamine dependence: an ERPs study. *Drug Alcohol Depend* (2016) 161:331–9.
30. Wang, D., Zhou, C., & Chang, Y. K. Acute exercise ameliorates craving and inhibitory deficits in methamphetamine: an ERP study. *Physiol Behav* (2015) 147:38–46.
31. Folstein JR, Van Petten C. Influence of cognitive control and mismatch on the N2 component of the ERP: a review. *Psychophysiology* (2008) 45(1):152–70. doi: 10.1111/j.1469-8986.2007.00602.x
32. Janse Van Rensburg K, Taylor AH. The effects of acute exercise on cognitive functioning and cigarette cravings during temporary abstinence from smoking. *Hum Psychopharmacol* (2008) 23(3):193–9. doi: 10.1002/hup.925
33. Janse Van Rensburg K, Taylor A, Hodgson T, Benattayallah A. Acute exercise modulates cigarette cravings and brain activation in response to smoking-related images: an fMRI study. *Psychopharmacology* (2009) 203(3):589–98. doi: 10.1007/s00213-008-1405-3
34. Janse Van Rensburg K, Taylor A, Benattayallah A, Hodgson T. The effects of exercise on cigarette cravings and brain activation in response to smoking-related images. *Psychopharmacology* (2012) 221(4):659–66. doi: 10.1007/s00213-011-2610-z
35. Da Costa KG, Rachetti VS, Da Silva WQA, Cabral DAR, da Silva Machado DG, Costa, E. C. et al. (2017) Drug abusers have impaired cerebral oxygenation and cognition during exercise. *PLoS One* (2017) 12(11):e0188030.
36. da Costa KG, Barbieri JF, Hohl R, Costa EC, Fontes EB. Exercise training improves cardiorespiratory fitness and cognitive function in individuals with substance use disorders: a pilot study. *Sport Sci Health* (2016), 1–5. doi: 10.1007/s11332-016-0338-1
37. Cabral DA, da Costa KG, Okano AH, Elsangedy HM, Rachetti VP, Fontes EB. Improving cerebral oxygenation, cognition and autonomic nervous system control of a chronic alcohol abuser through a three-month running program. *Addict Behav Rep* (2017) 6(Supplement C):83–9. doi: 10.1016/j.abrep.2017.08.004
38. Wang D, Zhu T, Zhou C, Chang Y-K. Aerobic exercise training ameliorates craving and inhibitory control in methamphetamine dependencies: a randomized controlled trial and event-related potential study. *Psychol Sport Exerc* (2017) 30:82–90. doi: 10.1016/j.psychsport.2017.02.001
39. Cabral D, Tavares V, Costa K, Nascimento P, Faro H, Elsangedy H, et al. The benefits of high intensity exercise on the brain of a drug abuser. *Global J Health Sci* (2018) 10(6):123. doi: 10.5539/gjhs.v10n6p123
40. Klinsophon T, Thaveeratitham P, Sitthipornvorakul E, Janwantanakul P. Effect of exercise type on smoking cessation: a meta-analysis of randomized controlled trials. *BMC Res Notes* (2017) 10(1):442. doi: 10.1186/s13104-017-2762-y
41. Colledge F, Gerber M, Pühse U, Ludyga S. Anaerobic exercise training in the therapy of substance use disorders: a systematic review. *Front Psychiatry* (2018) 9:644. doi: 10.3389/fpsyt.2018.00644

42. Liebenberg L. The relevance of persistence hunting to human evolution. *J Hum Evol* (2008) 55(6):1156–9. doi: 10.1016/j.jhevol.2008.07.004
43. Lieberman Daniel E. *The story of the human body: evolution, health, and disease.* Vintage Books (2014).
44. Blair SN. Physical inactivity: the biggest public health problem of the 21st century. *Br J Sports Med* (2009) 43(1):1–2.
45. Ekkekakis P, Parfitt G, Petruzzello SJ. The pleasure and displeasure people feel when they exercise at different intensities: decennial update and progress towards a tripartite rationale for exercise intensity prescription. *Sports Med* (2011) 41(8):641–71. doi: 10.2165/11590680-000000000-00000
46. Ekkekakis P. Let them roam free? Physiological and psychological evidence for the potential of self-selected exercise intensity in public health. *Sports Med* (2009) 39(10):857–88. doi: 10.2165/11315210-000000000-00000
47. Parfitt G, Rose EA, Burgess WM. The psychological and physiological responses of sedentary individuals to prescribed and preferred intensity exercise. *Br J Health Psychol* 11(Pt (2006) 1:39–53. doi: 10.1348/135910705X43606
48. Mama SK, McNeill LH, McCurdy SA, Evans AE, Diamond PM, Adamus-Leach HJ, et al. Psychosocial factors and theory in physical activity studies in minorities. *Am J Health Behav* (2015) 39(1):68–76. doi: 10.5993/AJHB.39.1.8
49. Robertson CV, Marino FE. A role for the prefrontal cortex in exercise tolerance and termination. *J Appl Physiol (1985)* (2016) 120(4):464–6. doi: 10.1152/japplphysiol.00363.2015
50. Damasio A, Carvalho GB. The nature of feelings: evolutionary and neurobiological origins. *Nat Rev Neurosci* (2013) 14(2):143–52. doi: 10.1038/nrn3403
51. Noakes T, St C, Lambert E. From catastrophe to complexity: a novel model of integrative central neural regulation of effort and fatigue during exercise in humans. *Br J Sports Med* (2004) 38(4):511–4. doi: 10.1136/bjsm.2003.009860
52. Tucker R, Lambert MI, Noakes TD. An analysis of pacing strategies during men's world-record performances in track athletics. *Int J Sports Physiol Perform* (2006) 1(3):233–45. doi: 10.1123/ijspp.1.3.233
53. St Clair Gibson A, Lambert EV, Rauch LHG, Tucker R, Baden DA, Foster C, et al. The role of information processing between the brain and peripheral physiological systems in pacing and perception of effort. *Sports Med* (2006) 36(8):705–22. doi: 10.2165/00007256-200636080-00006
54. Martin K, Staiano W, Menaspà P, Hennessey T, Marcora S, Keegan R, et al. Superior inhibitory control and resistance to mental fatigue in professional road cyclists. *PLoS ONE* (2016) 11(7). doi: 10.1371/journal.pone.0159907
55. Hardy J, Hall CR, Alexander MR. Exploring self-talk and affective states in sport. *J Sports Sci* (2001) 19(7):469–75. doi: 10.1080/026404101750238926
56. Buchanan TW, Tranel D. Central and peripheral nervous system interactions: from mind to brain to body. *Int J Psychophysiol* (2009) 72(1):1–4. doi: 10.1016/j.ijpsycho.2008.09.002
57. Taylor AG, Goehler LE, Galper DI, Innes KE, Bourguignon C. Top-down and bottom-up mechanisms in mind-body medicine: development of an integrative framework for psychophysiological research. *Explore (NY)* (2010) 6(1):29–41. doi: 10.1016/j.explore.2009.10.004
58. Hanlon CA, Dowdle LT, Gibson NB, Li X, Hamilton S, Canterberry M, et al. Cortical substrates of cue-reactivity in multiple substance dependent populations: transdiagnostic relevance of the medial prefrontal cortex. *Transl Psychiatry* (2018) 8. doi: 10.1038/s41398-018-0220-9
59. Prisciandaro JJ, Myrick H, Henderson S, McRae-Clark AL, Brady KT. Prospective associations between brain activation to cocaine and no-go cues and cocaine relapse. *Drug Alcohol Depend* (2013) 131(0):44–9. doi: 10.1016/j.drugalcdep.2013.04.008

4

# Effects of Opioid Dependence on Visuospatial Memory and its Associations with Depression and Anxiety

***Serenella Tolomeo[1,2*], Fleur Davey[3], J. Douglas Steele[4] and Alexander Mario Baldacchino[4,5]***

*[1] Department of Psychology, National University of Singapore, Singapore, Singapore, [2] Centre for Family and Population Research, National University of Singapore, Singapore, Singapore, [3] NHS Fife, Queen Margaret Hospital, Dunfermline, United Kingdom, [4] School of Medicine, University of Dundee, Ninewells Hospital and Medical School, Dundee, United Kingdom, [5] Division of Population and Behavioural Science, Medical School, University of St Andrews, St Andrews, United Kingdom*

***Correspondence:**
*Serenella Tolomeo*
*fasst@nus.edu.sg*

**Introduction:** The cognitive impact of opioid dependence is rarely measured systematically in everyday clinical practice even though both patients and clinicians accept that cognitive symptoms often occur in the opioid-dependent population. There are only a few publications which utilized computerized neuropsychological tests to assess possible impairments of visuospatial memory in opioid-dependent individuals either receiving opioid replacement therapy (ORT) or during subsequent short-term abstinence and the effects of anxiety and depression.

**Methods:** We assessed a cohort of 102 participants, comprising i) a stable opioid-dependent group receiving methadone maintenance treatment (MMT) (n = 22), ii) a stable opioid-dependent group receiving buprenorphine (BMT) (n = 20), iii) a current abstinent but previously opioid-dependent group (ABS) (n = 8), and iv) a control group who have never been dependent on opioids. The Cambridge Neuropsychological Automated Test Battery (CANTAB) neuropsychological tasks undertaken by participants included: Delayed Matching to Sample (DMS), Pattern Recognition Memory (PRM), Spatial Recognition Memory (SRM), and Paired Associate Learning (PAL) tasks. Three clinical measures were used to assess the severity of anxiety and depressive illness: Hospital Anxiety Scale-Hospital Anxiety Depression (HADA)-(HADD), Beck Depression Inventory (BDI), and Inventory of Depressive Symptomatology (self-report) (ISD-SR).

**Results:** The methadone- and buprenorphine-treated groups showed significant impairments ($p < 0.001$) in visuospatial memory tasks but not the abstinent group. Impairments in visuospatial memory strongly correlated with higher mood and anxiety symptom severity scores ($p < 0.001$).

**Discussion:** These results are broadly consistent with previous studies. Uniquely, though, here we report a strong relationship between visuospatial memory and depression and anxiety scores, which might suggest common illness mechanisms.

**Keywords: memory, opioid dependence, heroin, methadone, buprenorphine, depression, anxiety**

# INTRODUCTION

Substance misuse is a chronic condition often characterized by remissions and relapses (1). Individuals with a history of long-term opioid dependence may demonstrate cognitive impairments, primarily within the executive functioning domains (2–8).

These impairments have been linked to grey matter reductions in the prefrontal cortex, anterior mid-cingulate cortex, and basal ganglia (9), brain regions thought responsible for the regulation of cravings, pain, and emotional experience. In addition, other studies have reported how opioids affect memory, learning, and emotional disturbances (2, 3, 10, 11). Depression has long been associated with widespread cognitive deficits (12) which tend to worsen over a life span (13).

Specific memory tasks have shown to be sensitive and useful in detecting brain dysfunction in the temporal and amygdalo-hippocampal regions (14), which are consistently reported as functionally abnormal in mood disorders and sensation-seeking behaviors (15–17).

Importantly, these brain regions are also relevant to the neurobiology of substance misuse (18) with similar symptoms such as mood, anhedonia, and anxiety associated with drug dependence (19). These symptoms may represent a risk factor for the development of dependence and also may constitute a specific factor by which dependence is maintained, as well as strongly associated with major depressive disorder (MDD). However, depressive and anxiety symptoms have rarely been investigated in opioid dependence within a clinical environment.

Previous studies showed impairments in episodic memory (20), visual memory, verbal memory, information processing, problem solving (21), and spatial, tactile, and verbal memory (2) in heroin-, morphine-, and methadone-dependent participants. Curran and colleagues showed that a single dose of methadone could negatively impact on episodic memory in opiate users (20).

Previously, we have shown that visuospatial memory was impaired in chronic heroin and methadone-dependent participants, those maintained on methadone as part of opioid replacement therapy (ORT), or patients prescribed opioids for chronic pain (10). However, to our knowledge, there are no previous studies reporting the impact of opioid dependence on memory during short-term abstinence from opioids.

Here, we tested the following hypotheses:

(i) Visuospatial memory impairments are associated with current opioid exposure. Conversely, we therefore predicted that abstinence would be associated with no significant impairments.
(ii) Cognitive impairments would correlate with mood and anxiety ratings. Specifically, we predicted that participants with higher depression and anxiety symptoms would have greater visuospatial memory impairments.

# METHODS

Study approval was granted by the East of Scotland Research Ethics Committee (REC reference number: 06/S1401/32) and written informed consent obtained from all participants. National Health Service (NHS) Scotland Research Governance approval was provided by the NHS Fife Research and Development Department.

A total of 102 participants were *opportunistically* enrolled in this study with four groups: (i) a stable opioid-dependent group receiving methadone maintenance treatment (MMT) (n = 22), (ii) a stable opioid-dependent group receiving buprenorphine (BMT) (n = 20), (iii) a current abstinent but previously opioid-dependent group (ABS) (n = 8), and (iv) controls, with no history of illicit heroin, methadone, or buprenorphine use (n = 52). Patients had a diagnosis of *Diagnostic and Statistical Manual of Mental Disorders, Fourth Edition* (*DSM-IV*), Opioid Dependence and a history of poly-substance misuse with heroin as the primary "drug of choice" preceding initiation of MMT.

An extensive detailed screening was assessed by two clinicians (A.B. or F.D.), which included sociodemographic information collection and a semi-structured interview to obtain detailed previous histories of drug and alcohol use and current opioid dependence status (**Table 1** and **Supplementary Table 1**). Clinical histories and diagnoses were obtained using the structured Mini International Neuropsychiatric Interview (MINI Plus v 5.0) (22) together with a detailed review of individual clinical care records. The latter included recording the dose of methadone and buprenorphine that each participant received at the time of testing. A morphine equivalent calculation was performed in accordance to a previous publication by Vieweg et al. (23). Each methadone dose was multiplied by 20, and each buprenorphine dose was multiplied by 12 (23). Ongoing abstinence from illicit drug use was also objectively confirmed just prior to scanning with a urine drug test (24) using automated enzyme-mediated immunoassay to classify any detected drug (25). The Clinical Opioid Withdrawal Scale (COWS) was used to quantify the level of opioid withdrawal if present (26). Previous care records from Addiction Services, psychiatric notes, and general practitioners' records confirmed the absence of hepatitis B and C and HIV. Other exclusion criteria included: past or current histories of psychotic disorders; post-traumatic stress disorder (PTSD); antisocial and borderline personality disorders; neurological and neurodevelopmental disorders; significant head injury; confirmed history of non-fatal overdose episodes; and co-occurring benzodiazepine, stimulant, and/or alcohol dependence.

Current and premorbid intelligence was estimated using the Wechsler Abbreviated Scale of Intelligence (WASI) and National Adult Reading Test (NART) (27, 28).

## Visuospatial Memory Tasks

The Cambridge Neuropsychological Automated Test Battery (CANTAB, www.camcog.com) comprises a series of computerized memory tasks (29). As previously reported, the following tasks have shown specificity to detect impairments in *visual memory performance* [Delayed Matching to Sample (DMS), Pattern Recognition Memory (PRM), Spatial Recognition

**TABLE 1** | Demographic, clinical, and substance use history data.

| | MMT (N = 22) | BMT (N = 20) | ABS (N = 8) | HC (N = 52) | Statistics |
|---|---|---|---|---|---|
| Number | 22 | 20 | 8 | 51 | |
| Age in years | 33.6. | 37.4 | 37.6 | 28.0 | P < 0.001<br>MMT, BMT, ABS > HC*** |
| NART | 114.3 (5.2) | 98.0 (13.5) | 106.4 (15.6) | 117.5 (6) | P < 0.001<br>BMT, ABS < HC*** |
| HADA | 6.0 (4.3) | 4.8 (2.7) | 4.0 (2.3) | 3.5 (3.4) | P = 0.04 |
| HADD | 4.4 (3.5) | 4.4 (2.9) | 8.0 (1.5) | 1.2 (2.3) | P < 0.001 |
| BDI | 12.4 (10) | 9.9 (6.3) | 9.0 (1.8) | 3.7 (5.2) | P = 0.02 |
| IDS-SR | 17.8 (12) | 12.6 (6.6) | 14.0 (3.2) | 7.9 (7.3) | P < 0.001 |
| Fagerstrom (total score) | 3.4 (2.3) | 3.9 (2.3) | 3.5 (2.8) | | ns |
| OD (methadone or buprenorphine in mg) | 73.4 (60.8) | 11.0 (6.7) | – | – | P < 0.001<br>MMT > BMT*** |
| Daily intake expressed as morphine equivalent dose in mg | 1,835.5 (1,277) | 888.0 (533) | – | – | P < 0.001<br>MMT > BMT*** |
| Age when first used heroin in years | 20.2 (4.4) | 21.7 (5.4) | 20.0 (4.7) | – | ns |
| Age when dependent on opioids in years | 20.2 (4.4) | 23.6 (5.9) | 22.9 (8.5) | – | ns |
| Age when injecting opioids in years | 21.8 (4.2) | 24.8 (6) | 22.7 (6.9) | – | ns |
| Years of opioid use | 12.9 (4.4) | 13.4 (6.7) | 13.4 (7.6) | – | ns |
| Age when first used benzodiazepine in years | 17.2 (5.8) | 21.7 (7.7) | 15.6 (6.6) | | P < 0.04<br>MMT < BMT* |
| Days of benzodiazepine use in the last 30 days | – | – | – | – | – |
| Age when first used cocaine in years | 17.3 (1) | 21.9 (6.6) | 18.3 (4.2) | – | ns |
| Days of cocaine use in last 30 days | – | – | – | – | – |
| Age when first used cannabis in years | 13.3 (3.8) | 15.8 (5.3) | 13.1 (1.2) | – | ns |
| Days of cannabis use in last 30 days | – | – | – | – | – |
| Age when first used alcohol in years | 10.5 (7.9) | 15.1 (3) | 13.0 (1.9) | – | 0.04<br>MMT < BMT* |
| Days of alcohol use in last 30 days | – | – | – | – | – |
| Duration abstinence (days) | – | – | 102.2 (61.3) | – | – |

*Values are mean (SD); MMT, methadone maintenance treatment group; BMT, buprenorphine maintenance treatment group; ABS, abstinent group; HC, healthy control group; N, total number; HADA, Hospital Anxiety Scale; HADD, Hospital Anxiety Depression; BDI, Beck Depression Inventory; IDS-SR, Inventory of Depressive Symptomatology (self-report); NART, National Adult Reading Test; significance * = p = 0.05, *** = p < 0.001; ns, non-significant; mg, milligrams; OD, opioid dose (methadone or buprenorphine).*

Memory (SRM), and Paired Associate Learning (PAL)] and *spatial memory performance* [Spatial Span Task (SSP) and Spatial Working Memory (SWM)] (10).

## Depression and Anxiety Rating Scales

Three clinical measures were used to assess the severity of anxiety and depressive illness: the Hospital Anxiety and Depression Scale (HADS) (30), Beck Depression Inventory (BDI) (23), and Inventory of Depressive Symptomatology (IDS): clinician (IDS-C) and self-report (IDS-SR) (31).

HADS is commonly used to determine depression and anxiety. It is a 14-item scale with 7 items that relate to depression (HADD) and 7 items to anxiety (HADA) (30). BDI and IDS are self-report inventories, and they have been mostly used to assess depression and anhedonia (32, 33). BDI demonstrated high internal consistency, with an alpha coefficient of 0.82 (34). Similarly, IDS demonstrated strong internal consistency, with an alpha coefficient of 0.88 (35).

## Statistical Analysis

Data meeting assumptions of normality and homogeneity of variance were analyzed using analysis of variance (ANOVA) (36). All other data were compared using Mann–Whitney test. Preliminary analysis of all the experimental and control groups separately indicated that the samples did not come from normally distributed populations with the same standard deviation. We used a *post hoc Bonferroni* correction in order to control for family-wise error for unplanned tests. Mann–Whitney U tests established that NART, age, and smoking history needed to be used as covariates for hypothesis testing.

A general linear model was performed with "groups" as a factor and "visuospatial memory task performances" as dependent variables using analysis of covariance (ANCOVA). To explore the potential contribution of the impact of depression and anxiety scores on memory task performance, we added an additional correlational analysis within the ANCOVA.

Data were analyzed using the Statistical Package for the Social Science (SPSS) version 24 (SPSS Inc.) in Windows 10 on a PC computer. P values < 0.05 were considered significant.

# RESULTS

## Demographic Characteristics

Demographic and clinical characteristics are presented in **Table 1**. Participants and controls were matched on the basis of gender (all males). The MMT, BMT, and ABS groups were older than the healthy controls (HCs) ($p < 0.001$). The HC group had higher estimated premorbid IQ ($p < 0.001$) according to the NART than the BMT and ABS groups. The mean morphine equivalent daily dose for the MMT group was significantly higher than the BMT ($p < 0.001$). Urine analyses confirmed complete absence of recent heroin, amphetamine, benzodiazepine, and cocaine prior to neuropsychological testing. The MMT group reported they first drank alcohol and consumed benzodiazepine approximately 4.5 years prior to the BMT cohort ($p < 0.04$). There were no significant group differences identified on several clinical substance history data such as: age when they first used heroin ($p = 0.6$), age when dependent on heroin ($p = 0.2$), or age when injecting opioids ($p = 0.3$). The MMT, BMT, and ABS were well matched with regard to age when they first used cocaine ($p = 0.15$) and cannabis ($p = 0.13$).

## Visual Memory

### Performance on DMS

There was a significant effect of group on the percentage of correct responses for DMS [$F(4, 78) = 7.5$, $p < 0.001$]. *Post hoc* Bonferroni comparisons showed that participants from the MMT and BMT groups made significantly more errors than the ABS and HC groups ($p = 0.03$ and $p < 0.001$, respectively). There was a significant effect of group on the percentage of correct responses for DMS [$F(4, 78) = 7.4$, $p < 0.001$]. *Post hoc* Bonferroni comparisons showed that participants from the MMT and BMT groups made significantly more errors than the ABS and HC groups ($p = 0.02$ and $p < = .001$, respectively).

More details are reported in **Table 2** and **Figure 1**.

### Performance on PRM, SRM, and PAL

There was a significant effect of group on the percentage of correct responses for the PRM task [$F(4, 60) = 9.3$, $p < 0.001$] and on the mean correct latency for the SRM task [$F(4, 60) = 6.4$, $p < 0.001$]. Similarly, there was a significant effect of group on the total adjusted errors on the PAL task [$F(4, 75) = 6.1$, $p < 0.001$] and on PAL first trial memory [$F(4, 75) = 5.7$, $p < 0.001$] (see **Figure 2**).

**TABLE 3 |** Correlations between depression and anxiety and visuospatial performance.

| | HADA | BDI | IDS-SR |
|---|---|---|---|
| PAL (total error adjusted) | 0.3** | 0.25* | 0.3** |
| PAL (first trial memory score) | 0.3** | 0.28* | 0.4*** |
| DMS (% correct) | – | 0.3** | – |

** indicates p < 0.05, ** indicates p < 0.01, *** indicates p < 0.001.*

## Spatial Memory

### Performance on SSP and SWM

There was a significant effect of group on the SSP task (span length) [$F(4, 75) = 10.5$, $p < 0.001$]. The BMT and ABS groups (a) made significantly more errors (between errors) [$F(4, 75) = 5$, $p < 0.003$] and (b) presented with a poorer strategy on the SWM task [$F(4, 75) = 9.8$, $p < 0.001$].

## Depression and Anxiety and Visuospatial Memory Performance

Higher HADA anxiety, BDI, and IDS-SR depression scores were significantly correlated with PAL (total error adjusted [$r(66) = 0.3$, $p = 0.01$, $r(66) = 0.25$, $p = 0.04$, $r(64) = 0.3$, $p < 0.005$, respectively]). Similarly, higher HADA, BDI, and IDS-SR scores were significantly associated with PAL (first trial memory score) [$r(66) = 0.3$, $p = 0.007$, $r(66) = 0.28$, $p = 0.02$, $r(64) = 0.4$, $p = 0.001$, respectively]. DMS (% correct) significantly correlated with BDI [$r(66) = 0.3$, $p = 0.01$] (see **Table 3**).

**TABLE 2 |** Summary of neuropsychological findings for visual and spatial memory.

| Memory and learning measures | MMT (N = 22) | BMT (N = 20) | ABS (N = 8) | HC (N = 52) | Statistics |
|---|---|---|---|---|---|
| Visual Memory | | | | | |
| DMS % correct | 84.5 (11.6) | 80.0 (15) | 92.8 (2.1) | 92.5 (5.9) | P < 0.001, MMT, BMT < ABS, HC*** |
| DMS % correct (all delays) | 80.2 (14.8) | 75.6 (18.5) | 91.6 (3.9) | 90.7 (7.6) | P < 0.001, MMT, BMT < ABS, HC*** |
| PRM % correct | 83.8 (10.1) | 80.1 (11.7) | 90.2(0.09) | 93.2 (4.3) | P < 0.001, MMT, BMT < ABS, HC*** |
| SRM mean correct latency | 1,997 (377) | 2,743 (1,138) | 2,150 (454) | 1,882 (555) | P = 0.001, BMT > HC*** |
| PAL total errors adjusted | 125.7 (101) | 29.9 (34.6) | 11.0 (9) | 57.0 (90) | P = 0.001, MMT, BMT > ABS, HC*** |
| PAL first trial memory score | 8.5 (0.8) | 17.9 (4.5) | 19.7 (3) | 16.4 (9) | P = 0.001, MMT < HC, ABS*** |
| Spatial Memory | | | | | |
| SWM between errors | 8.8 (15.9) | 33.4 (21.4) | 22.7 (16.2) | 16.6 (21.9) | P = 0.003, BMT > MMT, HC*** |
| SWM strategy | 13.1 (14.9) | 32.9 (6.9) | 31.7 (6) | 21.3 (13.4) | P < 0.001, MMT < BMT, ABS*** |

*Values are mean (SD); significance *** = P < 0.001; DMS, Delayed Matching to Sample; PRM, Pattern Recognition Memory, SRM, Spatial Recognition Memory; PAL, Paired Associate Learning; SWM, Spatial Working Memory; N, total number.*

## DISCUSSION

In this clinically well-characterized study, we have demonstrated that memory for visually presented patterns and spatial locations was impaired in individuals on ORT. This is consistent with previous studies utilizing computerized CANTAB assessment with individuals on ORT and HCs. These studies revealed that individuals on ORT exhibited impairments in comparison to controls on the PRM task (2, 3) and on the PAL task (21). In a recent meta-analysis by Baldacchino and colleagues (37), short-term memory impairments were not present in the abstinence cohorts. This is consistent with our present results, as cognitive impairments were not present in the abstinent group for both visual and spatial memory tasks.

We previously reported that cognitive processes particularly associated with the prefrontal cortex are disrupted during chronic opioid use but not during abstinence (9). Our results could be explained by frontal lobe dysfunction (9, 38–40), which can potentially cause impairments on tasks requiring optimal memory function with patients receiving ORT. In addition, the identified impairments within the opioid-dependent groups on ORT point to specific correlations with depression and anxiety, particularly with tasks sensitive to the anatomical location of the medial temporal lobe.

This is consistent with numerous studies in healthy volunteers identifying the medial temporal lobe, such as the hippocampus and amygdala, as the area where memory-sensitive tasks are encoded (41, 42). Of specific interest, the medial temporal lobe regions have been reported 1) as structurally abnormal in depressive disorder (16) and 2) as one of the main putative candidate regions for both the development and the maintenance of dependence (18) and depression (43).

Regarding possible limitations of the present study, we recruited only males, so these findings shouldn't be generalized to females (44). Drug use and clinical histories were collected based upon self-report, and no blood, hair, or saliva samples were available to confirm the accuracy of the information given; however, our study did acquire urine drug screen analysis to confirm the absence of recent illicit drug use prior to every session. Additionally, the present study recruited well-matched subjects with regard to their previous drug history in the experimental groups and excluded regular and dependent users of most psychoactive substances, such as alcohol and benzodiazepines, as they have been shown to profoundly impact neuropsychological performance (18). We couldn't control the effect of nicotine, which may have influenced our results due to its known neuropsychological effects on visual and spatial memory (45). The burprenorphine group had a significant lower morphine equivalent dose than the methadone group, which may impact our findings; however, no statistically significant correlations were present. Larger studies with long-term abstinence are required to fully validate the observed reversibility and possible extinction of these impairments.

### Clinical Relevance

Patients' questions about the effects of opioid dependence on memory and its impact during abstinence cannot comprehensively be answered, due to a current lack of research in this area (10). More data are required on the consequences of opioid dependence on memory in order to evaluate the acceptability of differential treatments, such as methadone and buprenorphine, and perhaps maximize abstinence periods (46). Previous studies have indicated the importance of detecting memory impairments using highly structured and extensive neuropsychological batteries. This is further highlighted in the present study, indicating that opioid-dependent individuals have memory loss in both visual and spatial domains. Early identification of memory impairments associated with opioid dependence could improve the current standard clinical method of assessment. Elucidating the cognitive and neural mechanisms responsible for the formation and maintenance of opioid-related associative dependence has the

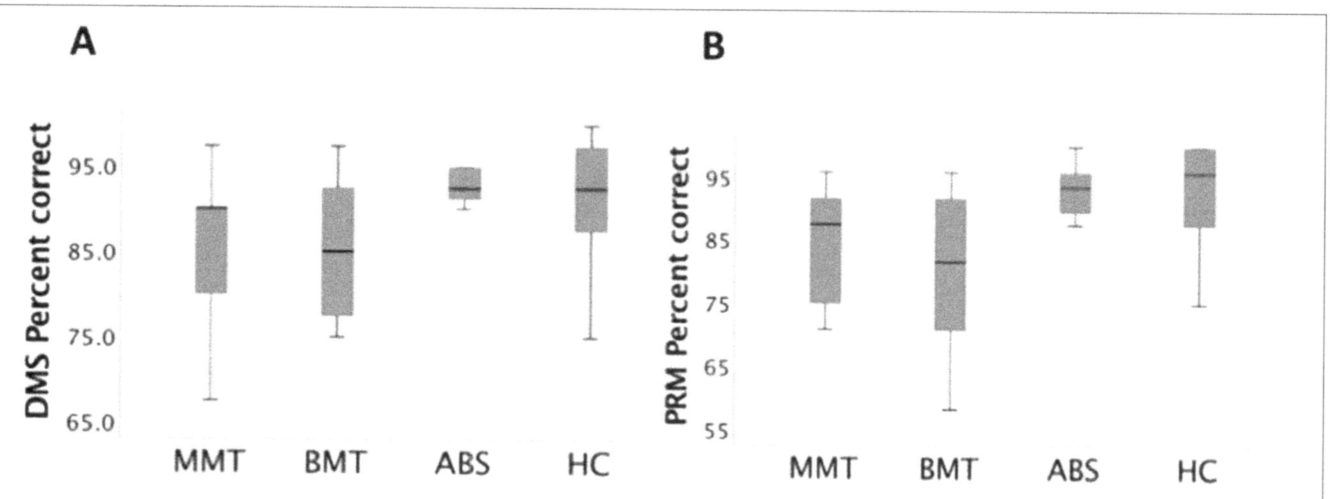


**FIGURE 1 | (A)** Delayed Matching to Sample (DMS) task (% correct) box plots: the stable opioid-dependent group receiving methadone maintenance treatment (MMT) and that receiving buprenorphine (BMT) made significantly more errors than the abstinent but previously opioid-dependent group (ABS) and healthy controls (HCs) ($p < 0.001$) groups. **(B)** Pattern Recognition Memory (PRM) task (% correct) box plots: the MMT and BMT made significantly more errors than the ABS and HC ($p < 0.001$) groups.

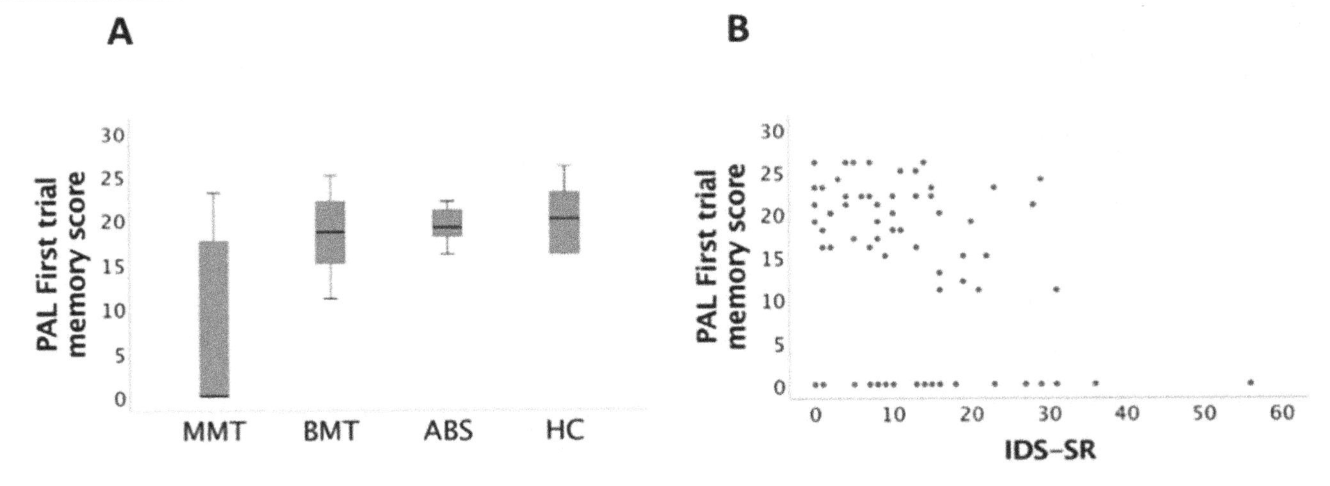


**FIGURE 2 | (A)** Paired Associate Learning (PAL) (first trial memory score) box plots: those in the MMT group were significant more impaired than the ABS and HC groups ($p < 0.001$). **(B)** PAL (first trial memory score) task significantly correlated with Inventory of Depressive Symptomatology (self-report) (IDS-SR) ($p = 0.005$).

potential for opening up new therapeutic trajectories during both the prevention and/or reversal of the significant effects on memory and learning, which may be a vulnerability for development and maintenance of opioid dependence. Notably, our results highlight the possibility that opioid-dependent individuals may benefit from focused treatments for depression and anxiety symptoms during ORT.

In particular, understanding the underlying neurocognitive and brain substrates linked to a dual close relationship between comorbid substance misuse and mood states may (a) reveal potential new interventions for the treatment of protracted opioid dependence and/or relapse (18) and (b) provide the required biomarkers to create predictive algorithms to detect early dependence and abstinence (6, 7).

## CONCLUSION

In summary, our results found that opioid-dependent participants exhibited visuospatial memory impairments closely associated with depression and anxiety scores. These impairments were not present in short-term abstinence, suggesting reversible impairments. Further studies need to explore the effect that mood plays in cognitive impairments observed in this and other dependent populations (e.g. nicotine and alcohol). Indeed, identifying and characterizing the visuospatial memory abilities and their potential mechanisms of action may be of crucial importance in identifying potential common mechanisms controlling the switch from the non-dependent to substance-dependent states and ultimately achieving abstinence in the opioid-dependent population.

## AUTHOR CONTRIBUTIONS

ST wrote the first draft of the manuscript with AB's input and created the figures and tables. FD and JS provided revisions to versions of the draft manuscript. ST formatted the manuscript for publication.

## ACKNOWLEDGMENTS

We thank the NHS Fide Research and Development Department and NHS Fife Addiction Services for their support. We thank Mairi Stirling, Sarah Gray, and Sawn Stewart for their help in the recruitment of the initial cohort data. Finally, we thank all participants in this study.

## REFERENCES

1. Wolf JP, Ponicki WR, Kepple NJ, Gaidus A. Are community level prescription opioid overdoses associated with child harm? A spatial analysis of California zip codes, 2001–2011. *Drug Alcohol Depend* (2016) 166:202–8. doi: 10.1016/j.drugalcdep.2016.07.014
2. Ornstein TJ, Iddon JL, Baldacchino AM, Sahakian BJ, London M, Everitt BJ, et al. Profiles of cognitive dysfunction in chronic amphetamine and heroin abusers. *Neuropsychopharmacology* (2000) 23(2):113. doi: 10.1016/S0893-133X(00)00097-X
3. Ersche KD, Clark L, London M, Robbins TW, Sahakian BJ. Profile of executive and memory function associated with amphetamine and opiate dependence. *Neuropsychopharmacology* (2006) 31(5):1036. doi: 10.1038/sj.npp.1300889
4. Ersche KD, Sahakian BJ. The neuropsychology of amphetamine and opiate dependence: implications for treatment. *Neuropsychol Rev* (2007) 17(3):317–36. doi: 10.1007/s11065-007-9033-y
5. Baldacchino A, Balfour DJK, Matthews K. Impulsivity and opioid drugs: differential effects of heroin, methadone and prescribed analgesic medication. *Psychol Med* (2015) 45(6):1167–79. doi: 10.1017/S0033291714002189
6. Verdejo-García A, Pérez-García M. Profile of executive deficits in cocaine and heroin polysubstance users: common and differential effects on separate executive components. *Psychopharmacology* (2007) 190(4):517–30. doi: 10.1007/s00213-006-0632-8

7. Tolomeo S, Gray S, Matthews K, Steele JD, Baldacchino A. Multifaceted impairments in impulsivity and brain structural abnormalities in opioid dependence and abstinence. *Psychol Med* (2016a) 46(13):2841–53. doi: 10.1017/S0033291716001513
8. Tolomeo S, Matthews K, Steele D, Baldacchino A. Compulsivity in opioid dependence. *Prog Neuropsychopharmacol Biol Psychiatry* (2018) 81:333–9. doi: 10.1016/j.pnpbp.2017.09.007
9. Tolomeo S, Christmas D, Jentzsch I, Johnston B, Sprengelmeyer R, Matthews K, et al. A causal role for the anterior mid-cingulate cortex in negative affect and cognitive control. *Brain* (2016b) 139(6):1844–54. doi: 10.1093/brain/aww069
10. Baldacchino A, Tolomeo S, Balfour DJ, Matthews K. Profiles of visuospatial memory dysfunction in opioid-exposed and dependent populations. *Psychol Med* (2018) 1–11. doi: 10.1017/S0033291718003318
11. Kutlu MG, Gould TJ. Effects of drugs of abuse on hippocampal plasticity and hippocampus-dependent learning and memory: contributions to development and maintenance of addiction. *Learn Mem* (2016) 23(10):515–33. doi: 10.1101/lm.042192.116
12. Austin MP, Mitchell P, Goodwin GM. Cognitive deficits in depression: possible implications for functional neuropathology. *Br J Psychiatry Suppl* (2001) 178(3):200–6. doi: 10.1192/bjp.178.3.200
13. Albert KM, Potter GG, McQuoid DR, Taylor WD. Cognitive performance in antidepressant-free recurrent major depressive disorder. *Depression and Anxiety* (2018) 35(8):694–9.
14. Owen AM, Sahakian BJ, Semple J, Polkey CE, Robbins TW. Visuo-spatial short-term recognition memory and learning after temporal lobe excisions, frontal lobe excisions or amygdalo-hippocampectomy in man. *Neuropsychologia* (1995) 33(1):1–24. doi: 10.1016/0028-3932(94)00098-A
15. Johnston BA, Tolomeo S, Gradin V, Christmas D, Matthews K, Douglas Steele J. Failure of hippocampal deactivation during loss events in treatment-resistant depression. *Brain* (2016) 138(9):2766–76. doi: 10.1093/brain/awv177
16. Schmaal L, Veltman DJ, van Erp TG, Sämann PG, Frodl T, Jahanshad N, et al. Subcortical brain alterations in major depressive disorder: findings from the ENIGMA major depressive disorder working group. *Mol Psychiatry* (2016) 21(6):806. https://doi.org/10.1038/mp.2015.69
17. Fornaro M, Ventriglio A, De Pasquale C, Pistorio ML, De Berardis D, Cattaneo CI, et al. Sensation seeking in major depressive patients: relationship to sub-threshold bipolarity and cyclothymic temperament. *J Affect Dis* (2013) 148(2–3):375–83.
18. Koob GF, Volkow ND. Neurocircuitry of addiction. *Neuropsychopharmacology* (2010) 35(1):217. doi: 10.1038/npp.2009.110
19. Koob GF. The dark side of emotion: the addiction perspective. *Eur J Pharmacol* (2015) 753:73–87. doi: 10.1016/j.ejphar.2014.11.044
20. Curran HV, Kleckham J, Bearn J, Strang J, Wanigaratne S. Effects of methadone on cognition, mood and craving in detoxifying opiate addicts: a dose-response study. *Psychopharmacology* (2001) 154(2):153–60.
21. Darke S, Sims J, McDonald S, Wickes W. Cognitive impairment among methadone maintenance patients. *Addiction* (2000) 95(5):687–95.
22. Sheehan DV, Lecrubier Y, Sheehan KH, Amorim P, Janavs J, Weiller E, et al. The Mini-International Neuropsychiatric Interview (MINI): the development and validation of a structured diagnostic psychiatric interview for DSM-IV and ICD-10. *J Clin Psychiatry* (1998) 59:22–23. doi: 10.1037/t18597-000
23. Vieweg WVR, Lipps WFC, Fernandez A. Opioids and methadone equivalents for clinicians. *Prim Care Companion J Clin Psychiatry* (2005) 7(3):86. doi: 10.4088/PCC.v07n0301
24. Armbruster DA, Krolak JM. Screening for drugs of abuse with the Roche ONTRAK assays. *J Anal Toxicol* (1992) 16(3):172–5. doi: 10.1093/jat/16.3.172
25. Wilson JF, Smith BL, Toseland PA, Williams J, Burnett D, Hirst AD. External quality assessment of techniques for the detection of drugs of abuse in urine. *Annal Clin Biochem* (1994) 31(4):335–42.
26. Wesson DR, Ling W. The Clinical Opiate Withdrawal Scale (COWS). *J Psychoactive Drugs* (2003) 35(2):253–9. doi: 10.1080/02791072.2003.10400007
27. Nelson HE, Willison J. *National Adult Reading Test (NART)*. Windsor: Nfer-Nelson (1991).
28. Woerner C, Overstreet K. *Wechsler Abbreviated Scale of Intelligence (WASI)*. San Antonio, TX: The Psychological Corporation (1999).
29. Robbins TW, James M, Owen AM, Sahakian BJ, Lawrence AD, McInnes L, et al. A study of performance on tests from the CANTAB battery sensitive to frontal lobe dysfunction in a large sample of normal volunteers: implications for theories of executive functioning and cognitive aging. *J Int Neuropsychol Soc* (1998) 4(5):474–90. doi: 10.1017/S1355617798455073
30. Zigmond AS, Snaith RP. The hospital anxiety and depression scale. *Acta Psychiatr Scand* (1983) 67(6):361–70. doi: 10.1111/j.1600-0447.1983.tb09716.x
31. Beck AT, Ward C, Mendelson M, Mock J, Erbaugh J. Beck Depression Inventory (BDI). *Arch Gen Psychiatry* (1961) 4(6):561–71. doi: 10.1001/archpsyc.1961.01710120031004
32. Rush AJ, Carmody T, Reimitz PE. The Inventory of Depressive Symptomatology (IDS): clinician (IDS-C) and self-report (IDS-SR) ratings of depressive symptoms. *Int J Methods Psychiatr Res* (2000) 9(2):45–59. doi: 10.1002/mpr.79
33. Deakin JFW. The origins of '5-HT and mechanisms of defence' by Deakin and Graeff: a personal perspective. *J Psychopharmacol* (2013) 27(12):1084–9. doi: 10.1177/0269881113503508
34. Beck AT, Steer RA, Carbin MG. Psychometric properties of the Beck Depression Inventory: Twenty-five years of evaluation. *Clin Psychol Rev* (1988) 8(1):77–100.
35. Rush AJ, Giles DE, Schlesser MA, Fulton CL, Weissenburger J, Burns C. The inventory for depressive symptomatology (IDS): preliminary findings. *Psychiatry Res* (1986) 18(1):65–87.
36. Winer BJ, Brown DR, Michels KM. *Statistical principles in experimental design*. 3rd ed. New York: McGraw Hill (1991).
37. Baldacchino A, Armanyous M, Balfour DJ, Humphris G, Matthews K. Neuropsychological functioning and chronic methadone use: a systematic review and meta-analysis. *Neuroscience & Biobehavioral Reviews* (2017) 73:23–38.
38. Lyoo IK, Pollack MH, Silveri MM, Ahn KH, Diaz CI, Hwang J, et al. Prefrontal and temporal gray matter density decreases in opiate dependence. *Psychopharmacology* (2006) 184(2):139–44.
39. Liu H, Hao Y, Kaneko Y, Ouyang X, Zhang Y, Xu L, et al. Frontal and cingulate gray matter volume reduction in heroin dependence: Optimized voxel-based morphometry. *Psychiatry Clin Neurosci* (2009) 63(4):563–8.
40. Yuan Y, Zhu Z, Shi J, Zou Z, Yuan F, Liu Y, Lee TM, Weng X. Gray matter density negatively correlates with duration of heroin use in young lifetime heroin-dependent individuals. *Brain and Cognition* (2009) 71(3):223–8.
41. Maguire EA, Frackowiak RS, Frith CD. Learning to find your way: a role for the human hippocampal formation. *Proc R Soc Lond B Biol Sci* (1996) 263(1377):1745–50. doi: 10.1098/rspb.1996.0255
42. Owen AM, Morris RG, Sahakian BJ, Polkey CE, Robbins TW. Double dissociations of memory and executive functions in working memory tasks following frontal lobe excisions, temporal lobe excisions or amygdalo-hippocampectomy in man. *Brain* (1996) 119(5):1597–615.
43. Hill D, Garner D, Baldacchino AM. Comparing neurocognitive function in individuals receiving chronic methadone or buprenorphine for the treatment of opioid dependence: a systematic review. *Heroin Addict Relat Clin Probl* (2018) 20(5):35–49.
44. Ardila A, Rosselli M, Matute E, Inozemtseva O. Gender differences in cognitive development. *Develop Psychol* (2011) 47(4):984.
45. Conti AA, McLean L, Tolomeo S, Steele JD, Baldacchino A. Chronic tobacco smoking and neuropsychological impairments: a systematic review and meta-analysis. *Neurosci Biobehav Rev* (2018).
46. Verdejo-García AJ, Perales JC, Pérez-García M. Cognitive impulsivity in cocaine and heroin polysubstance abusers. *Addict Behav* (2007) 32(5):950–66. doi: 10.1016/j.addbeh.2006.06.032

# 5

# The Neural Correlates of Implicit Cognitive Bias toward Internet-Related Cues in Internet Addiction: An ERP Study

*Limin Chen*[1†]*, Hongliang Zhou*[2†]*, Yue Gu*[3]*, Shuai Wang*[1]*, Jun Wang*[1]*, Lin Tian*[1]*,*
*Hongmei Zhu*[1] *and Zhenhe Zhou*[1*]

[1] *Wuxi Mental Health Center, Wuxi, China,* [2] *Nanjing Brain Hospital Affiliated to Nanjing Medical University, Wuxi, China,*
[3] *Basic Medicine College of Nanjing Medical University, Nanjing, China*

***Correspondence:***
*Zhenhe Zhou*
*scoatt@163.com*

*† These authors share co-first authorship*

Internet addiction is a sort of non-psychoactive substance dependence. The Implicit Association Test (IAT) is used to measure implicit cognition. Event-related potential (ERP) is one of the most widely used methods in cognitive neuroscience research to investigate the physiological correlates of cognitive activity associated with processing information. Further investigating the ERP characteristics of implicit cognitive bias in Internet addiction would be helpful in understanding the nature of Internet addiction. This study investigated the ERP characteristics of implicit cognitive bias in Internet addiction. The participants included 60 Internet-addicted individuals (IAG) and 60 normal controls (NCG). All participants were measured with ERPs using the IAT. The results showed that there was a significant difference in the Internet-related IAT effect for reaction times between IAG and NCG, and there were stronger positive implicit associations toward Internet related cues in IAG than NCG. Using P1, N2, P3, and N4 as dependent variables, a mixed repeated-measures analysis of variance (ANOVA) on the mean latencies and mean amplitudes revealed a significant interaction between the groups (IAG vs. NCG) and stimulus condition (compatible trials vs. incompatible trials) for the N2 and P3 amplitudes; the simple effects analysis showed that the N2 and P3 amplitudes were larger under the IAG-compatible trial conditions than under the IAG-incompatible trial conditions. In the IAG group, the positive implicit associations with Internet-related cues elicited larger N2 and P3 amplitudes at the occipital lobe sites. These results indicated that Internet addictive individuals show stronger positive implicit associations toward Internet-related cues, and the positive implicit associations toward Internet-related cues elicited ERP changes at occipital lobe sites.

**Keywords: internet addiction, implicit cognition, the implicit association test, event-related potentials, internet-related cues**

## INTRODUCTION

Internet addiction refers to excessive Internet use that has a highly adverse effect on individuals' daily lives. Based on previous studies using neuropsychological and neuroimaging methods, Internet addiction is a sort of non-psychoactive substance dependence (i.e., a type of behavioral addiction) (1–4). To date, there has been an agreement that Internet addiction include four subtypes: Internet gaming, online social networking, Internet pornography, and Internet shopping (5, 6); however, the psychopathological or aetiological mechanism of Internet addiction has been unclear. Using neuropsychological measurements and neuroimaging methods might clarify the nature of Internet addiction.

Implicit cognition is a key term in cognitive psychology; it primarily refers to the perceptual, comprehension, memory, understanding, reasoning, and performance processes that occur through unconscious awareness (7). Previous studies have indicated that some behavior-related associations might be appraised with authenticated associative memory evaluations that get close to and activate pre-existing associations in memory system (8, 9). The Implicit Association Test (IAT) is used to measure implicit cognition. IAT refers to a reaction time-based categorization task that examines the differential associative strength between bipolar targets and appraising attribute concepts as an approach to indexing implicit biases (10). IAT is a commonly used indirect test of association in memory (11, 12). Many studies have reported that implicit cognition is a predictor for some mental disorders, such as alcohol dependence and tobacco dependence (13, 14). For example, previous studies, which have used the IAT to evaluate implicit associations in tobacco, alcohol, marijuana, and cocaine use, have demonstrated that the IAT effectively differentiated substance users from non-users (15–18).

Because of the potential role for psychopathology or etiology, research of implicit cognition has increased, particularly within many mental disorders. A recent study reported that negative associations between Internet addiction and implicit learning abilities (19). To identify the potential mechanisms of dyscontrolled Internet use in individuals with Internet gaming addiction, a study investigated the positive motivational implicit response to Internet gaming cues and concluded that individuals with Internet gaming addiction had a positive motivational implicit response to screenshots of online games; implicit cognition might also be associated with dyscontrolled online gaming (20).

In the past decades, the mechanisms of implicit cognition basis in substance addiction has been evaluated with neuroimaging methods, such as functional magnetic resonance imaging (fMRI) and event-related potentials (ERPs). For example, a previous study assessed activation in the neural substrates involved in implicit associative processes through fMRI of an alcohol-IAT focused on positive outcomes of alcohol use, and the results showed that the striatum is responsible for the mediation of implicit associations underlying habit, and the prefrontal cortex is responsible for the mediation of the controlled behaviors (9). Another study used ERPs to investigate the responses of binge drinkers to alcohol-related pictures and showed that the P100 amplitudes elicited by the alcohol-related pictures were significantly larger than those elicited by the non-alcohol pictures (21).

ERP is one of the most widely used methods in cognitive neuroscience research to investigate the physiological correlates of cognitive activity associated with processing information. In particular, ERP is suited to study item on the speed of neural activity. Further investigating the ERP characteristic of implicit cognitive bias in Internet addiction would be helpful in understanding the nature of Internet addiction. To date, there have been no reported studies examining the ERP characteristics of implicit cognitive bias in Internet addiction. In this study, the participants included an Internet addiction individual group (IAG) and a normal control group (NCG). All participants were measured with ERPs using an Internet information-related IAT. The study investigated the ERP characteristics of implicit cognitive bias in Internet addiction.

# METHODS

## Time and Setting

This study was conducted at Wuxi Mental Health Center, Jiangsu Province, China, from January 2015 to February 2018.

## Characteristics of the Samples

### Internet Addiction Group

The diagnostic criteria used for Internet addiction consist of the following five items: (I) individuals with Internet addiction should meet the criteria of the modified Diagnostic Questionnaire for Internet Addiction (22); (II) 18 years of age or older; (III) did not meet the criteria of any of the Diagnostic and Statistical Manual of Mental Disorders-5 (DSM-5) axis I disorders or personality disorders; (IV) not diagnosed with tobacco or alcohol dependence; and (V) not diagnosed with some central nervous systemic diseases. Clinical assessments of all subjects were conducted by two psychiatric residents to collect patient medication and sociodemographic data and to confirm or exclude a DSM-5 diagnostic criterion for any mental illness and a diagnostic criterion for Internet addiction; the duration of each individual's Internet addiction was determined through a retrospective diagnosis. Researchers required the Internet addictive individuals to recall their lifestyles. IAG participants were recruited from the Wuxi Mental Health Center, China. A total of 60 Internet addictive individuals were recruited into the IAG group, including 51 outpatients and 9 inpatients. The reliability of these self-reports from the individuals with Internet addiction was determined by visiting their roommates and intimate friends. Individuals with Internet addiction spent 11.48 h/day (standard deviation = 2.07) on online activities. The duration of being online each week was 6.29 days (standard deviation = 0.57).

### Normal Control Group

Normal controls were selected from the local community through local advertisements. All normal controls underwent clinical assessments by two psychiatric residents to collect patient medication and sociodemographic data and to confirm or exclude a DSM-5 diagnostic criterion for any mental illness. Normal controls were tested with the modified Diagnostic Questionnaire for Internet Addiction to exclude a diagnosis of Internet Addiction. Normal controls were excluded from the research if they were substance dependants or were diagnosed with some central nervous systemic diseases. Sixty individuals were matched by sex and age with IAG participants and served as the NCG. Referring to the previous Internet addiction study (3), only normal controls who spent less than 2 h/day on the Internet were placed in the NCG.

Prior to the experiment, a psychiatric associate chief physician re-checked the participants' profiles. All participants' emotional states were tested with the Hamilton Depression Scale (HAMD, 17-item version) and Hamilton Anxiety Scale (HAMA). The Annett handedness scale (3) was used to evaluate all participants' handedness.

The subjects and normal controls received written informed consent forms and provided their own written informed consent to participate in this research. All participants were paid $48.39 plus travel costs. The Ethics Committee of Wuxi Mental Health Center, China, approved the protocol for the research project.

## NEUROPSYCHOLOGICAL TEST

### Internet-Related Implicit Association Test

The subjects and normal controls performed an Internet-related IAT. The Internet-related IAT was referred from an alcohol-IAT that was employed in a previous study by Ames et al. (9). Neither the subjects nor the normal controls received any instructions during the experiment. All participants were asked to go as fast as they could (correctly). The stimuli to be categorized were randomly presented target categories (Internet-related pictures vs. mammal pictures) and attribute categories (positive words vs. neutral words). The target categories (prime stimuli) were six Internet-related pictures and six mammal pictures, and the attribute categories were six positive and six neutral word (two Chinese character words) categories, which were identified through open-ended questionnaires from 180 undergraduate students (40 senior high school students, 101 undergraduate students, and 39 graduate students). Six Internet-related pictures, six mammal pictures, six positive, and six neutral word categories were selected, according to their frequency. Thirty students used a 7-point Likert response format to rate the six Internet-related pictures on their perceived relevance to Internet, and the average score was 6.09 (standard deviation = 0.51). The Internet-related pictures included the WeChat icon, King of Glory (online-game) icon, Taobao icon, Google Chrome icon, Internet explorer icon, and Tencent QQ icon; the mammal pictures included a Dog, Monkey, Horse, Pig, Sheep, and Dolphin. Positive words included Happy, Attractive, Relaxed, Excited, Friendly and Sociable, and neutral words included Common, Calmness, Impartial, Brown, Stationary, and Objective. Thirty students used a 7-point scale ranging from 1 (very approved) to 7 (very disapproved) to rate the affective intensity of six positive and six neutral words; the average score of the Positive words was 6.33 (standard deviation = 0.71), the average score of Neutral words was 3.55 (standard deviation = 0.30).

Combinations of Internet-related picture + positive word vs. mammal + neutral word were compatible trials, while combinations of mammal picture + positive word vs. Internet-related picture + neutral word were incompatible trials.

The target categories (prime stimuli) and the attribute categories were presented on a 17-inch computer monitor using E-Prime 2.0 software. The attribute words (Size 40) and the red "+" (1.0 × 1.0 cm) were presented centrally on the screen.

In this IAT, there were 80 exposures in compatible blocks and 80 in incompatible blocks. Blocks of compatible trials and incompatible trials were counterbalanced, and trials within the blocks were randomly ordered. Fixation point trials were baseline. A red "+" was used in the presentation of the fixation with onset timing ranging from 1.0 to 4.5 s, followed by stimuli presentation. Maximum exposure of test stimuli was for 2 s. There was an intertribal interval (2 s) after a participant pressed a response key, and then the trial was over and followed by the next trial.

Referred from Ames et al. (9), the Internet-related IAT consisted of the following blocks: (I) a target category practice (20 trials), during the experiment, all participants were requested to press the A key for the Internet-related picture and press the L key for the mammal picture; (II) an attribute category practice (20 trials), during the experiment, all participants were requested to press the A key for the positive word and press the L key for the neutral word; (III) a compatible block with both target and attribute category practice (20 trials), during the experiment, all participants were requested to press the A key for combinations of the Internet-related picture + the positive word and press the L key for the mammal + neutral word; (IV) a compatible block with both target and attribute category tests (60 trials), during the experiment, all participants were requested to press the A key for combinations of the Internet-related picture + the positive word and press the L key for the mammal + neutral word; (V) a target category only used in the reversed positions practice (20 trials); (VI) an incompatible block with both a reversed target category and the attribute category practice (20 trials); and (VII) an incompatible block with both the reversed target category and the attribute category test (60 trials) (**Figure 1**). Only the data from block IV and block VII were used for the analysis. According to the previous algorithm used for D-600 measurements (23), the IAG and NCG response latencies were calculated separately.

### Event-Related Potential Measurements

Referencing the international 10/20 system, electroencephalograms were recorded with the Stellate Harmonie Electroencephalogram device (Physiotec Electronics Ltd., Canada) using Electro-Cap Electrode System (ECITM Electro-Caps, Electro-cap International, INL, USA). Combined ear electrodes served as a reference, and the ground electrode was attached to the forehead. Vertical and horizontal electrooculograms were recorded from above and below the right eye and at the right and left outer canthi. The inter-electrode impedance was below 5 kΩ. The band-pass filter was 0.05–100 Hertz (Hz), and the sample rate was 250 Hz. Electroencephalogram and electrooculogram waveforms were filtered with bandpass filter 0.01–40 Hz, 24 dB/oct. The stimulus conditions of the ERPs included following two trials: compatible trials (combinations of the Internet-related picture + positive word vs. mammal + neutral word) and incompatible trials (combinations of the mammal picture + positive word vs. Internet-related picture + Neutral word). The trials in blocks 3, 4,

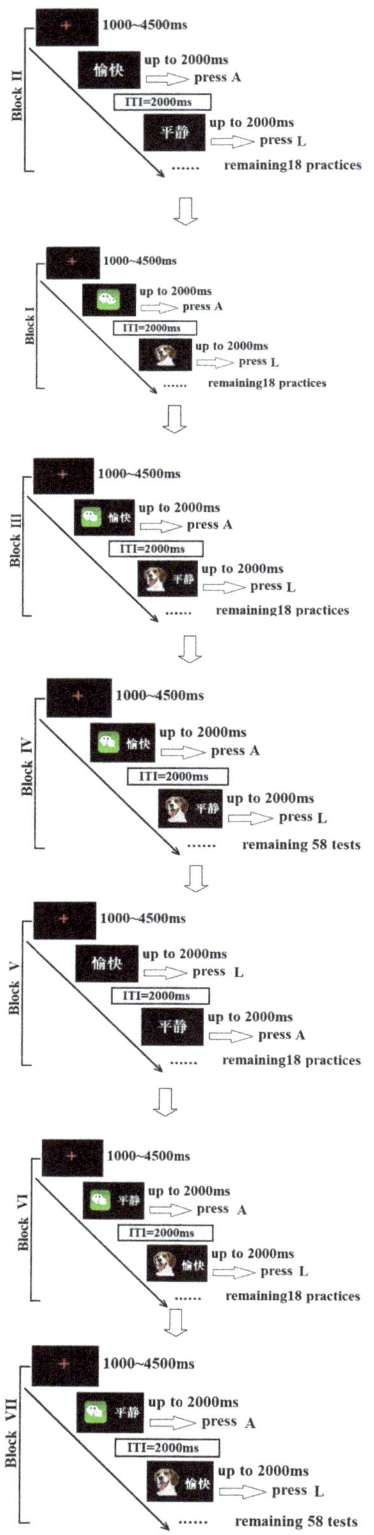


**FIGURE 1 |** A cartoon illustrating the Internet-related IAT. 愉快, happy; 平静, calmness. ITI, intertribal interval; ms, millisecond.

6, and 7 for Internet-related IAT were used for ERP analysis. The confirmation of ERP components depended on the latency after the stimulus onset, and the ERP components included the peak amplitudes of P1, N2, P3, and N4. ERP data from the following six scalp regions, 14 electrode sites altogether, were analyzed: frontal lobe sites (F3, Fz, and F4); parietal lobe sites (P3, Pz, and P4); central lobe sites (C3, Cz, and C4); left temporal lobe sites (T3) and right temporal lobe sites (T4); and occipital lobe sites (O1, Oz, and O2). The ERP epoch in each stimulus condition was 1000 milliseconds (ms) (including 200 ms before the stimulus onset and 800 ms after the stimulus onset). ERP component P1 was defined as the peak negativity within a 0–150 ms latency window, N2 was defined as the peak negativity within a 150–250 ms latency window, P3 was defined as the peak positivity within a 250–350 ms latency window, and N4 was defined as the peak negativity within a 350–450 ms latency window.

## Statistical Analysis

All data were analyzed with Statistical Product and Service Solution 18.0 statistical software (SPSS 18.0, WIN version, Inc., Chicago, IL, USA). Comparisons of the demographic and clinical characteristics (education years, HAMA scores and HAMD scores) between IAG and NCG were performed using independent-sample *t*-tests. Comparisons of handedness between IAG and NCG were performed using chi-squared tests. Comparisons of ERP data between IAG and NCG were performed using mixed repeated measures analysis of variance (ANOVA). The degrees of freedom of the F ratio were corrected, according to the Greenhouse-Geisser method. Least square difference tests were performed as *post-hoc* analyses, if indicated.

# RESULTS

## The Demographic and Clinical Characteristics of the Samples

The demographic characteristics of all samples are described in **Table 1**. There were no significant differences in the sex ratio, mean age, age range, mean education years, and handedness between the two groups. Although the mean scores of HAMA

**TABLE 1 |** Demographic and clinical characteristics of the samples.

| | IAG | NCG | Test statistic |
|---|---|---|---|
| Sex ratio (M/F) | 60 (32/28) | 60 (32/28) | – |
| Mean age (SD) | 23 (5) | 23 (5) | – |
| Handedness (R/M/L) | 23/15/22 | 22/17/21 | $x^2$ =3.60, $p = 0.18$, NS |
| Age range | 18–28 | 18–28 | – |
| Education years (SD) | 10.3 (2.2) | 10.1 (2.2) | $t = 0.585$, $p = 0.560$, NS |
| Dependence duration (month, SD) | 35.1 (11.0) | – | – |
| HAMA (SD) | 9.4 (3.2) | 8.4 (2.8) | $t = 1.762$, $p = 0.081$, NS |
| HAMD (SD) | 15.2 (4.8) | 13.5 (5.1) | $t = 1.928$, $p = 0.056$, NS |

*IAG, Internet addition group; NCG, Normal control group; M, male; F, female; SD, standard deviation; HAMA, Hamilton Anxiety Scale; HAMD, Hamilton Depression Scale; NS, not significant.*

and HAMD of IAG were higher than those of NCG, no significant differences were observed between the two groups.

## Internet-Related IAT Effect

The mean D-600 measure for IAG was 0.3152 (standard deviation = 0.3440), and the mean D-600 measure for NCG was 0.0625 (standard deviation = 0.2063). Accord to an independent sample $t$-test, there was a significant difference in the Internet-related IAT effect for the reaction times between IAG and NCG, and it showed stronger positive implicit associations toward Internet-related cues in IAG than in NCG ($t = 6.901$, $p = 0.001$).

The error rate for IAG was 0.0251 (standard deviation = 0.0187), and the error rates for NCG was 0.0260 (standard deviation = 0.0191). According to an independent sample $t$-test, no significant differences in the error rates for the Internet-related IAT were observed between IAG and NCG ($t = -0.356$, $p = 0.672$).

## Analysis of Event-Related Potential Data

The mean latencies and mean amplitudes of ERP component (P1, N2, P3, and N4) of all participants are shown in **Tables 2–5** and **Figures 2–5**. The sketch map of grand average waveforms elicited by IAG-compatible trial stimuli, IAG-incompatible trial

**TABLE 2 |** All participants' ERP P1 mean latencies [mean (SD), ms] and mean amplitudes [mean (SD), μV] *.

| Scalp regions | IAG | | | | NCG | | | |
|---|---|---|---|---|---|---|---|---|
| | Compatible trials | | Incompatible trials | | Compatible trials | | Incompatible trials | |
| | Latencies | Amplitudes | Latencies | Amplitudes | Latencies | Amplitudes | Latencies | Amplitudes |
| Frontal lobe | 136 (10) | 3.5 (0.4) | 133 (10) | 3.4 (0.4) | 135 (10) | 3.3 (0.4) | 139 (12) | 3.5 (0.3) |
| Parietal lobe | 130 (15) | 3.5 (0.5) | 134 (9) | 3.5 (0.6) | 138 (11) | 3.5 (0.5) | 136 (11) | 3.7 (0.6) |
| Central lobe | 137 (12) | 3.6 (0.5) | 136 (16) | 3.3 (0.6) | 141 (12) | 3.6 (0.4) | 133 (11) | 3.6 (0.6) |
| Temporal lobe (T3) | 130 (15) | 3.4 (0.5) | 140 (13) | 3.5 (0.5) | 134 (12) | 3.4 (0.5) | 136 (10) | 3.3 (0.8) |
| Temporal lobe (T4) | 135 (10) | 3.5 (0.4) | 135 (10) | 3.6 (0.5) | 133 (13) | 3.5 (0.6) | 135 (11) | 3.7 (0.6) |
| Occipital lobe | 134 (11) | 3.6 (0.7) | 132 (11) | 3.5 (0.6) | 138 (10) | 3.3 (0.5) | 132 (12) | 3.6 (0.6) |

*The sum of all corresponding scalp region latencies and amplitudes divided by the number of electrode sites are the mean latencies and mean ampl'tudes, respectively.*

**TABLE 3 |** All participants' ERP N2 mean latencies [mean (SD), ms] and mean amplitudes [mean (SD), μV] *.

| Scalp regions | IAG | | | | NCG | | | |
|---|---|---|---|---|---|---|---|---|
| | Compatible trials | | Incompatible trials | | Compatible trials | | Incompatible trials | |
| | Latencies | Amplitudes | Latencies | Amplitudes | Latencies | Amplitudes | Latencies | Amplitudes |
| Parietal lobe | 196 (14) | −3.6 (0.7) | 200 (12) | −3.7 (0.6) | 201 (8) | −3.6 (0.7) | 195 (13) | −4.2 (0.6) |
| Central lobe | 203 (16) | −3.5 (0.9) | 199 (10) | −4.0 (0.8) | 197 (11) | −3.7 (0.5) | 197 (13) | −3.7 (0.8) |
| Temporal lobe (T3) | 195 (11) | −3.8 (0.5) | 198 (10) | −3.9 (0.9) | 199 (16) | −3.8 (0.7) | 202 (8) | −3.9 (0.9) |
| Temporal lobe (T4) | 194 (15) | −4.0 (0.8) | 195 (16) | −3.8 (0.6) | 201 (12) | −4.0 (0.4) | 198 (14) | −4.0 (0.8) |
| Occipital lobe | 197 (13) | −6.2 (0.9) | 196 (15) | −4.1 (0.5) | 197 (10) | −3.6 (0.6) | 194 (16) | −4.2 (0.8) |

*The sum of all corresponding scalp region latencies and amplitudes divided by the number of electrode sites are the mean latencies and mean amplitudes, respectively.*

**TABLE 4 |** All participants' ERP P3 mean latencies [mean (SD), ms] and mean amplitudes [mean (SD), μV] *.

| Scalp regions | IAG | | | | NCG | | | |
|---|---|---|---|---|---|---|---|---|
| | Compatible trials | | Incompatible trials | | Compatible trials | | Incompatible trials | |
| | Latencies | Amplitudes | Latencies | Amplitudes | Latencies | Amplitudes | Latencies | Amplitudes |
| Frontal lobe | 297 (18) | 4.5 (0.6) | 296 (15) | 4.4 (0.7) | 296 (18) | 4.5 (0.8) | 300 (9) | 4.8 (1.0) |
| Parietal lobe | 296 (19) | 4.6 (0.8) | 302 (12) | 4.7 (0.9) | 301 (11) | 4.6 (0.7) | 305 (17) | 4.9 (0.6) |
| Central lobe | 301 (16) | 4.5 (0.9) | 299 (17) | 4.7 (0.8) | 297 (15) | 4.7 (0.6) | 297 (13) | 4.7 (0.7) |
| Temporal lobe (T3) | 295 (14) | 4.8 (0.7) | 298 (13) | 4.9 (0.9) | 304 (16) | 4.8 (0.7) | 302 (18) | 4.9 (0.9) |
| Temporal lobe (T4) | 294 (17) | 4.5 (1.0) | 303 (16) | 4.8 (0.6) | 301 (12) | 5.0 (0.6) | 298 (16) | 5.0 (0.6) |
| Occipital lobe | 299 (16) | 6.8 (0.9) | 302 (17) | 4.8 (0.8) | 297 (18) | 4.6 (0.9) | 306 (16) | 4.8 (0.8) |

*The sum of all corresponding scalp region latencies and amplitudes divided by numbers of electrode sites are the mean latencies and mean amplitudes, respectively.*

**TABLE 5 |** All participants' ERP N4 mean latencies [mean (SD), ms] and mean amplitudes [mean (SD), μV]*.

| Scalp regions | IAG | | | | NCG | | | |
|---|---|---|---|---|---|---|---|---|
| | Compatible trials | | Incompatible trials | | Compatible trials | | Incompatible trials | |
| | Latencies | Amplitudes | Latencies | Amplitudes | Latencies | Amplitudes | Latencies | Amplitudes |
| Frontal lobe | 405 (14) | −4.0 (0.6) | 403 (15) | −3.9 (0.7) | 403 (15) | −4.1 (0.8) | 400 (19) | −4.3 (1.0) |
| Parietal lobe | 400 (19) | −4.1 (0.8) | 402 (19) | −4.2 (0.9) | 401 (11) | −4.1 (0.7) | 405 (17) | −4.5 (0.8) |
| Central lobe | 401 (17) | −4.0 (0.5) | 402 (17) | −4.2 (0.6) | 400 (19) | −4.3 (0.6) | 406 (14) | −4.6 (0.7) |
| Temporal lobe (T3) | 406 (15) | −4.3 (0.6) | 401 (13) | −4.1 (0.5) | 404 (16) | −4.2 (0.8) | 402 (18) | −4.1 (0.9) |
| Temporal lobe (T4) | 399 (17) | −4.1 (1.0) | 407 (18) | −4.2 (0.5) | 401 (17) | −4.0 (0.6) | 400 (16) | −4.0 (0.6) |
| Occipital lobe | 402 (18) | −4.3 (0.8) | 402 (17) | −4.0 (0.6) | 405 (18) | −4.1 (0.8) | 406 (16) | −4.2 (0.6) |

*The sum of all corresponding scalp region latencies and amplitudes divided by the number of electrode sites are the mean latencies and mean amplitudes, respectively.

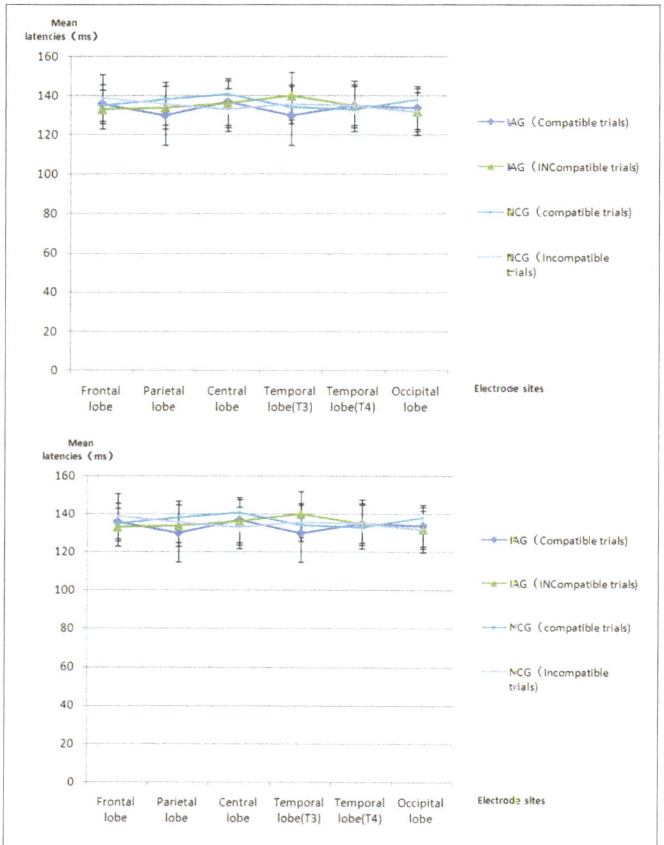


**FIGURE 2 |** ERP P1 component the latencies and amplitudes.

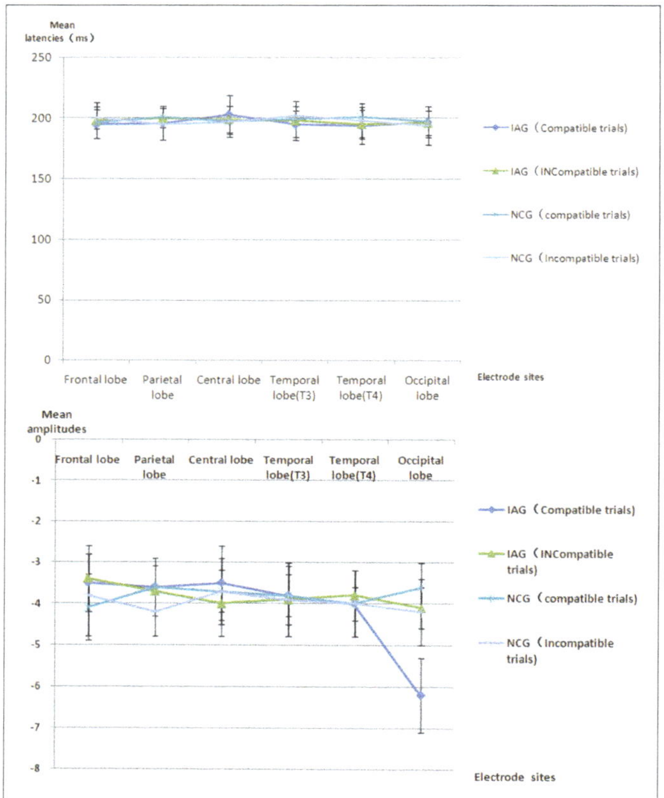


**FIGURE 3 |** ERP N2 component the latencies and amplitudes.

stimuli, NCG-compatible trial stimuli, and NCG-incompatible trial stimuli at Fz, Cz, Pz, T3, T4, Oz, O1, and O2 is shown as **Figure 6**.

Using P1, N2, P3, and N4 as dependent variables, a 2 × 2 × 6 mixed repeated measures ANOVA on the mean latencies and mean amplitudes, with group (IAG vs. NCG) as a between-subject factor and stimulus condition (compatible trials vs. incompatible trials) and scalp regions (frontal lobe, parietal lobe, central lobe, temporal lobe (T3), temporal lobe (T4), and occipital lobe) as within-subjects factors, was performed.

## P1 Component

There were no significant effects for P1 latency and amplitude.

## N2 Component

There were no significant effects for N2 latency. The results revealed a significant interaction between group (IAG vs. NCG) and stimulus condition (compatible trials vs. incompatible trials) [$F_{(1, 119)} = 32.76$, $p = 0.000$]. The simple effects analysis

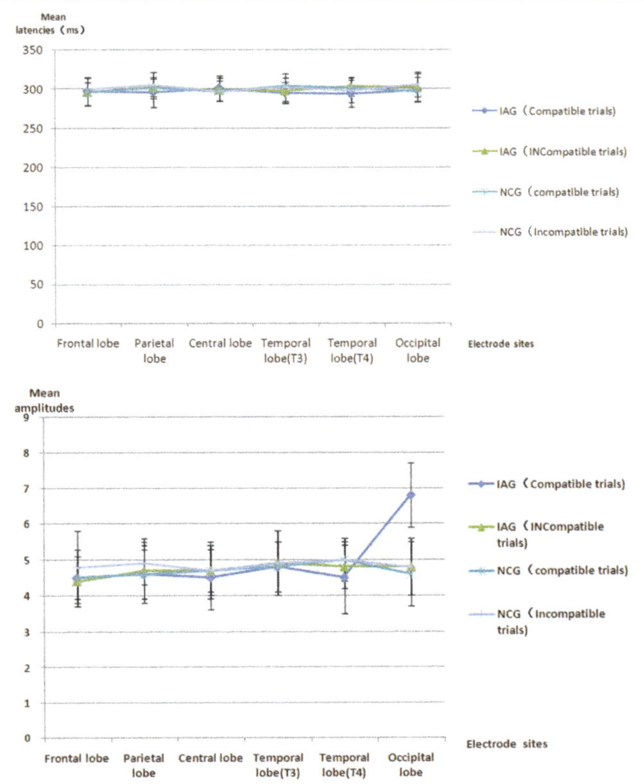


**FIGURE 4 |** ERP P3 component the latencies and amplitudes.

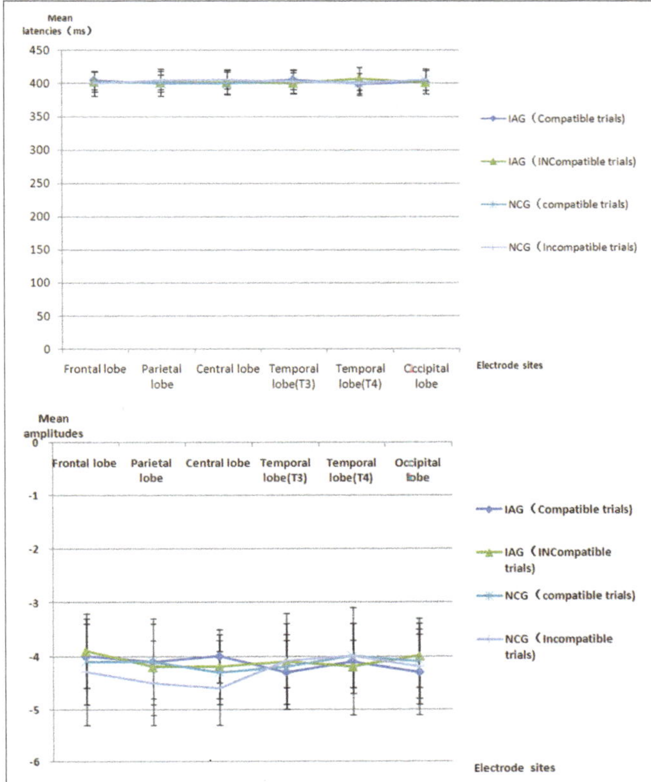


**FIGURE 5 |** ERP N4 component the latencies and amplitudes.

showed that N2 amplitudes were larger under the IAG-compatible trial conditions than under the IAG-incompatible trial conditions [$F_{(1, 119)} = 5.10, p = 0.018$]. In IAG, the positive implicit associations toward Internet related cues elicited larger N2 amplitudes. There was a significant three-way interaction between group (IAG vs. NCG), stimulus condition (compatible trials vs. incompatible trials) and scalp regions (frontal lobe, parietal lobe, central lobe, temporal lobe (T3), temporal lobe (T4), and occipital lobe) [$F_{(4, 236)} = 9.35$, $p = 0.000$]. The simple effects analysis showed a significant interaction between group (IAG vs. NCG) and stimulus condition (compatible trials vs. incompatible trials) on the occipital lobe sites [$F_{(1, 119)} = 29.78$, $p = 0.000$]. At the occipital lobe sites, IAG-compatible trials evoked larger N2 amplitudes than IAG-incompatible trials. There were no significant effects in the frontal lobe, parietal lobe, central lobe, temporal lobe (T3), and temporal lobe (T4) sites.

## P3 Component

There were no significant effects for P3 latency. The results revealed a significant interaction between group (IAG vs. NCG) and stimulus condition (compatible trials vs. incompatible trials) [$F_{(1, 119)} = 35.86$, $p = 0.000$]. The simple effects analysis showed that the P3 amplitudes were larger under the IAG-compatible trial conditions than under the IAG-incompatible trial conditions [$F_{(1, 119)} = 6.47, p = 0.025$]. In IAG, the positive implicit associations with Internet-related cues elicited larger P3 amplitudes. There was a significant three-way interaction between group (IAG vs. NCG), stimulus condition (compatible trials vs. incompatible trials) and scalp regions (frontal lobe, parietal lobe, central lobe, temporal lobe (T3), temporal lobe (T4), and occipital lobe) [$F_{(4, 236)} = 8.65, p = 0.000$]. The simple effects analysis showed a significant interaction between group (IAG vs. NCG) and stimulus condition (compatible trials vs. incompatible trials) at the occipital lobe sites [$F_{(1, 119)} = 30.42$, $p = 0.000$]. At the Occipital lobe sites, IAG-compatible trials evoked larger p3 amplitudes than the IAG-incompatible trials. There were no significant effects in the frontal lobe, parietal lobe, central lobe, temporal lobe (T3), and temporal lobe (T4) sites.

## N4 Component

There were no significant effects for N4 latency and amplitude.

# DISCUSSION

This study is the first to use ERPs to investigate the neural correlates of implicit cognitive bias toward Internet-related cues in Internet addiction. Our study results showed stronger positive implicit associations toward Internet-related cues in IAG than in NCG, and in IAG, the positive implicit associations toward Internet-related

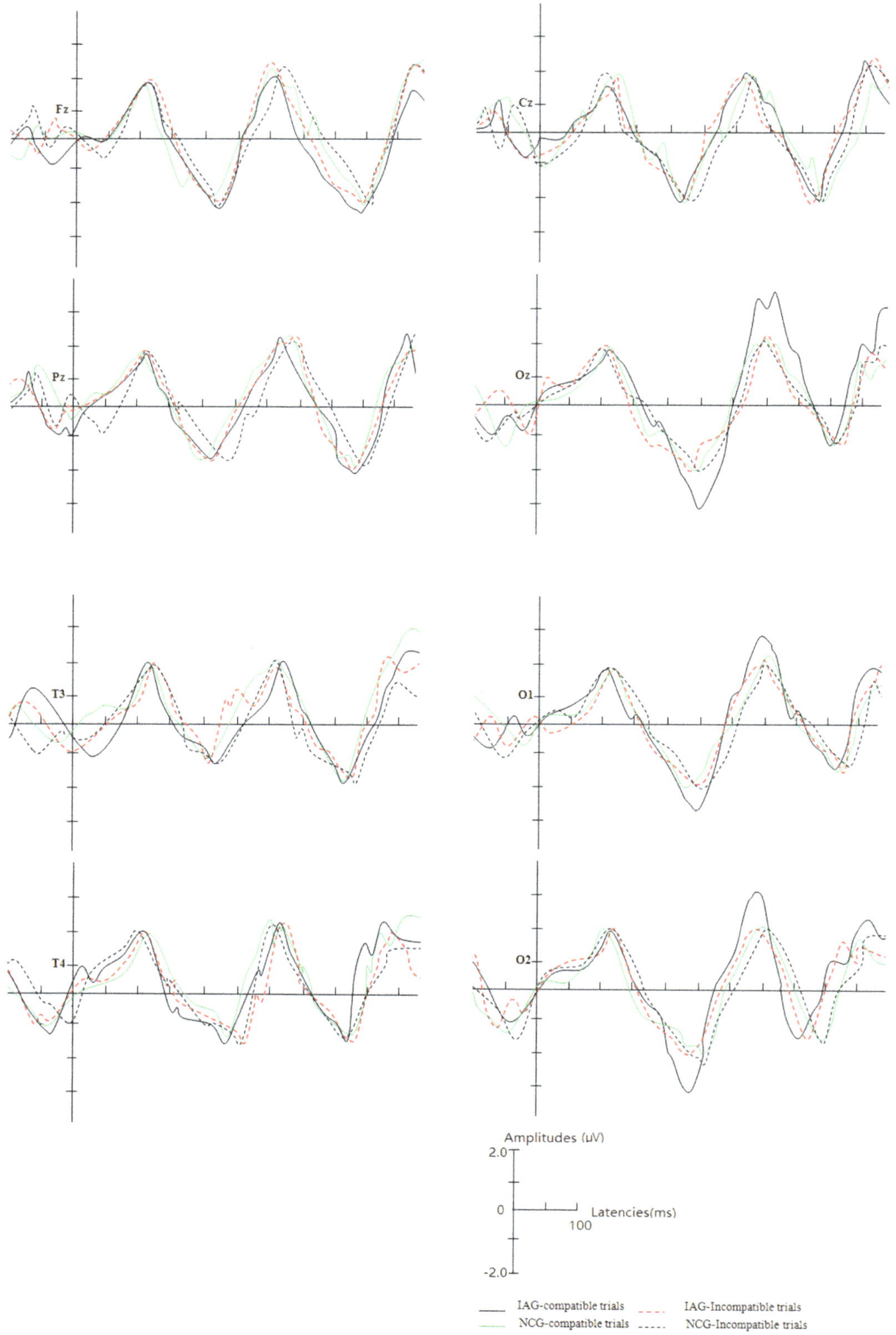


**FIGURE 6 |** The sketch map of grand average waveforms elicited by IAG-compatible trial stimuli, IAG-incompatible trial stimuli, NCG-compatible trial stimuli, and NCG-incompatible trial stimuli at Fz, Cz, Pz, T3, T4, Oz, O1, and O2. In IAG, at the Oz, O1, and O2 sites, the positive implicit associations with Internet-related cues elicited larger N2 and P3 amplitudes.

cues elicited larger N2 and P3 amplitudes at occipital lobe sites.

Previous studies have indicated that, as a sort of behavioral addiction, Internet addiction shares many psychopathological features with substance dependence (1, 24). Studies of substance dependence have demonstrated that key processes related to reinforcement and cognition in the development and maintenance of substance dependence, particularly the cognition process, represent viable treatment targets for psychosocial and pharmacological interventions (25).

Many scholars have suggested that implicit associations play a crucial role in substance and behavioral addiction (26). In the past decades, many studies, using IAT, have verified whether substance or behavioral addiction present implicit cognition bias. For example, a study used the IAT-Recoding Free (IAT-RF) to measure the predictive validity of recoding-free implicit alcohol associations with positive arousal (27); another previous study, which used IAT modified with pornographic pictures, investigated whether heterosexual male participants have tendencies toward cybersex addiction (26). The above two studies have demonstrated that implicit associations with positive arousal may play a key role in substance and behavioral addiction.

Consistent with a previous study, our results indicated that Internet addictive individuals have tendencies toward Internet related cues.

Event-related potential is a sort of high temporal resolution measures of human brain processing. Because ERPs present the rapid fluctuations associated with the key neurocognitive processes, it is suited to expand our understanding of the underlying neural mechanisms of change during the onset of substance and behavioral addiction (25).

Many studies have investigated the ERP characters when subjects were engaged in an IAT task. In a previous study, two positively valenced stimuli and two negatively valenced stimuli were used as category labels. The results displayed shorter response latencies for compatible trials compared to incompatible trials, and compatible trials tended to generate more positive waveforms in the central and parietal areas compared to incompatible trials (28). A study showed that when the participants performed an IAT task, the recorded ERPs presented an N2 that was larger in the incompatible stimuli, and they deduced that the ERP N2 amplitude reflected greater response monitoring (29). Another study displayed that many brain regions, including medial frontal, cingulate, insular, left-temporal, and parietal cortex, were responsible for ERP N2- and P3-related activity during performed IAT (10).

In this study, under the stimulus conditions of compatible trials, the positive implicit associations toward Internet-related cues elicited larger N2 and P3 amplitudes at occipital lobe sites in Internet addictive individuals. Although the ERP is poor in spatial resolution, it may provide evidence that some cerebral cortices (such as the posterior cingulate cortex) at occipital lobe sites are responsible for the implicit bias toward Internet-related cues in Internet addictive individuals.

Summary, individuals with Internet addiction present stronger positive implicit associations toward Internet-related cues, and the positive implicit associations toward Internet-related cues elicited changes in ERPs (i.e., larger N2 and P3 amplitudes at occipital lobe sites).

Determining the ERP characteristics of implicit cognitive bias in Internet addiction would be helpful in understanding the nature of Internet addiction; furthermore, the results can provide a theoretical basis for the development of possible prevention and treatment strategies for Internet addiction.

This study has some limitations. On the one hand, using the modified Diagnostic Questionnaire for Internet Addiction as a diagnostic tool for Internet addiction is not accurate because its validity as a diagnostic instrument has been not confirmed. On the other hand, to determine the neurotic mechanism of implicit cognitive bias toward Internet-related cues in Internet addiction depends on the integration between temporal resolution and spatial resolution in neuroimaging; however, ERP only provides an excellent temporal resolution. Future studies should use the reliable diagnostic instrument for Internet addiction and fMRI to measure the neurotic mechanism of implicit cognitive bias in Internet addiction.

## AUTHOR CONTRIBUTIONS

ZZ and HZhou designed the study. LC, HZhou, YG, SW, JW, LT, HZhu, and ZZ performed the experiment. LC, HZhou, YG, SW, JW, LT, HZhu, and ZZ analyzed the data and wrote the manuscript. All authors approved the final version of the manuscript for publication.

## ACKNOWLEDGMENTS

This study was supported by the National Natural Science Foundation, China (No. 81471354) and Key Talents Project Foundation for Medical and Health Services, Jiangsu Province (No. ZDRCC2016019).

## REFERENCES

1. Zhou ZH, Yuan GZ, Yao JJ, Li C, Cheng ZH. An event-related potential investigation of deficient inhibitory control in individuals with pathological Internet use. *Acta Neuropsychiatr.* (2010). 22:228–36. doi: 10.1111/j.1601-5215.2010.00444.x
2. Zhou ZH, Yuan GZ, Yao JJ. Cognitive biases toward Internet game-related pictures and executive deficits in individuals with an Internet game addiction. *PLoS ONE* (2012) 7:e48961. doi: 10.1371/journal.pone.0048961
3. Zhou ZH, Li C, Zhu HM. An error-related negativity potential investigation of response monitoring function in individuals with Internet addiction disorder. *Front Behav Neurosci.* (2013) 7:1–8. doi: 10.3389/fnbeh.2013.00131
4. Brand M, Laier C, Young KS. Internet addiction: coping styles, expectancies, and treatment implications. *Front Psychol.* (2014) 5:1256. doi: 10.3389/fpsyg.2014.01256
5. Kuss DJ, Lopezfernandez O. Internet addiction and problematic Internet use: a systematic review of clinical research. *World J Psychiatry* (2016) 6:143–76. doi: 10.5498/wjp.v6.i1.143

6. Moreno MA, Arseniev-Koehler A, Selkie E. Development and testing of a 3-item screening tool for problematic internet use. *J Pediatr.* (2016) 176:167–172.e1. doi: 10.1016/j.jpeds.2016.05.067
7. Schnabel K, Asendorpf JB, Greenwald AG. Assessment of individual differences in implicit cognition: a review of IAT measures. *Eur J Psychol Assess.* (2016) 24:210–7. doi: 10.1027/1015-5759.24.4.210
8. Stacy AW, Ames SL, Knowlton BJ. Neurologically plausible distinctions in cognition relevant to drug use etiology and prevention. *Subst Use Misuse* (2004) 39:1571–623. doi: 10.1081/JA-200033204
9. Ames SL, Grenard JL, He Q, Stacy AW, Wong SW, Xiao L, et al. Functional imaging of an alcohol-implicit association test (IAT). *Addict Biol.* (2014) 19:467–81. doi: 10.1111/adb.12071
10. Healy GF, Boran L, Smeaton AF. Neural patterns of the implicit association test. *Front Hum Neurosci.* (2015) 9:229. doi: 10.3389/fnhum.2015.00605
11. Greenwald AG, Mcghee DE, Schwartz JL. Measuring individual differences in implicit cognition: the implicit association test. *J Pers Soc Psychol.* (1998) 74:1464–80. doi: 10.1037/0022-3514.74.6.1464
12. Greenwald AG, Poehlman TA, Uhlmann EL, Banaji MR. Understanding and using the implicit association test: iii. Meta-analysis of predictive validity. *J Pers Soc Psychol.* (2009) 97:17–41. doi: 10.1037/a0015575
13. Stacy AW, Wiers RW. Implicit cognition and addiction: a tool for explaining paradoxical behavior. *Annu Rev Clin Psychol.* (2010) 6:551–75. doi: 10.1146/annurev.clinpsy.121208.131444
14. Wiers RW, Boelema SR, Nikolaou K, Gladwin TE. On the development of implicit and control processes in relation to substance use in adolescence. *Curr Addict Rep.* (2015) 2:141–55. doi: 10.1007/s40429-015-0053-z
15. Macy JT, Chassin L, Presson CC. The association between implicit and explicit attitudes toward smoking and support for tobacco control measures. *Nicotine Tob Res.* (2013) 15:291–6. doi: 10.1093/ntr/nts117
16. Wiers RW, Beckers L, Houben K, Hofmann W. A short fuse after alcohol: implicit power associations predict aggressiveness after alcohol consumption in young heavy drinkers with limited executive control. *Pharmacol Biochem Behav.* (2009) 93:300–5. doi: 10.1016/j.pbb.2009.02.003
17. Ames SL, Grenard JL, Stacy AW, Xiao L, He Q, Wong SW, et al. Functional imaging of implicit marijuana associations during performance on an implicit association test (IAT). *Behav Brain Res.* (2013) 256:494–502. doi: 10.1016/j.bbr.2013.09.013
18. Vargo EJ, Petróczi A. Detecting cocaine use? The autobiographical implicit association test (aiat) produces false positives in a real-world setting. *Subst Abuse Treat Prev Policy* (2013) 8:22. doi: 10.1186/1747-597X-8-22
19. Sariyska R, Lachmann B, Markett S, Reuter M, Montag C. Individual differences in implicit learning abilities and impulsive behavior in the context of Internet addiction and Internet Gaming Disorder under the consideration of gender. *Addict Behav Rep.* (2017) 5:19–28. doi: 10.1016/j.abrep.2017.02.002
20. Yen JY, Yen CF, Chen CS, Tang TC, Huang TH, Ko CH. Cue-induced positive motivational implicit response in young adults with Internet gaming addiction. *Psychiatry Res.* (2011) 190:282–6. doi: 10.1016/j.psychres.2011.07.003
21. Petit G, Kornreich C, Maurage P, Noël X, Letesson C, Verbanck P, et al. Early attentional modulation by alcohol-related cues in young binge drinkers: an event-related potentials study. *Clin Neurophysiol.* (2012) 123:925–36. doi: 10.1016/j.clinph.2011.10.042
22. Beard KW, Wolf EM. Modification in the proposed diagnostic criteria for internet addiction. *Cyberpsychol Behav.* (2001) 4:377–83. doi: 10.1089/109493101300210286
23. Greenwald AG, Nosek BA, Banaji MR. Understanding and using the Implicit Association Test: I. An improved scoring algorithm. *J Pers Soc Psychol.* (2003) 85:197–216. doi: 10.1037/0022-3514.85.2.197
24. Zhou Z, Zhu H, Li C, Wang J. Internet addictive individuals share impulsivity and executive dysfunction with alcohol-dependent patients. *Front Behav Neurosci.* (2014) 8:288. doi: 10.3389/fnbeh.2014.00288
25. Houston RJ, Schlienz N. Event-related potentials as biomarkers of behavior change mechanisms in substance use disorder treatment. *Biol Psychiatry Cogn Neurosci Neuroimaging* (2018) 3:30–40. doi: 10.1016/j.bpsc.2017.09.006
26. Snagowski J, Wegmann E, Pekal J, Laier C, Brand M. Implicit associations in cybersex addiction: adaption of an Implicit Association Test with pornographic pictures. *Addict Behav.* (2015). 49:7–12. doi: 10.1016/j.addbeh.2015.05.009
27. Houben K, Rothermund K, Wiers RW. Predicting alcohol use with a recoding-free variant of the Implicit Association Test. *Addict Behav.* (2009) 34:487–9. doi: 10.1016/j.addbeh.2008.12.012
28. O'Toole C, Barnes-Holmes D. Electrophysiological activity generated during the implicit association test: a study using event-related potentials. *Psychol Rec.* (2009) 59:207–19. doi: 10.1007/BF03395659
29. Coates MA, Campbell KB. Event-related potential measures of processing during an Implicit Association Test. *Neuroreport* (2010) 21:1029–33. doi: 10.1097/WNR.0b013e32833f5e7d

# 6

# State-Dependent Effects of Ventromedial Prefrontal Cortex Continuous Theta Burst Stimulation on Cocaine Cue Reactivity in Chronic Cocaine Users

*Tonisha E. Kearney-Ramos[1], Logan T. Dowdle[2,3], Oliver J. Mithoefer[2], William Devries[2], Mark S. George[2,3,4,5] and Colleen A. Hanlon[2,3,4]**

*[1] Division on Substance Use Disorders, Columbia University Irving Medical Center, New York, NY, United States, [2] Department of Psychiatry, Medical University of South Carolina, Charleston, SC, United States, [3] Department of Neurosciences, Medical University of South Carolina, Charleston, SC, United States, [4] Center for Biomedical Imaging, Medical University of South Carolina, Charleston, SC, United States, [5] Ralph S. Johnson VA Medical Center, Charleston, SC, United States*

***Correspondence:***
*Colleen A. Hanlon*
*hanlon@musc.edu*

Cue-induced craving is a significant barrier to obtaining abstinence from cocaine. Neuroimaging research has shown that cocaine cue exposure evokes elevated activity in a network of frontal-striatal brain regions involved in drug craving and drug seeking. Prior research from our laboratory has demonstrated that when targeted at the medial prefrontal cortex (mPFC), continuous theta burst stimulation (cTBS), an inhibitory form of non-invasive brain stimulation, can decrease drug cue-related activity in the striatum in cocaine users and alcohol users. However, it is known that there are individual differences in response to repetitive transcranial magnetic stimulation (rTMS), with some individuals being responders and others non-responders. There is some evidence that state-dependent effects influence response to rTMS, with baseline neural state predicting rTMS treatment outcomes. In this single-blind, active sham-controlled crossover study, we assess the striatum as a biomarker of treatment response by determining if baseline drug cue reactivity in the striatum influences striatal response to mPFC cTBS. The brain response to cocaine cues was measured in 19 cocaine-dependent individuals immediately before and after real and sham cTBS (110% resting motor threshold, 3600 total pulses). Group independent component analysis (ICA) revealed a prominent striatum network comprised of bilateral caudate, putamen, and nucleus accumbens, which was modulated by the cocaine cue reactivity task. Baseline drug cue reactivity in this striatal network was inversely related to change in striatum reactivity after real (vs. sham) cTBS treatment ($\rho = -.79$; $p < .001$; $R^2_{Adj} = .58$). Specifically, individuals with a *high* striatal response to cocaine cues at baseline had significantly *attenuated* striatal activity after real but not sham cTBS ($t_9 = -3.76$; $p \leq .005$). These data demonstrate that the effects of mPFC cTBS on the neural circuitry of craving are not uniform and may depend on an individual's baseline frontal-striatal reactivity to cues. This underscores the importance of assessing individual variability as we develop brain stimulation treatments for addiction.

**Keywords: addiction, functional magnetic resonance imaging, repetitive transcranial magnetic stimulation, inhibitory, neural circuit, independent component analysis**

# INTRODUCTION

Substance dependence is a chronic, relapsing brain disease characterized by compulsive drug seeking and use behaviors, despite harmful consequences (1). Cocaine use disorder (CUD) is among the most difficult substance use disorders to treat. The lack of FDA-approved pharmacotherapies, and limited efficacy of conventional psychotherapies, means that as many as 70% of treatment-seeking cocaine users relapse within the first 3 months (1). This leaves cocaine-dependent individuals with limited support for overcoming their chronic illness. Consequently, there is a pressing need for innovative treatment development, including approaches that specifically target the neural circuits associated with continued, habitual use in this population.

One of the strongest precipitants of relapse is drug cue-induced craving (1–4). Craving is associated with activity in reward-motivation brain regions, including the medial prefrontal cortex (mPFC) and striatum (1, 5, 6). Chronic cocaine users exhibit elevated activity in reward-motivation circuitry when exposed to drug-related cues (1, 5, 7). Functional neuroimaging studies have shown that the level of activity in this circuit is related to the intensity of craving (8, 9),and can reliably predict relapse in treatment-seeking substance users (1, 4, 10). Thus, one way to effectively treat CUD may be through a more targeted neurobiological approach, such as by directly modulating activity in this mPFC-striatal craving circuit.

Repetitive transcranial magnetic stimulation (rTMS) is a non-invasive brain stimulation technique that can be used to selectively modulate cortical and subcortical brain activity. Theta burst stimulation (TBS) is a patterned variant of rTMS that mimics endogenous neuronal firing patterns associated with learning and memory (11, 12). Depending on the TBS delivery pattern, either long-term potentiation-like (LTP-like) (intermittent TBS, iTBS) or long-term depression-like (LTD-like) [continuous TBS (cTBS)] effects can be induced in a circuit-specific way (13, 14). A recent study from our laboratory has shown that in cocaine and alcohol users, respectively, mPFC cTBS can lead to a decrease in drug cue reactivity in the mPFC and downstream subcortical targets, including the striatum (15).

However, it is also known that there are individual differences in responses to rTMS treatment, with some individuals responding as expected and others responding less or not at all (16–19). We recently showed that white matter integrity between the mPFC and putamen was one factor that influences individual differences in striatal response to mPFC cTBS (20). In addition, there is some evidence of state-dependent effects, where baseline neural state influences individual differences in response to rTMS (21–23). The objective of the present study was to assess the striatum as a biomarker of treatment response by determining if baseline drug cue reactivity in the striatum influences striatal response to mPFC cTBS. To accomplish this goal, striatal network activity during the cocaine-cue exposure task was extracted using group independent component analysis (ICA) before and after real and sham cTBS, and baseline striatal cue reactivity was related to striatal treatment response.

# METHODS

## Participants and Procedures

Twenty-five nontreatment-seeking chronic cocaine users [13 females; mean (SD) age = 42 (9) years] were recruited from the Charleston, SC, metropolitan area using digital and print media (i.e., Craigslist, bus ads) to participate in this single-blind, active sham-controlled crossover study. Following informed consent procedures approved by the Medical University of South Carolina Institutional Review Board, participants completed assessments related to protocol safety, mental status, and drug use to determine study eligibility (see **Supplemental Materials, Methods** for detailed inclusion/exclusion information).

Eligible participants completed two MRI/rTMS visits (each ~1 h). A multi-panel urine drug screen (Quikvue 6-panel urine drug screen, Quidel, San Diego, CA) was given to ensure participants were not under the influence of cocaine, [meth]amphetamine, opiates, benzodiazepines, and marijuana during study sessions. A breathalyzer was given to ensure that participants were not under the influence of alcohol. All participants received real cTBS (FP1 landmark based on electroencephalogram (EEG) 10–20 system, 110% resting motor threshold) and sham cTBS (order counterbalanced across participants, six 600-pulse sessions of cTBS on each visit, 60-s break after 1,800 pulses). Functional MRI (fMRI) data were collected immediately before and after exposure to cTBS (see **Supplemental Materials Figure S1** for study design). Visit 2 occurred 7 to 14 days after visit 1. The second cue reactivity fMRI scan was initiated within 10 min of receiving cTBS and completed no later than 30 min after cTBS to maximize presumed effects of cTBS on cortical activity (11). Self-reported cocaine craving was assessed upon visit initiation, before the baseline fMRI scan, before the cTBS session, immediately after cTBS, and immediately after the second fMRI scan.

**Clinical Assessments.** Self-report assessments included the Structured Clinical Interview for the Diagnostic and Statistical Manual of Mental Disorders IV (SCID for DSM-IV) (SCID) (24), Timeline Follow-back (TLFB; for cocaine, alcohol, marijuana, and nicotine) (25), Alcohol Use Disorders Identification Test (AUDIT) (26), Fagerstrom Smoking Inventory (27), Beck's Depression Inventory (BDI-II) (28), and Spielberger State-Trait Anxiety Inventory (STAI) (29). TLFB was used to evaluate past week's substance use at screening and both MRI/rTMS visits. In addition, a brief cocaine craving assessment (scale 1–10: 1, no craving; 10, high craving) was administered at five time points during both MRI/rTMS visits to monitor craving levels throughout the study (see **Figure S1**). As typically done in cue-induced craving studies, study personnel ensured craving levels were at or below baseline before participants were dismissed from each visit. Participants received monetary compensation for their time and effort and travel to and from the university.

**Cocaine Cue Reactivity fMRI Task.** The cocaine cue reactivity task was administered in the MRI scanner as a block design using E-Prime software (Psychology Software Tools, Inc.; 30). The total task time was approximately 12 min and consisted of six 120-s epochs. Each epoch included alternating 24-s blocks of four task conditions: *Drug, Neutral, Blur,* and *Rest*, with each block followed by a 6-s cocaine craving inquiry where participants were asked to rate their current cocaine craving level on a 1 to 5 rating scale (1, none and 5, high). The task conditions included images of cocaine-related stimuli (e.g., crack pipe; users snorting cocaine), neutral stimuli (e.g., cooking utensils; people eating dinner), blurred stimuli acting as visual controls by matching cocaine images in color and hue, and a fixation cross for alert rest periods. During each task block, five images were presented (4.8 s). Task blocks were counterbalanced across epochs.

**Neuroimaging.** Participants were scanned using a Siemens 3.0T Tim Trio (Siemens Medical, Erlangen, Germany) MRI scanner with a 32-channel head coil. High-resolution T1-weighted structural images were acquired using a magnetization prepared gradient echo (MPRAGE) sequence (repetition time/echo time = 1,900 ms/2.34 ms; field of view = 220 mm; matrix = 256 × 256 voxels; 192 slices; slice thickness = 1.0 mm with no gap; final resolution = 1 $mm^3$ voxels). Functional images were acquired with a multislice gradient-echo echo planar imaging (EPI) sequence (repetition time/echo time = 2,200 ms/35 ms; field of view = 192 mm; matrix = 64 x 64 voxels; 36 slices; slice thickness = 3 mm with no gap; final resolution = 3 $mm^3$ voxels). Each functional run consisted of 328 time points.

**cTBS Protocol — Real and Sham cTBS.** Coil position was determined using standardized coordinates from the EEG International 10–20 system (with FP1 corresponding to the left mPFC stimulation target). The location and orientation of each participant's coil placement was indicated on a nylon cap that participants wore throughout visit 1 and both MRI/rTMS sessions. Participants' resting motor threshold (rMT; stimulation intensity applied over left motor cortex to produce 50% motor evoked potential response rate in contralateral abductor pollicis brevis) was identified using the standardized PEST procedure (31). The stimulation dose applied to the mPFC was set to be 110% rMT due to the larger scalp-to-cortex distance for PFC versus motor cortex requiring a larger dose to attain equivalent effects (32). The cTBS treatment was administered with a figure-of-eight MagPro Cool-B65 A/P coil (MagVenture, Farum, Denmark). Participants received two 2-min trains of cTBS over FP1 (1 train = 120 s; 3 pulse bursts at 5 Hz; 15 pulses/s; 1,800 pulses/train; 60-s intertrain interval). To enhance tolerability, stimulation intensity was gradually escalated in 5% increments (from 80% to 110% rMT) over the first 30 s of each train.

The Magventure MagPro system includes an integrated active sham. When the coil was oriented in the treatment position, real cTBS was administered, and the scalp electrodes placed on the left frontalis muscle under the coil were not active. When the coil was flipped 180°, the active side of the coil faced *away* from the scalp. In this configuration, the sound and pressure of the coil remained constant and the scalp electrodes became active, thus mimicking the multi-sensory experience of real cTBS, without the CNS stimulation. Previous studies in our laboratory have demonstrated that participants are unable to differentiate real from sham stimulation, with participants exhibiting ~48% accuracy (i.e., ~chance) in identifying whether they received real or sham cTBS in a given session (33). However, for continued assurance, participants were surveyed after each session to routinely assess the integrity of the blinded study.

**Cue Recollection During cTBS Administration.** Before cTBS administration, participants were asked to recall the last time they used cocaine, and using a series of standardized questions from traditional Narrative Exposure Therapy practice (34), they were asked to describe the place they were using, a visual description of the scene, and a description of the sensory properties of the drug including taste, smell, and sensation. During cTBS administration, the participants were primed every 20 s to "Think about that scene you described wherein you were last using cocaine/crack" (paraphrased such that this was tailored to the participant's description).

## Data Analysis

**Neuroimaging Preprocessing.** MRI data were preprocessed using SPM12 (Wellcome Department of Cognitive Neurology, London, UK) implemented in Matlab 7.14 (MathWorks, Inc., Natick, MA; see **Supplemental Materials, Methods** for preprocessing details). Of the 25 recruited participants, 6 participants were excluded for excessive head motion artifact (>3 mm in any plane; x, y, z, roll, pitch, yaw; see **Supplemental Materials, Methods** for details). Data analyses were conducted on the remaining 19 participants [11 males; mean (SD) age = 41 (10) years; range, 21–54 years; see **Table 1** for demographics].

**Independent Component Analysis.** To accomplish the primary objective of the present study, which was to assess the impact of baseline striatal network drug cue reactivity on cTBS treatment response, the temporal dynamics of the striatal network as a whole were isolated using group-level ICA. Specifically, group spatial ICA was conducted on all 76 cue reactivity task fMRI data sets [4 per participant (pre/post-real, pre/post-sham) × 19 participants] using Matlab's Group ICA of fMRI toolbox (GIFT) (35) (see **Supplemental Materials, Methods** for detailed spatial ICA methods). Briefly, the GIFT ICA procedure uses a two-step data reduction approach. In the first step, principal component analysis (PCA) reduced each subject's data set into 100 subject-specific principal components. For the second step, subject-specific principal components were concatenated and further reduced into 50 group-level principal components, which were then entered into the final group ICA for identification of the 50 group-level independent components. The component reliability was determined by a stability index (20 iterations of ICASSO, Infomax algorithm). Each independent component's subject-specific representation (i.e., unique spatial map and time course) was computed *via* back-reconstruction of the group independent components. These data were normalized to *z* scores to enable comparison across subjects.

**General Linear Modeling (GLM) of ICA Network Time Courses.** Each subject-specific striatal network time course was entered into a general linear regression [Analysis of Functional Neuroimages' (AFNI's) 3dDeconvolve] with five task conditions (*drug, neutral, blur, rate_craving_drug, rate_craving_other*) and six movement parameters as regressors. For each subject, a mean beta weight value (β) was estimated for the striatal network, which provided a single measure of the level of task-related activity for the network as a whole during each of the task conditions (35–38). Striatal network drug cue reactivity was computed by contrasting network activity during drug cue versus neutral cue conditions. Network drug cue reactivity *after* real/sham cTBS was compared with engagement *before* real/sham cTBS using a factorial design and *post hoc* paired *t* tests.

## Linear Regression to Identify Predictors of Neural Response to mPFC cTBS Treatment

***Baseline Striatum Drug Cue Reactivity.*** Robust linear regression was used to determine the association between baseline striatum drug cue reactivity and changes in drug cue reactivity after real (vs. sham) mPFC cTBS. Robust regression was performed in Matlab using iteratively reweighted least squares with a Huber weighting function (default weighting parameter, 1.345). Robust regression was preferred over standard least-squares linear regression due to its minimization of the influence of response variable outliers (39, 40). The regression included baseline striatum network drug cue reactivity as the predictor variable and change in striatum network reactivity after real (vs. sham) cTBS as the outcome variable.

***Clinical, Demographic, and Drug Use History Variables.*** To determine whether clinical and demographic variables influenced or predicted cTBS treatment outcomes, hierarchical multiple linear regressions were conducted with clinical and demographic variables of interest as the predictors and covariate predictors and striatum network reactivity after real (vs. sham) cTBS as the outcome variable.

***Scalp-to-Cortex Distance.*** Given that the effects of TMS on cortical excitability are proportional to the distance between the skull and cortex (32, 41), we calculated the distance from the scalp to cortex on the transverse plane of MPRAGE images for each participant (see **Supplemental Materials, Results**). The average distance from participant-specific placement of FP1 to the cortex was 18 mm (±3.7 mm). These distances were incorporated into the analyses as covariates.

# RESULTS

**Identification of Striatum ICA Component.** Of the 50 components identified by ICA, 17 were classified as noise components (i.e., corresponding to motion and/or other signal artifacts). The 33 non-noise components were comprised of several canonical functional networks commonly associated with sensory, motor, cognitive, and affective processing (42, 43). However, given our focus on evaluating striatum craving circuitry, we focused on the striatum network component, which encompassed bilateral caudate, putamen, and nucleus accumbens (**Figure 1**). Evaluation of the back reconstruction of the striatum component onto the 76 participant data sets confirmed that all participant data sets exhibited a robust striatum network component, including a subject-specific striatum spatial map and time course.

## Effect of mPFC cTBS Treatment on Striatum Network Activity During Drug Cue Exposure

***Group Analysis.*** Across all subjects, there was no significant elevation of striatal network activity during drug cue exposure at any time point (**Figure 2A**). Additionally, across all subjects, there was no significant attenuation of striatal network cue reactivity following real versus sham cTBS ($F_{1,68} = 0.17$; $p > 0.05$; **Figure 2A**).

***Individual Differences Analysis.*** Analysis of individual differences, however, revealed that real cTBS *did* strongly alter striatum drug cue reactivity but was modulated by participants' baseline striatum network cue reactivity (**Figure 2B**). Specifically, "cue-sensitive" participants who were responsive to cue induction and initially exhibited *elevated* drug cue reactivity ($t_9 = 4.34$; $p \leq 0.005$), revealed significantly *attenuated* activity after real (vs. sham) cTBS ($t_9 = -3.76$; $p \leq 0.005$; **Figure 2B**, *black bars*). "Cue-insensitive" participants, who were not responsive to cue induction and initially exhibited *suppressed* drug cue reactivity ($t_8 = -4.09$; $p \leq 0.005$), revealed significantly *enhanced* activity after real (vs. sham) cTBS ($t_8 = 4.01$; $p \leq 0.005$; **Figure 2B**, *gray triangles*). These strongly opposing neural responses canceled each other out in the group-level analysis, at both time points, thus causing the group-level analyses to appear non-significant. Conversely, no statistically distinct response patterns were identified for sham stimulation (**Figure 2B**; *striped bars/triangles*). Thus, these data convey a bimodal neural response profile for real (vs. sham) mPFC cTBS (paired $t$ test for cue-sensitive vs. cue-insensitive subjects: $t_{17} = -5.36$; $p < 0.005$) and an overall significant three-way interaction between treatment type (real/sham), time (pre/post), and baseline cue reactivity (cue-sensitive/cue-insensitive) ($F_{1,68} = 11.83$, $p = 0.001$). These results are not likely to reflect regression to the mean, as this bimodal

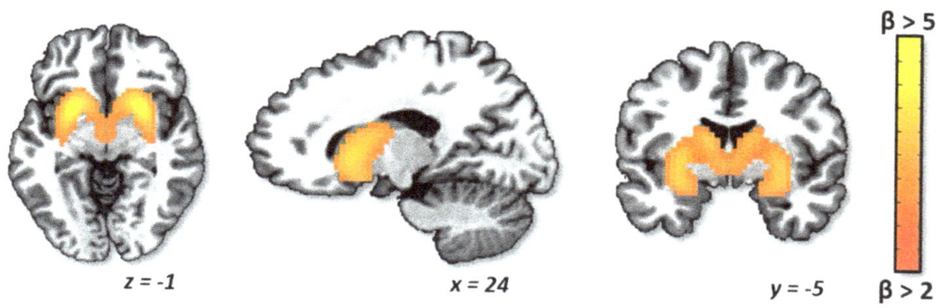


**FIGURE 1** | Striatum independent component analysis (ICA) network. Axial, sagittal, and coronal planes are shown, respectively, for the group average striatum network component, which includes the bilateral caudate, putamen, and nucleus accumbens. The network is depicted in neurological convention (left = left) in Montreal Neurological Institute (MNI) coordinate space with cluster-level threshold at β > 2 and minimum cluster size = 50 voxels.

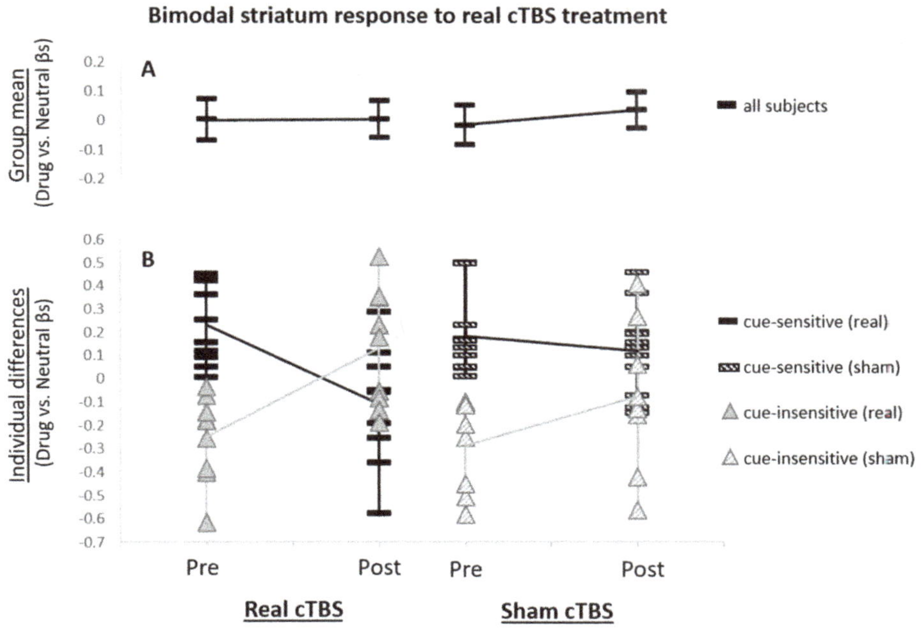


**FIGURE 2 |** Striatum network drug cue reactivity before and after real and sham continuous theta burst stimulation (cTBS). **(A)** For the group, striatum network did not exhibit significantly elevated drug cue reactivity for any of the functional magnetic resonance imaging (fMRI) scans ($p > 0.05$ for pre- and post-real cTBS and sham, respectively). **(B)** Individual differences analysis revealed a bimodal neural response to real cTBS. Participants, who had initially exhibited elevated striatum network drug cue reactivity ($t_9 = 4.34$; $p \leq 0.005$), revealed significantly attenuated activity after real cTBS ($t_9 = -3.76$; $p \leq 0.005$; black bars). Subjects, who had initially exhibited suppressed network drug cue reactivity ($t_8 = -4.09$; $p \leq 0.005$), revealed significantly enhanced activity after real cTBS ($t_8 = 4.01$; $p \leq 0.005$; gray triangles). No significant differences were found for sham (striped bars/triangles).

response pattern was only seen for the real cTBS condition and not for sham, whereas in the case of regression to the mean, this pattern would be expected for both conditions. In addition, in a *post hoc* analysis, we assessed whether treatment order (real or sham first in this crossover design) influenced treatment response and found no effect.

**Baseline Striatum Drug Cue Reactivity Predicts Changes in Striatum Network Response to Real Versus Sham mPFC cTBS.** Baseline striatum network drug cue reactivity was strongly inversely related to striatum network reactivity following real (vs. sham) mPFC cTBS (ρ = -0.79; $p < 0.001$; $R^2_{Adj} = 0.58$; **Figure 3**).

***Influence of Clinical, Demographic, and Drug Use History Variables.*** Analysis of the influence of clinical and demographic variables on treatment outcomes (see **Table 1** for variables assessed) revealed that only the total years of cocaine use was a significant modulator of striatum drug cue reactivity—for both baseline and treatment-related changes (**Figure 4**). Specifically, hierarchical multiple linear regression showed that the years of cocaine use was strongly positively related to baseline striatum cue reactivity (ρ = 0.67; $p < 0.01$; $R^2_{Adj} = 0.45$; when controlling for route of drug administration and Fagerström nicotine dependence; **Figure 4A**) and strongly inversely related to changes in striatum cue reactivity after real (vs. sham) cTBS treatment (ρ = -0.57; $p < 0.01$; $R^2_{Adj} = 0.32$; **Figure 4B**). However, despite strong correlations between baseline striatum cue reactivity and years of cocaine use, these variables each explained unique variance in striatum network response to real (vs. sham) cTBS treatment.

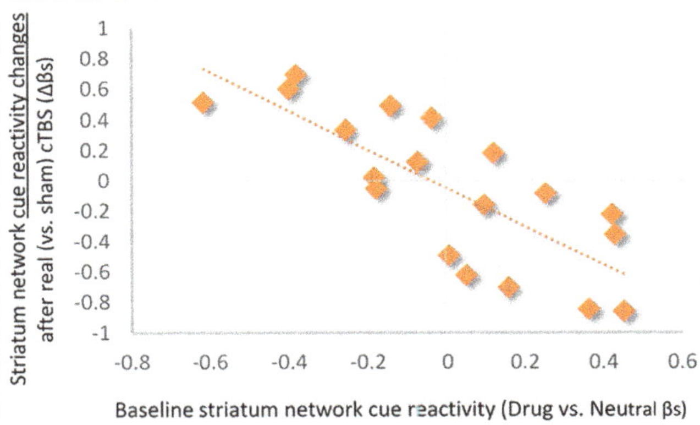


**FIGURE 3 |** Relationship between baseline striatum network drug cue reactivity and change in drug cue reactivity after real (vs. sham) cTBS treatment. Baseline striatum drug cue reactivity was strongly inversely related to striatum network response to real (vs. sham) cTBS (ρ = −0.79; $p < 0.001$; $R^2_{Adj} = 0.58$).

## DISCUSSION

In our previous study, we showed that mPFC cTBS could attenuate drug cue reactivity in both the mPFC and striatum in cocaine and alcohol users (15, 20). The present study extends these data by demonstrating that individual variability in the effect of mPFC cTBS on striatal circuitry may be related to baseline

**TABLE 1** | Descriptive demographic, clinical, and drug use statistics.

| | *n* = 19 Total sample | *n* = 10 cue-sensitive | *n* = 9 cue-insensitive | Cue-sensitive vs. cue-insensitive |
|---|---|---|---|---|
| **Demographics** | | | | |
| Sex | 11 M, 8 F | 6 M, 4 F | 5 M, 4 F | $\chi^2$ 0.04 |
| Age | 41.2 (± 9.5) years | 42.7 (± 8.7) years | 39.4 (± 10.0) years | *t* 0.72 |
| Ethnicity | 18 AA, 1 C | 9 AA, 1 C | 9 AA | $\chi^2$ 0.95 |
| Education | 12.2 (± 1.4) years | 12.2 (± 1.8) years | 12.1 (± 0.7) years | *t* 0.13 |
| **Cocaine use** | | | | |
| Preferred drug administration | 10 smoke, 8 snort, 1 both | 5 smoke, 4 snort, 1 both | 5 smoke, 4 snort | $\chi^2$ 0.95 |
| Age of first cocaine use | 22.4 (± 5.7) years | 20.3 (± 4.3) years | 24.7 (± 6.2) years | *t* -1.71 |
| Total duration of cocaine use | 18.8 (± 9.4) years | 22.4 (± 9.8) years | 14.8 (± 7.1) years | *t* 1.82 |
| Amount $ spent per week | $136.71 (± $98.70) | $147.80 (± 110.00) | $124.40 (± 82.70) | *t* 0.49 |
| Days used in last 30 days | 11.3 (± 6.9) days | 10.5 (± 4.8) days | 12.1 (± 8.5) days | *t* -0.49 |
| Time since last use (at visit) | 2.4 (± 1.0) days | 2.3 (± 1.1) days | 2.6 (± 1.0) days | *t* -0.51 |
| **Other substance use** | | | | |
| Nicotine smokers | 17 (89%) | 9 (90%) | 8 (89%) | $\chi^2$ 0.39 |
| Nicotine severity (Fagerström) | 3.1 (± 1.9) | 2.8 (± 2.1) | 3.1 (± 1.9) | *t* -0.32 |
| Marijuana smokers | 14 (74%) | 7 (70%) | 7 (78%) | $\chi^2$ 0.15 |
| Days MJ used in last 30 days | 4.4 (± 9.0) days | 3.4 (± 6.8) days | 5.3 (± 10.2) days | *t* -0.37 |
| Alcohol use severity (AUDIT) | 9.2 (± 5.3) | 10.6 (± 3.8) | 7.7 (± 6.2) | *t* 1.18 |
| Age first alcohol use | 17.0 (± 3.3) years | 17.7 (± 4.5) years | 17.1 (± 1.5) years | *t* 0.34 |
| **Mental status** | | | | |
| Depressive symptoms (BDI) | 10.6 (± 9.1) | 12.3 (± 10.9) | 8.8 (± 6.0) | *t* 0.82 |
| State Anxiety (STAI-S) | 37.4 (± 12.3) | 34.0 (± 12.2) | 41.2 (± 11.2) | *t* -1.26 |
| Trait Anxiety (STAI-T) | 40.7 (± 12.2)[+] | 41.4 (± 13.4)[+] | 39.9 (± 10.8) | *t* 0.26[+] |
| **Treatment-related measures** | | | | |
| Scalp-to-cortex distance (mm)[¥] | 17.9 (± 3.7) mm | 17.3 (± 3.9) mm | 18.9 (± 3.1) mm | *t* -0.84 |
| Mean absolute cTBS dose[%] | 57% (± 9%) | 61% (± 9%) | 52% (± 8%) | *t* -0.25 |
| Baseline cocaine craving | 3.3 (± 2.0) | 3.9 (± 2.3) | 2.7 (± 1.6) | *t* 1.30 |
| Change in cocaine craving[o] | -0.6 (± 1.9) | -0.6 (± 1.3) | -0.5 (± 2.4) | *t* -0.11 |
| Baseline striatum reactivity (β) | 0.0 (± 0.3) | 0.2 (± 0.2)* | -0.3 (± 0.2)* | *t* 5.96** |
| Change striatum reactivity (Δβ) | -0.1 (± 0.5) | -0.4 (± 0.4)* | 0.5 (± 0.3)* | *t* -5.36** |

*M, males; F, females; AA, African-American; C, Caucasian; MJ, marijuana; AUDIT, Alcohol Use Disorders Identification Test; BDI, Beck's Depression Inventory; STAI, Spielberger State-Trait Anxiety Inventory. Values either indicate mean (± standard deviation) or count (percent%). [+]Missing STAI-T score for one participant. [¥]Scalp-to-cortex distance (mm) for mPFC coil placement at EEG 10-20 FP1. [%]Mean absolute dose of cTBS administered (% total machine output to achieve 110% rMT, averaged over both stimulation sessions). [o]Change in craving values given by: Δafter real cTBS - Δafter sham. Significance after multiple comparison adjustment (adjusted p < .05*; p < .005**).*

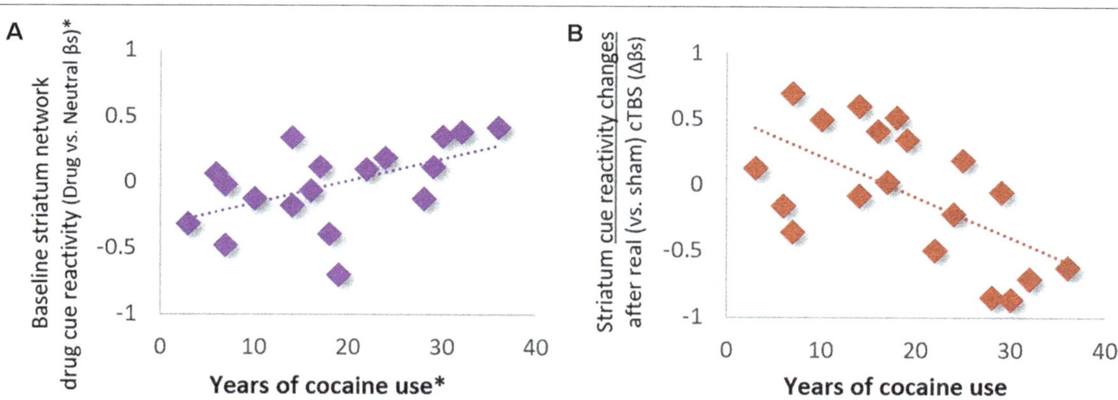


**FIGURE 4** | Years of cocaine use was **(A)** positively related to baseline striatum network reactivity to drug cues ($\rho = 0.67$; $p < 0.01$; $R^2_{Adj} = 0.45$; *Controlling for route of drug administration and nicotine dependence), and **(B)** inversely related to network response to real (vs. sham) cTBS treatment ($\rho = -0.57$; $p < 0.01$; $R^2_{Adj} = 0.32$).

striatal reactivity to cues. Thus, our preliminary findings in this small data set are a first glimpse into informing treatment by suggesting that cocaine users with the greatest striatum network reactivity to drug cues at baseline may "benefit" most from mPFC cTBS treatment and that individuals with low baseline striatal reactivity to drug cues may not make good treatment candidates.

**Individual Variability in Response to Theta Burst Stimulation.** Although, to date, there have only been a handful of therapeutic neurostimulation studies implementing mPFC-targeted rTMS [see Ref. (13) for review], individual variability observed in the present study is consistent with studies of dorsal mPFC (dmPFC) rTMS in major depression (17), eating disorders (18), and obsessive-compulsive disorder (19, 44). Using resting-state fMRI, Dunlop et al. (18) demonstrated that in patients with eating disorders, baseline fronto-striatal connectivity discriminated treatment responders from non-responders, with divergent treatment-related alterations in connectivity corresponding to either symptom improvement or worsening, respectively. This divergence has also been observed when rTMS is applied to other cortical targets (16, 17, 19, 45–51). Together, these studies demonstrate that 1) the effects of various rTMS interventions, especially TBS, can be highly variable within a patient population, but 2) baseline levels of neural activity may be useful biomarkers of an individual's predisposition to TMS-induced neuroplastic changes.

Individual variability in neural responsiveness to TBS may be related to differences in plasticity potential (aka metaplasticity) of a given neural circuit across individuals. This concept is often referred to as homeostatic metaplasticity, whereby changes in cortical excitability induced by rTMS depend on the history of neural activation (22, 52). Specifically, the Bienenstock–Cooper–Munro (BCM) theory of homeostatic plasticity (53) posits that a history of lower post-synaptic activity will lower the synaptic modification threshold for LTP and increase the threshold for LTD. Conversely, a history of high synaptic activity will shift the modification threshold toward favoring the induction of LTD and increase the threshold for LTP (54).

Therefore, metaplasticity—or the propensity of a neural circuit to experience a plastic change—may be related to the current state of that circuit's engagement. Several studies involving both animals and humans have provided strong evidence for this phenomenon by showing that the effects of brain stimulation are influenced by prior activation of a given circuit, whether through priming stimulation or physiologic activity (see 21–23 for reviews). Therefore, it is possible that the bimodal neural responses shown across many rTMS studies—where patients with higher baseline neural activity or connectivity show subsequent attenuation, and patients with lower baseline activity or connectivity show subsequent elevation (or facilitation)—are, in fact, evidence of system- or network-level homeostatic metaplasticity (21, 22).

This theory warrants further investigation in human brain stimulation studies (22, 23), particularly in substance abuse populations where other biologic and drug-related factors impact neuroplasticity (5, 13, 20). However, if metaplastic mechanisms do play a significant role in the direction and magnitude of neural response to brain stimulation, then not accounting for or understanding these phenomena may continue to lead to broad variation in rTMS study outcomes (21, 55). It is, therefore, clear that researchers implementing TBS as an intervention in psychiatry should exercise caution in interpreting their study outcomes without considering the role of individual differences in correlates and predictors of response to stimulation. Understanding individual variability and potential mechanisms of metaplasticity in the relevant neural circuits will enable us to optimize the efficacy of rTMS, and TBS in particular, as a treatment tool (22, 23). Therefore, considerations for future implementation of TBS research should involve a focus on identifying the neural, behavioral, and clinical markers that predict clinically relevant outcomes to treatment.

**The Utility of fMRI as a Biomarker.** In particular, studies like the present, which use functional neuroimaging to inform brain stimulation, are of critical importance to characterizing and developing therapeutic neuromodulation techniques (13, 17, 18). Specifically, the present fMRI task data revealed the neural predictors and correlates of mPFC cTBS response and provided support for homeostatic metaplasticity as a potential neural mechanism for divergent treatment outcomes. Thus, fMRI was of both clinical and neuroscientific relevance, indicating potential treatment candidacy while also illuminating avenues for investigating neuromodulatory mechanisms.

Given that the primary goal of this study was to assess the striatum (the primary projection of mPFC neurons) as a biomarker for treatment response to mPFC-targeted cTBS, we utilized a data-driven ICA to capture changes in the temporal dynamics of striatal network task engagement. ICA was used in the present study versus traditional univariate or Region-of-interest (ROI)-based methods for three primary reasons: 1) the data-driven basis of ICA enabled extraction of the intrinsic spatiotemporal structure of the striatum network in this population without relying on *a priori* input (35, 38, 56, 57); 2) ICA's multivariate statistical approach permitted the measurement of the engagement of the striatum network as a whole, such that the multifocal brain areas simultaneously activated during the cue reactivity task could be captured in their overall patterns of association, rather than being assessed voxelwise or as ROI pairs (38, 57, 58); and 3) increased sensitivity in detecting task-related changes in fMRI signal would result from ICA's ability to diminish noise in the final output by separating artifact from real fMRI signal (36, 59–61). As such, ICA was selected for identification and characterization of the striatum network to enable measurement of network-level task engagement in the subsequent task analysis. However, although focusing on the striatum network was appropriate to address our primary research question, it did not enable us to make conclusions about other brain regions, which may also be affected by the task and mPFC cTBS treatment protocol. As such, these questions could be addressed through further investigation of other relevant cognitive and affective networks, identified through ICA or through a whole-brain, general linear model approach. Although this was beyond the scope of the present research investigation, it would be a valuable approach for future investigation.

The primary limitation of the present study is that it only involves 1 day of cTBS treatment. Although the participants received six 600-pulse sessions of cTBS on that day, there is conflicting evidence as for whether a single day of brain stimulation is sufficient to induce sustainable neural changes (11, 12, 62, 63). Relatedly, we recently showed, in a subset of these subjects, that a single session of mPFC cTBS produced neural changes, but did not produce changes in drug cue-induced craving (15). However, it is generally recognized that a single day of rTMS is likely not sufficient to produce changes in complex behaviors, such as craving, because rTMS effects are cumulative, and it often takes multiple sessions of treatment for clinically meaningful responses in behavior to emerge (64–67). These data are, however, an important "proof of principle," demonstrating that it is not only possible to shift neural reactivity to cocaine cues in a single day using rTMS but also that individual differences in neural response to rTMS are state dependent, which is an important, foundational step toward determining the efficacy of mPFC cTBS as a treatment for substance abuse. Additionally, the sample size is relatively small compared with many clinical treatment studies in cocaine users. However, it is similar in size to many currently published rTMS studies in cocaine dependence (33, 68)—none of which have used neuroimaging as a predictor of response.

These preliminary findings provide the first demonstration that striatal network activity patterns during drug cue exposure fMRI tasks may be sensitive predictors of response to rTMS treatment and can be used to refine treatment selection and monitor outcomes. However, variability in neural response to treatment and lack of significant changes in cocaine craving indicate the need to further study the neurobiological and technical parameters of successful therapeutic stimulation in substance abuse.

## AUTHOR CONTRIBUTIONS

CH was responsible for the concept and design of the overall research study. OM and WD were responsible for study administration and data collection. LD preprocessed MRI data. TK-R designed and executed data analyses, interpreted results, and drafted the manuscript. CH and MG provided critical revision of the manuscript for intellectual content. All authors critically reviewed and approved the final version for publication.

## ACKNOWLEDGMENTS

We also thank James Purl and Jayce Doose for assistance in MRI scanner operation, and Alison Line for her assistance with data entry.

## REFERENCES

1. Sinha R. New findings on biological factors predicting addiction relapse vulnerability. *Curr Psychiatry Rep* (2011) 13(5):398–405. doi: 10.1007/s11920-011-0224-0
2. Drummond DC. What does cue-reactivity have to offer clinical research? *Addiction* (2000) 95:129–44. doi: 10.1046/j.1360-0443.95.8s2.2.x
3. Hartz DT, Frederick-Osborne SL, Galloway GP. Craving predicts use during treatment for methamphetamine dependence: a prospective, repeated-measures, within-subject analysis. *Drug Alcohol Depend* (2001) 63:269–76. doi: 10.1016/S0376-8716(00)00217-9
4. Paliwal P, Hyman SM, Sinha R. Craving predicts time to cocaine relapse: further validation of the now and brief versions of the cocaine craving questionnaire. *Drug Alcohol Depend* (2008) 93:252–9. doi: 10.1016/j.drugalcdep.2007.10.002
5. Jasinska AJ, Stein EA, Kaiser J, Naumer MJ, Yalachkov Y. Factors modulating neural reactivity to drug cues in addiction: a survey of human neuroimaging studies. *Neurosci Biobehav Rev* (2014) 38:1–16. doi: 10.1016/j.neubiorev.2013.10.013
6. Volkow ND, Morales M. The brain on drugs: from reward to addiction. *Cell* (2015) 162:712–25. doi: 10.1016/j.cell.2015.07.046
7. Garrison KA, Potenza MN. Neuroimaging and biomarkers in addiction treatment. *Curr Psychiatry Rep* (2014) 16(12):513. doi: 10.1007/s11920-014-0513-5
8. Volkow ND, Wang GJ, Telang F, Fowler JS, Logan J, Childress AR, et al. Cocaine cues and dopamine in dorsal striatum: mechanism of craving in cocaine addiction. *J Neurosci* (2006) 26(24):6583–8. doi: 10.1523/JNEUROSCI.1544-06.2006
9. Wong DF, Kuwabara H, Schretlen DJ, Bonson KR, Zhou Y, Nandi A, et al. Increased occupancy of dopamine receptors in human striatum during cue-elicited cocaine craving. *Neuropsychopharmacology* (2006) 31:2716–27. doi: 10.1038/sj.npp.1301194
10. Grüsser SM, Wrase J, Klein S, Hermann D, Smolka MN, Ruf M, et al. Cue-induced activation of the striatum and medial prefrontal cortex is associated with subsequent relapse in abstinent alcoholics. *Psychopharmacol Berl* (2004) 175(3):296–302. doi: 10.1007/s00213-004-1828-4
11. Huang YZ, Edwards MJ, Rounis E, Bhatia KP, Rothwell JC. Theta burst stimulation of the human motor cortex. *Neuron* (2005) 45(2):201–6. doi: 10.1016/j.neuron.2004.12.033
12. Huang YZ, Sommer M, Thickbroom G, Hamada M, Pascual-Leonne A, Paulus W, et al. Consensus: new methodologies for brain stimulation. *Brain Stimul* (2009) 2:2–13. doi: 10.1016/j.brs.2008.09.007
13. Dunlop K, Hanlon CA, Downar J. Noninvasive brain stimulation treatments for addiction and major depression. *Ann N Y Acad Sci* (2016) 1394(1):31–54. doi: 10.1111/nyas.12985
14. Hanlon CA, Beveridge TJ, Porrino LJ. Recovering from cocaine: insights from clinical and preclinical investigations. *Neurosci Biobehav Rev* (2013) 37(9):2037–46. doi: 10.1016/j.neubiorev.2013.04.007
15. Kearney-Ramos TE, Dowdle LT, Lench DH, Mithoefer OJ, Devries WH, George MS, et al. Transdiagnostic effects of ventromedial prefrontal cortex transcranial magnetic stimulation on cue reactivity. *Biol Psychiatry Cogn Neurosci Neuroimaging* (2018) 3:599–609. doi: 10.1016/j.bpsc.2018.03.016
16. Cárdenas-Morales L, Volz LJ, Michely J, Rehme AK, Pool E-M, Nettekoven C, et al. Network connectivity and individual responses to brain stimulation in the human motor system. *Cereb Cortex* (2014) 24(7):1697–707. doi: 10.1093/cercor/bht023
17. Downar J, Geraci J, Salomons TV, Dunlop K, Wheeler S, McAndrews MP, et al. Anhedonia and reward-circuit connectivity distinguish nonresponders from responders to dorsomedial prefrontal repetitive transcranial magnetic stimulation in major depression. *Biol Psychiatry* (2014) 76:176–85. doi: 10.1016/j.biopsych.2013.10.026
18. Dunlop K, Woodside B, Lam E, Olmsted M, Colton P, Giacobbe P, et al. Increases in frontostriatal connectivity are associated with response to dorsomedial repetitive transcranial magnetic stimulation in refractory binge/purge behaviors. *Neuroimage Clin* (2015) 8:611–8. doi: 10.1016/j.nicl.2015.06.008
19. Salomons TV, Dunlop K, Kennedy SH, Flint A, Geraci J, Giacobbe P, et al. Resting-state cortico-thalamic-striatal connectivity predicts response to dorsomedial prefrontal rTMS in major depressive disorder. *Neuropsychopharmacology* (2014) 39:488–98. doi: 10.1038/npp.2013.222
20. Kearney-Ramos TE, Lench DH, Hoffman M, Correia B, Dowdle LT, Hanlon CA. Gray and white matter integrity influence TMS signal propagation: a multimodal evaluation in cocaine-dependent individuals. *Sci Rep* (2018) 8:3253. doi: 10.1038/s41598-018-21634-0
21. Hoogendam JM, Ramakers GM, Di Lazzaro V. Physiology of repetitive transcranial magnetic stimulation of the human brain. *Brain Stimul* (2010) 3(2):95–118. doi: 10.1016/j.brs.2009.10.005
22. Karabanov A, Ziemann U, Hamada M, George MS, Quartarone A, Classen J, et al. Consensus paper: probing homeostatic plasticity of human cortex with non-invasive transcranial brain stimulation. *Brain Stimul* (2015) 8:442–54. doi: 10.1016/j.brs.2015.01.404
23. Suppa A, Huang YZ, Funke K, Ridding MC, Cheeran B, Di Lazzaro V, et al. Ten years of theta burst stimulation in humans: established knowledge, unknowns and prospects. *Brain Stimul* (2016) 9(3):323–35. doi: 10.1016/j.brs.2016.01.006

24. First MB, Spritzer RL, Gibbon M. *Structured Clinical Interview for DSM-IV-TR Axis 1 Disorders—Research Version.* New York: Nonpatient ed. Biometrics Research, New York State Psychiatric Institute (2001).
25. Sobell L, Sobell M. *Timeline Follow Back Manual.* Ontario: Addiction Research Foundation (1996).
26. Babor TF, de la Fuente JR, Saunders J, Grant M. *The Alcohol Use Disoders Identification Test: guidelines for use in primary health care.* WHO Publication No. 92.4. Geneva, Switzerland: World Health Organization (1992).
27. Heatherton TF, Kozlowski LT, Frecker RC, Fagerström KO. The Fagerström test for nicotine dependence: a revision of the Fagerström tolerance questionnaire. *Br J Addict* (1991) 86:1119–27. doi: 10.1111/j.1360-0443.1991.tb01879.x
28. Beck AT, Steer RA, Brown GK. *Manual for the Beck Depression Inventory—II.* San Antonio, TX: Psychological Corporation (1996). doi: 10.1037/t00742-000
29. Spielberger CD, Gorsuch RL, Lushene R, Vagg PR, Jacobs GA. *Manual for the State-Trait Anxiety Inventory.* Palo Alto, CA: Consulting Psychologists Press (1983).
30. Prisciandaro JJ, McRae-Clark AL, Myrick H, Henderson S, Brady KT. Brain activation to cocaine cues and motivation/treatment status. *Addict Biol* (2014) 19:240–9. doi: 10.1111/j.1369-1600.2012.00446.x
31. Borckardt JJ, Nahas Z, Koola J, George MS. Estimating resting motor thresholds in TMS research and practice: a computer simulation evaluation of best methods. *J ECT* (2006) 22(3):169–75. doi: 10.1097/01.yct.0000235923.52741.72
32. Stokes MG, Barker AT, Dervinis M, Verbruggen F, Maizey L, Adams RC, et al. Biophysical determinants of transcranial magnetic stimulation: effects of excitability and depth of targeted area. *J Neurophysiology* (2013) 109(2):437–44. doi: 10.1152/jn.00510.2012
33. Hanlon CA, Dowdle LT, Austelle CW, Devries W, Mithoefer O, Badran BW, et al. What goes up, can come down: novel brain stimulation paradigms may attenuate craving and craving-related neural circuitry in substance dependent individuals. *Brain Res* (2015) 1628(Pt A):199–209. doi: 10.1016/j.brainres.2015.02.053
34. Robjant K, Fazel M. The emerging evidence for narrative exposure therapy: a review. *Clin Psychol Rev* (2010) 30(8):1030–9. doi: 10.1016/j.cpr.2010.07.004
35. Calhoun VD, Adali T, Pearlson GD, Pekar JJ. A method for making group inferences from functional MRI data using independent component analysis. *Hum Brain Mapp* (2001) 14:140–51. doi: 10.1002/hbm.1048
36. Kearney-Ramos TE, Fausett JS, Gess JL, Reno A, Peraza J, Kilts CD, et al. Merging clinical neuropsychology and functional neuroimaging to evaluate the construct validity and neural network engagement of the n-back task. *J Int Neuropsychol Soc* (2014) 20(7):736–50. doi: 10.1017/S135561771400054X
37. Kilts CD, Kennedy A, Elton AL, Tripathi SP, Young J, Cisler JM, et al. Individual differences in attentional bias associated with cocaine dependence are related to varying engagement of neural processing networks. *Neuropsychopharmacology* (2014) 39(5):1135–47. doi: 10.1038/npp.2013.314
38. McKeown MJ, Makeig S, Brown GG, Jung TP, Kindermann SS, Bell AJ, et al. Analysis of fMRI data by blind separation into independent spatial components. *Hum Brain Mapp* (1998) 6:160–88. doi: 10.1002/(SICI)1097-0193(1998)6:3<160::AID-HBM5>3.3.CO;2-R
39. Huber PJ. *Robust Statistics.* New York: John Wiley and Sons (1981). doi: 10.1002/0471725250
40. Wager TD, Keller MC, Lacey SC, Jonides J. Increased sensitivity in neuroimaging analyses using robust regression. *Neuroimage* (2005) 26:99–113. doi: 10.1016/j.neuroimage.2005.01.011
41. Kozel AF, Nahas Z, deBrux C, Molloy M, Lorberbaum JP, Bohning D, et al. How coil–cortex distance relates to age, motor threshold, and antidepressant response to repetitive transcranial magnetic stimulation. *J Neuropsychiatry Clin Neurosci* (2000) 12(3):376–84. doi: 10.1176/jnp.12.3.376
42. Elton A, Young J, Smitherman S, Gross RE, Mletzko T, Kilts CD. Neural network activation during a stop-signal task discriminates cocaine-dependent from non-drug-abusing men. *Addict Biol* (2014) 19(3):427–38. doi: 10.1111/adb.12011
43. Smith SM, Fox PT, Miller KL, Glahn DC, Fox PM, Mackay CE, et al. Correspondence of the brain's functional architecture during activation and rest. *Proc Natl Acad Sci U S A* (2009) 106(31):13040–5. doi: 10.1073/pnas.0905267106
44. Dunlop K, Woodside B, Olmsted M, Colton P, Giacobbe P, Downar J. Reductions in cortico-striatal hyperconnectivity accompany successful treatment of obsessive-compulsive disorder with dorsomedial prefrontal rTMS. *Neuropsychopharmacology* (2015) 41(5):1395–403. doi: 10.1038/npp.2015.292
45. Eldaief MC, Halko MA, Buckner RL, Pascual-Leone A. Transcranial magnetic stimulation modulates the brain's intrinsic activity in a frequency-dependent manner. *Proc Natl Acad Sci U S A* (2011) 108(52):21229–34. doi: 10.1073/pnas.1113103109
46. Eschweiler GW, Wegerer C, Schlotter W, Spandl C, Stevens A, Bartels M, et al. Left prefrontal activation predicts therapeutic effects of repetitive transcranial magnetic stimulation (rTMS) in major depression. *Psychiatry Res* (2000) 99:161–72. doi: 10.1016/S0925-4927(00)00062-7
47. Fox MD, Buckner RL, White MP, Greicius MD, Pascual-Leone A. Efficacy of transcranial magnetic stimulation targets for depression is related to intrinsic functional connectivity with the subgenual cingulate. *Biol Psychiatry* (2012) 72(7):595–603 doi: 10.1016/j.biopsych.2012.04.028
48. Fox MD, Liu H, Pascual-Leone A. Identification of reproducible individualized targets for treatment of depression with TMS based on intrinsic connectivity. *Neuroimage* (2013) 66:151–60 doi: 10.1016/j.neuroimage.2012.10.082
49. Herremans SC, De Raedt R, Van Schuerbeek P, Marinazzo D, Matthys F, De Mey J, et al. Accelerated HF-rTMS protocol has a rate-dependent effect on dACC activation in alcohol-dependent patients: an open-label feasibility study. *Alcohol Clin Exp Res* (2016) 40:196–205. doi: 10.1111/acer.12937
50. Liston C, Chen AC, Zebley BD, Drysdale AT, Gordon R, Leuchter B, et al. Default mode network mechanisms of transcranial magnetic stimulation in depression. *Biol Psychiatry* (2014) 76(7):517–26. doi: 10.1016/j.biopsych.2014.01.023
51. Maeda F, Keenan JP, Tormos JM, Topka H, Pascual-Leone A. Interindividual variability of the modulatory effects of repetitive transcranial magnetic stimulation on cortical excitability. *Exp Brain Res* (2000) 133(4):425–30. doi: 10.1007/s002210000432
52. Abraham WC. Metaplasticity: tuning synapses and networks for plasticity. *Nat Rev Neurosci* (2008) 9:387. doi: 10.1038/nrn2356
53. Bienenstock EL, Cooper LN, Munro PW. Theory for the development of neuron selectivity: orientation specificity and binocular interaction in visual cortex. *J Neurosci* (1982) 2:32–48. doi: 10.1523/JNEUROSCI.02-01-00032.1982
54. Ziemann U, Siebner HR. Modifying motor learning through gating and homeostatic metaplasticity. *Brain Stimul* (2008) 1:60–6. doi: 10.1016/j.brs.2007.08.003
55. Hulme SR, Jones OD, Abraham WC. Emerging roles of metaplasticity in behaviour and disease. *Trends Neurosci* (2013) 36(6):353–62. doi: 10.1016/j.tins.2013.03.007
56. Calhoun VD, Liu J, Adali T. A review of group ICA for fMRI data and ICA for joint inference of imaging, genetic, and ERP data. *Neuroimage* (2009) 45:S163–72. doi: 10.1016/j.neuroimage.2008.10.057
57. McKeown MJ, Hansen LK, Sejnowski TJ. Independent component analysis of functional MRI: what is signal and what is noise? *Curr Opin Neurobiol* (2003) 13(5):620–29. doi: 10.1016/j.conb.2003.09.012
58. Xu J, Zhang S, Calhoun VD, Monterosso J, Li C-SR, Worhunsky PD, et al. Task-related concurrent but opposite modulations of overlapping functional networks as revealed by spatial ICA. *Neuroimage* (2013) 79:62–71. doi: 10.1016/j.neuroimage.2013.04.038
59. Aron AR, Poldrack RA. Cortical and subcortical contributions to stop signal response inhibition: role of the subthalamic nucleus. *J Neurosci* (2006) 26(9):2424–33. 10.1523/JNEUROSCI.4682-05.2006
60. Tie Y, Whalen S, Suarez RO, Golby AJ. Group independent component analysis of language fMRI from word generation tasks. *Neuroimage* (2008) 42(3):1214–25. doi: 10.1016/j.neuroimage.2008.05.028
61. Xu J, Potenza MN, Calhoun VD. Spatial ICA reveals functional activity hidden from traditional fMRI GLM-based analyses. *Front Neurosci* (2013) 7:154. doi: 10.3389/fnins.2013.00154
62. Di Lazzaro V, Pilato F, Saturno E, Oliviero A, Dileone M, Mazzone P. Theta-burst repetitive transcranial magnetic stimulation suppresses specific excitatory circuits in the human motor cortex. *J Physiol* (2005) 565:945–50. doi: 10.1113/jphysiol.2005.087288

63. George MS, Raman R, Benedek DM, Pelic CG, Grammer GG, Stokes KT, et al. A two-site pilot randomized 3 day trial of high dose left prefrontal repetitive transcranial magnetic stimulation (rTMS) for suicidal inpatients. *Brain Stimul* (2014) 7(3):421–31. doi: 10.1016/j.brs.2014.03.006
64. Berlim MT, van den Eynde F, Tovar-Perdomo S, Daskalakis ZJ. Response, remission and drop-out rates following high-frequency repetitive transcranial magnetic stimulation (rTMS) for treating major depression: a systematic review and meta-analysis of randomized, double-blind and sham-controlled trials. *Psychol Med* (2014) 44(2):225–39. doi: 10.1017/S0033291713000512
65. Dinur-Klein L, Dannon P, Hadar A, Rosenberg O, Roth Y, Kotler M, et al. Smoking cessation induced by deep repetitive transcranial magnetic stimulation of the prefrontal and insular cortices: a prospective, randomized controlled trial. *Biol Psychiatry* (2014) 76:742–9. doi: 10.1016/j.biopsych.2014.05.020
66. Mishra BR, Nizamie SH, Das B, Praharaj SK. Efficacy of repetitive transcranial magnetic stimulation in alcohol dependence: a sham-controlled study. *Addiction* (2010) 105(1):49–55. doi: 10.1111/j.1360-0443.2009.02777.x
67. Politi E, Fauci E, Santoro A, Smeraldi E. Daily sessions of transcranial magnetic stimulation to the left prefrontal cortex gradually reduce cocaine craving. *Am J Addict* (2008) 17(4):345–6. doi: 10.1080/10550490802139283
68. Camprodon JA, Martinez-Raga J, Alonso-Alonso M, Shih MC, Pascual-Leone A. One session of high frequency repetitive transcranial magnetic stimulation (rTMS) to the right prefrontal cortex transiently reduces cocaine craving. *Drug Alcohol Depend* (2007) 86:91–4 doi: 10.1016/j.drugalcdep.2006.06.002

# 7

# Brain and Cognition for Addiction Medicine: From Prevention to Recovery Neural Substrates for Treatment of Psychostimulant-Induced Cognitive Deficits

*Manoranjan S. D'Souza**

*Department of Pharmaceutical and Biomedical Sciences, The Raabe College of Pharmacy, Ohio Northern University, Ada, OH, United States*

***Correspondence:**
*Manoranjan S. D'Souza*
*m-dsouza@onu.edu*

Addiction to psychostimulants like cocaine, methamphetamine, and nicotine poses a continuing medical and social challenge both in the United States and all over the world. Despite a desire to quit drug use, return to drug use after a period of abstinence is a common problem among individuals dependent on psychostimulants. Recovery for psychostimulant drug-dependent individuals is particularly challenging because psychostimulant drugs induce significant changes in brain regions associated with cognitive functions leading to cognitive deficits. These cognitive deficits include impairments in learning/memory, poor decision making, and impaired control of behavioral output. Importantly, these drug-induced cognitive deficits often impact adherence to addiction treatment programs and predispose abstinent addicts to drug use relapse. Additionally, these cognitive deficits impact effective social and professional rehabilitation of abstinent addicts. The goal of this paper is to review neural substrates based on animal studies that could be pharmacologically targeted to reverse psychostimulant-induced cognitive deficits such as impulsivity and impairment in learning and memory. Further, the review will discuss neural substrates that could be used to facilitate extinction learning and thus reduce emotional and behavioral responses to drug-associated cues. Moreover, the review will discuss some non-pharmacological approaches that could be used either alone or in combination with pharmacological compounds to treat the above-mentioned cognitive deficits. Psychostimulant addiction treatment, which includes treatment for cognitive deficits, will help promote abstinence and allow for better rehabilitation and integration of abstinent individuals into society.

**Keywords: cocaine, nicotine, methamphetamine, memory, extinction, nucleus accumbens, prefrontal cortex**

## INTRODUCTION

Addiction to psychostimulant drugs such as cocaine, methamphetamine, and nicotine adds a significant burden on healthcare budgets in the form of premature morbidity and mortality. Alarmingly, the use and abuse of illicit psychostimulant drugs like cocaine and methamphetamine is showing a trend of steady increase than in the last decade (1). In addition to illicit stimulant use, use and abuse of licit weak stimulant like nicotine continues to increase especially in the form of e-cigarettes and vaping (2). In addition, abuse of prescription stimulants like amphetamine, which are used to treat patients with attention deficit hyperactivity (ADHD), also adds to the problem of psychostimulant addiction. While not all people who experiment with psychostimulants will get addicted, an increasing trend of initiation does not augur well for psychostimulant addiction rates. Importantly, factors that promote transition from use/abuse to addiction are not fully understood (3, 4).

Considerable progress has been made over the last few decades in understanding the brain circuitry and pathological changes that facilitate and promote abuse of drugs (5). Despite this progress, significant challenges remain in the treatment of psychostimulant drug addiction (6). For example, currently, among the different psychostimulants described above, the Food and Drug Administration (FDA) has approved treatments for only nicotine (7, 8). Current treatment protocol for psychostimulant addiction depends largely on managing withdrawal symptoms of dependent individuals, providing behavioral/psychotherapy and utilizing self-help support groups (6). The inadequacy of current psychostimulant drug addiction is supported by high rates of relapse among abstinent addicts.

The goal of behavioral/psychotherapy is to help prevent relapse among abstinent addicts by helping them develop coping strategies to deal with cravings and emotional disturbances occurring as a result of withdrawal from psychostimulant drugs (9). This requires engagement of various cognitive domains such as attention, learning, and memory. Ironically, research over the last two decades and more has demonstrated that abuse of psychostimulants results in several cognitive deficits such as impulsivity (i.e., inability to inhibit disadvantageous rapid behavioral responses), risky and/or poor decision making, impaired cognitive flexibility (i.e., impaired ability to alter behavioral responses based on changing environmental contingencies), deficits in learning and memory, and/or hyperattentiveness to drug-associated cues compared with non-drug associated cues (10–13). Interestingly, individuals with pre-existing deficits in cognition and/or suffering from psychiatric disease states that are associated with impaired cognitive function (e.g., schizophrenia and depression) are more vulnerable to abusing illicit and licit stimulants (14, 15). Importantly, recovering addicts with significant cognitive deficits are more vulnerable to relapse (12, 16). Thus, cognitive deficits in recovering drug addicts irrespective of whether they were pre-existing or drug induced need to be adequately treated to promote abstinence among drug addicts (**Figure 1**).

Among the different psychostimulant-induced cognitive deficits, this review will focus on psychostimulant-induced cognitive deficits such as impulsivity and impairments in learning and memory. The review will primarily identify neural substrates that could be pharmacologically targeted to alleviate psychostimulant-induced cognitive deficits. Finally, the review will discuss evidence from animal studies that support use of non-pharmacological approaches to alleviate the above-mentioned cognitive deficits.

## DRUG-INDUCED COGNITIVE DEFICITS

### Impulsivity

Impulsivity in the human literature is often conceptualized as a personality trait (17). However, in the cognitive neuroscience field and for the purpose of this article, we will refer to impulsivity as behavior resulting from impaired inhibition in specific brain regions that play a role in regulating behavioral output (18). Based on the specific cognitive domains that are disrupted, impulsivity can be divided broadly into behavioral and decisional impulsivity (19). Behavioral impulsivity as the name suggests usually involves a quick behavioral response without consideration to consequences of the behavioral response (19). In contrast, decisional impulsivity

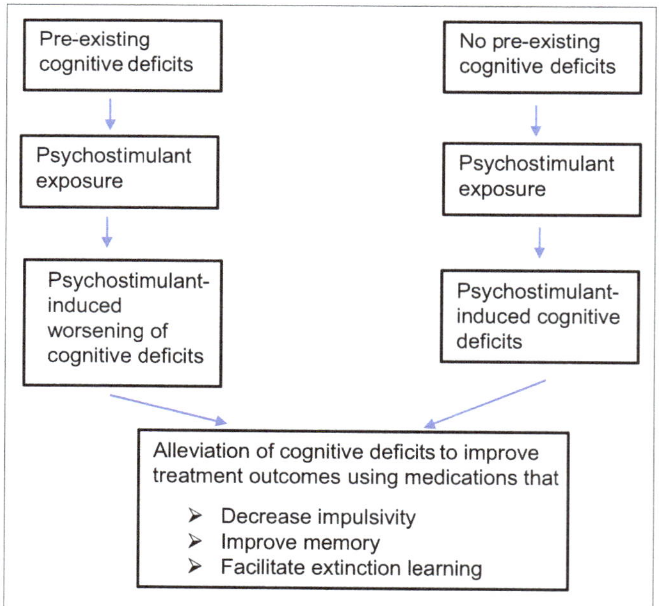


**FIGURE 1** | Figure shows overall hypothesis of the review and possible treatment strategies to improve outcomes of psychostimulant addiction treatment. Psychostimulant-induced cognitive deficits include impulsivity, learning/memory impairments, attentional impairment, and impairment in decision making. In this review, we mainly restrict ourselves to targets that could potentially alleviate impulsivity and/or learning/memory impairments and facilitate extinction learning. Patients with pre-existing cognitive deficits prior to drug abuse may need more aggressive treatment to break the vicious cycle of drug addiction.

**Abbreviations:** ACPC, 1-aminocyclopropanecarboxylic acid; AMPA, amino-3-hydroxy-5-methyl-4-isoxazolepropionate/kainate; AP-5, (2*R*)-amino-5-phosphonovaleric acid; AQP-4, aquaporin-4; CDPPB, 3-cyano-*N*-(1,3-diphenyl-1*H*-pyrazol-5-yl)benzamide; CPP, conditioned place preference; 5-CSRTT, 5-choice serial reaction time task; DBS, deep brain stimulation; DDT, delay discounting task; 5HT, serotonin; GABA, γ-aminobutyric acid; GLT, glutamate transporter; MDMA, 3,4-methylenedioxymethamphetamine; MK-801, (5*R*,10*S*)-(−)-5-methyl-10,11-dihydro-5*H*-dibenzo[*a*,*d*]cylcohepten-5,10-imine; mPFC, medial prefrontal cortex; mGlu, metabotropic glutamate; MPEP, 2-methyl-6-(phenylethynyl)pyridine; MTEP, 3-(2-methyl-1,3-thiazol-4-yl)ethynyl)pyridine; mRNA, microRNA; MOR, mu opioid receptor; NAcc, nucleus accumbens; NMDA, *N*-methyl-D-aspartate; OFC, orbitofrontal cortex; PAMs, positive allosteric modulators; Trk B, tropomyosin-related kinase B; VTA, ventral tegmental area; xCT, cystine–glutamate exchanger.

involves actions and decisions taken by the individual that are less advantageous to the individual.

Psychostimulant addicts show high levels of both behavioral and decisional impulsivity than do healthy controls (20–27). It is hypothesized that this impulsive behavior is responsible for high rates of relapse among these addicts during abstinence. Consistent with these data, a recent human study reported that smokers and polysubstance abusers who abused nicotine, cocaine, and alcohol were more impulsive than controls (28).

Impulsivity observed in drug-dependent individuals can exist prior to drug abuse and worsens with repeated drug use (**Figure 1**). In support of this hypothesis, several studies have shown that individuals who are impulsive have greater sensitivity to drugs of abuse, are more likely to experiment with drugs of abuse, and are more vulnerable to develop drug dependence (29–36). This hypothesis is also supported by animal studies. For example, animals showing poor inhibitory control prior to exposure to drugs of abuse (i.e., showed more impulsive behavior) acquired cocaine self-administration behavior much more rapidly than did animals that showed good inhibitory control (37). Additionally, animals that showed more risk-taking behavior as assessed using the rodent model of Iowa gambling task (rIGT) self-administered greater amount of cocaine than did animals that did not display high risk behavior in the same task (38). However, it is not known if repeated use of drugs of abuse induces impulsivity in humans. In animals, repeated administration of cocaine, methamphetamine, and nicotine increased impulsive behavior in animals (39–43). This increase in impulsivity was observed both when animals were challenged with the drug of abuse and during withdrawal from the drug (i.e., when animals were not under the influence of the drug). Thus, these studies support the hypothesis that exposure to drugs of abuse may *de novo* induce impulsivity.

Keeping with focus of this review, we will only discuss assessment of behavioral and decisional impulsivity in animals. Behavioral impulsivity in animals can be assessed by measuring either premature responding or the ability of an animal to stop already initiated action. In animals, premature responding is measured using the five-choice serial reaction time task (5-CSRTT), while ability of an animal to stop already initiated action is measured using the stop-signal reaction time (SSRT) (44, 45) (**Box 1**). Several brain regions such as the nucleus accumbens (NAcc), dorsal striatum, infralimbic prefrontal cortex

**BOX 1** | Tasks used to measure psychostimulant-induced impulsivity.

| Task | Parameter measured | Description |
|---|---|---|
| **5-Choice serial reaction time task (5-CSRTT)** | Behavioral impulsivity | The apparatus for the 5-CSRTT consists of five apertures. During a trial, a signal is presented in one of the apertures. Upon presentation of a signal, the animals must respond in the form of a nose poke into the aperture where the signal is presented. Nose poke in the aperture not presenting the signal is considered as an incorrect response. Similarly, response of the animal prior to presentation of a signal is considered as a premature response. Increase in premature responding is a measure of behavioral impulsivity. Lack of response by the animal is considered an omission and is indicative of impaired motor activity. Increase in incorrect responses is considered a manifestation of lack of attention. Every correct response of the animal is rewarded with a food pellet, which is collected by the animal from an aperture located on the opposite wall from the five apertures. |
| **Go/No-Go task** | Behavioral impulsivity | Each chamber is equipped with two retractable levers and tri-colored stimulus lights centered above each lever. The Go/No-Go trials consist of four alternating Go and No-Go components. Each component is usually 15 min long with a 5-s timeout between components for a 2-h session. During the Go component, the light on the active lever is illuminated, and a response on the active lever produces a food reward pellet on a variable interval of 30 s, and a press on the inactive lever has no consequence. Alternatively, the No-Go trial is indicated by a continuous flashing light on the active lever, and the animal must withhold a response on the active lever for a specific duration (e.g., 30 s). Responding on the active lever during the No-Go trial resets the time the animal must withhold their response (i.e., 30-s timer). The number of times the timer is reset is used as an index of behavioral impulsivity. |
| **Delay discounting task (DDT)** | Decisional impulsivity | The apparatus usually consists of three levers or apertures on one wall of the apparatus. Each lever or aperture usually has a light above it. The center aperture/lever and associated light are used to initiate trials. The two levers/apertures on either side of the center aperture are associated with rewards. Response on one of the apertures/levers is associated with immediate access to an assured small reward. In contrast, response on the other lever/aperture is associated with an assured larger reward. However, this larger reward is available after a delay. Preference of an animal for an immediate small reward compared with the delayed larger reward is suggestive of decisional impulsivity. |
| **Rodent version of Iowa gambling task (rIGT)** | Decisional impulsivity | The apparatus for the rIGT consists of five apertures like the 5-CSRTT. However, unlike the 5-CSRTT, during a trial, a signal light is presented in four apertures at the same time. Each aperture is associated with a different size of reward, and the probability of the reward is also different for each aperture. For example, responding on one of the apertures may earn the rat one pellet 90% of the time. In contrast, responding on an adjoining aperture may earn the rat four pellets, but only 40% of the time. The other two apertures may be associated with two pellets 80% or three pellets 50% of the time. Thus, the rat can choose the aperture for the amount of reward and hedge its luck. Because not all trials are rewarded, the unrewarded trials are considered punishment and are indicated by flashing light. Response of the animal prior to presentation of a signal is considered a premature response. Lack of response by the animal is considered an omission and could be indicative of impaired motor activity. Selection of aperture that is associated with larger reward but with lower probability is suggestive of risky choice and termed as "decisional impulsivity." |

(infralimbic PFC), insula, and hippocampus have been shown to mediate behavioral impulsivity (19, 46–49). In contrast, decisional impulsivity in animals is usually assessed by measuring either temporal discounting or probability discounting. Temporal discounting is assessed using the delay discounting task (DDT), which involves assessing the ability of animal to wait for a larger reward compared with opting for an immediate smaller reward (50) (**Box 1**). Several studies have identified the role of the basolateral amygdala, orbitofrontal cortex (OFC), and hippocampus in mediating the DDT (51–53). In contrast, probability discounting is assessed using a task known as rIGT or probability discounting task and involves choosing a smaller sure reward (i.e., 100% chance to obtain the reward) compared with a larger reward, which is not always assured (i.e., approximately 50% chance or risky choice) (54, 55) (**Box 1**). Research has shown that the OFC, amygdala, habenula, and prelimbic PFC play a role in mediating probability discounting (56–58). Despite identifying the role of specific brain regions in specific types of impulsive behavior, more work is required to identify specific signaling mechanisms between the different brain regions.

## Learning and Memory Deficits

Both learning and working memory deficits have been reported in abstinent psychostimulant addicts (21, 59–63). These learning/memory deficits are hypothesized to result in poor treatment outcomes among abstinent addicts. It is also hypothesized that working memory deficits prior to drug exposure increase vulnerability to drug addiction. Consistent with this hypothesis, individuals suffering from psychiatric disorders with significant learning and memory deficits such as depression and schizophrenia have high rates of stimulant addiction (14, 15, 64, 65). Also, a recent study reported that adolescents with weak working memory were more vulnerable to get addicted to drugs of abuse (66). In fact, acute administration of drugs like nicotine and cocaine enhances hippocampal function (67–69). Thus, individuals may compensate for memory deficits by abusing psychostimulants. Together, these findings suggest that use of psychostimulants induces memory deficits and that memory deficits present prior to drug use promote experimentation with stimulants leading to drug addiction.

Several models such as the Morris water maze, novel object recognition, and delayed match-to-sample task are used to assess learning/memory deficits in animals (**Box 2**) (70, 71). Similar to humans, chronic exposure and/or withdrawal from psychostimulants induced working memory deficits in animals. For example, animals with chronic extended-access cocaine self-administration experience showed working memory and learning deficits (72, 73). Further, animals undergoing withdrawal after chronic extended access to cocaine showed decreased functional activity of brain circuits mediating learning and memory such as the PFC, hippocampus, and striatum as measured by determining glucose utilization by these brain regions (74). Further memory deficits have been reported after withdrawal from nicotine, methamphetamine, and 3,4-methylenedioxymethamphetamine (MDMA) (75–79). Moreover, consistent with human studies, animals with memory deficits show significantly greater drug-seeking behavior than do controls. For example, neonatal ventral hippocampal lesions in rats, which lead to working memory deficits, resulted in increased reinstatement of nicotine seeking (80).

In abstinent addicts, exposure to stress, drug of abuse itself, and/or drug-associated environmental cues induces cravings, which promotes drug seeking often resulting in relapse (81–84). In humans, several behavioral and cognitive therapies, such as behavioral therapy, cue exposure therapy, motivational enhancement therapy, and contingency management, are used to

**BOX 2 |** Tasks used to measure psychostimulant-induced memory impairment and described in this review.

| Task | Parameter measured | Description |
|---|---|---|
| **Delayed match-to-sample (DMTS)** | Working memory | In this task, as the name suggests, animals are initially presented with a particular stimulus on a computer touchscreen. For example, the stimulus could be a triangle of a particular color, e.g., red. Once the animal touches the triangle, the triangle disappears from the screen. There is then predefined delay. At the end of the delay, the animal is presented with two stimuli. One of the stimuli is the previously presented red triangle. The other stimulus is new triangle of a different color, e.g., blue. Selection of the "red triangle" is considered as the correct response, while selection of the "blue triangle" is considered as the incorrect response. A high percentage of correct response is indicative of intact working memory. In contrast, a high percentage of incorrect responses is indicative of impaired working memory. |
| **Novel object recognition** | Episodic memory | In this task, the animal is exposed to two identical objects for a defined period of the time. The animal can explore these objects, and they are termed as familiar objects. After a period of time, which can range for 24 to 72 h, animals are again exposed to two objects. One of them is the previously exposed "familiar object," and the other object is termed as the "novel object." Retention of memory in the animal is determined by calculating the discrimination index, which is defined as the time spent on the novel object divided by the sum of the time spent on the novel and familiar objects. A higher discrimination index indicates intact memory. In contrast, a low discrimination index suggests impairment of memory. |
| **Morris water maze** | Spatial memory | The apparatus consists of black painted circular pool containing water and divided into four quadrants with four starting points. The pool contains a platform that is submerged (hidden) in the water in a particular quadrant. During training, animals are trained to locate the hidden submerged platform irrespective of the start position. During the test trials, the submerged platform is removed, and animals are placed in a quadrant opposite to the quadrant where the platform was previously hidden (quadrant of interest). The time taken for the animal to reach the quadrant of interest, the path taken to reach the quadrant of interest, and time spent in the quadrant of interest are suggestive of spatial memory. In case of impairment of spatial memory, the animal will either take longer time to reach the quadrant of interest or spend less time in the quadrant of interest or take circuitous path to reach the quadrant of interest. |

help abstinent addicts overcome craving (6, 85). The main goal of all these therapies is to decrease emotional and physiological responses to drug-associated cues among abstinent addicts. In animals, extinction learning is used to suppress learned responses to drug-associated cues (86–88). Extinction learning is a form of learning that involves exposure to drug-associated cues/contexts in the absence of the drug, which ultimately leads to decreased responses to drug-associated cues/contexts. In fact, reinstatement of drug seeking in response to drug-associated cues/environments after extinction training is a putative model of relapse in humans (89, 90). Several brain regions such as the infralimbic PFC, basolateral amygdala and NAcc shell, hypothalamus, and thalamus play a role in extinction learning (88). In fact, extinction learning resulted in decrease in activity of neurons in the prelimbic PFC and increase in activity of neurons in the infralimbic PFC (91–93). It has been hypothesized that facilitation of extinction learning could help in attenuating responses to drug-associated cues and prevent relapse (94, 95). Interestingly, there is significant overlap in pathways that mediate extinction of fear-associated memories and extinction of drug-associated memories (93). In fact, currently, behavioral therapies are being used to concurrently treat both substance abuse and post-traumatic stress disorder (96). Thus, in this review where direct evidence is lacking, we suggest neural substrates that play a role in extinction of fear-associated memories as possible targets for promoting extinction of drug-associated memories. It goes without saying that any such proposed targets will need to be assessed in models assessing extinction of drug-associated memories (**Box 3**). In summary, treatment of psychostimulant-dependent subjects must include procognitive agents that could alleviate working memory deficits and enhance learning/memory. Importantly, facilitation of extinction learning will help improve efficacy of cognitive behavioral therapies in humans especially cue exposure therapy.

## PHARMACOLOGICAL TARGETS TO TREAT PSYCHOSTIMULANT-INDUCED COGNITIVE IMPAIRMENTS

### Dopamine Receptors and Uptake Transporters

Changes in dopamine neurotransmission and dopamine receptors after exposure to psychostimulants like nicotine, cocaine, and methamphetamine have been previously described (97–100). Dopamine neurotransmission is primarily mediated *via* D1-like (D1 and D5) and D2-like (D2, D3, and D4) dopamine receptors. Most of the action of synaptic dopamine is terminated *via* uptake of dopamine by the dopamine uptake transporter (DAT). The dopamine uptake transporter is one of the primary targets for medications that are used to treat ADHD (101, 102). Thus, dopamine neurotransmission plays a role in both impulsivity and psychostimulant addiction. In this section, the role of D1- and D2-like dopamine receptors as possible targets for treatment of psychostimulant-induced cognitive deficits is discussed.

#### D1-Like Dopamine Receptors

Several studies have evaluated the role of D1-like dopamine receptors in impulsivity [see Jupp and Dalley (103) for review].

**BOX 3 |** Tasks used to assess facilitation of extinction learning.

| Task | Parameter measured | Description |
|---|---|---|
| **Extinction of drug-induced CPP** | Extinction of drug-associated memories | In this model, a conditioned place preference (CPP) apparatus consisting of two main chambers is used. The two chambers are distinct in terms of their walls and/or floors. First, preference of the animal to the two main chambers is assessed. Next, animals are conditioned to the effects of the drug and saline/vehicle. During conditioning, animals are administered the drug and restricted to one of the chambers. Subsequently, animals are administered the vehicle/saline and restricted to the other distinct chamber. The conditioning trials are conducted either on the same day separated by at least 4–6 h or on alternate days. Once the animals are conditioned, drug-induced CPP is determined by allowing animals to assess both chambers freely. Animals will spend more time in the drug-associated chamber, suggesting rewarding effects of the drug. Subsequently, animals undergo extinction trials when they are repeatedly exposed to both chambers without drug treatment. Over a period of a few days, the time spent by the animals in the drug-associated chamber decreases, suggesting extinction of drug-induced CPP. A treatment, compared with controls, is said to facilitate extinction if the time spent by the animal in the drug-associated chamber diminishes faster. |
| **Extinction of drug seeking** | Extinction of drug-associated memories | In this model, animals are first trained to intravenously self-administer the concerned drug in self-administration chambers. A typical chamber has two levers—one is called the active lever and the other is called the inactive lever. Responses on the active lever are associated with drug administration. Drug administration is also associated with visual cues such as illumination of a light located above the lever. Once the animals establish stable intravenous self-administration, they undergo extinction training. During extinction training, animals can respond on either the active or inactive levers. Responses on the active lever are accompanied by neither presentation of visual cues nor drug administration. With time, responses of the animal on the active lever decrease to a point where no further decrease occurs (asymptote). A treatment is said to facilitate extinction if the animal takes fewer days to reach the lowest asymptote levels and/or if the responses on the active lever are lower compared with those of controls. In this model, reinstatement of drug seeking can be assessed by presenting the animal with drug-associated cues and by measuring responses on the active/drug-associated lever. Reinstatement of drug seeking is a putative model of relapse in humans. |

Blockade of D1 receptors alone after systemic administration of a D1 receptor antagonist had no influence on decisional impulsivity (104). However, blockade of D1 receptors after systemic administration of a D1 receptor antagonist in mice lacking DAT attenuated behavioral impulsivity as assessed using the 5-CSRTT (105). Interestingly, D1 receptors in specific brain regions such as the NAcc and PFC play a differential role in impulsivity. For example, blockade of D1 receptors in the NAcc core and shell decreased behavioral impulsivity (106). Consistent with these data, blockade of D1-like receptors in the NAcc shell attenuated reinstatement of cocaine seeking in rats (107). In contrast, blockade of D1-like receptors in the medial PFC (mPFC) induced decisional impulsivity (108). Together, these data suggest that D1-like receptors in specific brain regions and circuits may play a differential role in impulsivity. A recent study reported that mice lacking D1 receptors compared with control did not show premature responding after morphine exposure (109). However, the effects of D1 receptor activation and blockade in psychostimulant-induced impulsivity have not been investigated.

D1-mediated dopamine neurotransmission in the PFC has been shown to play a role in extinction of drug-associated memories. For example, genetically induced overexpression of D1 dopamine receptors on glutamate neurons in the PFC facilitated extinction of cocaine-induced CPP in juvenile male rats compared with controls (110) (**Table 1**; **Figure 2**). Activation of dopamine D1-like receptors results in increase in activity of the cAMP/protein kinase A/cyclic AMP-dependent response binding element (CREB) pathway. Rolipram, a phosphodiesterase 4 (PDE-4) inhibitor, increases cAMP levels and PKA activation that resulted in facilitation of fear extinction (116). Moreover, rolipram *via* an increase in CREB levels alleviated working memory deficits associated with alcohol withdrawal (117). Withdrawal from psychostimulants is also associated with decreased activity in PKA/CREB pathway especially in brain regions mediating learning/memory such the hippocampus and PFC (118, 119). Therefore, it is possible that rolipram may help facilitate extinction learning and/or working memory deficits associated with psychostimulant withdrawal. In summary, targeting D1 receptors in specific brain regions and circuits may have utility in the treatment of psychostimulant-induced cognitive deficits especially learning and memory deficits.

### D2-Like Dopamine Receptors

Acute cocaine dose dependently decreased decisional impulsivity in rats as assessed using the DDT (120). The same study showed that systemic administration of D2 receptor antagonist, eticlopride, reversed acute cocaine-induced inhibition of decisional impulsivity, suggesting that the effects of cocaine on decisional impulsivity are mediated by D2 receptor activation. Further, the study showed that D2 receptors in the amygdala possibly mediate the inhibitory effect of acute cocaine on decisional impulsivity. Chronic cocaine exposure decreased striatal D2 receptor mRNA in both high and low impulsive rats and selectively decreased immediate early gene zif268 mRNA in the OFC and infralimbic cortices of high impulsive animals (121). Thus, impulsive behavior observed after chronic cocaine exposure was possibly due to decreased D2-mediated dopamine signaling in the above-described brain regions.

D2 dopamine receptors located in the NAcc, ventral tegmental area (VTA), and PFC also play a role in impulsive behavior. Specifically, D2/3 receptor availability was significantly decreased in the NAcc of high impulsive rats compared with low impulsive rats (122, 123). Further chronic methylphenidate treatment decreased impulsivity in high impulsive rats by increasing expression of D2 receptor availability in the dorsal striatum and NAcc (123). Similarly, decreased D2-mediated dopamine transmission in the PFC and VTA induced decisional impulsivity (124, 125). Interestingly, systemic administration of D2 agonist ropinirole induced decisional impulsivity as assessed using the rIGT (126). However, ex vivo analyses of brain slices revealed that chronic ropinirole treatment led to upregulation of the β-arrestin-AKT-GSK3β intracellular cascade, which usually suggests D2-mediated signaling under hyperdopaminergic conditions.

Interestingly, activation of D3 receptors induced decisional impulsivity as assessed using the rIGT (109, 127–129). In contrast, blockade of D3 receptors decreased decisional impulsivity. In addition, blockade of D3 receptors attenuated cocaine and methamphetamine seeking (130, 131). Together, the data suggest that blockade of D3 receptors may help to attenuate decisional impulsivity and drug seeking. Further studies are required to assess the effects of D3 antagonists on psychostimulant-induced impulsivity.

In summary, the above-described evidence suggests that D2-mediated dopamine neurotransmission in specific brain regions such as striatum and mPFC receptors may help to alleviate decisional impulsivity associated with psychostimulant addiction (**Box 4**). In contrast to D2 receptors, blockade of D3 dopamine receptors may help alleviate psychostimulant-induced decisional impulsivity. Overall, D2-like dopamine receptors are useful targets in the treatment of psychostimulant addiction.

## Adrenergic Receptors and Noradrenergic Reuptake Transporters

The role of noradrenaline in impulsivity is evident by use of medications that increase noradrenergic transmission in the treatment of ADHD (101, 102). Noradrenergic transmission is mediated by α (α1 and α2) and β (β1 and β2) adrenergic receptors, and the action of synaptic noradrenaline is terminated by the noradrenaline uptake transporter (NET). Several drugs approved by the FDA for ADHD treatment include α2 adrenergic receptor agonists (e.g., guanfacine and clonidine), NET and DAT inhibitors (e.g., amphetamine and methylphenidate), and selective NET inhibitor (e.g., atomoxetine). Importantly, exposure to psychostimulants like cocaine, nicotine, and methamphetamine alters noradrenergic neurotransmission in the brain (132–135). In this section the role of α2, β2, and NET in psychostimulant-induced cognitive deficits is discussed.

### α2 Adrenergic Receptors and NET

Like in humans, drugs that increase noradrenergic transmission decreased impulsivity in animal models (136–138). Guanfacine, a selective α2A adrenergic receptor agonist, attenuated cocaine-induced behavioral impulsivity and memory impairment in monkeys (139) (**Tables 2** and **3**). More recently, it was reported

**TABLE 1** | Brain region-specific manipulation on psychostimulant-induced cognitive deficits.

| Brain region | Manipulation | Species | Task | Reward | Findings | Reference |
|---|---|---|---|---|---|---|
| PFC (prelimbic) | D1 receptor overexpression | Rats | Extinction of cocaine-induced CPP | Cocaine | Facilitated extinction of cocaine-induced CPP | Brenhouse et al. (110) |
| PFC (infralimbic) | Blockade of β receptors | Mice | Extinction of cocaine-induced CPP | Cocaine | Inhibited extinction of cocaine-induced CPP | Huang et al. (111) |
| PFC (infralimbic) | β-Arrestin 2 knockdown | Mice | Extinction of cocaine-induced CPP | Cocaine | Inhibited extinction of cocaine-induced CPP | Huang et al. (111) |
| PFC (infralimbic) | β-Arrestin 2 overexpression | Mice | Extinction of cocaine-induced CPP | Cocaine | Facilitated extinction of cocaine-induced CPP | Huang et al. (111) |
| PFC (infralimbic) | BDNF | Rats | Extinction of cocaine-induced CPP | Cocaine | Facilitated extinction of cocaine-induced CPP | Otis et al. (112) |
| PFC (infralimbic) | TrkB receptor antagonist (ANA-12) | Rats | Extinction of cocaine-induced CPP | Cocaine | Inhibited extinction of cocaine-induced CPP | Otis et al. (112) |
| PFC (infralimbic) | GluN2B receptor antagonist ifenprodil | Rats | Extinction of cocaine-induced CPP | Cocaine | Inhibited extinction of cocaine-induced CPP | Otis et al. (112) |
| PFC (infralimbic) | HDAC3 deacetylase inhibitor | Rats | Extinction of cocaine-induced CPP | Cocaine | No effect on extinction of cocaine-induced CPP | Alaghband et al. (113) |
| PFC | CB1 antagonist (rimonabant) | Mice | Extinction of cocaine-induced CPP | Cocaine | Facilitated extinction of cocaine-induced CPP | Hu et al. (114) |
| NAcc shell | $GABA_A$ agonist (muscimol) | Rats | Morris water maze | Methamphetamine | Improved methamphetamine withdrawal induced spatial memory deficit | Heysieattalab et al. (115) |
| NAcc shell | $GABA_A$ antagonist (bicuculline) | Rats | Morris water maze | Methamphetamine | Worsened methamphetamine withdrawal induced spatial memory deficit | Heysieattalab et al. (115) |
| NAcc shell | NMDA antagonist (AP-5) | Rats | Morris water maze | Methamphetamine | Improved methamphetamine withdrawal induced spatial memory deficit | Heysieattalab et al. (115) |
| Dorsal hippocampus | HDAC3 deacetylase inhibitor | Rats | Extinction of cocaine-induced CPP | Cocaine | Facilitated extinction of cocaine-induced CPP | Alaghband et al. (113) |

*BDNF, brain-derived neurotrophic factor; Trk B, tropomyosin-related kinase B.*

**BOX 4** | Potential targets/approaches for alleviation of psychostimulant-induced impulsivity, memory impairment, and/or facilitation extinction of drug-associated memories. BDNF, brain-derived neurotrophic factor; CRF, corticotrophin-related factor; Trk B, tropomyosin-related kinase B; nACh, nicotinic acetylcholine; IGF, insulin growth factor; PAM, positive allosteric modulator; PPARγ, peroxisome proliferator agonist receptor gamma.

| Decreasing impulsivity | Reversing memory impairment | Facilitating extinction learning |
|---|---|---|
| α2 agonists | NMDA receptor antagonists | mGlu5 receptor PAM |
| NET blockers | mGlu5 receptor PAM | AMPA receptor agonist |
| Orexin receptor antagonists | *N*-Acetylcysteine, riluzole | Glycine receptor coagonist |
| CB1 receptor antagonists | α7 nACh receptor agonist/PAM | $GABA_B$ agonist |
| D3 receptor antagonists | CB1 antagonists | Phosphodiesterase inhibitors |
| α4β2 nACh receptor antagonists | Activation of PKCε | Orexin receptor antagonists |
| mGlu4 PAM | Insulin | Increase BDNF levels |
| mGlu2/3 agonists | PPARγ agonists | TrK B receptor activation |
| 5-HT3, 5-HT2A, and 5-HT2c antagonists | IGF-2 agonists | Increase in oxytocin levels |
| 5-HT1A agonist | Exercise | Increase in ghrelin levels |
| Progesterone | Brain stimulation | CRF receptor antagonists |
| Exercise | Neurogenesis | IGF-2 agonists |
| | | 17β-estradiol |
| | | Exercise |
| | | Brain stimulation |

that guanfacine improved inhibitory control in abstinent cocaine-dependent subjects (153). Also, α1 and α2 adrenergic receptor agonists decreased reinstatement of cocaine seeking (154). In contrast, α2 adrenergic receptor antagonist yohimbine is commonly used to pharmacologically induce reinstatement of psychostimulant drug seeking (155).

In addition, direct injection of atomoxetine in the NAcc shell, but not NAcc core or the PFC, reduced behavioral impulsivity as assessed using the 5-CSRTT (156). However, decisional impulsivity as measured using DDT was not altered by atomoxetine injections into either the mPFC or OFC (125). Importantly, relevant to this review, atomoxetine reduced decisional impulsivity for cocaine rewards using the DDT in male rats [(144) (**Table 2**), but see Ref. (157)]. In contrast, atomoxetine alone did not attenuate decisional impulsivity associated with cocaine rewards in female rats. However, decisional impulsivity for cocaine rewards in females was attenuated after treatment with either progesterone alone or progesterone in combination

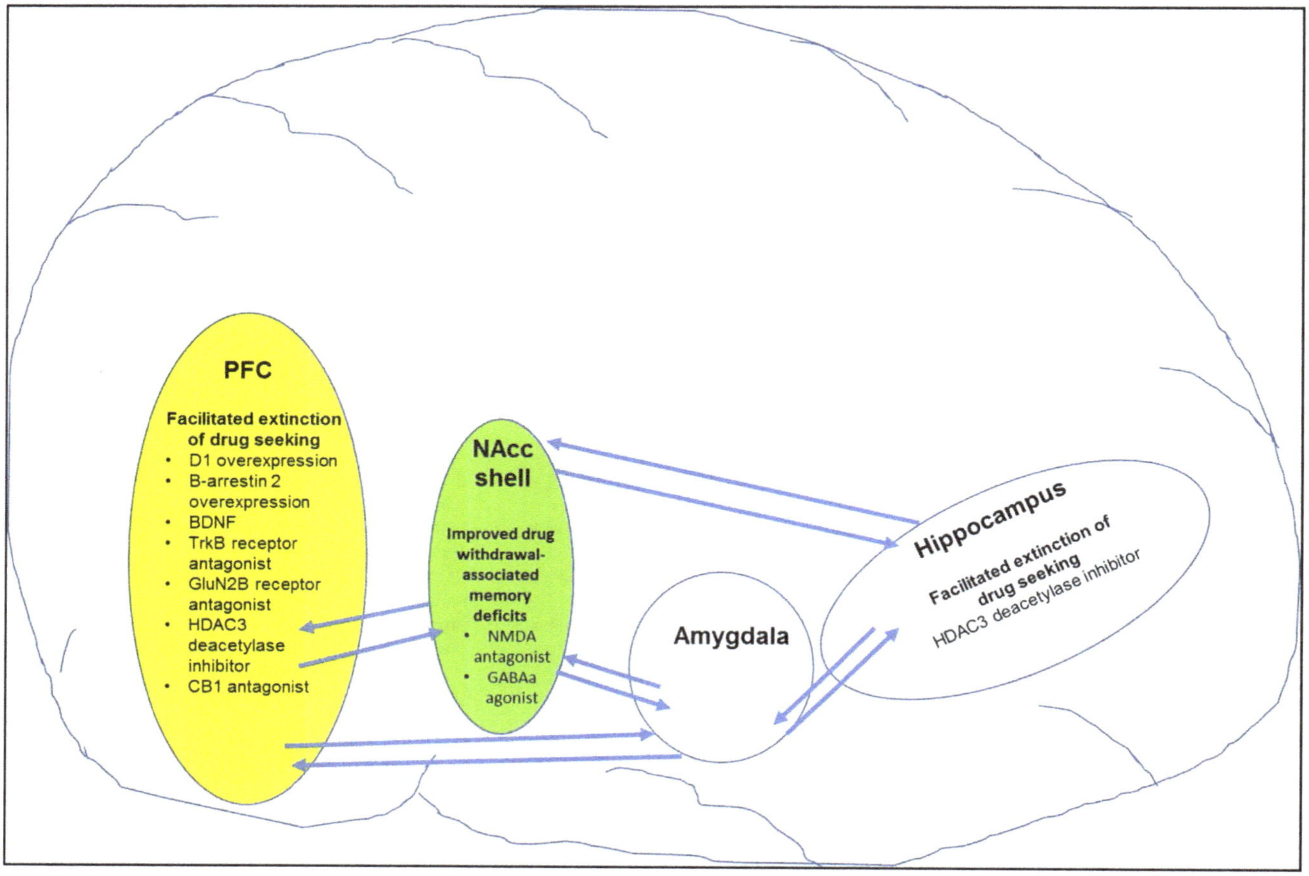


**FIGURE 2 |** Figure shows specific targets in brain regions that play a role in improving drug-induced cognitive deficits (also see **Table 3** for more details). For example, pharmacological manipulation of targets in the prefrontal cortex (PFC) and hippocampus facilitated extinction of drug-seeking behavior. In addition, pharmacological manipulation of targets in the nucleus accumbens shell (NAcc shell) improved drug-withdrawal associated memory.

**TABLE 2 |** Pharmacological alleviation of psychostimulant-induced impulsivity in animals.

| Target | Task | Species | Drug | Findings | Reference |
|---|---|---|---|---|---|
| α2A adrenergic receptor agonists (guanfacine) | 5-CSRTT | Rats | Acute cocaine | Dose-dependent decrease in behavioral impulsivity | Terry et al. (139) |
| Orexin receptor antagonist (suvorexant) | 5-CSRTT | Rats | Acute cocaine | Decreased behavioral impulsivity but had no effect on decisional impulsivity | Gentile et al. (140) |
| Progesterone | Go/No-Go task | Rats | Acute cocaine | Decreased behavioral impulsivity in female but not male rats | Swalve et al. (141) |
| NET uptake blocker (atomoxetine) | DDT | Rats | Acute cocaine | Decreased decisional impulsivity in male rats compared with controls; no effect of atomoxetine alone in females | Smethelss et al. (142) |
| CB1 antagonists (rimonabant) | DDT | Rats | Repeated cocaine exposure | Both prevented and reversed cocaine-induced decisional impulsivity | Hernandez et al. (39) |

*5-CSRTT, 5-choice serial reaction time task; DDT, delay discounting task.*

with atomoxetine. Together, the data suggest atomoxetine may not be as effective in female compared with male cocaine abusers, suggesting a role for gender in psychostimulant-induced impulsivity treatment (discussed later). Systemic administration of atomoxetine also attenuated reinstatement of cocaine seeking (157–159). Overall, the data support the role of α2 adrenergic receptor agonists and/or selective NET inhibitors in the treatment of psychostimulant-induced impulsivity (**Box 4**).

## β Adrenergic Receptors

The role of noradrenergic neurotransmission *via* β adrenergic receptors has been explored in both consolidation of drug-associated memory and extinction learning. Specifically, administration of β receptor antagonist propranolol immediately after nicotine administration attenuated reinstatement of nicotine seeking in animals (160). Consistent with these findings, administration of propranolol attenuated craving among abstinent

**TABLE 3 |** Pharmacological alleviation of psychostimulant-induced memory impairment and/or facilitation of extinction learning.

| Compounds | Task | Species | Drug treatment | Findings | Reference |
|---|---|---|---|---|---|
| α2A adrenergic receptor agonists (guanfacine) | Delayed match-to-sample (DMTS) | Monkeys | Acute cocaine | Alleviated cocaine-induced impairment in accuracy in the DMTS task suggesting improvement in working memory | Terry et al. (140) |
| NMDA antagonist (memantine) | Novel object recognition | Rats | Amphetamine withdrawal | Attenuated amphetamine withdrawal-induced impairment in memory | Marszalek-Grabska et al. (145) |
| CB1 antagonist (rimonabant) | Novel object recognition | Mice | Nicotine withdrawal | Attenuated nicotine withdrawal-induced impairment in memory | Saravia et al. (146) |
| Glycine site partial agonist (D-cycloserine) | Extinction of cocaine-induced CPP | Rats | Cocaine | Facilitated extinction of cocaine-induced CPP | Botreau et al. (147) |
| mGlu5 PAM (CDPPB) | Extinction of cocaine-induced CPP | Rats | Cocaine | Facilitated extinction of cocaine-induced CPP | Gas and Olive (148) |
| | Extinction of cocaine seeking | Rats | Cocaine | Facilitated extinction of cocaine seeking | Cleva et al. (149) |
| PD4 inhibitor (rolipram) | Extinction of cocaine-induced CPP | Mice | Cocaine | Facilitated extinction of cocaine-induced CPP | Liddie et al. (150) |
| PD9 inhibitor (BAY-73-6691) | Extinction of cocaine-induced CPP | Mice | Cocaine | Facilitated extinction of cocaine-induced CPP | Liddie et al. (150) |
| TrK B agonist | Extinction of cocaine-induced CPP | Rats | Cocaine | Facilitated extinction of cocaine-induced CPP | Otis at al. (112, 113) |
| 17β estradiol | Extinction of cocaine-induced CPP | Rats | Cocaine | Facilitated extinction of cocaine-induced CPP | Twining et al. (151) |
| Vagal nerve stimulation | Extinction of cocaine seeking | Rats | Cocaine | Facilitated extinction of cocaine seeking | Childs et al. (152) |
| $GABA_B$ agonist (baclofen) | Extinction of methamphetamine-induced CPP | Rats | Methamphetamine | Facilitated extinction of methamphetamine-induced CPP | Voigt et al. (153) |

*DMTS, delayed matching to sample task; CPP, conditioned place preference.*

smokers for a novel conditioned stimulus associated with nicotine. Inhibition of hippocampal β receptors attenuated expression of cocaine-associated memory as assessed using the cocaine-induced CPP model (113). Importantly, propranolol facilitated extinction of fear in rabbits (162). However, a recent study has reported that direct injections of propranolol in the infralimbic PFC attenuated extinction learning of cocaine-induced CPP *via* inhibition of ERK-signaling pathway (111) (**Table 1**; **Figure 2**). In fact, the study also reported that overexpression of β-arrestin 2 in the infralimbic PFC promoted extinction of cocaine-induced CPP. Further, knockout of β-arrestin 2 in the infralimbic PFC impaired extinction of cocaine-induced CPP. Taken together, the data suggest a role for β-adrenergic receptors in facilitating extinction of drug-associated memories. Further, development of β-adrenergic ligands that selectively promote signaling *via* β-arrestin 2 pathway will help in better understanding the role of β-adrenergic receptors in extinction learning. In summary, α2 and β adrenergic receptors and NET are very viable targets for treatment of cognitive impairments associated with psychostimulant addiction. Future work must focus on determining specific circuits that are targeted by α2 and β adrenergic receptor agonists and/or selective NET inhibitors to decrease impulsivity and facilitate working memory and/or extinction of drug-associated cues.

## Serotoninergic Receptors

Alteration in serotoninergic neurotransmission after chronic exposure to cocaine and other psychostimulants has been previously described (163). Serotoninergic tone in the brain plays an important role in inhibitory control (164). Several lines of evidence suggest that a decrease in brain serotonin (5-HT) increases impulsivity, while elevation of brain 5-HT levels decreased impulsivity (165–167). Interestingly, increased 5-HT release in the PFC was found to be associated with higher levels of behavioral impulsivity as assessed using the 5-CSRTT (168, 169). Overall, a majority of the data suggest that elevation of serotoninergic transmission improves impulsive behavior.

In addition to 5-HT, several studies support a role of both 5-HT2A and 5-HT2C receptors in impulsive behavior. For example, 5-HT2A receptor expression in the mPFC was higher in high compared with low impulsive animals (170). Further, activation of 5-HT2A receptors induced behavioral impulsivity, while blockade of 5-HT2A receptors inhibited behavioral impulsivity (170, 171). Moreover, 5-HT2A receptor activation in the OFC induced decisional impulsivity (172). Future work needs to assess the effects of 5-HT2A receptor antagonists in psychostimulant-induced impulsivity. Similar to 5-HT2A, 5-HT2C receptor expression was significantly greater in the OFC in high compared with low impulsive animals (122). In contrast, no difference in 5-HT2C receptor expression was reported in the striatum between high and low impulsive animals. Blockade of 5-HT2C receptors selectively improved decisional impulsivity in the rIGT (173). Chronic cocaine self-administration decreased 5-HT2C receptor expression in the NAcc shell in the high impulsive animals but decreased 5-HT2C receptor expression in the infralimbic PFC in the low impulsive animals (122). Together, the data suggest that cocaine differentially influences 5-HT2C receptor expression in different brain regions depending on the impulsivity in the animals prior to cocaine exposure. Based on the above data, it is hypothesized that 5-HT2C receptor antagonists will attenuate psychostimulant-induced impulsivity.

5-HT3 antagonists, granisetron and ondansetron, decreased decisional impulsivity in the DDT (173) (**Box 4**). This decrease in decisional impulsivity was not observed after administration of the 5-HT reuptake blocker (paroxetine) or the 5-HT1A receptor agonist (8-OH-DPAT). Interestingly, infusion of 5-HT1A receptor agonist 8-OH-DPAT into the OFC decreased decisional impulsivity (124). Together, 5-HT3 receptor antagonists and 5-HT1A receptor agonists could be potentially useful in treating psychostimulant-induced impulsivity. In summary, establishing serotoninergic tone in psychostimulant-dependent subjects may help ameliorate cognitive deficits induced by abuse of psychostimulants. Further, 5-HT1A, 5-HT2A, 5-HT2C, and 5-HT3 receptors are possible targets that need to be further explored for the treatment of psychostimulant-induced impulsivity.

## GABA Receptors

Exposure to psychostimulants like cocaine, nicotine, and methamphetamine alters GABAergic neurotransmission (174–176). GABA also plays a role in both impulsivity and learning/memory (177–179). Activation of $GABA_A$ receptors in the mPFC induced behavioral impulsivity, while blockade of $GABA_A$ receptors in the same region reduced behavioral impulsivity (180–182). Moreover, activation of $GABA_A$ receptors in the lateral habenula increased cue-induced cocaine seeking, suggesting lack of inhibitory control in response to drug-associated cues (183). Importantly, activation of $GABA_A$ receptors in the NAcc shell improved methamphetamine-induced working memory deficit as measured using the Morris water maze (115). Together, the data suggest that $GABA_A$-mediated neurotransmission in different brain regions plays a differential role in psychostimulant-induced impulsivity and memory deficits (**Box 4**).

In addition to $GABA_A$ receptors, $GABA_B$ receptors play a role in drug seeking. For example, $GABA_B$ agonists and positive allosteric modulators (PAMs) attenuated reinstatement of nicotine and cocaine seeking (174, 184, 185). Importantly, activation of $GABA_B$ receptors facilitated extinction of methamphetamine-induced CPP (152) (**Table 3**). In summary, both $GABA_A$ and $GABA_B$ receptors mediate psychostimulant-induced cognitive deficits. However, further work is required to fully exploit the potential of $GABA_A$ and $GABA_B$ receptors in the treatment of psychostimulant-induced cognitive deficits.

## Glutamate Neurotransmission

Dysregulation in glutamate transmission has been reported after exposure to psychostimulants (174, 186–188). Further, research has shown that both ionotropic and metabotropic glutamate (mGlu) receptors play a role in impulsivity, memory deficits, and extinction of drug-associated memories (189, 190) (**Box 4**).

### NMDA Receptors

Systemically administered GluN2B antagonists Ro 63-1908 and traxoprodil increased premature responses in the 5-CSRTT, suggesting behavioral impulsivity (191). Similarly, systemic administration of NMDA antagonists induced decisional impulsivity as assessed using the DDT [(192, 193); but also see Higgins et al. (191)]. Together, the data suggest that blockade of NMDA-mediated glutamate transmission after systemic administration of NMDA antagonists induced behavioral and decisional impulsivity. However, blockade of NMDA receptors in specific brain regions had a differential effect on behavioral and decisional impulsivity. For example, blockade of NMDA receptors in the infralimbic PFC induced behavioral impulsivity (181). In contrast, blockade of GluN2B-containing NMDA receptors in the NAcc core induced decisional impulsivity in rats (194). Together, these data suggest that NMDA-mediated glutamate transmission in the infralimbic PFC and NAcc core plays a role in behavioral and decisional impulsivity, respectively. The effects of NMDA-antagonists and specifically GluN2B antagonists in psychostimulant-induced impulsivity still need to be assessed.

The role of NMDA-mediated glutamate transmission in learning and memory including extinction learning is well documented (189, 195, 196). Relevant to this review, systemic administration of NMDA antagonist memantine improved amphetamine withdrawal-induced memory deficit as assessed using the novel object recognition test (143) (**Table 3**). Similarly, blockade of NMDA receptors in the NAcc using NMDA antagonist AP-5 improved methamphetamine-induced working memory deficit as measured using the Morris water maze (115) (**Table 1**; **Figure 2**). Interestingly, increasing activity of NMDA-mediated glutamate transmission *via* manipulation of the glycine site facilitated extinction of fear- and cocaine-associated memories (145, 197, 198) (**Table 3**). In addition, increased NMDA-mediated transmission especially *via* GluN2B-containing NMDA receptors facilitated extinction of fear memories (199). Consistent with these findings, increasing glutamate transmission *via* GluN2B-containing NMDA receptors in the infralimbic cortex facilitated extinction of cocaine-associated memory (112) (**Table 1**; **Figure 2**). More recently, it was reported that aquaporin-4 (AQP-4) deletion increased GluN2B-mediated glutamate transmission in the CA3–CA1 hippocampal pathway (200). AQP-4 is the predominant water channel primarily expressed in astrocytes and plays a role in regulating synaptic plasticity. Importantly, deficiency of AQP-4 facilitated fear memory extinction (200). Future work must investigate if AQP-4 may be a potential target for facilitating extinction of psychostimulant drug-associated memories. In summary, NMDA receptors could serve as targets for alleviation of psychostimulant-induced impulsivity and memory deficits. Furthermore, NMDA receptors could be targeted to facilitate extinction of drug-associated memories.

### AMPA Receptors

The AMPA receptors are also involved in extinction learning. For example, AMPA receptor activation facilitated extinction of fear-associated memories (199, 201). Activation of AMPA receptors in the infralimbic PFC facilitated extinction of heroin-associated memories (202). However, the effects of AMPA receptor activation on extinction of psychostimulant-associated memories have not been evaluated. Surface expression of AMPA receptors can be regulated by a process called ubiquitination. Ubiquitination of AMPA receptors results in internalization of AMPA receptors, which indirectly decreases AMPA-mediated glutamate transmission. More recent work has shown that ubiquitination of AMPA receptors is partially regulated by epidermal growth factor receptor substrate 15 (Eps15). Decreased expression of Eps15 resulted in decreased internalization of GluA1-containing AMPA receptors possibly by decreased ubiquitination of GluA1 subunits of the AMPA receptors (204). However, further work is required to determine if knockdown of Eps15 facilitates extinction learning *via* decreased internalization of AMPA receptors. In summary, Eps15 *via* AMPA-mediated glutamate transmission could be a potential target to facilitate extinction learning of psychostimulant-associated memories.

### Metabotropic Glutamate (mGlu) Receptors

Several experimental studies support the role of mGlu receptors in cognitive deficits. For example, blockade of mGlu1 receptors resulted in decisional impulsivity (195). These data suggest that PAMs of the mGlu1 receptors may help to reduce decisional impulsivity, although this hypothesis needs to be experimentally tested in psychostimulant-induced impulsivity. In addition to mGlu1 receptors, mGlu2/3 receptors also mediate behavioral and decisional impulsivity. Pretreatment with the mGlu2/3 agonist LY379268 attenuated 5-HT2A agonist-induced behavioral impulsivity (205). Furthermore, direct injections of mGlu2/3 agonist in the OFC and mPFC attenuated intra-OFC and intra-PFC 5-HT2A agonist-induced decisional and behavioral impulsivity, respectively (172). Moreover, systemic administration of mGlu4 PAM, 4-((*F*)-styryl)-pyrimidin-2-ylamine (Cpd11), induced behavioral impulsivity but decreased decisional impulsivity (206). In contrast to mGlu4 receptors, blockade of mGlu5 receptors, using a mGlu5 negative allosteric modulator (NAM), attenuated behavioral impulsivity (207). In addition, activation of mGlu5 receptors, using a mGlu5 receptor PAM, attenuated NMDA antagonist MK-801-induced behavioral impulsivity. Interestingly, no effects of mGlu5 receptor modulation on decisional impulsivity were observed (207). Importantly, systemic administration of mGlu5 PAM, CDPPB, facilitated extinction of fear- and cocaine-associated memories (148, 149, 208) (**Table 3**). Consistent with these findings, decreased glutamate transmission *via* mGlu1 and mGlu5 receptors in the mPFC facilitated resistance to extinction of cocaine-associated memories in animals with chronic cocaine self-administration experience (209). Taken together, the data suggest that mGlu5 receptors have a role in behavioral impulsivity and can also be targeted to facilitate extinction of psychostimulant-associated memories. Based on the above-described data, mGlu1, mGlu2/3, mGlu4, and mGlu5 receptors can serve as potential targets in psychostimulant-induced impulsivity.

### Drugs That Restore Glutamatergic Tone

As described above, dysregulation in glutamate transmission has been reported after exposure to psychostimulants. Thus, agents that restore glutamatergic tone may help to treat psychostimulant addiction. Administration of riluzole, a pharmacological compound that reestablishes glutamatergic tone, decreased activity of the prelimbic PFC and increased activity of the infralimbic PFC (210). Also, direct injections of riluzole in the amygdala facilitated extinction of fear-associated memories, possibly due to the increase infralimbic PFC activity (211). Importantly, riluzole attenuated reinstatement of cocaine seeking (210). Like riluzole, *N*-acetylcysteine, a cystine–glutamate antiporter that helps restore glutamatergic tone, attenuated reinstatement of cocaine and nicotine seeking (212, 213). *N*-Acetylcysteine also reduced reinstatement of nicotine seeking observed in animals with neonatal ventral hippocampal lesions (80, 214). As described above, animals with neonatal ventral hippocampal lesions show memory deficits and higher nicotine seeking than do controls. It is hypothesized that memory deficits associated with ventral hippocampal lesions are partially responsible for this increased nicotine seeking. Together, the data suggest that *N*-acetylcysteine helps animals overcome memory deficits and thus possibly helps reduce drug seeking. Overall, the above data with riluzole and *N*-acetylcysteine suggest that correcting the dysregulation in glutamate transmission can improve memory deficits and/or facilitate extinction learning. Future work needs to determine if these drugs can facilitate extinction of drug-associated memories. In summary, both ionotropic and metabotropic glutamate receptors are viable targets for treatment of psychostimulant-induced cognitive deficits. However, more work is required to understand glutamate dysregulation in specific brain circuits after psychostimulant exposure to fully exploit the various glutamate targets for treatment of psychostimulant-induced cognitive deficits.

## Nicotinic Acetylcholine Receptors (nAChRs)

The role of nAChRs in impulsive behavior has been discussed previously (215). In humans, polymorphism in the α4 subunits of the nAChRs (CHRNA4) was associated with pathological gambling in Korean gamblers (216). Also, systemic administration of varenicline, a partial agonist of α4β2 nAChRs, induced behavioral impulsivity in animals (217). Importantly, blockade of α4β2 nAChRs in the infralimbic PFC attenuated varenicline-induced behavioral impulsivity, suggesting that the effects of varenicline are mediated by α4β2 nAChRs in the infralimbic PFC (218). Also, intra-cerebroventricular injection of α4β2 nAChR antagonist decreased behavioral impulsivity in animals (219). Together, the data highlight that the role of α4β2 nAChRs in behavioral impulsivity and α4β2 nAChR antagonists may help to alleviate behavioral impulsivity. More recently, compounds that decrease signaling *via* α4β2 nAChRs attenuated cocaine and methamphetamine seeking (220). In addition, systemic administration of partial agonists of the α7-containing nAChRs decreased behavioral impulsivity and improved attention as assessed using the five choice-continuous performance task (5-CCPT) (221). The decrease was specifically observed in female rats that had been classified as animals with low attention at baseline. α7 nAChR agonists have also been shown to improve memory (222, 223). Together, the data suggest a possible role for α4- and α7-containing nAChRs in cognitive deficits such as impulsivity and impairment of memory. However, the role of the different nAChR subunits in psychostimulant-induced cognitive deficits is yet to be evaluated.

## Opioid Receptors

Several lines of evidence support the role of endogenous opioids in impulsive behavior. For example, human imaging studies suggest upregulation of μ opioid receptor (MORs) in the mPFC and OFC in individuals with traits suggestive of impulsivity (223). Further, pathological gamblers, who are known to be impulsive and impaired in making rational decisions, show decreased endogenous opioid release in the brain than do healthy volunteers (224). Consistent with these findings, administration of MOR antagonist decreased pathological gambling (225, 226). MORs and opioid peptides are extensively found in PFC and regulate PFC neuronal activity (227). Activation of MORs in the PFC induced behavioral impulsivity (228). In addition, mice lacking MORs showed markedly decreased behavioral impulsivity (229). In contrast, the same study showed that mice lacking delta opioid receptors (DORs) showed increased behavioral impulsivity. More recently, it was reported that α2 agonist yohimbine-induced increase in behavioral impulsivity was attenuated by blockade of kappa opioid receptors (KORs) (230). Interestingly, KOR activation on its own decreased behavioral impulsivity possibly due to impairment of motor activity. Together, the data from these pharmacological and genetic studies suggest a differential role for MORs, DORs, and KORs in behavioral impulsivity. Further, the data suggest that MOR and KOR antagonists may help to reduce impulsivity.

Chronic cocaine administration is associated with upregulation of MORs and KORs in the PFC (231). Furthermore, upregulation of MORs in the anterior cingulate cortex predicts both severity of craving and relapse in cocaine users (232, 233). Similarly, dysregulation of endogenous opioid neurotransmission occurs after exposure to nicotine (234). However, much work needs to be done in determining the role of MORs, MOR antagonists, and other opioid receptors in psychostimulant-induced cognitive deficits especially impulsivity (**Box 4**). Moreover, most of the research on the role of opioid receptors in impulsivity has focused on the PFC. However, further work must be carried out in other brain regions to determine the role of endogenous opioids in psychostimulant-induced impulsivity.

## Cannabinoid Receptors

The endogenous cannabinoid system is altered after exposure to psychostimulant drugs. For example, exposure to cocaine administration during adolescence increased expression of CB1 receptors and decreased expression of CB2 receptors in the PFC and hippocampus (235). In contrast in adult rats, chronic cocaine self-administration resulted in decreased CB1 and CB2 receptor expression in the PFC, dorsal striatum, and amygdala (236). Further, blockade of CB1 receptors attenuated both cocaine intake and reinstatement of cocaine seeking (237). Importantly, blockade of CB1 receptors prevented cocaine-induced impairment in decisional impulsivity as assessed using the DDT (39) (**Table 2**). In addition, acute administration of CB1 antagonists prior to DDT in cocaine-treated rats reversed cocaine-induced decisional impulsivity. Together, these data support a role for endogenous cannabinoids in both preventing and reversing cocaine-induced impulsivity. Consistent with the findings of this study, activation of CB1 receptors using cannabidiol (CBD) did not improve impulsivity during tobacco abstinence in human smokers (238).

In addition, CB1 receptors located in the amygdala and hippocampus play a role in learning and memory. For example, blockade of CB1 receptors attenuated nicotine withdrawal-induced memory deficits (144) (**Table 3**). Interestingly, the same study also showed that selective deletion of CB1 receptors in the GABA neurons also mitigated nicotine withdrawal-induced memory deficits. Overall, these data suggest that CB1 receptor antagonists may have therapeutic utility in promoting smoking cessation by decreasing memory deficits associated with nicotine withdrawal. Importantly, systemic or intra-mPFC administration of CB1 receptor antagonist rimonabant enhanced extinction of cocaine-associated memories (114) (**Table 1**; **Figure 2**). Together, these data suggest that CB1 receptor antagonists could be potentially used to treat psychostimulant-induced impulsivity and memory impairment (**Box 4**). However, further research is required to fully exploit the potential of the endocannabinoid system as a potential treatment for psychostimulant-induced cognitive deficits.

## Phosphodiesterase Inhibitors

The role of cAMP/protein kinase A/cyclic-AMP response element binding (CREB) protein pathway plays an important role in both memory and reinforcing effects of psychostimulant drugs (239–241). The enzyme phosphodiesterase (PDE) plays a role in breakdown of cAMP and thus indirectly decreases CREB formation. Phosphodiesterase inhibitors, which increase CREB formation, facilitate learning and memory (242). For example, subchronic administration of rolipram, a PDE4 inhibitor, using osmotic pumps facilitated learning of conditioned fear (243). Importantly, more recently it has been reported that rolipram facilitated extinction of fear-associated memory in mice (116). Interestingly, PDE4 inhibitors did not facilitate extinction of cocaine-induced CPP (148) (**Table 3**). However, the same study showed that PDE9 inhibitor BAY-73-6691 facilitated extinction of cocaine-induced CPP (**Table 3**). This effect of PDE9 inhibitor was possibly mediated by an increase in cGMP levels in the hippocampus and amygdala. Further work is required to assess the effects of PDE9 inhibitors and other PDE inhibitors in facilitation of extinction of drug-associated memories. In summary, the various isoforms of the PDE enzyme continue to be viable targets for treatment of psychostimulant addiction.

## Orexin

Orexin neurons (also referred to as hypocretin) are found in the hypothalamus and release the neuropeptides orexin A and orexin B (also referred to as hypocretins 1 and 2) throughout the CNS (244). With its widespread targets, the orexin system is involved in a number of functions including stress, reward, wakefulness, and food seeking (245). The hypocretin/orexin system plays an important role in the reinforcing effects of cocaine. For example, suvorexant, a dual orexin receptor antagonist, attenuated both the rewarding and motivational effects of cocaine (141). Also, knockdown of hypocretin/orexin neurons in the dorsal hypothalamus attenuated cocaine self-administration (246). Further knockdown of orexin 1 receptor in the VTA both altered dopamine signaling in the NAcc and attenuated cocaine-induced increase in NAcc DA (248). The hypocretin/orexin system also plays a role in opioid- and alcohol-dependent behaviors (249, 250).

Increased activation of medial hypothalamic orexin neurons, but not lateral hypothalamic neurons, was reported during a Go/No-Go task involving food reward, suggesting a role for medial hypothalamic orexin neurons in behavioral impulsivity (251). More recently, systemic or intra-VTA administration of suvorexant, a dual orexin receptor antagonist, attenuated cocaine-induced behavioral impulsivity (140) (**Table 2**). Interestingly, neither suvorexant nor orexin 1 (SB334867) nor orexin 2 (TCS-OX2-29) receptor-selective compounds altered decisional impulsivity. Taken together, the data suggest that orexin receptor antagonists may be useful in reducing psychostimulant-induced behavioral impulsivity.

The hypocretin/orexin receptors are also found in brain regions that play a role in memory especially the hippocampus. Administration of orexin peptides increased firing of hippocampal neurons and facilitated learning and memory (252–256). The orexin-induced facilitation of learning is mediated by increasing neurogenesis in the hippocampus (257). The hypocretin/orexin system also plays a role in extinction learning. For example, blockade of orexin 1 receptor facilitated extinction of fear-associated memories possibly by increasing amygdalar input to the infralimbic PFC during extinction learning (258). However, the role of the orexin system in facilitation of extinction of drug-associated memories has not been explored. In summary, blocking orexin-mediated signaling decreased behavioral impulsivity and facilitated extinction learning (**Box 4**). The hypocretin/orexin system is a very promising target, but further work is required to fully exploit the orexin system for the treatment of psychostimulant-induced cognitive deficits.

## Brain-Derived Neurotrophic Factor (BDNF)

BDNF, a neurotrophin, is extensively distributed in the brain (259). BDNF plays a role in psychostimulant-induced behavioral effects. Inhibition of BDNF signaling and/or decreased expression of BDNF attenuated the rewarding effects of cocaine and cocaine-seeking behaviors (260–262). Methamphetamine withdrawal was associated with elevated BDNF levels in the dorsal striatum (263). In addition, genetically induced depletion of BDNF expression resulted in social cognitive deficits after chronic methamphetamine treatment compared with controls (264). Impaired BDNF signaling in the frontal and striatal regions during nicotine withdrawal was also associated with cognitive deficits (265). Together, the data suggest that decreased BDNF signaling possibly mediates psychostimulant-induced cognitive deficits.

Importantly, increase in BDNF signaling plays a role in consolidation of both recognition and spatial memory (266). Intracerebroventicular injection of antibodies to BDNF attenuated spatial learning in rats (267). Increase in BDNF signaling was also associated with extinction of fear-associated memories (268, 269). Interestingly, infusing BDNF into the ventral hippocampus increased the firing rate of neurons in the infralimbic PFC, which plays an important role in extinction learning (270). Importantly, increased BDNF signaling *via* stimulating tropomyosin-related kinase B (Trk B) receptors in the infralimbic PFC facilitated extinction of cocaine-induced CPP (112) (**Table 1; Figure 2**). Also, the study showed that systemic administration of Trk B receptor agonist facilitated extinction of cocaine-associated memories (**Table 3**). Overall, receptors mediating BDNF signaling are promising targets for facilitation of extinction of drug-associated memories and could be used for advancing treatment of psychostimulant addiction (**Box 4**). However, further work is required to understand BDNF signaling in specific circuits to maximally exploit its receptors as a therapeutic target.

## Corticotrophin Releasing Factor (CRF) Receptors

The role of CRF receptors in the behavioral and rewarding effects of psychostimulants has been previously reviewed (271–273). Blockade of CRF1 and CRF2 receptors in the VTA attenuated the reinforcing effects of cocaine (274). Interestingly, the rewarding effects of cocaine were enhanced in mice lacking CRF1 receptors compared with wild-type controls (275). Importantly, chronic cocaine administration induced memory deficits in wild-type mice but not in CRF1 deficient mice (276). In addition, cocaine withdrawal-induced memory deficits were observed in CRF2-deficient mice compared with wild-type controls (277). These data suggest that CRF receptors mediate cocaine withdrawal-induced impairment of memory and other cocaine-dependent effects.

CRF receptors are extensively distributed in brain regions that play a role in learning and memory (278). Blockade of CRF receptors, using CRF antagonist D-Phe-CRF, improved cognitive performance (279). Further, the study also showed that blockade of CRF1 receptors using CRF1 selective antagonist NBI 35965 improved memory in PFC-dependent tasks. Taken together, the data suggest that CRF receptors can be targeted to alleviate psychostimulant-induced memory deficits.

Importantly, CRF receptors in the VTA play a role in reinstatement of cocaine seeking (280). In addition, the same study showed that after cocaine self-administration and extinction training, stimulation of CRF2 receptors in brain slices resulted in increased glutamate release and decreased GABA release as compared in cocaine-naïve animals. These data suggest that extinction training and cocaine exposure altered CRF2-mediated transmission. Importantly, infusions of the CRF receptor antagonist α-helical CRF(9-41) into the basolateral amygdala enhanced extinction of fear-associated memories (281). However, further work needs to be carried out to determine if CRF receptors play a role in extinction of psychostimulant drug-associated memories. In summary, CRF receptors could serve as a potential target to alleviate psychostimulant-induced memory deficits and/or promote extinction of drug-associated memories.

# NON-PHARMACOLOGICAL APPROACHES FOR TREATMENT OF PSYCHOSTIMULANT-INDUCED COGNITIVE DEFICITS

## Brain Stimulation

Brain stimulation can be achieved using a variety of different approaches such as transcranial magnetic stimulation, deep brain stimulation (DBS) using intracranial electrodes, transcranial direct current stimulation, and vagus nerve stimulation (282). Evidence from both human and animal studies supports use of brain stimulation to ameliorate cognitive deficits and improve learning and memory. For example, in humans, increase in verbal working memory accuracy was observed following transcranial magnetic stimulation (283). Similarly, DBS of the ventromedial PFC resulted in improvement in novel object recognition memory compared with that in controls in animals (284). Intracranial DBS also improved spatial memory in rats as assessed using the Morris water maze task (285). Also, DBS facilitated extinction of fear-associated memories (286, 287).

More importantly, DBS using intracranial electrodes attenuated reinstatement of cocaine seeking (288). Also, low-frequency DBS, but not high-frequency DBS, of the ventral striatum strengthened extinction of morphine-associated memories in rats (289). In addition, low-frequency stimulation of the ventral striatum was accompanied by an increase in immediate early gene c-fos synthesis in brain regions associated with extinction such as the infralimbic PFC and amygdala, suggesting increased activity of these regions. Importantly, vagal nerve stimulation during extinction training improved rates of extinction and reduced reinstatement of cocaine seeking in rats (151) (**Table 3**). Interestingly, DBS of subthalamic nucleus and vagal nerve stimulation also helped in decreasing decisional impulsivity in "risk preferring" rats compared with controls (290, 291).

Together, these data suggest that brain stimulation can help in both decreasing impulsivity and facilitating extinction of psychostimulant-associated memories. Thus, brain stimulation has the potential to alleviate multiple cognitive deficits. Future work must focus on identifying precise neural substrates and brain stimulation parameters to fully exploit the benefits of brain stimulation in psychostimulant addiction treatment. Furthermore, identification of pharmacological compounds that will help in improving efficacy of brain stimulation in addiction treatment will also be very useful.

### Exercise

Exercise in animals influences psychostimulant-dependent behavioral effects. For example, exercise attenuated reinstatement of cocaine seeking after a period of abstinence (292, 293). In addition, reinstatement of cocaine seeking in high impulsive rats was attenuated when animals were treated with a combination of atomoxetine and exercise during withdrawal from cocaine compared with either treatment alone (294). Importantly, post-extinction exercise training was more effective than extinction alone in attenuating reinstatement of cocaine seeking (295).

Exercise in the form of wheel running and swimming has been shown to improve learning and memory (296). Consistent with these findings, exercise using a treadmill attenuated morphine withdrawal-induced memory deficit in rats (297). Also, exercise facilitated extinction of fear-associated memories (298, 299). However, it is not known if exercise facilitates extinction of psychostimulant-associated drug memories. Further, effects of exercise on amelioration of psychostimulant withdrawal-associated memory deficits have not been explored. Several questions such as intensity and duration of exercise, neural changes as a consequence of exercise, and optimal combination of exercise with pharmacological medications need to be determined to use exercise most efficaciously as a tool for psychostimulant addiction treatment.

### Promoting Neurogenesis

Psychostimulant exposure impairs neurogenesis in the hippocampus in adult animals. For example, chronic exposure to nicotine, methamphetamine, and cocaine altered/blunted neurogenesis in the hippocampus (300–303). In addition, cocaine withdrawal-induced memory deficits were associated with blunted neurogenesis in the hippocampus (304). Hippocampal neurogenesis has been shown to play a role in consolidation of memory (305). Also, disruption of adult hippocampal neurogenesis impaired short- and long-term memory formation (306).

Relevant to this review, enhancing neurogenesis facilitated extinction of fear-associated memories (307, 308). Furthermore, pharmacological facilitation of neurogenesis facilitated extinction of morphine-associated memory (309). Importantly, increasing hippocampal neurogenesis in adult animals using chronic intracerebroventricular infusions of lysophosphatidic acid (LPA; an endogenous lysophospholipid with pro-neurogenesis effects) facilitated extinction of cocaine-associated memories (310). In contrast, suppression of neurogenesis using cranial irradiation resulted in resistance to extinction of cocaine seeking (311). Together, the above data suggest that pharmacological manipulation of adult hippocampal neurogenesis could facilitate extinction of drug-associated memories (**Box 4**). In summary, promoting neurogenesis can serve as an important strategy to treat psychostimulant addiction. However, future research must focus on understanding cellular mechanisms that underlie psychostimulant-induced impairment of hippocampal neurogenesis and identify pathways that can promote neurogenesis. Together, both of the above-described approaches will help to effectively treat psychostimulant-induced cognitive deficits.

## FUTURE DIRECTIONS

### Ghrelin

Ghrelin is an orexigenic peptide hormone acting on receptors in both the brain and periphery (312). Modulation of ghrelin altered effects of psychostimulants. For example, administration of ghrelin enhanced the rewarding effects of cocaine (313). Consistent with these findings, blockade of ghrelin-mediated transmission attenuated behavioral effects of cocaine, amphetamine, and nicotine (314, 315). In cocaine-experienced animals, during early withdrawal, ghrelin levels were elevated possibly in anticipation of cocaine (316). Similarly, in abstinent smokers, elevated ghrelin levels were associated with increased craving and relapse (317).

More importantly, ghrelin is neuroprotective, promotes hippocampal neurogenesis, and enhances learning and memory (318–320). Elevation of ghrelin levels as a consequence of food deprivation facilitated extinction of fear-associated memories, possibly by inhibition of long-term depression in the lateral amygdala (321). Consistent with these findings, a human clinical study reported facilitated extinction of fear-associated memories in subjects that had increased ghrelin levels as a result of overnight fasting (322). Based on these data, it is hypothesized here that increasing ghrelin-mediated signaling during extinction training may facilitate extinction of drug-associated memories. However, experimental data supporting this hypothesis are currently lacking. Besides, the precise mechanism of how ghrelin facilitates learning still needs to be explored. Nevertheless, there exists strong rationale for assessing the effects of ghrelin in extinction of drug-associated memories. Finally, based on the above data, it appears that elevated ghrelin levels are associated with craving in abstinent drug-dependent individuals, facilitation of extinction learning, and neuroprotection/neurogenesis. It is possible that ghrelin in different brain regions may have a differential role. Future work may need to understand the role of ghrelin in specific brain circuitries to fully exploit the therapeutic potential of ghrelin.

## Oxytocin

Oxytocin is synthesized by hypothalamic nuclei such as the supraoptic, parvocellular, and accessory nuclei. Oxytocin-containing neurons from these nuclei primarily project to posterior pituitary, but they also innervate brain regions mediating reward and emotion such as the PFC and amygdala (323). Systemic administration of oxytocin attenuated reinstatement of cocaine and methamphetamine seeking (324, 325). Consistent with this study, direct injection of oxytocin in the NAcc attenuated methamphetamine-induced CPP (326). Together, these data suggest that activation of oxytocin receptors attenuated drug-associated memories. Additionally, cocaine withdrawal was associated with increased oxytocin receptor binding in the piriform cortex, lateral septum, and amygdala (327).

Oxytocin receptors are extensively found in the PFC (328). Interestingly, activation of oxytocin receptors in the infralimbic PFC facilitated extinction of fear-associated memories (329, 330). Further social cues, such as presence of an animal, during extinction learning increased PFC oxytocin transmission (330). Overall, the data suggest that oxytocin receptor activation in the PFC facilitated extinction learning. However, the effects of increased oxytocin transmission on extinction of drug-associated memories have not been investigated. Together, these findings suggest that changes in oxytocin transmission may mediate some of the emotional and cognitive deficits associated with cocaine use. Based on the above-described findings, oxytocin receptors may serve as useful targets for the treatment of psychostimulant addiction, especially in promoting extinction of drug-associated memories (**Box 4**).

## Vasopressin

Vasopressin and its receptors play a role in psychostimulant-dependent behavioral effects. For example, elevated levels of vasopressin mRNA in the amygdala were observed in animals during withdrawal from cocaine (331). Additionally, blockade of vasopressin 1a receptors in the NAcc during conditioning attenuated expression of cocaine-induced CPP. Blockade of vasopressin 1b receptor also attenuated reinstatement of methamphetamine-induced CPP (332). Finally, blockade of vasopressin 1a receptors reversed oxytocin-induced attenuation of reinstatement of methamphetamine seeking (325). Together, the above evidence suggests a role for vasopressin in cocaine- and methamphetamine-dependent behavioral effects.

Vasopressin neurons and receptors are extensively found in brain regions involved in learning and memory such as the hippocampus, PFC, and amygdala (333–335). Knockout of vasopressin 1b receptor impaired hippocampal-dependent memory tasks (336). Vasopressin also plays an important role in social memory (337). Furthermore, blockade of vasopressin 1b receptor attenuated stress-induced impairment of memory (338). Elevated levels of vasopressin mRNA in the amygdala were also reported in animals showing high predisposition to stress-induced reinstatement of heroin seeking (339). A recent study has suggested that vasopressin may be involved in risky behaviors in humans, which suggest that it may have a role in impulsivity (340). In summary, the above data suggest that vasopressin-mediated neurotransmission is involved in memory and drug-dependent effects. Although still early, vasopressin receptors may serve as targets for treatment of psychostimulant-induced cognitive deficits.

## Protein Kinase Cε

PKCε is extensively found in the brain and is a downstream mediator of G-protein receptor signaling (341). Recent studies suggest that PKCε possibly mediates the reinforcing effects of psychostimulants like nicotine and cocaine. For example, mice lacking PKCε showed reduced mRNA levels of α6 and β3 nAChR subunits in brain regions associated with drug reward such as the VTA and striatum (342). Consistent with these findings, knockout of PKCε reduced nicotine-induced CPP and attenuated nicotine self-administration compared with wild-type controls. Relevant to this review, the infralimbic PFC showed elevated levels of PKCε after with withdrawal from extended cocaine self-administration experience (343). More importantly, inhibition of PKCε in the infralimbic PFC attenuated reinstatement of cocaine seeking. However, the effects of PKCε expression in the infralimbic PFC on extinction learning have not been assessed.

Activation of PKCε facilitates learning and memory (344, 345). In fact, inhibition of PKCε using peptides that directly bind to PKCε attenuated recognition memory as assessed using novel object recognition task (345). It is postulated that the memory-enhancing effects of PKCε activation are mediated *via* increased activity of ERK1/2 in the hippocampus. Together, the above data suggest that activation of PKCε could be useful in facilitating extinction of drug-associated memories. Based on the role of PKCε in memory and cocaine-dependent behaviors, it is hypothesized that PKCε may be an attractive target for treating psychostimulant addiction by promoting extinction learning.

## Peroxisome Proliferator-Activated Receptor γ (PPARγ) Receptors and Insulin

Insulin and PPARγ agonists influence the behavioral and psychological effects of drugs of abuse. For example, a recent double-blind randomized study reported that patients receiving PPARγ agonist pioglitazone compared with placebo reduced cocaine craving and improved brain white matter integrity in cocaine-dependent patients (346). In animals with cocaine self-administration experience, insulin levels were reduced by approximately 40–70% during cocaine self-administration (316). In addition, intra-VTA injections of insulin attenuated cocaine-induced increase in NAcc dopamine and decreased cocaine-induced increase in locomotor activity (347).

Additionally, insulin and PPARγ agonists play a role in alleviating memory deficits. For example, systemic administration of insulin and insulin-growth factor 2 (IGF-2) facilitated learning and memory (348, 349). Additionally, intranasal insulin administration improved memory in patients with either mild cognitive impairment or early Alzheimer's disease (350). Further, PPARγ agonists improved memory in some humans with early Alzheimer's disease (351). These memory-enhancing effects of PPARγ agonists are possibly mediated by actions of PPARγ agonists on hippocampal dentate neurons (352, 353). In summary, both insulin and PPARγ play a role in cognition and memory and could influence the behavioral effects of psychostimulants.

Importantly, PPARγ agonist pioglitazone attenuated alcohol-induced spatial memory deficit as assessed using the Morris water maze (354). Additionally, pioglitazone attenuated drug-induced heroin seeking (355). Finally, increased IGF-2-mediated transmission in the hippocampus facilitated extinction of fear-associated memories (356). It is hypothesized that this IGF-2-mediated facilitation of extinction occurs *via* stimulation of neurogenesis (357). However, it is not known if insulin and PPARγ agonists could facilitate extinction of drug-associated memories? Could insulin and PPARγ agonists be used to ameliorate psychostimulant withdrawal-induced memory impairment? Future work will need to address these and other questions.

## Enzymes Involved in Epigenetic Changes

Epigenetic changes occur as a consequence of behavioral activity, learning, and/or drug exposure (358). In fact, enzymes involved in epigenetic DNA changes are involved in psychostimulant and non-psychostimulant drug-associated memories. For example, DNA methylation *via* chronic L-methionine (MET) attenuated reinstatement of cocaine seeking (359). Also, knockdown of histone methyltransferase PR containing domain 2 (PRDM2) in the dorsomedial PFC using viral vectors enhanced stress-induced reinstatement of alcohol seeking (360). Genetically induced loss of histone acetyltransferase CREB-binding protein (CBP) in the NAcc attenuated cocaine-induced CPP.

Activity-dependent epigenetic changes play an important role in learning and memory consolidation (361). Importantly, the enzymes that mediate these epigenetic changes could be targeted to facilitate learning and memory. For example, blocking of histone deacetylase (HDAC3) enzyme activity in the dorsal hippocampus enhanced long-term memory for object location (114). Additionally, manipulation of enzymes involved in epigenetic changes facilitated extinction learning. For example, inhibition of histone acetyltransferase (HAT) p300 enzyme, which is highly expressed in pyramidal neurons of the infralimbic PFC, facilitated extinction of fear-associated memories (362). Importantly, blocking of HDAC3 deacetylase activity in the dorsal hippocampus, but not the infralimbic PFC, facilitated extinction of cocaine-associated memories (114) (**Table 1; Figure 2**). Overall, these data suggest that enzymes involved in epigenetic changes could play a role in facilitation of extinction of psychostimulant-associated memories. More generally, they could also play a role in the treatment of cognitive deficits associated with psychostimulants such as impulsivity and memory impairments. However, much work remains to not only identify specific enzymes but also to identify specific brain regions where these enzymes are actively involved in psychostimulant-induced cognitive deficits.

## MicroRNAs (miRs)

The role of non-coding microRNAs (miRs) has been implicated in psychostimulant-dependent behaviors. For example, methyl CpG binding protein 2 (MeCP2) and miR-212 in the dorsal striatum play a role in regulating escalation of cocaine intake in rats with extended access to cocaine (363). Further, upregulation of miR-212 and miR-132 in the dorsal striatum persisted for approximately 10 days after withdrawal of cocaine (364). Similarly, miR-496-3p, miR-194-5p, miR-200b-3p, and miR-181a-5p were upregulated significantly following methamphetamine exposure (365). Together, the data suggest that exposure to psychostimulants alters expression of microRNAs.

The role of non-coding miRs has been implicated in cognitive processes such as impulsivity, learning, and memory. For example, several miRs in the amygdala such as miR-190b, miR-28a, miR-340, miR-219a, and miR-491 have been reported to correlate with inhibitory control (366). Thus, theoretically decreased expression of these miRs could result in impulsive behaviors, although direct experimental evidence for this hypothesis is currently lacking. Similarly, miR-641, which binds to SNAP-25 gene, has been implicated in impulsive behaviors (367). In addition, miR-183-96-182 has been associated with comorbid ADHD and drug addiction (368). Together, these data suggest that miRs play a role in regulating impulsive behavioral traits.

miRs also play a role in memory (369). For example, inhibition of miR-9-3p resulted in deficits in hippocampal-dependent tasks (370). Overexpression of miR-144-3p in the basolateral amygdala facilitated extinction of fear-associated memories in C57BL/6 mice (371). In addition, the same study showed that overexpression of miR-144-3p in the basolateral amygdala rescued extinction of fear memories in S1 mice, which show resistance to extinction of fear memories. Similarly, extinction training after fear conditioning trials resulted in increase in expression of miR-128b in the infralimbic PFC, and overexpression of miR-128b in the infralimbic PFC facilitated extinction of fear-associated memories (372). Importantly, significant increases in the expression of miR-101b, miR-137, miR-212, and miR-132 in NAcc shell and miR-137 in the dorsal striatum were observed after extinction training and reinstatement of cocaine seeking in rats (373). Future studies must focus on brain regions associated with extinction learning such as the basolateral amygdala and infralimbic PFC to identify miRs that are involved in extinction of drug-associated memories. Although currently data are lacking, based on the above data, non-coding miRs could be targeted to facilitate extinction of drug-associated memories and to reduce psychostimulant-associated impulsivity.

## Gender and Sex Gonadal Hormones

Both gender and sex gonadal hormones influence cognition. For example, behavioral impulsivity was greater in males compared with females (374). In contrast, females compared with males showed more decisional impulsivity, preferring small immediate rewards compared with larger delayed rewards. Treatment with progesterone attenuated decisional impulsivity for food reward in both males and females (375). Interestingly, progesterone alone attenuated both behavioral and decisional impulsivity for cocaine rewards in female but not male rats (141, 142) (**Table 2**). These data suggest that sex gonadal hormones influence impulsive behaviors. Also, amphetamine worsened impulsive behavior in females compared with males (376). Together, the above data suggest that gender and sex gonadal hormones influence psychostimulant-induced impulsive behaviors.

With respect to extinction of fear-associated memories, differential electrophysiological responses in the infralimbic and prelimbic PFC have been reported between males and females. For example, female rats compared with male rats showed persistent activity in the prelimbic PFC during extinction training, and there was lack of activity in the infralimbic PFC during extinction recall (377). Additionally, the role of estrogen and progesterone in extinction of fear-associated memories has been evaluated. In ovariectomized female rats, estrogen alone or in combination with progesterone facilitated extinction of fear-associated memories (378). Several other studies support the role of estrogen in extinction of fear-associated memories (379, 380). Together, the data suggest that gender and sex gonadal hormones may influence extinction learning.

Gender and sex gonadal hormones also influence psychostimulant drug-associated memories. Extinction of cocaine-induced CPP took longer in male compared with female adolescent rats (110). More recent work has shown that after similar extinction training, context-induced reinstatement of methamphetamine seeking was more pronounced in male compared with female rats (381). Further, the study showed that this difference in methamphetamine seeking between male and female rats was possibly mediated by differential plasticity in the dentate gyrus in the hippocampus. Together, the data suggest differential gender-dependent responses to extinction of psychostimulant drug-associated memories. Treatment with 17β estradiol compared with controls facilitated extinction of cocaine-induced CPP in female rats (150) (**Table 3**). Allopregnanolone, a steroid synthesized from progesterone, attenuated reinstatement of drug-induced cocaine seeking in female but not male rats (382). Allopregnanolone also attenuated reinstatement of cocaine seeking in low impulsive female rats but not in high impulsive female rats, classified as such on baseline performance prior to cocaine exposure (383). However, further studies are required to fully exploit the role of estrogen and progesterone in facilitation of extinction of psychostimulant drug-associated memories. In summary, the above data suggest that gender and sex-gonadal hormones could play an important role in cognitive deficits associated with psychostimulant drugs. However, further work is required to develop more efficacious gender-based treatments for cognitive deficits in human drug-dependent subjects.

## CONCLUSION

Addiction to psychostimulant drugs continues to be a challenge, and current treatment options available for psychostimulant addiction are not adequate. Targeting cognitive deficits in patients dependent on psychostimulants provides an excellent opportunity to improve retention and clinical outcomes of addiction treatment programs. Cognitive deficits should especially be targeted in psychostimulant-dependent patients with a history of prenatal drug exposure and patients with comorbid psychiatric disorders known to be associated with cognitive deficits. In this review, several neural substrates mediating psychostimulant-induced cognitive deficits and identified using preclinical animal models have been discussed. It remains to be seen if these could be translated into viable pharmacological targets for medications to be used in humans to improve clinical outcomes of patients dependent on drugs of abuse. However, the main question is which of the described targets would be most ideal to carry forward into the clinic. Among the various targets described, it will be important to focus on targets that could help alleviate multiple psychostimulant-induced cognitive deficits such as impulsivity and memory impairment (e.g., orexin and cannabinoid receptors). Further, drugs that facilitate/strengthen extinction of drug-associated memories should be an essential strategy of addiction treatment programs.

Future studies must focus on identifying specific circuits mediating psychostimulant-induced cognitive deficits. Better understanding of the role of non-coding miRs, neurogenesis, and enzymes involved in epigenetic changes will greatly help in developing highly selective treatments. Finally, combining non-pharmacological strategies such as brain stimulation and exercise with pharmacological compounds will enhance alleviation of psychostimulant-induced cognitive deficits. In this review, the focus has been on targeting specific psychostimulant-induced cognitive deficits such as impulsivity and impairment of learning/memory. However, psychostimulant-induced cognitive deficits include other deficits such as impairment in attention, lack of cognitive flexibility, and impaired decision making, which have not been discussed in this review but need to be therapeutically addressed. In conclusion, a multipronged strategy targeting behavioral, emotional, and cognitive deficits in recovering abstinent addicts will greatly improve outcomes of psychostimulant addiction treatment.

## AUTHOR CONTRIBUTIONS

This paper was conceived, researched, and written by MD'S.

## REFERENCES

1. S.A.M.H.S.A. *Key substance use and mental health indicators in the United States: results from the 2017 National Survey on Drug Use and Health* (ed). Hhs. Rockville, MD: Center for Behavioral Health Statistics and Quality, Substance Abuse and Mental Health Services Administration (2018).

2. Johnson M, Pennington N. Adolescent use of electronic cigarettes: an emergent health concern for pediatric nurses. *J Pediatr Nurs* (2015) 30:611–5. doi: 10.1016/j.pedn.2014.11.006
3. Koob GF, Ahmed SH, Boutrel B, Chen SA, Kenny PJ, Markou A, et al. Neurobiological mechanisms in the transition from drug use to drug dependence. *Neurosci Biobehav Rev* (2004) 27:739–49. doi: 10.1016/j.neubiorev.2003.11.007
4. Everitt BJ, Robbins TW. Drug addiction: updating actions to habits to compulsions ten years on. *Annu Rev Psychol* (2016) 67:23–50. doi: 10.1146/annurev-psych-122414-033457
5. Koob GF, Volkow ND. Neurocircuitry of addiction. *Neuropsychopharmacology* (2010) 35:217–38. doi: 10.1038/npp.2009.110
6. Phillips KA, Epstein DH, Preston KL. Psychostimulant addiction treatment. *Neuropharmacology* (2014) 87:150–60. doi: 10.1016/j.neuropharm.2014.04.002
7. D'souza MS, Markou A. Neuronal mechanisms underlying development of nicotine dependence: implications for novel smoking-cessation treatments. *Addict Sci Clin Pract* (2011) 6:4–16.
8. Prochaska JJ, Benowitz NL. The past, present, and future of nicotine addiction therapy. *Annu Rev Med* (2016) 67:467–86. doi: 10.1146/annurev-med-111314-033712
9. An H, He RH, Zheng YR, Tao R. Cognitive-behavioral therapy. *Adv Exp Med Biol* (2017) 1010:321–9. doi: 10.1007/978-981-10-5562-1_16
10. Stevens L, Verdejo-Garcia A, Goudriaan AE, Roeyers H, Dom G, Vanderplasschen W. Impulsivity as a vulnerability factor for poor addiction treatment outcomes: a review of neurocognitive findings among individuals with substance use disorders. *J Subst Abuse Treat* (2014) 47:58–72. doi: 10.1016/j.jsat.2014.01.008
11. Stevens L, Verdejo-Garcia A, Roeyers H, Goudriaan AE, Vanderplasschen W. Delay discounting, treatment motivation and treatment retention among substance-dependent individuals attending an in inpatient detoxification program. *J Subst Abuse Treat* (2015) 49:58–64. doi: 10.1016/j.jsat.2014.08.007
12. Dominguez-Salas S, Diaz-Batanero C, Lozano-Rojas OM, Verdejo-Garcia A. Impact of general cognition and executive function deficits on addiction treatment outcomes: systematic review and discussion of neurocognitive pathways. *Neurosci Biobehav Rev* (2016) 71:772–801. doi: 10.1016/j.neubiorev.2016.09.030
13. Mizoguchi H, Yamada K. Methamphetamine use causes cognitive impairment and altered decision-making. *Neurochem Int* (2019) 124:106–13. doi: 10.1016/j.neuint.2018.12.019
14. Khantzian EJ. The self-medication hypothesis of addictive disorders: focus on heroin and cocaine dependence. *Am J Psychiatry* (1985) 142:1259–64. doi: 10.1176/ajp.142.11.1259
15. D'souza MS, Markou A. Neural substrates of psychostimulant withdrawal-induced anhedonia. *Curr Top Behav Neurosci* (2010) 3:119–78. doi: 10.1007/7854_2009_20
16. Bell RP, Garavan H, Foxe JJ. Neural correlates of craving and impulsivity in abstinent former cocaine users: towards biomarkers of relapse risk. *Neuropharmacology* (2014) 85:461–70. doi: 10.1016/j.neuropharm.2014.05.011
17. Eysenck SB, Eysenck HJ. The place of impulsiveness in a dimensional system of personality description. *Br J Soc Clin Psychol* (1977) 16:57–68. doi: 10.1111/j.2044-8260.1977.tb01003.x
18. Aron AR. The neural basis of inhibition in cognitive control. *Neuroscientist* (2007) 13:214–28. doi: 10.1177/1073858407299288
19. Dalley JW, Robbins TW. Fractionating impulsivity: neuropsychiatric implications. *Nat Rev Neurosci* (2017) 18:158–71. doi: 10.1038/nrn.2017.8
20. Harris M, Penfold RB, Hawkins A, Maccombs J, Wallace B, Reynolds B. Dimensions of impulsive behavior and treatment outcomes for adolescent smokers. *Exp Clin Psychopharmacol* (2014) 22:57–64. doi: 10.1037/a0034403
21. Potvin S, Stavro K, Rizkallah E, Pelletier J. Cocaine and cognition: a systematic quantitative review. *J Addict Med* (2014) 8:368–76. doi: 10.1097/ADM.0000000000000066
22. Smith JL, Mattick RP, Jamadar SD, Iredale JM. Deficits in behavioural inhibition in substance abuse and addiction: a meta-analysis. *Drug Alcohol Depend* (2014) 145:1–33. doi: 10.1016/j.drugalcdep.2014.08.009
23. Jones HW, Dean AC, Price KA, London ED. Increased self-reported impulsivity in methamphetamine users maintaining drug abstinence. *Am J Drug Alcohol Abuse* (2016) 42:500–6. doi: 10.1080/00952990.2016.1192639
24. Hess ARB, Menezes CB, De Almeida RMM. Inhibitory control and impulsivity levels in women crack users. *Subst Use Misuse* (2018) 53:972–9. doi: 10.1080/10826084.2017.1387568
25. Kale D, Stautz K, Cooper A. Impulsivity related personality traits and cigarette smoking in adults: a meta-analysis using the UPPS-P model of impulsivity and reward sensitivity. *Drug Alcohol Depend* (2018) 185:149–67. doi: 10.1016/j.drugalcdep.2018.01.003
26. Mashhoon Y, Betts J, Farmer SL, Lukas SE. Early onset tobacco cigarette smokers exhibit deficits in response inhibition and sustained attention. *Drug Alcohol Depend* (2018) 184:48–56. doi: 10.1016/j.drugalcdep.2017.11.020
27. Moallem NR, Courtney KE, Ray LA. The relationship between impulsivity and methamphetamine use severity in a community sample. *Drug Alcohol Depend* (2018) 187:1–7. doi: 10.1016/j.drugalcdep.2018.01.034
28. Schulte MHJ, Kaag AM, Wiers RW, Schmaal L, Van Den Brink W, Reneman L, et al. Prefrontal Glx and GABA concentrations and impulsivity in cigarette smokers and smoking polysubstance users. *Drug Alcohol Depend* (2017) 179:117–23. doi: 10.1016/j.drugalcdep.2017.06.025
29. Martin CA, Kelly TH, Rayens MK, Brogli BR, Brenzel A, Smith WJ, et al. Sensation seeking, puberty, and nicotine, alcohol, and marijuana use in adolescence. *J Am Acad Child Adolesc Psychiatry* (2002) 41:1495–502. doi: 10.1097/00004583-200212000-00022
30. Moeller FG, Barratt ES, Fischer CJ, Dougherty DM, Reilly EL, Mathias CW, et al. P300 event-related potential amplitude and impulsivity in cocaine-dependent subjects. *Neuropsychobiology* (2004) 50:167–73. doi: 10.1159/000079110
31. Verdejo-Garcia AJ, Perales JC, Perez-Garcia M. Cognitive impulsivity in cocaine and heroin polysubstance abusers. *Addict Behav* (2007) 32:950–66. doi: 10.1016/j.addbeh.2006.06.032
32. Verdejo-Garcia A, Lawrence AJ, Clark L. Impulsivity as a vulnerability marker for substance-use disorders: review of findings from high-risk research, problem gamblers and genetic association studies. *Neurosci Biobehav Rev* (2008) 32:777–810. doi: 10.1016/j.neubiorev.2007.11.003
33. Albein-Urios N, Martinez-Gonzalez JM, Lozano O, Clark L, Verdejo-Garcia A. Comparison of impulsivity and working memory in cocaine addiction and pathological gambling: implications for cocaine-induced neurotoxicity. *Drug Alcohol Depend* (2012) 126:1–6. doi: 10.1016/j.drugalcdep.2012.03.008
34. Moreno-Lopez L, Catena A, Fernandez-Serrano MJ, Delgado-Rico E, Stamatakis EA, Perez-Garcia M, et al. Trait impulsivity and prefrontal gray matter reductions in cocaine dependent individuals. *Drug Alcohol Depend* (2012) 125:208–14. doi: 10.1016/j.drugalcdep.2012.02.012
35. Kirkpatrick MG, Johanson CE, De Wit H. Personality and the acute subjective effects of d-amphetamine in humans. *J Psychopharmacol* (2013) 27:256–64. doi: 10.1177/0269881112472564
36. Van Wel JH, Spronk DB, Kuypers KP, Theunissen EL, Toennes SW, Verkes RJ, et al. Psychedelic symptoms of cannabis and cocaine use as a function of trait impulsivity. *J Psychopharmacol* (2015) 29:324–34. doi: 10.1177/0269881114563633
37. Cervantes MC, Laughlin RE, Jentsch JD. Cocaine self-administration behavior in inbred mouse lines segregating different capacities for inhibitory control. *Psychopharmacology (Berl)* (2013) 229:515–25. doi: 10.1007/s00213-013-3135-4
38. Ferland JN, Winstanley CA. Risk-preferring rats make worse decisions and show increased incubation of craving after cocaine self-administration. *Addict Biol* (2017) 22:991–1001. doi: 10.1111/adb.12388
39. Hernandez G, Oleson EB, Gentry RN, Abbas Z, Bernstein DL, Arvanitogiannis A, et al. Endocannabinoids promote cocaine-induced impulsivity and its rapid dopaminergic correlates. *Biol Psychiatry* (2014) 75:487–98. doi: 10.1016/j.biopsych.2013.09.005
40. Kayir H, Semenova S, Markou A. Baseline impulsive choice predicts the effects of nicotine and nicotine withdrawal on impulsivity in rats. *Prog Neuropsychopharmacol Biol Psychiatry* (2014) 48:6–13. doi: 10.1016/j.pnpbp.2013.09.007
41. Kolokotroni KZ, Rodgers RJ, Harrison AA. Trait differences in response to chronic nicotine and nicotine withdrawal in rats. *Psychopharmacology (Berl)* (2014) 231:567–80. doi: 10.1007/s00213-013-3270-y
42. Furlong TM, Leavitt LS, Keefe KA, Son JH. Methamphetamine-, d-amphetamine-, and *p*-chloroamphetamine-induced neurotoxicity differentially effect impulsive responding on the stop-signal task in rats. *Neurotox Res* (2016) 29:569–82. doi: 10.1007/s12640-016-9605-9

43. Broos N, Van Mourik Y, Schetters D, De Vries TJ, Pattij T. Dissociable effects of cocaine and yohimbine on impulsive action and relapse to cocaine seeking. *Psychopharmacology (Berl)* (2017) 234:3343–51. doi: 10.1007/s00213-017-4711-9
44. Robbins TW. The 5-choice serial reaction time task: behavioural pharmacology and functional neurochemistry. *Psychopharmacology (Berl).* (2002) 163:362–80. doi: 10.1007/s00213-002-1154-7
45. Logan GD, Van Zandt T, Verbruggen F, Wagenmakers EJ. On the ability to inhibit thought and action: general and special theories of an act of control. *Psychol Rev* (2014) 121:66–95. doi: 10.1037/a0035230
46. Belin-Rauscent A, Daniel ML, Puaud M, Jupp B, Sawiak S, Howett D, et al. Impulsivity is predicted by the thinness of the insular cortex in rats. *Mol Psychiatry* (2016) 21:445. doi: 10.1038/mp.2016.32
47. Tsutsui-Kimura I, Ohmura Y, Izumi T, Matsushima T, Amita H, Yamaguchi T, et al. Neuronal codes for the inhibitory control of impulsive actions in the rat infralimbic cortex. *Behav Brain Res* (2016) 296:361–72. doi: 10.1016/j.bbr.2015.08.025
48. Rotge JY, Cocker PJ, Daniel ML, Belin-Rauscent A, Everitt BJ, Belin D. Bidirectional regulation over the development and expression of loss of control over cocaine intake by the anterior insula. *Psychopharmacology (Berl)* (2017) 234:1623–31. doi: 10.1007/s00213-017-4593-x
49. Naaijen J, Lythgoe DJ, Zwiers MP, Hartman CA, Hoekstra PJ, Buitelaar JK, et al. Anterior cingulate cortex glutamate and its association with striatal functioning during cognitive control. *Eur Neuropsychopharmacol* (2018) 28:381–91. doi: 10.1016/j.euroneuro.2018.01.002
50. Ho MY, Mobini S, Chiang TJ, Bradshaw CM, Szabadi E. Theory and method in the quantitative analysis of "impulsive choice" behaviour: implications for psychopharmacology. *Psychopharmacology (Berl)* (1999) 146:362–72. doi: 10.1007/PL00005482
51. Cardinal RN, Winstanley CA, Robbins TW, Everitt BJ. Limbic corticostriatal systems and delayed reinforcement. *Ann N Y Acad Sci* (2004) 1021:33–50. doi: 10.1196/annals.1308.004
52. Winstanley CA, Theobald DE, Cardinal RN, Robbins TW. Contrasting roles of basolateral amygdala and orbitofrontal cortex in impulsive choice. *J Neurosci* (2004) 24:4718–22. doi: 10.1523/JNEUROSCI.5606-03.2004
53. Cheung TH, Cardinal RN. Hippocampal lesions facilitate instrumental learning with delayed reinforcement but induce impulsive choice in rats. *BMC Neurosci* (2005) 6:36. doi: 10.1186/1471-2202-6-36
54. Mobini S, Chiang TJ, Ho MY, Bradshaw CM, Szabadi E. Effects of central 5-hydroxytryptamine depletion on sensitivity to delayed and probabilistic reinforcement. *Psychopharmacology (Berl)* (2000) 152:390–7. doi: 10.1007/s002130000542
55. Zeeb FD, Robbins TW, Winstanley CA. Serotonergic and dopaminergic modulation of gambling behavior as assessed using a novel rat gambling task. *Neuropsychopharmacology* (2009) 34:2329–43. doi: 10.1038/npp.2009.62
56. St Onge JR, Floresco SB. Prefrontal cortical contribution to risk-based decision making. *Cereb Cortex* (2010) 20:1816–28. doi: 10.1093/cercor/bhp250
57. Stopper CM, Floresco SB. What's better for me? Fundamental role for lateral habenula in promoting subjective decision biases. *Nat Neurosci* (2014) 17:33–5. doi: 10.1038/nn.3587
58. Stopper CM, Green EB, Floresco SB. Selective involvement by the medial orbitofrontal cortex in biasing risky, but not impulsive, choice. *Cereb Cortex* (2014) 24:154–62. doi: 10.1093/cercor/bhs297
59. Berry J, Van Gorp WG, Herzberg DS, Hinkin C, Boone K, Steinman L, et al. Neuropsychological deficits in abstinent cocaine abusers: preliminary findings after two weeks of abstinence. *Drug Alcohol Depend* (1993) 32:231–7. doi: 10.1016/0376-8716(93)90087-7
60. Pompili M, Lester D, Girardi P, Tatarelli R. High suicide risk after the development of cognitive and working memory deficits caused by cannabis, cocaine and ecstasy use. *Subst Abus* (2007) 28:25–30. doi: 10.1300/J465v28n01_04
61. Fernandez-Serrano MJ, Perez-Garcia M, Perales JC, Verdejo-Garcia A. Prevalence of executive dysfunction in cocaine, heroin and alcohol users enrolled in therapeutic communities. *Eur J Pharmacol* (2010) 626:104–2. doi: 10.1016/j.ejphar.2009.10.019
62. Almeida PP, De Araujo Filho GM, Malta SM, Laranjeira RR, Marques A, Bressan RA, et al. Attention and memory deficits in crack-cocaine users persist over four weeks of abstinence. *J Subst Abuse Treat* (2017) 81:73–8. doi: 10.1016/j.jsat.2017.08.002
63. Wunderli MD, Vonmoos M, Furst M, Schadelin K, Kraemer T, Baumgartner MR, et al. Discrete memory impairments in largely pure chronic users of MDMA. *Eur Neuropsychopharmacol* (2017) 27:987–99. doi: 10.1016/j.euroneuro.2017.08.425
64. Kilbey MM, Breslau N, Andreski P. Cocaine use and dependence in young adults: associated psychiatric disorders and personality traits. *Drug Alcohol Depend* (1992) 29:283–90. doi: 10.1016/0376-8716(92)90103-J
65. Falck RS, Wang J, Carlson RG, Eddy M, Siegal HA. The prevalence and correlates of depressive symptomatology among a community sample of crack-cocaine smokers. *J Psychoactive Drugs* (2002) 34:281–8. doi: 10.1080/02791072.2002.10399964
66. Khurana A, Romer D, Betancourt LM, Hurt H. Working memory ability and early drug use progression as predictors of adolescent substance use disorders. *Addiction* (2017) 112:1220–8. doi: 10.1111/add.13792
67. Thompson AM, Swant J, Wagner JJ. Cocaine-induced modulation of long-term potentiation in the CA1 region of rat hippocampus. *Neuropharmacology* (2005) 49:185–94. doi: 10.1016/j.neuropharm.2005.03.005
68. Stramiello M, Wagner JJ. Cocaine enhancement of long-term potentiation in the CA1 region of rat hippocampus: lamina-specific mechanisms of action. *Synapse* (2010) 64:644–8. doi: 10.1002/syn.20764
69. Kutlu MG, Gould TJ. Nicotinic modulation of hippocampal cell signaling and associated effects on learning and memory. *Physiol Behav* (2016) 155:162–71. doi: 10.1016/j.physbeh.2015.12.008
70. Chudasama Y. Animal models of prefrontal-executive function. *Behav Neurosci* (2011) 125:327–43. doi: 10.1037/a0023766
71. Floresco SB, Jentsch JD. Pharmacological enhancement of memory and executive functioning in laboratory animals. *Neuropsychopharmacology* (2011) 36:227–50. doi: 10.1038/npp.2010.158
72. Briand LA, Gross JP, Robinson TE. Impaired object recognition following prolonged withdrawal from extended-access cocaine self-administration. *Neuroscience* (2008) 155:1–6. doi: 10.1016/j.neuroscience.2008.06.004
73. George O, Mandyam CD, Wee S, Koob GF. Extended access to cocaine self-administration produces long-lasting prefrontal cortex-dependent working memory impairments. *Neuropsychopharmacology* (2008) 33:2474–82. doi: 10.1038/sj.npp.1301626
74. Calipari ES, Beveridge TJ, Jones SR, Porrino LJ. Withdrawal from extended-access cocaine self-administration results in dysregulated functional activity and altered locomotor activity in rats. *Eur J Neurosci* (2013) 38:3749–57. doi: 10.1111/ejn.12381
75. Ashare RL, Falcone M, Lerman C. Cognitive function during nicotine withdrawal: implications for nicotine dependence treatment. *Neuropharmacology* (2014) 76 Pt B:581–91. doi: 10.1016/j.neuropharm.2013.04.034
76. Krall DM, Lim SL, Cooper AM, Burleson PW, Rhoades DJ, Jacquemin SJ, et al. Withdrawal effect of chronic amphetamine exposure during adolescence on complex maze performance. *Addict Biol* (2014) 19:634–42. doi: 10.1111/adb.12029
77. Janetsian SS, Linsenbardt DN, Lapish CC. Memory impairment and alterations in prefrontal cortex gamma band activity following methamphetamine sensitization. *Psychopharmacology (Berl)* (2015) 232:2083–95. doi: 10.1007/s00213-014-3840-7
78. Garcia-Pardo MP, De La Rubia Orti JE, Aguilar Calpe MA. Differential effects of MDMA and cocaine on inhibitory avoidance and object recognition tests in rodents. *Neurobiol Learn Mem* (2017) 146:1–11. doi: 10.1016/j.nlm.2017.10.013
79. Gobin C, Schwendt M. The effects of extended-access cocaine self-administration on working memory performance, reversal learning and incubation of cocaine-seeking in adult male rats. *J Addict Prev* (2017) 5. doi: 10.13188/2330-2178.1000035
80. Rao KN, Sentir AM, Engleman EA, Bell RL, Hulvershorn LA, Breier A, et al. Toward early estimation and treatment of addiction vulnerability: radial arm maze and *N*-acetyl cysteine before cocaine sensitization or nicotine self-administration in neonatal ventral hippocampal lesion rats. *Psychopharmacology (Berl)* (2016) 233:3933–45. doi: 10.1007/s00213-016-4421-8
81. Wallace BC. Psychological and environmental determinants of relapse in crack cocaine smokers. *J Subst Abuse Treat* (1989) 6:95–106. doi: 10.1016/0740-5472(89)90036-6

82. O'Brien CP, Childress AR, Ehrman R, Robbins SJ. Conditioning factors in drug abuse: can they explain compulsion? *J Psychopharmacol* (1998) 12:15–22. doi: 10.1177/026988119801200103
83. Childress AR, Mozley PD, Mcelgin W, Fitzgerald J, Reivich M, O'Brien CP. Limbic activation during cue-induced cocaine craving. *Am J Psychiatry* (1999) 156:11–8. doi: 10.1176/ajp.156.1.11
84. Sinha R, Fuse T, Aubin LR, O'Malley SS. Psychological stress, drug-related cues and cocaine craving. *Psychopharmacology (Berl)* (2000) 152:140–8. doi: 10.1007/s002130000499
85. Perry CJ, Lawrence AJ. Addiction, cognitive decline and therapy: seeking ways to escape a vicious cycle. *Genes Brain Behav* (2017) 16:205–8. doi: 10.1111/gbb.12325
86. Quirk GJ, Mueller D. Neural mechanisms of extinction learning and retrieval. *Neuropsychopharmacology* (2008) 33:56–72. doi: 10.1038/sj.npp.1301555
87. Myers KM, Carlezon WA, Jr. Extinction of drug- and withdrawal-paired cues in animal models: relevance to the treatment of addiction. *Neurosci Biobehav Rev* (2010) 35:285–302. doi: 10.1016/j.neubiorev.2010.01.011
88. Mcnally GP. Extinction of drug seeking: neural circuits and approaches to augmentation. *Neuropharmacology* (2014) 76 Pt B:528–32. doi: 10.1016/j.neuropharm.2013.06.007
89. Shaham Y, Shalev U, Lu L, De Wit H, Stewart J. The reinstatement model of drug relapse: history, methodology and major findings. *Psychopharmacology (Berl)* (2003) 168:3–20. doi: 10.1007/s00213-002-1224-x
90. Crombag HS, Bossert JM, Koya E, Shaham Y. Review. Context-induced relapse to drug seeking: a review. *Philos Trans R Soc Lond B Biol Sci* (2008) 363:3233–43. doi: 10.1098/rstb.2008.0090
91. Morgan MA, Ledoux JE. Differential contribution of dorsal and ventral medial prefrontal cortex to the acquisition and extinction of conditioned fear in rats. *Behav Neurosci* (1995) 109:681–8. doi: 10.1037//0735-7044.109.4.681
92. Peters J, Lalumiere RT, Kalivas PW. Infralimbic prefrontal cortex is responsible for inhibiting cocaine seeking in extinguished rats. *J Neurosci* (2008) 28:6046–53. doi: 10.1523/JNEUROSCI.1045-08.2008
93. Peters J, Kalivas PW, Quirk GJ. Extinction circuits for fear and addiction overlap in prefrontal cortex. *Learn Mem* (2009) 16:279–88. doi: 10.1101/lm.1041309
94. Nic Dhonnchadha BA, Kantak KM. Cognitive enhancers for facilitating drug cue extinction: insights from animal models. *Pharmacol Biochem Behav* (2011) 99:229–44. doi: 10.1016/j.pbb.2011.01.018
95. Torregrossa MM, Taylor JR. Learning to forget: manipulating extinction and reconsolidation processes to treat addiction. *Psychopharmacology (Berl)* (2013) 226:659–72. doi: 10.1007/s00213-012-2750-9
96. Back SE, Killeen T, Badour CL, Flanagan JC, Allan NP, Ana ES, et al. Concurrent treatment of substance use disorders and PTSD using prolonged exposure: a randomized clinical trial in military veterans. *Addict Behav* (2019) 90:369–77. doi: 10.1016/j.addbeh.2018.11.032
97. Dani JA, De Biasi M. Cellular mechanisms of nicotine addiction. *Pharmacol Biochem Behav* (2001) 70:439–46. doi: 10.1016/S0091-3057(01)00652-9
98. Guilarte TR, Nihei MK, Mcglothan JL, Howard AS. Methamphetamine-induced deficits of brain monoaminergic neuronal markers: distal axotomy or neuronal plasticity. *Neuroscience* (2003) 122:499–513. doi: 10.1016/S0306-4522(03)00476-7
99. Edwards S, Whisler KN, Fuller DC, Orsulak PJ, Self DW. Addiction-related alterations in D1 and D2 dopamine receptor behavioral responses following chronic cocaine self-administration. *Neuropsychopharmacology* (2007b) 32:354–66. doi: 10.1038/sj.npp.1301062
100. Thomas MJ, Kalivas PW, Shaham Y. Neuroplasticity in the mesolimbic dopamine system and cocaine addiction. *Br J Pharmacol* (2008) 154:327–42. doi: 10.1038/bjp.2008.77
101. Sharma A, Couture J. A review of the pathophysiology, etiology, and treatment of attention-deficit hyperactivity disorder (ADHD). *Ann Pharmacother* (2014) 48:209–25. doi: 10.1177/1060028013510699
102. Caye A, Swanson JM, Coghill D, Rohde LA. Treatment strategies for ADHD: an evidence-based guide to select optimal treatment. *Mol Psychiatry* (2019) 24:390–408. doi: 10.1038/s41380-018-0116-3
103. Jupp B, Dalley JW. Convergent pharmacological mechanisms in impulsivity and addiction: insights from rodent models. *Br J Pharmacol* (2014) 171:4729–66. doi: 10.1111/bph.12787
104. Wade TR, De Wit H, Richards JB. Effects of dopaminergic drugs on delayed reward as a measure of impulsive behavior in rats. *Psychopharmacology (Berl)* (2000) 150:90–101. doi: 10.1007/s002130000402
105. Milienne-Petiot M, Groenink L, Minassian A, Young JW. Blockade of dopamine D1-family receptors attenuates the mania-like hyperactive, risk-preferring, and high motivation behavioral profile of mice with low dopamine transporter levels. *J Psychopharmacol* (2017) 31:1334–46. doi: 10.1177/0269881117731162
106. Pattij T, Janssen MC, Vanderschuren LJ, Schoffelmeer AN, Van Gaalen MM. Involvement of dopamine D1 and D2 receptors in the nucleus accumbens core and shell in inhibitory response control. *Psychopharmacology (Berl)* (2007) 191:587–98. doi: 10.1007/s00213-006-0533-x
107. Anderson SM, Bari AA, Pierce RC. Administration of the D1-like dopamine receptor antagonist SCH-23390 into the medial nucleus accumbens shell attenuates cocaine priming-induced reinstatement of drug-seeking behavior in rats. *Psychopharmacology (Berl)* (2003) 168:132–8. doi: 10.1007/s00213-002-1298-5
108. Loos M, Pattij T, Janssen MC, Counotte DS, Schoffelmeer AN, Smit AB, et al. Dopamine receptor D1/D5 gene expression in the medial prefrontal cortex predicts impulsive choice in rats. *Cereb Cortex* (2010) 20:1064–70. doi: 10.1093/cercor/bhp167
109. Wang Y, Yin F, Guo H, Zhang J, Yan P, Lai J. The role of dopamine D1 and D3 receptors in *N*-methyl-d-aspartate (NMDA)/glycineB site-regulated complex cognitive behaviors following repeated morphine administration. *Int J Neuropsychopharmacol* (2017) 20:562–74. doi: 10.1093/ijnp/pyx010
110. Brenhouse HC, Thompson BS, Sonntag KC, Andersen SL. Extinction and reinstatement to cocaine-associated cues in male and female juvenile rats and the role of D1 dopamine receptor. *Neuropharmacology* (2015) 95:22–8. doi: 10.1016/j.neuropharm.2015.02.017
111. Huang B, Li Y, Cheng D, He G, Liu X, Ma L. Beta-arrestin-biased beta-adrenergic signaling promotes extinction learning of cocaine reward memory. *Sci Signal* (2018) 11 (512): eaam 5402. doi: 10.1126/scisignal.aam5402
112. Otis JM, Fitzgerald MK, Mueller D. Infralimbic BDNF/TrkB enhancement of GluN2B currents facilitates extinction of a cocaine-conditioned place preference. *J Neurosci* (2014a) 34:6057–64. doi: 10.1523/JNEUROSCI.4980-13.2014
113. Alaghband Y, Kwapis JL, Lopez AJ, White AO, Aimiuwu OV, Al-Kachak A, et al. Distinct roles for the deacetylase domain of HDAC3 in the hippocampus and medial prefrontal cortex in the formation and extinction of memory. *Neurobiol Learn Mem* (2017) 145:94–104. doi: 10.1016/j.nlm.2017.09.001
114. Hu SS, Liu YW, Yu L. Medial prefrontal cannabinoid CB1 receptors modulate consolidation and extinction of cocaine-associated memory in mice. *Psychopharmacology (Berl)* (2015) 232:1803–15. doi: 10.1007/s00213-014-3812-y
115. Heysieattalab S, Naghdi N, Zarrindast MR, Haghparast A, Mehr SE, Khoshbouei H. The effects of GABAA and NMDA receptors in the shell-accumbens on spatial memory of METH-treated rats. *Pharmacol Biochem Behav* (2016) 142:23–35. doi: 10.1016/j.pbb.2015.12.008
116. Kinoshita KI, Muroi Y, Unno T, Ishii T. Rolipram improves facilitation of contextual fear extinction in the 1-methyl-4-phenyl-1,2,3,6-tetrahydropyridine-induced mouse model of Parkinson's disease. *J Pharmacol Sci* (2017) 134:55–8. doi: 10.1016/j.jphs.2017.04.002
117. Dominguez G, Dagnas M, Decorte L, Vandesquille M, Belzung C, Beracochea D, et al. Rescuing prefrontal cAMP-CREB pathway reverses working memory deficits during withdrawal from prolonged alcohol exposure. *Brain Struct Funct* (2016) 221:865–77. doi: 10.1007/s00429-014-0941-3
118. Edwards S, Graham DL, Bachtell RK, Self DW. Region-specific tolerance to cocaine-regulated cAMP-dependent protein phosphorylation following chronic self-administration. *Eur J Neurosci* (2007a) 25:2201–13. doi: 10.1111/j.1460-9568.2007.05473.x
119. Ru Q, Xiong Q, Zhou M, Chen L, Tian X, Xiao H, et al. Withdrawal from chronic treatment with methamphetamine induces anxiety and depression-like behavior in mice. *Psychiatry Res* (2018) 271:476–83. doi: 10.1016/j.psychres.2018.11.072
120. Li Y, Zuo Y, Yu P, Ping X, Cui C. Role of basolateral amygdala dopamine D2 receptors in impulsive choice in acute cocaine-treated rats. *Behav Brain Res* (2015b) 287:187–95. doi: 10.1016/j.bbr.2015.03.039
121. Besson M, Pelloux Y, Dilleen R, Theobald DE, Lyon A, Belin-Rauscent A, et al. Cocaine modulation of frontostriatal expression of Zif268, D2, and 5-HT2c receptors in high and low impulsive rats. *Neuropsychopharmacology* (2013) 38:1963–73. doi: 10.1038/npp.2013.95

122. Caprioli D, Hong YT, Sawiak SJ, Ferrari V, Williamson DJ, Jupp B, et al. Baseline-dependent effects of cocaine pre-exposure on impulsivity and D2/3 receptor availability in the rat striatum: possible relevance to the attention-deficit hyperactivity syndrome. *Neuropsychopharmacology* (2013) 38:1460–71. doi: 10.1038/npp.2013.44
123. Caprioli D, Jupp B, Hong YT, Sawiak SJ, Ferrari V, Wharton L, et al. Dissociable rate-dependent effects of oral methylphenidate on impulsivity and D2/3 receptor availability in the striatum. *J Neurosci* (2015) 35:3747–55. doi: 10.1523/JNEUROSCI.3890-14.2015
124. Yates JR, Perry JL, Meyer AC, Gipson CD, Charnigo R, Bardo MT. Role of medial prefrontal and orbitofrontal monoamine transporters and receptors in performance in an adjusting delay discounting procedure. *Brain Res* (2014) 1574:26–36. doi: 10.1016/j.brainres.2014.06.004
125. Bernosky-Smith KA, Qiu YY, Feja M, Lee YB, Loughlin B, Li JX, et al. Ventral tegmental area D2 receptor knockdown enhances choice impulsivity in a delay-discounting task in rats. *Behav Brain Res* (2018) 341:129–34. doi: 10.1016/j.bbr.2017.12.029
126. Cocker PJ, Tremblay M, Kaur S, Winstanley CA. Chronic administration of the dopamine D2/3 agonist ropinirole invigorates performance of a rodent slot machine task, potentially indicative of less distractible or compulsive-like gambling behaviour. *Psychopharmacology (Berl)* (2017) 234:137–53. doi: 10.1007/s00213-016-4447-y
127. Seeman P. Parkinson's disease treatment may cause impulse-control disorder *via* dopamine D3 receptors. *Synapse* (2015) 69:183–9. doi: 10.1002/syn.21805
128. Barrus MM, Winstanley CA. Dopamine D3 receptors modulate the ability of win-paired cues to increase risky choice in a rat gambling task. *J Neurosci* (2016) 36:785–94. doi: 10.1523/JNEUROSCI.2225-15.2016
129. Di Ciano P, Cormick PM, Stefan C, Wong E, Kim A, Remington G, et al. The effects of buspirone on occupancy of dopamine receptors and the rat gambling task. *Psychopharmacology (Berl)* (2017) 234:3309–20. doi: 10.1007/s00213-017-4715-5
130. Chen Y, Song R, Yang RF, Wu N, Li J. A novel dopamine D3 receptor antagonist YQA14 inhibits methamphetamine self-administration and relapse to drug-seeking behaviour in rats. *Eur J Pharmacol* (2014) 743:126–32. doi: 10.1016/j.ejphar.2014.09.026
131. Song R, Bi GH, Zhang HY, Yang RF, Gardner EL, Li J, et al. Blockade of D3 receptors by YQA14 inhibits cocaine's rewarding effects and relapse to drug-seeking behavior in rats. *Neuropharmacology* (2014) 77:398–405. doi: 10.1016/j.neuropharm.2013.10.010
132. Picciotto MR, Corrigall WA. Neuronal systems underlying behaviors related to nicotine addiction: neural circuits and molecular genetics. *J Neurosci* (2002) 22:3338–41. doi: 10.1523/JNEUROSCI.22-09-03338.2002
133. Howell LL, Kimmel HL. Monoamine transporters and psychostimulant addiction. *Biochem Pharmacol* (2008) 75:196–217. doi: 10.1016/j.bcp.2007.08.003
134. Smith RJ, Aston-Jones G. Noradrenergic transmission in the extended amygdala: role in increased drug-seeking and relapse during protracted drug abstinence. *Brain Struct Funct* (2008) 213:43–61. doi: 10.1007/s00429-008-0191-3
135. Sofuoglu M, Sewell RA. Norepinephrine and stimulant addiction. *Addict Biol* (2009) 14:119–29. doi: 10.1111/j.1369-1600.2008.00138.x
136. Fernando AB, Economidou D, Theobald DE, Zou MF, Newman AH, Spoelder M, et al. Modulation of high impulsivity and attentional performance in rats by selective direct and indirect dopaminergic and noradrenergic receptor agonists. *Psychopharmacology (Berl)* (2012) 219:341–52. doi: 10.1007/s00213-011-2408-z
137. Freund N, Jordan CJ, Lukkes JL, Norman KJ, Andersen SL. Juvenile exposure to methylphenidate and guanfacine in rats: effects on early delay discounting and later cocaine-taking behavior. *Psychopharmacology (Berl)* (2019) 236:685–698. doi: 10.1007/s00213-018-5096-0
138. Nishitomi K, Yano K, Kobayashi M, Jino K, Kano T, Horiguchi N, et al. Systemic administration of guanfacine improves food-motivated impulsive choice behavior primarily *via* direct stimulation of postsynaptic alpha2A-adrenergic receptors in rats. *Behav Brain Res* (2018) 345:21–9. doi: 10.1016/j.bbr.2018.02.022
139. Terry AV, Jr., Callahan PM, Schade R, Kille NJ, Plagenhoef M. Alpha 2A adrenergic receptor agonist, guanfacine, attenuates cocaine-related impairments of inhibitory response control and working memory in animal models. *Pharmacol Biochem Behav* (2014) 126:63–72. doi: 10.1016/j.pbb.2014.09.010
140. Gentile TA, Simmons SJ, Watson MN, Connelly KL, Brailoiu E, Zhang Y, et al. Effects of suvorexant, a dual orexin/hypocretin receptor antagonist, on impulsive behavior associated with cocaine. *Neuropsychopharmacology* (2018b) 43:1001–9. doi: 10.1038/npp.2017.158
141. Swalve N, Smethells JR, Younk R, Mitchell J, Dougen B, Carroll ME. Sex-specific attenuation of impulsive action by progesterone in a Go/No-Go task for cocaine in rats. *Psychopharmacology (Berl)* (2018) 235:135–43. doi: 10.1007/s00213-017-4750-2
142. Smethells JR, Swalve NL, Eberly LE, Carroll ME. Sex differences in the reduction of impulsive choice (delay discounting) for cocaine in rats with atomoxetine and progesterone. *Psychopharmacology (Berl)* (2016) 233:2999–3008. doi: 10.1007/s00213-016-4345-3
143. Marszalek-Grabska M, Gibula-Bruzda E, Jenda M, Gawel K, Kotlinska JH. Memantine improves memory impairment and depressive-like behavior induced by amphetamine withdrawal in rats. *Brain Res* (2016) 1642:389–96. doi: 10.1016/j.brainres.2016.04.026
144. Saravia R, Flores A, Plaza-Zabala A, Busquets-Garcia A, Pastor A, De La Torre R, et al. CB1 cannabinoid receptors mediate cognitive deficits and structural plasticity changes during nicotine withdrawal. *Biol Psychiatry* (2017) 81:625–34. doi: 10.1016/j.biopsych.2016.07.007
145. Botreau F, Paolone G, Stewart J. d-Cycloserine facilitates extinction of a cocaine-induced conditioned place preference. *Behav Brain Res* (2006) 172:173–8. doi: 10.1016/j.bbr.2006.05.012
146. Gass JT, Olive MF. Positive allosteric modulation of mGluR5 receptors facilitates extinction of a cocaine contextual memory. *Biol Psychiatry* (2009) 65:717–20. doi: 10.1016/j.biopsych.2008.11.001
147. Cleva RM, Hicks MP, Gass JT, Wischerath KC, Plasters ET, Widholm JJ, et al. mGluR5 positive allosteric modulation enhances extinction learning following cocaine self-administration. *Behav Neurosci* (2011) 125:10–9. doi: 10.1037/a0022339
148. Liddie S, Anderson KL, Paz A, Itzhak Y. The effect of phosphodiesterase inhibitors on the extinction of cocaine-induced conditioned place preference in mice. *J Psychopharmacol* (2012) 26:1375–82. doi: 10.1177/0269881112447991
149. Otis JM, Fitzgerald MK, Mueller D. Inhibition of hippocampal beta-adrenergic receptors impairs retrieval but not reconsolidation of cocaine-associated memory and prevents subsequent reinstatement. *Neuropsychopharmacology* (2014b) 39:303–10. doi: 10.1038/npp.2013.187
150. Twining RC, Tuscher JJ, Doncheck EM, Frick KM, Mueller D. 17Beta-estradiol is necessary for extinction of cocaine seeking in female rats. *Learn Mem* (2013) 20:300–6. doi: 10.1101/lm.030304.113
151. Childs JE, Deleon J, Nickel E, Kroener S. Vagus nerve stimulation reduces cocaine seeking and alters plasticity in the extinction network. *Learn Mem* (2017) 24:35–42. doi: 10.1101/lm.043539.116
152. Voigt RM, Herrold AA, Napier TC. Baclofen facilitates the extinction of methamphetamine-induced conditioned place preference in rats. *Behav Neurosci* (2011) 125:261–7. doi: 10.1037/a0022893
153. Fox H, Sofuoglu M, Sinha R. Guanfacine enhances inhibitory control and attentional shifting in early abstinent cocaine-dependent individuals. *J Psychopharmacol* (2015) 29:312–23. doi: 10.1177/0269881114562464
154. Smith RJ, Aston-Jones G. Alpha(2) adrenergic and imidazoline receptor agonists prevent cue-induced cocaine seeking. *Biol Psychiatry* (2011) 70:712–9. doi: 10.1016/j.biopsych.2011.06.010
155. Feltenstein MW, See RE. Potentiation of cue-induced reinstatement of cocaine-seeking in rats by the anxiogenic drug yohimbine. *Behav Brain Res* (2006) 174:1–8. doi: 10.1016/j.bbr.2006.06.039
156. Economidou D, Theobald DE, Robbins TW, Everitt BJ, Dalley JW. Norepinephrine and dopamine modulate impulsivity on the five-choice serial reaction time task through opponent actions in the shell and core sub-regions of the nucleus accumbens. *Neuropsychopharmacology* (2012) 37:2057–66. doi: 10.1038/npp.2012.53
157. Broos N, Loonstra R, Van Mourik Y, Schetters D, Schoffelmeer AN, Pattij T, et al. Subchronic administration of atomoxetine causes an enduring reduction in context-induced relapse to cocaine seeking without affecting impulsive decision making. *Addict Biol* (2015) 20:714–23. doi: 10.1111/adb.12168
158. Economidou D, Pelloux Y, Robbins TW, Dalley JW, Everitt BJ. High impulsivity predicts relapse to cocaine-seeking after punishment-induced abstinence. *Biol Psychiatry* (2009) 65:851–6. doi: 10.1016/j.biopsych.2008.12.008
159. Economidou D, Cippitelli A, Stopponi S, Braconi S, Clementi S, Ubaldi M, et al. Activation of brain NOP receptors attenuates acute and protracted

alcohol withdrawal symptoms in the rat. *Alcohol Clin Exp Res* (2011) 35:747–55. doi: 10.1111/j.1530-0277.2010.01392.x

160. Xue YX, Deng JH, Chen YY, Zhang LB, Wu P, Huang GD, et al. Effect of selective inhibition of reactivated nicotine-associated memories with propranolol on nicotine craving. *JAMA Psychiatry* (2017) 74:224–32. doi: 10.1001/jamapsychiatry.2016.3907
161. Burhans LB, Smith-Bell CA, Schreurs BG. Propranolol produces short-term facilitation of extinction in a rabbit model of post-traumatic stress disorder. *Neuropharmacology* (2018) 135:386–98. doi: 10.1016/j.neuropharm.2018.03.029
162. Muller CP, Homberg JR. The role of serotonin in drug use and addiction. *Behav Brain Res* (2015) 277:146–92. doi: 10.1016/j.bbr.2014.04.007
163. Pattij T, Schoffelmeer AN. Serotonin and inhibitory response control: focusing on the role of 5-HT(1A) receptors. *Eur J Pharmacol* (2015) 753:140–5. doi: 10.1016/j.ejphar.2014.05.064
164. Marek GJ, Li AA, Seiden LS. Evidence for involvement of 5-hydroxytryptamine1 receptors in antidepressant-like drug effects on differential-reinforcement-of-low-rate 72-second behavior. *J Pharmacol Exp Ther* (1989) 250:60–71.
165. Homberg JR, Pattij T, Janssen MC, Ronken E, De Boer SF, Schoffelmeer AN, et al. Serotonin transporter deficiency in rats improves inhibitory control but not behavioural flexibility. *Eur J Neurosci* (2007) 26:2066–73. doi: 10.1111/j.1460-9568.2007.05839.x
166. Baarendse PJ, Vanderschuren LJ. Dissociable effects of monoamine reuptake inhibitors on distinct forms of impulsive behavior in rats. *Psychopharmacology (Berl)* (2012) 219:313–26. doi: 10.1007/s00213-011-2576-x
167. Puumala T, Sirvio J. Changes in activities of dopamine and serotonin systems in the frontal cortex underlie poor choice accuracy and impulsivity of rats in an attention task. *Neuroscience* (1998) 83:489–99. doi: 10.1016/S0306-4522(97)00392-8
168. Dalley JW, Theobald DE, Eagle DM, Passetti F, Robbins TW. Deficits in impulse control associated with tonically-elevated serotonergic function in rat prefrontal cortex. *Neuropsychopharmacology* (2002) 26:716–28. doi: 10.1016/S0893-133X(01)00412-2
169. Fink LH, Anastasio NC, Fox RG, Rice KC, Moeller FG, Cunningham KA. Individual differences in impulsive action reflect variation in the cortical serotonin 5-HT2A receptor system. *Neuropsychopharmacology* (2015) 40:1957–68. doi: 10.1038/npp.2015.46
170. Sholler DJ, Stutz SJ, Fox RG, Boone EL, Wang Q, Rice KC, et al. The 5-HT2A receptor (5-HT2AR) regulates impulsive action and cocaine cue reactivity in male Sprague–Dawley rats. *J Pharmacol Exp Ther* (2019) 368:41–9. doi: 10.1124/jpet.118.251199
171. Wischhof L, Hollensteiner KJ, Koch M. Impulsive behaviour in rats induced by intracortical DOI infusions is antagonized by co-administration of an mGlu2/3 receptor agonist. *Behav Pharmacol* (2011) 22:805–13. doi: 10.1097/FBP.0b013e32834d6279
172. Adams WK, Barkus C, Ferland JN, Sharp T, Winstanley CA. Pharmacological evidence that 5-HT2C receptor blockade selectively improves decision making when rewards are paired with audiovisual cues in a rat gambling task. *Psychopharmacology (Berl)* (2017a) 234:3091–104. doi: 10.1007/s00213-017-4696-4
173. Mori M, Tsutsui-Kimura I, Mimura M, Tanaka KF. 5-HT3 antagonists decrease discounting rate without affecting sensitivity to reward magnitude in the delay discounting task in mice. *Psychopharmacology (Berl)* (2018) 235:2619–29. doi: 10.1007/s00213-018-4954-0
174. Li X, Semenova S, D'Souza MS, Stoker AK, Markou A. Involvement of glutamatergic and GABAergic systems in nicotine dependence: implications for novel pharmacotherapies for smoking cessation. *Neuropharmacology* (2014) 76 Pt B:554–65. doi: 10.1016/j.neuropharm.2013.05.042
175. Mccreary AC, Muller CP, Filip M. Psychostimulants: basic and clinical pharmacology. *Int Rev Neurobiol* (2015) 120:41–83. doi: 10.1016/bs.irn.2015.02.008
176. Berro LF, Andersen ML, Tufik S, Howell LL. GABAA receptor positive allosteric modulators modify the abuse-related behavioral and neurochemical effects of methamphetamine in rhesus monkeys. *Neuropharmacology* (2017) 123:299–309. doi: 10.1016/j.neuropharm.2017.05.010
177. Hayes DJ, Jupp B, Sawiak SJ, Merlo E, Caprioli D, Dalley JW. Brain gamma-aminobutyric acid: a neglected role in impulsivity. *Eur J Neurosci* (2014) 39:1921–32. doi: 10.1111/ejn.12485
178. Heaney CF, Kinney JW. Role of GABA(B) receptors in learning and memory and neurological disorders. *Neurosci Biobehav Rev* (2016) 63:1–28. doi: 10.1016/j.neubiorev.2016.01.007
179. Mick I, Ramos AC, Myers J, Stokes PR, Chandrasekera S, Erritzoe D, et al. Evidence for GABA-A receptor dysregulation in gambling disorder: correlation with impulsivity. *Addict Biol* (2017) 22:1601–09. doi: 10.1111/adb.12457
180. Paine TA, Slipp LE, Carlezon WA, Jr.. Schizophrenia-like attentional deficits following blockade of prefrontal cortex GABAA receptors. *Neuropsychopharmacology* (2011) 36:1703–13. doi: 10.1038/npp.2011.51
181. Murphy ER, Fernando AB, Urcelay GP, Robinson ES, Mar AC, Theobald DE, et al. Impulsive behaviour induced by both NMDA receptor antagonism and GABAA receptor activation in rat ventromedial prefrontal cortex. *Psychopharmacology (Berl)* (2012) 219:401–10. doi: 10.1007/s00213-011-2572-1
182. Feja M, Koch M. Ventral medial prefrontal cortex inactivation impairs impulse control but does not affect delay-discounting in rats. *Behav Brain Res* (2014) 264:230–9. doi: 10.1016/j.bbr.2014.02.013
183. Zapata A, Hwang EK, Lupica CR. Lateral habenula involvement in impulsive cocaine seeking. *Neuropsychopharmacology* (2017) 42:1103–12. doi: 10.1038/npp.2016.286
184. Froger-Colleaux C, Castagne V. Effects of baclofen and raclopride on reinstatement of cocaine self-administration in the rat. *Eur J Pharmacol* (2016) 777:147–55. doi: 10.1016/j.ejphar.2016.03.008
185. Li X, Sturchler E, Kaczanowska K, Cameron M, Finn MG, Griffin P, et al. KK-92A, a novel GABAB receptor positive allosteric modulator, attenuates nicotine self-administration and cue-induced nicotine seeking in rats. *Psychopharmacology (Berl)* (2017b) 234:1633–44. doi: 10.1007/s00213-017-4594-9
186. Kalivas PW. The glutamate homeostasis hypothesis of addiction. *Nat Rev Neurosci* (2009) 10:561–72. doi: 10.1038/nrn2515
187. D'souza MS. Glutamatergic transmission in drug reward: implications for drug addiction. *Front Neurosci* (2015) 9:404. doi: 10.3389/fnins.2015.00404
188. Bobadilla AC, Heinsbroek JA, Gipson CD, Griffin WC, Fowler CD, Kenny PJ, et al. Corticostriatal plasticity, neuronal ensembles, and regulation of drug-seeking behavior. *Prog Brain Res* (2017) 235:93–112. doi: 10.1016/bs.pbr.2017.07.013
189. Myers KM, Carlezon WA, Jr., Davis M. Glutamate receptors in extinction and extinction-based therapies for psychiatric illness. *Neuropsychopharmacology* (2011) 36:274–93. doi: 10.1038/npp.2010.88
190. Yates JR, Batten SR, Bardo MT, Beckmann JS. Role of ionotropic glutamate receptors in delay and probability discounting in the rat. *Psychopharmacology (Berl)* (2015) 232:1187–96. doi: 10.1007/s00213-014-3747-3
191. Higgins GA, Silenieks LB, Macmillan C, Sevo J, Zeeb FD, Thevarkunnel S. Enhanced attention and impulsive action following NMDA receptor GluN2B-selective antagonist pretreatment. *Behav Brain Res* (2016) 311:1–14. doi: 10.1016/j.bbr.2016.05.025
192. Floresco SB, Tse MT, Ghods-Sharifi S. Dopaminergic and glutamatergic regulation of effort- and delay-based decision making. *Neuropsychopharmacology* (2008) 33:1966–79. doi: 10.1038/sj.npp.1301565
193. Cottone P, Iemolo A, Narayan AR, Kwak J, Momaney D, Sabino V. The uncompetitive NMDA receptor antagonists ketamine and memantine preferentially increase the choice for a small, immediate reward in low-impulsive rats. *Psychopharmacology (Berl)* (2013) 226:127–38. doi: 10.1007/s00213-012-2898-3
194. Yates JR, Bardo MT. Effects of intra-accumbal administration of dopamine and ionotropic glutamate receptor drugs on delay discounting performance in rats. *Behav Neurosci* (2017) 131:392–405. doi: 10.1037/bne0000214
195. Mcentee WJ, Crook TH. Glutamate: its role in learning, memory, and the aging brain. *Psychopharmacology (Berl)* (1993) 111:391–401. doi: 10.1007/BF02253527
196. Riedel G, Platt B, Micheau J. Glutamate receptor function in learning and memory. *Behav Brain Res* (2003) 140:1–47. doi: 10.1016/S0166-4328(02)00272-3
197. Paolone G, Botreau F, Stewart J. The facilitative effects of D-cycloserine on extinction of a cocaine-induced conditioned place preference can be long lasting and resistant to reinstatement. *Psychopharmacology (Berl)* (2009) 202:403–9. doi: 10.1007/s00213-008-1280-y
198. Wu IT, Tang TH, Ko MC, Chiu CY, Lu KT. Amygdaloid zif268 participated in the d-cycloserine facilitation effect on the extinction of conditioned fear. *Psychopharmacology (Berl)* (2015) 232:3809–19. doi: 10.1007/s00213-015-4042-7
199. Trent S, Barnes P, Hall J, Thomas KL. AMPA receptors control fear extinction through an Arc-dependent mechanism. *Learn Mem* (2017) 24:375–80. doi: 10.1101/lm.045013.117

200. Wu X, Zhang JT, Li D, Zhou J, Yang J, Zheng HL, et al. Aquaporin-4 deficiency facilitates fear memory extinction in the hippocampus through excessive activation of extrasynaptic GluN2B-containing NMDA receptors. *Neuropharmacology* (2017) 112:124–34. doi: 10.1016/j.neuropharm.2016.06.031
201. Yamada D, Wada K, Sekiguchi M. Facilitating actions of an AMPA receptor potentiator upon extinction of contextually conditioned fear response in stressed mice. *Neurosci Lett* (2011) 488:242–6. doi: 10.1016/j.neulet.2010.11.038
202. Chen W, Wang Y, Sun A, Zhou L, Xu W, Zhu H, et al. Activation of AMPA receptor in the infralimbic cortex facilitates extinction and attenuates the heroin-seeking behavior in rats. *Neurosci Lett* (2016) 612:126–31. doi: 10.1016/j.neulet.2015.11.024
203. Lin A, Man HY. Endocytic adaptor epidermal growth factor receptor substrate 15 (Eps15) is involved in the trafficking of ubiquitinated alpha-amino-3-hydroxy-5-methyl-4-isoxazolepropionic acid receptors. *J Biol Chem* (2014) 289:24652–64. doi: 10.1074/jbc.M114.582114
204. Wischhof L, Koch M. Pre-treatment with the mGlu2/3 receptor agonist LY379268 attenuates DOI-induced impulsive responding and regional c-Fos protein expression. *Psychopharmacology (Berl)* (2012) 219:387–400. doi: 10.1007/s00213-011-2441-y
205. Isherwood SN, Robbins TW, Nicholson JR, Dalley JW, Pekcec A. Selective and interactive effects of D2 receptor antagonism and positive allosteric mGluR4 modulation on waiting impulsivity. *Neuropharmacology* (2017) 123:249–60. doi: 10.1016/j.neuropharm.2017.05.006
206. Isherwood SN, Pekcec A, Nicholson JR, Robbins TW, Dalley JW. Dissociable effects of mGluR5 allosteric modulation on distinct forms of impulsivity in rats: interaction with NMDA receptor antagonism. *Psychopharmacology (Berl)* (2015) 232:3327–44. doi: 10.1007/s00213-015-3984-0
207. Sethna F, Wang H. Pharmacological enhancement of mGluR5 facilitates contextual fear memory extinction. *Learn Mem* (2014) 21:647–50. doi: 10.1101/lm.035857.114
208. Ben-Shahar O, Sacramento AD, Miller BW, Webb SM, Wroten MG, Silva HE, et al. Deficits in ventromedial prefrontal cortex group 1 metabotropic glutamate receptor function mediate resistance to extinction during protracted withdrawal from an extensive history of cocaine self-administration. *J Neurosci* (2013) 33:495–506a. doi: 10.1523/JNEUROSCI.3710-12.2013
209. Sepulveda-Orengo MT, Healey KL, Kim R, Auriemma AC, Rojas J, Woronoff N, et al. Riluzole impairs cocaine reinstatement and restores adaptations in intrinsic excitability and GLT-1 expression. *Neuropsychopharmacology* (2018) 43:1212–23. doi: 10.1038/npp.2017.244
210. Sugiyama A, Yamada M, Saitoh A, Oka JI, Yamada M. Administration of riluzole to the basolateral amygdala facilitates fear extinction in rats. *Behav Brain Res* (2018) 336:8–14. doi: 10.1016/j.bbr.2017.08.031
211. Kupchik YM, Moussawi K, Tang XC, Wang X, Kalivas BC, Kolokithas R, et al. The effect of *N*-acetylcysteine in the nucleus accumbens on neurotransmission and relapse to cocaine. *Biol Psychiatry* (2012) 71:978–86. doi: 10.1016/j.biopsych.2011.10.024
212. Ramirez-Nino AM, D'Souza MS, Markou A. *N*-Acetylcysteine decreased nicotine self-administration and cue-induced reinstatement of nicotine seeking in rats: comparison with the effects of *N*-acetylcysteine on food responding and food seeking. *Psychopharmacology (Berl)* (2013) 225:473–82. doi: 10.1007/s00213-012-2837-3
213. Chambers RA, Moore J, Mcevoy JP, Levin ED. Cognitive effects of neonatal hippocampal lesions in a rat model of schizophrenia. *Neuropsychopharmacology* (1996) 15:587–94. doi: 10.1016/S0893-133X(96)00132-7
214. Ohmura Y, Tsutsui-Kimura I, Yoshioka M. Impulsive behavior and nicotinic acetylcholine receptors. *J Pharmacol Sci* (2012) 118:413–22. doi: 10.1254/jphs.11R06CR
215. Jeong JE, Rhee JK, Kim TM, Kwak SM, Bang SH, Cho H, et al. The association between the nicotinic acetylcholine receptor alpha4 subunit gene (CHRNA4) rs1044396 and Internet gaming disorder in Korean male adults. *PLoS One* (2017) 12:e0188358. doi: 10.1371/journal.pone.0188358
216. Fletcher PJ, Li Z, Silenieks LB, Macmillan C, Delannoy I, Higgins GA. Preclinical evidence for combining the 5-HT2C receptor agonist lorcaserin and varenicline as a treatment for nicotine dependence. *Addict Biol* (2019) 24:376–87. doi: 10.1111/adb.12602
217. Ohmura Y, Sasamori H, Tsutsui-Kimura I, Izumi T, Yoshida T, Yoshioka M. Varenicline provokes impulsive action by stimulating alpha4beta2 nicotinic acetylcholine receptors in the infralimbic cortex in a nicotine exposure status-dependent manner. *Pharmacol Biochem Behav* (2017) 154:1–10. doi: 10.1016/j.pbb.2017.01.002
218. Tsutsui-Kimura I, Ohmura Y, Izumi T, Yamaguchi T, Yoshida T, Yoshioka M. Endogenous acetylcholine modulates impulsive action *via* alpha4beta2 nicotinic acetylcholine receptors in rats. *Eur J Pharmacol* (2010) 641:148–53. doi: 10.1016/j.ejphar.2010.05.028
219. Levin ED, Rezvani AH, Wells C, Slade S, Yenugonda VM, Liu Y, et al. Alpha4beta2 nicotinic receptor desensitizing compounds can decrease self-administration of cocaine and methamphetamine in rats. *Eur J Pharmacol* (2018) 845:1–7. doi: 10.1016/j.ejphar.2018.12.010
220. Hayward A, Adamson L, Neill JC. Partial agonism at the alpha7 nicotinic acetylcholine receptor improves attention, impulsive action and vigilance in low attentive rats. *Eur Neuropsychopharmacol* (2017) 27:325–35. doi: 10.1016/j.euroneuro.2017.01.013
221. Levin ED, Bradley A, Addy N, Sigurani N. Hippocampal alpha 7 and alpha 4 beta 2 nicotinic receptors and working memory. *Neuroscience* (2002) 109:757–65. doi: 10.1016/S0306-4522(01)00538-3
222. Nikiforuk A, Kos T, Potasiewicz A, Popik P. Positive allosteric modulation of alpha 7 nicotinic acetylcholine receptors enhances recognition memory and cognitive flexibility in rats. *Eur Neuropsychopharmacol* (2015) 25:1300–13. doi: 10.1016/j.euroneuro.2015.04.018
223. Love TM, Stohler CS, Zubieta JK. Positron emission tomography measures of endogenous opioid neurotransmission and impulsiveness traits in humans. *Arch Gen Psychiatry* (2009) 66:1124–34. doi: 10.1001/archgenpsychiatry.2009.134
224. Mick I, Myers J, Ramos AC, Stokes PR, Erritzoe D, Colasanti A, et al. Blunted endogenous opioid release following an oral amphetamine challenge in pathological gamblers. *Neuropsychopharmacology* (2016) 41:1742–50. doi: 10.1038/npp.2015.340
225. Kim SW, Grant JE, Adson DE, Shin YC. Double-blind naltrexone and placebo comparison study in the treatment of pathological gambling. *Biol Psychiatry* (2001) 49:914–21. doi: 10.1016/S0006-3223(01)01079-4
226. Yoon G, Kim SW. Monthly injectable naltrexone for pathological gambling. *Am J Psychiatry* (2013) 170:682–3. doi: 10.1176/appi.ajp.2013.12111469
227. Baldo BA. Prefrontal cortical opioids and dysregulated motivation: a network hypothesis. *Trends Neurosci* (2016) 39:366–77. doi: 10.1016/j.tins.2016.03.004
228. Selleck RA, Lake C, Estrada V, Riederer J, Andrzejewski M, Sadeghian K, et al. Endogenous opioid signaling in the medial prefrontal cortex is required for the expression of hunger-induced impulsive action. *Neuropsychopharmacology* (2015) 40:2464–74. doi: 10.1038/npp.2015.97
229. Olmstead MC, Ouagazzal AM, Kieffer BL. Mu and delta opioid receptors oppositely regulate motor impulsivity in the signaled nose poke task. *PLoS One* (2009) 4:e4410. doi: 10.1371/journal.pone.0004410
230. Funk D, Tamadon S, Coen K, Fletcher PJ, Le AD. Kappa opioid receptors mediate yohimbine-induced increases in impulsivity in the 5-choice serial reaction time task. *Behav Brain Res* (2019) 359:258–65. doi: 10.1016/j.bbr.2018.11.006
231. Unterwald EM, Rubenfeld JM, Kreek MJ. Repeated cocaine administration upregulates kappa and mu, but not delta, opioid receptors. *Neuroreport* (1994) 5:1613–16. doi: 10.1097/00001756-199408150-00018
232. Ghitza UE, Fabbricatore AT, Prokopenko V, Pawlak AP, West MO. Persistent cue-evoked activity of accumbens neurons after prolonged abstinence from self-administered cocaine. *J Neurosci.* (2003) 23:7239–45. doi: 10.1523/JNEUROSCI.23-19-07239.2003
233. Gorelick DA, Kim YK, Bencherif B, Boyd SJ, Nelson R, Copersino M, et al. Imaging brain mu-opioid receptors in abstinent cocaine users: time course and relation to cocaine craving. *Biol Psychiatry* (2005) 57:1573–82. doi: 10.1016/j.biopsych.2005.02.026
234. Norman H, D'Souza MS. Endogenous opioid system: a promising target for future smoking cessation medications. *Psychopharmacology (Berl)* (2017) 234:1371–94. doi: 10.1007/s00213-017-4582-0
235. Garcia-Cabrerizo R, Garcia-Fuster MJ. Opposite regulation of cannabinoid CB1 and CB2 receptors in the prefrontal cortex of rats treated with cocaine during adolescence. *Neurosci Lett* (2016) 615:60–5. doi: 10.1016/j.neulet.2016.01.018
236. Bystrowska B, Frankowska M, Smaga I, Pomierny-Chamiolo L, Filip M. Effects of cocaine self-administration and its extinction on the rat brain cannabinoid CB1 and CB2 receptors. *Neurotox Res* (2018) 34:547–58. doi: 10.1007/s12640-018-9910-6

237. Mcreynolds JR, Doncheck EM, Vranjkovic O, Ganzman GS, Baker DA, Hillard CJ, et al. CB1 receptor antagonism blocks stress-potentiated reinstatement of cocaine seeking in rats. *Psychopharmacology (Berl)* (2016) 233:99–109. doi: 10.1007/s00213-015-4092-x
238. Hindocha C, Freeman TP, Grabski M, Stroud JB, Crudgington H, Davies AC, et al. Cannabidiol reverses attentional bias to cigarette cues in a human experimental model of tobacco withdrawal. *Addiction* (2018). doi: 10.1111/add.14243
239. Silva AJ, Kogan JH, Frankland PW, Kida S. CREB and memory. *Annu Rev Neurosci* (1998) 21:127–48. doi: 10.1146/annurev.neuro.21.1.127
240. Nestler EJ. Molecular neurobiology of addiction. *Am J Addict* (2001) 10:201–17. doi: 10.1080/105504901750532094
241. Kandel ER. The molecular biology of memory: cAMP, PKA, CRE, CREB-1, CREB-2, and CPEB. *Mol Brain* (2012) 5:14. doi: 10.1186/1756-6606-5-14
242. Gurney ME, D'Amato EC, Burgin AB. Phosphodiesterase-4 (PDE4) molecular pharmacology and Alzheimer's disease. *Neurotherapeutics* (2015) 12:49–56. doi: 10.1007/s13311-014-0309-7
243. Monti B, Berteotti C, Contestabile A. Subchronic rolipram delivery activates hippocampal CREB and arc, enhances retention and slows down extinction of conditioned fear. *Neuropsychopharmacology* (2006) 31:278–86. doi: 10.1038/sj.npp.1300813
244. Yeoh JW, Campbell EJ, James MH, Graham BA, Dayas CV. Orexin antagonists for neuropsychiatric disease: progress and potential pitfalls. *Front Neurosci* (2014) 8:36. doi: 10.3389/fnins.2014.00036
245. James MH, Campbell EJ, Dayas CV. Role of the orexin/hypocretin system in stress-related psychiatric disorders. *Curr Top Behav Neurosci* (2017) 33:197–219. doi: 10.1007/7854_2016_56
246. Gentile TA, Simmons SJ, Barker DJ, Shaw JK, Espana RA, Muschamp JW. Suvorexant, an orexin/hypocretin receptor antagonist, attenuates motivational and hedonic properties of cocaine. *Addict Biol* (2018a) 23:247–55. doi: 10.1111/adb.12507
247. Schmeichel BE, Matzeu A, Koebel P, Vendruscolo LF, Sidhu H, Shahryari R, et al. Knockdown of hypocretin attenuates extended access of cocaine self-administration in rats. *Neuropsychopharmacology* (2018) 43:2373–82. doi: 10.1038/s41386-018-0054-4
248. Bernstein DL, Badve PS, Barson JR, Bass CE, Espana RA. Hypocretin receptor 1 knockdown in the ventral tegmental area attenuates mesolimbic dopamine signaling and reduces motivation for cocaine. *Addict Biol* (2017) 23:1032–45. doi: 10.1111/adb.12553
249. Alijanpour S, Tirgar F, Zarrindast MR. Role of dorsal hippocampal orexin-1 receptors in memory restoration induced by morphine sensitization phenomenon. *Neuroscience* (2016) 312:215–26. doi: 10.1016/j.neuroscience.2015.11.023
250. Moorman DE, James MH, Kilroy EA, Aston-Jones G. Orexin/hypocretin-1 receptor antagonism reduces ethanol self-administration and reinstatement selectively in highly-motivated rats. *Brain Res* (2017) 1654:34–42. doi: 10.1016/j.brainres.2016.10.018
251. Freeman LR, Aston-Jones G. Activation of medial hypothalamic orexin neurons during a Go/No-Go task. *Brain Res* (2018). doi: 10.1016/j.brainres.2018.08.031
252. Deadwyler SA, Porrino L, Siegel JM, Hampson RE. Systemic and nasal delivery of orexin-A (hypocretin-1) reduces the effects of sleep deprivation on cognitive performance in nonhuman primates. *J Neurosci* (2007) 27:14239–47. doi: 10.1523/JNEUROSCI.3878-07.2007
253. Fronczek R, Van Geest S, Frolich M, Overeem S, Roelandse FW, Lammers GJ, et al. Hypocretin (orexin) loss in Alzheimer's disease. *Neurobiol Aging* (2012) 33:1642–50. doi: 10.1016/j.neurobiolaging.2011.03.014
254. Aitta-Aho T, Pappa E, Burdakov D, Apergis-Schoute J. Cellular activation of hypothalamic hypocretin/orexin neurons facilitates short-term spatial memory in mice. *Neurobiol Learn Mem* (2016) 136:183–8. doi: 10.1016/j.nlm.2016.10.005
255. Chen XY, Chen L, Du YF. Orexin-A increases the firing activity of hippocampal CA1 neurons through orexin-1 receptors. *J Neurosci Res* (2017) 95:1415–26. doi: 10.1002/jnr.23975
256. Mavanji V, Butterick TA, Duffy CM, Nixon JP, Billington CJ, Kotz CM. Orexin/hypocretin treatment restores hippocampal-dependent memory in orexin-deficient mice. *Neurobiol Learn Mem* (2017) 146:21–30. doi: 10.1016/j.nlm.2017.10.014
257. Ito N, Yabe T, Gamo Y, Nagai T, Oikawa T, Yamada H, et al. I.c.v. administration of orexin-A induces an antidepressive-like effect through hippocampal cell proliferation. *Neuroscience* (2008) 157:720–32. doi: 10.1016/j.neuroscience.2008.09.042
258. Flores A, Herry C, Maldonado R, Berrendero F. Facilitation of contextual fear extinction by orexin-1 receptor antagonism is associated with the activation of specific amygdala cell subpopulations. *Int J Neuropsychopharmacol* (2017) 20:654–9. doi: 10.1093/ijnp/pyx029
259. Hofer M, Pagliusi SR, Hohn A, Leibrock J, Barde YA. Regional distribution of brain-derived neurotrophic factor mRNA in the adult mouse brain. *EMBO J* (1990) 9:2459–64. doi: 10.1002/j.1460-2075.1990.tb07423.x
260. Hall FS, Drgonova J, Goeb M, Uhl GR. Reduced behavioral effects of cocaine in heterozygous brain-derived neurotrophic factor (BDNF) knockout mice. *Neuropsychopharmacology* (2003) 28:1485–90. doi: 10.1038/sj.npp.1300192
261. St Laurent R, Helm SR, Glenn MJ. Reduced cocaine-seeking behavior in heterozygous BDNF knockout rats. *Neurosci Lett* (2013) 544:94–9. doi: 10.1016/j.neulet.2013.03.050
262. Verheij MM, Vendruscolo LF, Caffino L, Giannotti G, Cazorla M, Fumagalli F, et al. Systemic delivery of a brain-penetrant TrkB antagonist reduces cocaine self-administration and normalizes TrkB signaling in the nucleus accumbens and prefrontal cortex. *J Neurosci* (2016) 36:8149–59. doi: 10.1523/JNEUROSCI.2711-14.2016
263. Li X, Rubio FJ, Zeric T, Bossert JM, Kambhampati S, Cates HM, et al. Incubation of methamphetamine craving is associated with selective increases in expression of Bdnf and trkb, glutamate receptors, and epigenetic enzymes in cue-activated fos-expressing dorsal striatal neurons. *J Neurosci* (2015a) 35:8232–44. doi: 10.1523/JNEUROSCI.1022-15.2015
264. Manning EE, Van Den Buuse M. Altered social cognition in male BDNF heterozygous mice and following chronic methamphetamine exposure. *Behav Brain Res* (2016) 305:181–5. doi: 10.1016/j.bbr.2016.03.014
265. Parikh V, Cole RD, Patel PJ, Poole RL, Gould TJ. Cognitive control deficits during mecamylamine-precipitated withdrawal in mice: possible links to frontostriatal BDNF imbalance. *Neurobiol Learn Mem* (2016) 128:110–6. doi: 10.1016/j.nlm.2016.01.003
266. Ozawa T, Yamada K, Ichitani Y. Hippocampal BDNF treatment facilitates consolidation of spatial memory in spontaneous place recognition in rats. *Behav Brain Res* (2014) 263:210–6. doi: 10.1016/j.bbr.2014.01.034
267. Mu JS, Li WP, Yao ZB, Zhou XF. Deprivation of endogenous brain-derived neurotrophic factor results in impairment of spatial learning and memory in adult rats. *Brain Res* (1999) 835:259–65. doi: 10.1016/S0006-8993(99)01592-9
268. Heldt SA, Stanek L, Chhatwal JP, Ressler KJ. Hippocampus-specific deletion of BDNF in adult mice impairs spatial memory and extinction of aversive memories. *Mol Psychiatry* (2007) 12:656–70. doi: 10.1038/sj.mp.4001957
269. Peters J, Dieppa-Perea LM, Melendez LM, Quirk GJ. Induction of fear extinction with hippocampal–infralimbic BDNF. *Science* (2010) 328:1288–90. doi: 10.1126/science.1186909
270. Rosas-Vidal LE, Do-Monte FH, Sotres-Bayon F, Quirk GJ. Hippocampal–prefrontal BDNF and memory for fear extinction. *Neuropsychopharmacology* (2014) 39:2161–9. doi: 10.1038/npp.2014.64
271. Roberto M, Cruz MT, Gilpin NW, Sabino V, Schweitzer P, Bajo M, et al. Corticotropin releasing factor-induced amygdala gamma-aminobutyric acid release plays a key role in alcohol dependence. *Biol Psychiatry* (2010) 67(9):831–9. doi: 10.1016/j.biopsych.2009.11.007
272. Zorrilla EP, Logrip ML, Koob GF. Corticotropin releasing factor: a key role in the neurobiology of addiction. *Front Neuroendocrinol* (2014) 35:234–44. doi: 10.1016/j.yfrne.2014.01.001
273. Bruijnzeel AW. Neuropeptide systems and new treatments for nicotine addiction. *Psychopharmacology (Berl)* (2017) 234:1419–37. doi: 10.1007/s00213-016-4513-5
274. Boyson CO, Holly EN, Shimamoto A, Albrecht-Souza L, Weiner LA, Debold JF, et al. Social stress and CRF-dopamine interactions in the VTA: role in long-term escalation of cocaine self-administration. *J Neurosci* (2014) 34:6659–67. doi: 10.1523/JNEUROSCI.3942-13.2014
275. Contarino A, Kitchener P, Vallee M, Papaleo F, Piazza PV. CRF1 receptor-deficiency increases cocaine reward. *Neuropharmacology* (2017) 117:41–8. doi: 10.1016/j.neuropharm.2017.01.024
276. Morisot N, Millan MJ, Contarino A. CRF1 receptor-deficiency induces anxiety-like vulnerability to cocaine. *Psychopharmacology (Berl)* (2014b) 231:3965–72. doi: 10.1007/s00213-014-3534-1
277. Morisot N, Le Moine C, Millan MJ, Contarino A. CRF(2) receptor-deficiency reduces recognition memory deficits and vulnerability to stress induced by

cocaine withdrawal. *Int J Neuropsychopharmacol* (2014a) 17:1969–79. doi: 10.1017/S1461145714000625

278. Swanson LW, Sawchenko PE, Rivier J, Vale WW. Organization of ovine corticotropin-releasing factor immunoreactive cells and fibers in the rat brain: an immunohistochemical study. *Neuroendocrinology* (1983) 36:165–86. doi: 10.1159/000123454
279. Hupalo S, Berridge CW. Working memory impairing actions of corticotropin-releasing factor (CRF) neurotransmission in the prefrontal cortex. *Neuropsychopharmacology* (2016) 41:2733–40. doi: 10.1038/npp.2016.85
280. Williams CL, Buchta WC, Riegel AC. CRF-R2 and the heterosynaptic regulation of VTA glutamate during reinstatement of cocaine seeking. *J Neurosci* (2014) 34:10402–14. doi: 10.1523/JNEUROSCI.0911-13.2014
281. Abiri D, Douglas CE, Calakos KC, Barbayannis G, Roberts A, Bauer EP. Fear extinction learning can be impaired or enhanced by modulation of the CRF system in the basolateral nucleus of the amygdala. *Behav Brain Res* (2014) 271:234–9. doi: 10.1016/j.bbr.2014.06.021
282. Salling MC, Martinez D. Brain stimulation in addiction. *Neuropsychopharmacology* (2016) 41:2798–809. doi: 10.1038/npp.2016.80
283. Shields J, Mock J, Devier D, Foundas A. Unilateral repetitive transcranial magnetic stimulation differentially affects younger and older adults completing a verbal working memory task. *J Neurol Sci* (2018) 384:15–20. doi: 10.1016/j.jns.2017.10.021
284. Liu A, Jain N, Vyas A, Lim LW. Ventromedial prefrontal cortex stimulation enhances memory and hippocampal neurogenesis in the middle-aged rats. *Elife* (2015) 4. doi: 10.7554/eLife.04803
285. Garcia-Brito S, Morgado-Bernal I, Biosca-Simon N, Segura-Torres P. Intracranial self-stimulation also facilitates learning in a visual discrimination task in the Morris water maze in rats. *Behav Brain Res* (2017) 317:360–6. doi: 10.1016/j.bbr.2016.09.069
286. Rodriguez-Romaguera J, Do Monte FH, Quirk GJ. Deep brain stimulation of the ventral striatum enhances extinction of conditioned fear. *Proc Natl Acad Sci U S A* (2012) 109:8764–9. doi: 10.1073/pnas.1200782109
287. Rodriguez-Romaguera J, Do-Monte FH, Tanimura Y, Quirk GJ, Haber SN. Enhancement of fear extinction with deep brain stimulation: evidence for medial orbitofrontal involvement. *Neuropsychopharmacology* (2015) 40:1726–33. doi: 10.1038/npp.2015.20
288. Guercio LA, Schmidt HD, Pierce RC. Deep brain stimulation of the nucleus accumbens shell attenuates cue-induced reinstatement of both cocaine and sucrose seeking in rats. *Behav Brain Res* (2015) 281:125–30. doi: 10.1016/j.bbr.2014.12.025
289. Martinez-Rivera FJ, Rodriguez-Romaguera J, Lloret-Torres ME, Do Monte FH, Quirk GJ, Barreto-Estrada JL. Bidirectional modulation of extinction of drug seeking by deep brain stimulation of the ventral striatum. *Biol Psychiatry* (2016) 80:682–90. doi: 10.1016/j.biopsych.2016.05.015
290. Cao B, Wang J, Shahed M, Jelfs B, Chan RH, Li Y. Vagus nerve stimulation alters phase synchrony of the anterior cingulate cortex and facilitates decision making in rats. *Sci Rep* (2016) 6:35135. doi: 10.1038/srep35135
291. Adams WK, Vonder Haar C, Tremblay M, Cocker PJ, Silveira MM, Kaur S, et al. Deep-brain stimulation of the subthalamic nucleus selectively decreases risky choice in risk-preferring rats. *eNeuro* (2017b) 4(4):ENEURO.0094-17. doi: 10.1523/ENEURO.0094-17.2017
292. Zlebnik NE, Carroll ME. Prevention of the incubation of cocaine seeking by aerobic exercise in female rats. *Psychopharmacology (Berl)* (2015b) 232:3507–13. doi: 10.1007/s00213-015-3999-6
293. Beiter RM, Peterson AB, Abel J, Lynch WJ. Exercise during early, but not late abstinence, attenuates subsequent relapse vulnerability in a rat model. *Transl Psychiatry* (2016) 6:e792. doi: 10.1038/tp.2016.58
294. Zlebnik NE, Carroll ME. Effects of the combination of wheel running and atomoxetine on cue- and cocaine-primed reinstatement in rats selected for high or low impulsivity. *Psychopharmacology (Berl)* (2015a) 232:1049–59. doi: 10.1007/s00213-014-3744-6
295. Ogbonmwan YE, Schroeder JP, Holmes PV, Weinshenker D. The effects of post-extinction exercise on cocaine-primed and stress-induced reinstatement of cocaine seeking in rats. *Psychopharmacology (Berl)* (2015) 232:1395–403. doi: 10.1007/s00213-014-3778-9
296. Nasehi M, Nasehi M, Rahmani-Nia F, Mirzaei B, Torabi-Nami M, Zarrindast MR. Swimming improves the emotional memory deficit by scopolamine *via* mu opioid receptors. *Physiol Behav* (2014) 128:237–46. doi: 10.1016/j.physbeh.2014.02.011
297. Mokhtari-Zaer A, Ghodrati-Jaldbakhan S, Vafaei AA, Miladi-Gorji H, Akhavan MM, Bandegi AR, et al. Effects of voluntary and treadmill exercise on spontaneous withdrawal signs, cognitive deficits and alterations in apoptosis-associated proteins in morphine-dependent rats. *Behav Brain Res* (2014) 271:160–70. doi: 10.1016/j.bbr.2014.05.061
298. Bouchet CA, Lloyd BA, Loetz EC, Farmer CE, Ostrovskyy M, Haddad N, et al. Acute exercise enhances the consolidation of fear extinction memory and reduces conditioned fear relapse in a sex-dependent manner. *Learn Mem* (2017) 24:358–68. doi: 10.1101/lm.045195.117
299. Faria RS, Bereta ALB, Reis GHT, Santos LBB, Pereira MSG, Cortez PJO, et al. Effects of swimming exercise on the extinction of fear memory in rats. *J Neurophysiol* (2018) 120:2649–53. doi: 10.1152/jn.00586.2018
300. Mandyam CD, Koob GF. The addicted brain craves new neurons: putative role for adult-born progenitors in promoting recovery. *Trends Neurosci* (2012) 35:250–60. doi: 10.1016/j.tins.2011.12.005
301. Cohen A, Soleiman MT, Talia R, Koob GF, George O, Mandyam CD. Extended access nicotine self-administration with periodic deprivation increases immature neurons in the hippocampus. *Psychopharmacology (Berl)* (2015) 232:453–63. doi: 10.1007/s00213-014-3685-0
302. Garcia-Fuster MJ, Parsegian A, Watson SJ, Akil H, Flagel SB. Adolescent cocaine exposure enhances goal-tracking behavior and impairs hippocampal cell genesis selectively in adult bred low-responder rats. *Psychopharmacology (Berl)* (2017) 234:1293–305. doi: 10.1007/s00213-017-4566-0
303. Takashima Y, Mandyam CD. The role of hippocampal adult neurogenesis in methamphetamine addiction. *Brain Plast* (2018) 3:157–68. doi: 10.3233/BPL-170058
304. Ladron De Guevara-Miranda D, Millon C, Rosell-Valle C, Perez-Fernandez M, Missiroli M, Serrano A, et al. Long-lasting memory deficits in mice withdrawn from cocaine are concomitant with neuroadaptations in hippocampal basal activity, GABAergic interneurons and adult neurogenesis. *Dis Model Mech* (2017) 10:323–36. doi: 10.1242/dmm.026682
305. Koyanagi I, Akers KG, Vergara P, Srinivasan S, Sakurai T, Sakaguchi M. Memory consolidation during sleep and adult hippocampal neurogenesis. *Neural Regen Res* (2019) 14:20–3. doi: 10.4103/1673-5374.243695
306. Pristera A, Saraulli D, Farioli-Vecchioli S, Strimpakos G, Costanzi M, Di Certo MG, et al. Impact of N-tau on adult hippocampal neurogenesis, anxiety, and memory. *Neurobiol Aging* (2013) 34:2551–63. doi: 10.1016/j.neurobiolaging.2013.05.010
307. Ishikawa R, Fukushima H, Frankland PW, Kida S. Hippocampal neurogenesis enhancers promote forgetting of remote fear memory after hippocampal reactivation by retrieval. *Elife* (2016) 5:e17464. doi: 10.7554/eLife.17464
308. Li J, Han Z, Cao B, Cai CY, Lin YH, Li F, et al. Disrupting nNOS-PSD-95 coupling in the hippocampal dentate gyrus promotes extinction memory retrieval. *Biochem Biophys Res Commun* (2017a) 493:862–8. doi: 10.1016/j.bbrc.2017.09.003
309. Zhang Y, Kibaly C, Xu C, Loh HH, Law PY. Temporal effect of manipulating neuroD1 expression with the synthetic small molecule KHS101 on morphine contextual memory. *Neuropharmacology* (2017) 126:58–69. doi: 10.1016/j.neuropharm.2017.08.030
310. Ladron De Guevara-Miranda D, Moreno-Fernandez RD, Gil-Rodriguez S, Rosell-Valle C, Estivill-Torrus G, Serrano A, et al. Lysophosphatidic acid-induced increase in adult hippocampal neurogenesis facilitates the forgetting of cocaine-contextual memory. *Addict Biol* (2019) 24:458–70. doi: 10.1111/adb.12612
311. Noonan MA, Bulin SE, Fuller DC, Eisch AJ. Reduction of adult hippocampal neurogenesis confers vulnerability in an animal model of cocaine addiction. *J Neurosci* (2010) 30:304–15. doi: 10.1523/JNEUROSCI.4256-09.2010
312. Panagopoulos VN, Ralevski E. The role of ghrelin in addiction: a review. *Psychopharmacology (Berl)* (2014) 231:2725–40. doi: 10.1007/s00213-014-3640-0
313. Davis KW, Wellman PJ, Clifford PS. Augmented cocaine conditioned place preference in rats pretreated with systemic ghrelin. *Regul Pept* (2007) 140:148–52. doi: 10.1016/j.regpep.2006.12.003
314. Jerlhag E, Egecioglu E, Dickson SL, Engel JA. Ghrelin receptor antagonism attenuates cocaine- and amphetamine-induced locomotor stimulation, accumbal dopamine release, and conditioned place preference. *Psychopharmacology (Berl)* (2010) 211:415–22. doi: 10.1007/s00213-010-1907-7
315. Jerlhag E, Engel JA. Ghrelin receptor antagonism attenuates nicotine-induced locomotor stimulation, accumbal dopamine release and conditioned place preference in mice. *Drug Alcohol Depend* (2011) 117:126–31. doi: 10.1016/j.drugalcdep.2011.01.010

316. You ZB, Wang B, Gardner EL, Wise RA. Cocaine and cocaine expectancy increase growth hormone, ghrelin, GLP-1, IGF-1, adiponectin, and corticosterone while decreasing leptin, insulin, GIP, and prolactin. *Pharmacol Biochem Behav* (2019) 176:53–6. doi: 10.1016/j.pbb.2018.11.001
317. Al'absi M, Lemieux A, Nakajima M. Peptide YY and ghrelin predict craving and risk for relapse in abstinent smokers. *Psychoneuroendocrinology* (2014) 49:253–9. doi: 10.1016/j.psyneuen.2014.07.018
318. Toth K, Laszlo K, Lukacs E, Lenard L. Intraamygdaloid microinjection of acylated-ghrelin influences passive avoidance learning. *Behav Brain Res* (2009) 202:308–11. doi: 10.1016/j.bbr.2009.03.031
319. Chen L, Xing T, Wang M, Miao Y, Tang M, Chen J, et al. Local infusion of ghrelin enhanced hippocampal synaptic plasticity and spatial memory through activation of phosphoinositide 3-kinase in the dentate gyrus of adult rats. *Eur J Neurosci* (2011) 33:266–75. doi: 10.1111/j.1460-9568.2010.07491.x
320. Beck B, Pourie G. Ghrelin, neuropeptide Y, and other feeding-regulatory peptides active in the hippocampus: role in learning and memory. *Nutr Rev* (2013) 71:541–61. doi: 10.1111/nure.12045
321. Huang CC, Chou D, Yeh CM, Hsu KS. Acute food deprivation enhances fear extinction but inhibits long-term depression in the lateral amygdala *via* ghrelin signaling. *Neuropharmacology* (2016) 101:36–45. doi: 10.1016/j.neuropharm.2015.09.018
322. Shi L, Deng J, Chen S, Que J, Sun Y, Wang Z, et al. Fasting enhances extinction retention and prevents the return of fear in humans. *Transl Psychiatry* (2018) 8:214. doi: 10.1038/s41398-018-0260-1
323. Bowen MT, Neumann ID. Rebalancing the addicted brain: oxytocin interference with the neural substrates of addiction. *Trends Neurosci* (2017) 40:691–708. doi: 10.1016/j.tins.2017.10.003
324. Zhou L, Sun WL, Young AB, Lee K, Mcginty JF, See RE. Oxytocin reduces cocaine seeking and reverses chronic cocaine-induced changes in glutamate receptor function. *Int J Neuropsychopharmacol* (2014) 18 (1):pyu009. doi: 10.1093/ijnp/pyu009
325. Everett NA, Mcgregor IS, Baracz SJ, Cornish JL. The role of the vasopressin V1A receptor in oxytocin modulation of methamphetamine primed reinstatement. *Neuropharmacology* (2018) 133:1–11. doi: 10.1016/j.neuropharm.2017.12.036
326. Baracz SJ, Rourke PI, Pardey MC, Hunt GE, Mcgregor IS, Cornish JL. Oxytocin directly administered into the nucleus accumbens core or subthalamic nucleus attenuates methamphetamine-induced conditioned place preference. *Behav Brain Res* (2012) 228:185–93. doi: 10.1016/j.bbr.2011.11.038
327. Georgiou P, Zanos P, Hourani S, Kitchen I, Bailey A. Cocaine abstinence induces emotional impairment and brain region-specific upregulation of the oxytocin receptor binding. *Eur J Neurosci* (2016) 44:2446–54. doi: 10.1111/ejn.13348
328. Skuse DH, Gallagher L. Dopaminergic–neuropeptide interactions in the social brain. *Trends Cogn Sci* (2009) 13:27–35. doi: 10.1016/j.tics.2008.09.007
329. Lahoud N, Maroun M. Oxytocinergic manipulations in corticolimbic circuit differentially affect fear acquisition and extinction. *Psychoneuroendocrinology* (2013) 38:2184–95. doi: 10.1016/j.psyneuen.2013.04.006
330. Brill-Maoz N, Maroun M. Extinction of fear is facilitated by social presence: synergism with prefrontal oxytocin. *Psychoneuroendocrinology* (2016) 66:75–81. doi: 10.1016/j.psyneuen.2016.01.003
331. Zhou Y, Bendor JT, Yuferov V, Schlussman SD, Ho A, Kreek MJ. Amygdalar vasopressin mRNA increases in acute cocaine withdrawal: evidence for opioid receptor modulation. *Neuroscience* (2005) 134:1391–7. doi: 10.1016/j.neuroscience.2005.05.032
332. Subiah CO, Mabandla MV, Phulukdaree A, Chuturgoon AA, Daniels WM. The effects of vasopressin and oxytocin on methamphetamine-induced place preference behaviour in rats. *Metab Brain Dis* (2012) 27:341–50. doi: 10.1007/s11011-012-9297-7
333. Paban V, Alescio-Lautier B, Devigne C, Soumireu-Mourat B. Fos protein expression induced by intracerebroventricular injection of vasopressin in unconditioned and conditioned mice. *Brain Res* (1999) 825:115–31. doi: 10.1016/S0006-8993(99)01232-9
334. Brunnlieb C, Munte TF, Tempelmann C, Heldmann M. Vasopressin modulates neural responses related to emotional stimuli in the right amygdala. *Brain Res* (2013) 1499:29–42. doi: 10.1016/j.brainres.2013.01.009
335. Caldwell HK, Aulino EA, Rodriguez KM, Witchey SK, Yaw AM. Social context, stress, neuropsychiatric disorders, and the vasopressin 1b receptor. *Front Neurosci* (2017) 11:567. doi: 10.3389/fnins.2017.00567
336. Devito LM, Konigsberg R, Lykken C, Sauvage M, Young WS, 3rd, Eichenbaum H. Vasopressin 1b receptor knock-out impairs memory for temporal order. *J Neurosci* (2009) 29:2676–83. doi: 10.1523/JNEUROSCI.5488-08.2009
337. Stevenson EL, Caldwell HK. The vasopressin 1b receptor and the neural regulation of social behavior. *Horm Behav* (2012) 61:277–82. doi: 10.1016/j.yhbeh.2011.11.009
338. Barsegyan A, Atsak P, Hornberger WB, Jacobson PB, Van Gaalen MM, Roozendaal B. The vasopressin 1b receptor antagonist a-988315 blocks stress effects on the retrieval of object-recognition memory. *Neuropsychopharmacology* (2015) 40:1979–89. doi: 10.1038/npp.2015.48
339. Zhou Y, Leri F, Cummins E, Kreek MJ. Individual differences in gene expression of vasopressin, D2 receptor, POMC and orexin: vulnerability to relapse to heroin-seeking in rats. *Physiol Behav* (2015) 139:127–35. doi: 10.1016/j.physbeh.2014.11.002
340. Brunnlieb C, Nave G, Camerer CF, Schosser S, Vogt B, Munte TF, et al. Vasopressin increases human risky cooperative behavior. *Proc Natl Acad Sci U S A* (2016) 113:2051–6. doi: 10.1073/pnas.1518825113
341. Chen Y, Tian Q. The role of protein kinase C epsilon in neural signal transduction and neurogenic diseases. *Front Med* (2011) 5:70–6. doi: 10.1007/s11684-011-0119-9
342. Lee AM, Messing RO. Protein kinase C epsilon modulates nicotine consumption and dopamine reward signals in the nucleus accumbens. *Proc Natl Acad Sci U S A* (2011) 108:16080–5. doi: 10.1073/pnas.1106277108
343. Miller BW, Wroten MG, Sacramento AD, Silva HE, Shin CB, Vieira PA, et al. Cocaine craving during protracted withdrawal requires PKCepsilon priming within vmPFC. *Addict Biol* (2017) 22:629–39. doi: 10.1111/adb.12354
344. Hongpaisan J, Xu C, Sen A, Nelson TJ, Alkon DL. PKC activation during training restores mushroom spine synapses and memory in the aged rat. *Neurobiol Dis* (2013) 55:44–62. doi: 10.1016/j.nbd.2013.03.012
345. Zisopoulou S, Asimaki O, Leondaritis G, Vasilaki A, Sakellaridis N, Pitsikas N, et al. PKC-epsilon activation is required for recognition memory in the rat. *Behav Brain Res* (2013) 253:280–9. doi: 10.1016/j.bbr.2013.07.036
346. Schmitz JM, Green CE, Hasan KM, Vincent J, Suchting R, Weaver MF, et al. PPAR-gamma agonist pioglitazone modifies craving intensity and brain white matter integrity in patients with primary cocaine use disorder: a double-blind randomized controlled pilot trial. *Addiction* (2017) 112:1861–8. doi: 10.1111/add.13868
347. Naef L, Seabrook L, Hsiao J, Li C, Borgland SL. Insulin in the ventral tegmental area reduces cocaine-evoked dopamine in the nucleus accumbens *in vivo*. *Eur J Neurosci*. (2018). doi: 10.1111/ejn.14291
348. Stern SA, Chen DY, Alberini CM. The effect of insulin and insulin-like growth factors on hippocampus- and amygdala-dependent long-term memory formation. *Learn Mem* (2014a) 21:556–63. doi: 10.1101/lm.029348.112
349. Stern SA, Kohtz AS, Pollonini G, Alberini CM. Enhancement of memories by systemic administration of insulin-like growth factor II. *Neuropsychopharmacology* (2014b) 39:2179–90. doi: 10.1038/npp.2014.69
350. Avgerinos KI, Kalaitzidis G, Malli A, Kalaitzoglou D, Myserlis PG, Lioutas VA. Intranasal insulin in Alzheimer's dementia or mild cognitive impairment: a systematic review. *J Neurol* (2018) 265:1497–510. doi: 10.1007/s00415-018-8768-0
351. Read S, Wu P, Biscow M. Sustained 4-year cognitive and functional response in early Alzheimer's disease with pioglitazone. *J Am Geriatr Soc* (2014) 62:584–6. doi: 10.1111/jgs.12722
352. Nenov MN, Laezza F, Haidacher SJ, Zhao Y, Sadygov RG, Starkey JM, et al. Cognitive enhancing treatment with a PPARgamma agonist normalizes dentate granule cell presynaptic function in Tg2576 APP mice. *J Neurosci* (2014) 34:1028–36. doi: 10.1523/JNEUROSCI.3413-13.2014
353. Nenov MN, Tempia F, Denner L, Dineley KT, Laezza F. Impaired firing properties of dentate granule neurons in an Alzheimer's disease animal model are rescued by PPARgamma agonism. *J Neurophysiol* (2015) 113:1712–26. doi: 10.1152/jn.00419.2014
354. Cippitelli A, Domi E, Ubaldi M, Douglas JC, Li HW, Demopulos G, et al. Protection against alcohol-induced neuronal and cognitive damage by the PPARgamma receptor agonist pioglitazone. *Brain Behav Immun* (2017) 64:320–9. doi: 10.1016/j.bbi.2017.02.001
355. De Guglielmo G, Kallupi M, Scuppa G, Demopulos G, Gaitanaris G, Ciccocioppo R. Pioglitazone attenuates the opioid withdrawal and vulnerability

to relapse to heroin seeking in rodents. *Psychopharmacology (Berl)* (2017) 234:223–34. doi: 10.1007/s00213-016-4452-1

356. Agis-Balboa RC, Arcos-Diaz D, Wittnam J, Govindarajan N, Blom K, Burkhardt S, et al. A hippocampal insulin-growth factor 2 pathway regulates the extinction of fear memories. *EMBO J* (2011) 30:4071–83. doi: 10.1038/emboj.2011.293
357. Agis-Balboa RC, Fischer A. Generating new neurons to circumvent your fears: the role of IGF signaling. *Cell Mol Life Sci* (2014) 71:21–42. doi: 10.1007/s00018-013-1316-2
358. Sen N. Epigenetic regulation of memory by acetylation and methylation of chromatin: implications in neurological disorders, aging, and addiction. *Neuromolecular Med* (2015) 17:97–110. doi: 10.1007/s12017-014-8306-x
359. Wright KN, Hollis F, Duclot F, Dossat AM, Strong CE, Francis TC, et al. Methyl supplementation attenuates cocaine-seeking behaviors and cocaine-induced c-Fos activation in a DNA methylation-dependent manner. *J Neurosci* (2015) 35:8948–58. doi: 10.1523/JNEUROSCI.5227-14.2015
360. Barbier E, Johnstone AL, Khomtchouk BB, Tapocik JD, Pitcairn C, Rehman F, et al. Dependence-induced increase of alcohol self-administration and compulsive drinking mediated by the histone methyltransferase PRDM2. *Mol Psychiatry* (2017) 22:1746–58. doi: 10.1038/mp.2016.131
361. Woldemichael BT, Bohacek J, Gapp K, Mansuy IM. Epigenetics of memory and plasticity. *Prog Mol Biol Transl Sci* (2014) 122:305–40. doi: 10.1016/B978-0-12-420170-5.00011-8
362. Marek R, Coelho CM, Sullivan RK, Baker-Andresen D, Li X, Ratnu V, et al. Paradoxical enhancement of fear extinction memory and synaptic plasticity by inhibition of the histone acetyltransferase p300. *J Neurosci* (2011) 31:7486–91. doi: 10.1523/JNEUROSCI.0133-11.2011
363. Im HI, Hollander JA, Bali P, Kenny PJ. MeCP2 controls BDNF expression and cocaine intake through homeostatic interactions with microRNA-212. *Nat Neurosci* (2010) 13:1120–7. doi: 10.1038/nn.2615
364. Sadakierska-Chudy A, Frankowska M, Miszkiel J, Wydra K, Jastrzebska J, Filip M. Prolonged induction of miR-212/132 and REST expression in rat striatum following cocaine self-administration. *Mol Neurobiol* (2017) 54:2241–54. doi: 10.1007/s12035-016-9817-2
365. Sim MS, Soga T, Pandy V, Wu YS, Parhar IS, Mohamed Z. MicroRNA expression signature of methamphetamine use and addiction in the rat nucleus accumbens. *Metab Brain Dis* (2017) 32:1767–83. doi: 10.1007/s11011-017-0061-x
366. Pietrzykowski AZ, Spijker S. Impulsivity and comorbid traits: a multi-step approach for finding putative responsible microRNAs in the amygdala. *Front Neurosci* (2014) 8:389. doi: 10.3389/fnins.2014.00389
367. Nemeth N, Kovacs-Nagy R, Szekely A, Sasvari-Szekely M, Ronai Z. Association of impulsivity and polymorphic microRNA-641 target sites in the SNAP-25 gene. *PLoS One* (2013) 8:e84207. doi: 10.1371/journal.pone.0084207
368. Sanchez-Mora C, Ramos-Quiroga JA, Garcia-Martinez I, Fernandez-Castillo N, Bosch R, Richarte V, et al. Evaluation of single nucleotide polymorphisms in the miR-183-96-182 cluster in adulthood attention-deficit and hyperactivity disorder (ADHD) and substance use disorders (SUDs). *Eur Neuropsychopharmacol* (2013) 23:1463–73. doi: 10.1016/j.euroneuro.2013.07.002
369. Schratt G. microRNAs at the synapse. *Nat Rev Neurosci* (2009) 10:842–9. doi: 10.1038/nrn2763
370. Sim SE, Lim CS, Kim JI, Seo D, Chun H, Yu NK, et al. The brain-enriched microRNA miR-9-3p regulates synaptic plasticity and memory. *J Neurosci* (2016) 36:8641–52. doi: 10.1523/JNEUROSCI.0630-16.2016
371. Murphy CP, Li X, Maurer V, Oberhauser M, Gstir R, Wearick-Silva LE, et al. MicroRNA-mediated rescue of fear extinction memory by miR-144-3p in extinction-impaired mice. *Biol Psychiatry* (2017) 81:979–9. doi: 10.1016/j.biopsych.2016.12.021
372. Lin Q, Wei W, Coelho CM, Li X, Baker-Andresen D, Dudley K, et al. The brain-specific microRNA miR-128b regulates the formation of fear-extinction memory. *Nat Neurosci* (2011) 14:1115–7. doi: 10.1038/nn.2891
373. Quinn RK, James MH, Hawkins GE, Brown AL, Heathcote A, Smith DW, et al. Temporally specific miRNA expression patterns in the dorsal and ventral striatum of addiction-prone rats. *Addict Biol* (2018) 23:631–42. doi: 10.1111/adb.12520
374. Weafer J, De Wit H. Sex differences in impulsive action and impulsive choice. *Addict Behav* (2014) 39:1573–9. doi: 10.1016/j.addbeh.2013.10.033
375. Swalve N, Smethells JR, Carroll ME. Progesterone attenuates impulsive action in a Go/No-Go task for sucrose pellets in female and male rats. *Horm Behav* (2016) 85:43–7. doi: 10.1016/j.yhbeh.2016.08.001
376. Hammerslag LR, Waldman AJ, Gulley JM. Effects of amphetamine exposure in adolescence or young adulthood on inhibitory control in adult male and female rats. *Behav Brain Res* (2014) 263:22–33 doi: 10.1016/j.bbr.2014.01.015
377. Fenton GE, Halliday DM, Mason R, Bredy TW, Stevenson CW. Sex differences in learned fear expression and extinction involve altered gamma oscillations in medial prefrontal cortex. *Neurobiol Learn Mem* (2016) 135:66–72. doi: 10.1016/j.nlm.2016.06.019
378. Graham BM, Daher M. Estradiol and progesterone have opposing roles in the regulation of fear extinction in female rats. *Neuropsychopharmacology* (2016) 41:774–80. doi: 10.1038/npp.2015.202
379. Milad MR, Igoe SA, Lebron-Milad K, Novales JE. Estrous cycle phase and gonadal hormones influence conditioned fear extinction. *Neuroscience* (2009) 164:887–95. doi: 10.1016/j.neuroscience.2009.09.011
380. Zeidan MA, Igoe SA, Linnman C, Vitalo A, Levine JB, Klibanski A, et al. Estradiol modulates medial prefrontal cortex and amygdala activity during fear extinction in women and female rats. *Biol Psychiatry* (2011) 70:920–7. doi: 10.1016/j.biopsych.2011.05.016
381. Takashima Y, Tseng J, Fannon MJ, Purohit DC, Quach LW, Terranova MJ, et al. Sex differences in context-driven reinstatement of methamphetamine seeking is associated with distinct neuroadaptations in the dentate gyrus. *Brain Sci* (2018) 8. doi: 10.3390/brainsci8120208
382. Anker JJ, Carroll ME. Sex differences in the effects of allopregnanolone on yohimbine-induced reinstatement of cocaine seeking in rats. *Drug Alcohol Depend* (2010) 107:264–7. doi: 10.1016/j.drugalcdep.2009.11.002
383. Regier PS, Claxton AB, Zlebnik NE, Carroll ME. Cocaine-, caffeine-, and stress-evoked cocaine reinstatement in high vs. low impulsive rats: treatment with allopregnanolone. *Drug Alcohol Depend* (2014) 143:58–64. doi: 10.1016/j.drugalcdep.2014.07.001

8

# Integrating Preclinical and Clinical Models of Negative Urgency

*Meredith Halcomb*[1]*, *Evangelia Argyriou*[2] *and Melissa A. Cyders*[2]

[1] *Department of Radiology and Imaging Sciences, Indiana University School of Medicine Indianapolis, Indianapolis, IN, United States,* [2] *Department of Psychology, Indiana University–Purdue University, Indianapolis, IN, United States*

***Correspondence:***
*Meredith Halcomb*
*mheighto@iupui.edu*

Overwhelming evidence suggests that negative urgency is robustly associated with rash, ill-advised behavior, and this trait may hamper attempts to treat patients with substance use disorder. Research applying negative urgency to clinical treatment settings has been limited, in part, due to the absence of an objective, behavioral, and translational model of negative urgency. We suggest that development of such a model will allow for determination of prime neurological and physiological treatment targets, the testing of treatment effectiveness in the preclinical and the clinical laboratory, and, ultimately, improvement in negative-urgency-related treatment response and effectiveness. In the current paper, we review the literature on measurement of negative urgency and discuss limitations of current attempts to assess this trait in human models. Then, we review the limited research on animal models of negative urgency and make suggestions for some promising models that could lead to a translational measurement model. Finally, we discuss the importance of applying objective, behavioral, and translational models of negative urgency, especially those that are easily administered in both animals and humans, to treatment development and testing and make suggestions on necessary future work in this field. Given that negative urgency is a transdiagnostic risk factor that impedes treatment success, the impact of this work could be large in reducing client suffering and societal costs.

**Keywords: negative urgency, animal model, delay discounting, Impulsive behavior, internalizing disorder, transitional, UPPS Impulsive Behavior Scale**

## INTRODUCTION

Negative urgency is an impulsive personality trait reflecting the tendency to act rashly when experiencing extreme negative emotional states, included in the UPPS-P Model of Impulsive Behavior (1, 2). Overwhelming evidence suggests that negative urgency is robustly associated with rash, ill-advised behavior, and this trait may hamper attempts to treat patients with substance use disorder [e.g., Refs. (3, 4)]. However, a systematic investigation of negative urgency in the context of treatment has been limited, in part, due to the lack of a valid objective, behavioral, and translational model of negative urgency. The goal of the current paper is to review the current human and animal approaches to the measurement of negative urgency and to make suggestions on how an objective translational model could be developed. We review the existing literature and make suggestions for prime models that can be explored as translational approaches in negative urgency. We also review the neural and psychopharmacological correlates of negative urgency, suggesting potential novel targets of intervention within a translational model. We suggest that the development of a translational model easily administered in animals and human would allow for better characterization of the neuroscientific correlates of negative urgency, determination of prime neurological and physiological treatment targets, and the validation of an objective measure of treatment effectiveness in the preclinical and clinical laboratory.

## NEGATIVE URGENCY IN THE BROADER CONSTRUCT OF IMPULSIVITY AND PERSONALITY

Impulsivity is broadly defined as traits and behaviors that predispose individuals to rash action (or ill-advised inaction) (5–7). The UPPS-P model integrated existing personality-based measures of impulsivity into five traits, using the Five-Factor Model as a theoretical framework. The five traits include negative urgency, positive urgency (i.e., a tendency to act rashly in response to extreme positive emotional states), lack of premeditation (i.e., a tendency to act without thinking), lack of perseverance (i.e., an inability to stay focused on a task), and sensation seeking (i.e., tendency to seek novel and exciting experiences). These traits are best described as separate, though related, tendencies toward rash action (8). Research supports a multidimensional nature of impulsivity, and extensions of the UPPS-P model have been suggested (9). There is increasing consensus that impulsive personality consists of traits that are affect-free and traits that have a strong affective component (9, 10). The distinction between affect-based and affect-free impulsigenic traits is further supported by the fact that they share little common variance (0–13%) (10).

Negative urgency is well placed in the personality literature. It shares conceptual overlap with the Impulsiveness facet of the NEO-PI-R (11); however, a factor analysis by Peterson and Smith (2008) found that negative urgency loaded onto the Neuroticism, Conscientiousness, and Agreeableness factors, suggesting that negative urgency is not represented by one domain or facet of the NEO-PI-R, but rather assesses a trait characterized by high distress, low conscientiousness, and low agreeableness (2). Some have suggested that negative urgency (along with the positive mood variant of positive urgency) is quite similar to one of the two higher-order dimensions of the Five-Factor Model (alpha, representing high levels of emotional instability, disagreeableness, and disinhibition) (12, 13).

What differentiates negative urgency from other constructs pertaining to responses to emotions, such as emotion regulation and emotional lability, is that it reflects a disposition to reflexive reactions in response to intense negative emotion. Emotion regulation involves efforts, either reflexive or effortful, to modify the intensity of the experienced emotion that varies across situations and across time, and emotion dysregulation can occur in the absence of intense emotion (14, 15). Negative urgency captures the between-person variability in the capacity to control intense emotion-driven urges (10). Effects of negative urgency are not explained by additive or interactive combinations of negative affective traits (e.g., neuroticism, emotional lability) combined with general disinhibition (2, 8). Similarly, negative urgency is only moderately correlated with measures of emotion regulation, which signifies that these are related, but separate, constructs with distinct contributions to psychopathology (16). In fact, the majority of the reliable variance in negative urgency is not explained by other related traits (2).

## NEGATIVE URGENCY AS A TRANSDIAGNOSTIC RISK AND TREATMENT FACTOR

Accumulating evidence suggests that negative urgency is one of the most robust predictors of a wide range of maladaptive behaviors and psychopathology, including alcohol use and dependence (3, 5, 17, 18), tobacco use and dependence (19–21), and problematic cannabis use (22–24). The fact that negative urgency developmentally precedes substance use and addictive disorders (25, 26) indicates that negative urgency is likely a contributor to the development and maintenance of addictive disorders. This is further bolstered by empirical evidence showing that decreases in impulsivity are associated with decreases in substance use across the lifespan (27). This accumulating evidence supports the notion that negative urgency is a transdiagnostic endophenotype for problematic levels of behaviors associated with risk (28). This includes not only addictive behaviors, but also disorders highly comorbid with these conditions, such as depression, anxiety, and bipolar disorders (5, 28, 29). Negative urgency is represented in broad diagnostic criteria of the *Diagnostic and Statistical Manual of Mental Disorders, Fifth Edition* (*DSM-5*) (29).

Despite the substantial amount of research implicating negative urgency in the development and maintenance of addictive behaviors, only a small body of empirical work has systematically studied its application to treatment (29, 30). There are no specific behavioral or pharmacological treatments for negative urgency, although some have been suggested (31). A meta-analysis conducted by Hershberger et al. (30) examined the effect of negative urgency on substance use disorder psychotherapy outcomes and how this trait changes during treatment. The findings showed that increased levels of negative urgency at baseline are related with poorer treatment outcomes, suggesting that this trait potentially inhibits substance use symptom improvement (30). Additionally, the authors identified only small decreases in negative urgency ($g = -0.25$) from the beginning to the end of treatment. This suggests that current substance use treatments are not changing negative urgency notably, which increases the risk for subsequent substance use re-initiation or relapse (30). They explain one way in which negative urgency lowers treatment efficacy: Most existing therapies for addictive disorders are focused on the modification of proximal factors related to addiction, such as substance use motives or environments that facilitate use, rather than the distal factors, such as negative urgency, that underlie them (32, 33). For example, negative urgency is a predictor of the development of substance use motives (34) and likely contributes to individuals seeking out and selecting environments that facilitate use, consistent with personality–environment transaction theories (35).

Although addressing proximal risk factors of addiction might improve current symptoms, if distal risk factors remain unchanged, relapse or treatment nonresponse becomes more likely (29), as the distal factors can impart risk independent of the modified proximal factor. The authors suggest that the integration of negative urgency in case conceptualization, treatment planning, and goal setting would significantly improve substance use treatment outcomes (30).

Although negative urgency-targeted interventions have not been systematically developed or investigated, there is promising evidence for their potential success. Zapolski et al. (31) provided recommendations for strategies to target negative urgency in treatment. Their recommended strategies include training in emotion regulation, distress tolerance, interpersonal effectiveness, training in modifying emotional reactions based on the context, relaxation techniques, identification of precipitating events and triggers to emotional reactivity and use of adaptive alternatives, and the use of medications, such as selective serotonin reuptake inhibitors (31, 36). Many of these strategies have been successfully incorporated in several clinical interventions in different contexts, including substance use, and their effectiveness has been tested and supported (5, 26, 36–40) with some exceptions (41, 42). Because negative urgency increases the risk of a wide range of addictive behaviors and other clinical disorders, negative-urgency-targeted interventions could have wide and broad benefit. Additionally, such interventions are easily adopted by addiction medicine practitioners and would improve their daily practice in prevention, treatment, and rehabilitation of addictive disorders and accompanying conditions.

We propose that an important and viable long-term goal is to design and test pharmacological, psychological, behavioral, and physiological treatments that specifically aim to reduce negative urgency. This would allow the application of these treatment strategies transdiagnostically, which would be fruitful to reduce not only the target disorder (e.g., alcohol use disorder), but also maladaptive coping related to comorbid disorders (e.g., depression). Thus, one intervention could be effective for treatment of multiple disorders or behaviors. In the current paper, we focus specifically on the role of negative urgency in addictive disorders, although the implications would likely apply to any disorder in which negative urgency is implicated (29).

## CURRENT MEASUREMENT OF NEGATIVE URGENCY IN HUMANS

Negative urgency is most commonly measured using the UPPS-P Impulsive Behavior Scale. The UPPS-P is a 59-item self-report questionnaire originally created by Whiteside and Lynam (1) with four subscales (negative urgency, lack of premeditation, lack of perseverance, and sensation seeking). The positive urgency subscale was added later (43, 44). Individuals rate their general tendencies on a four-point scale from *Agree Strongly* to *Disagree Strongly.* Individual item scores are reverse coded (as needed) and averaged together to approximate a mean level of each trait, with higher scores indicating higher levels of rash action. The negative urgency subscale includes items assessing the disposition of respondents to act without careful consideration of the consequences when faced with negative affect. Example items for the scale include "When I feel bad, I will often do things I later regret in order to make myself feel better now" and "When I am upset, I often act without thinking." The UPPS-P has been shown to produce valid and reliable data across men and women, different age groups, and clinical and community samples (43, 45–47).

Although there are no behavioral tasks developed specifically to assess negative urgency, there are many behavioral tasks measuring state-like rash action in general (48, 49). Both self-report and behavioral task measures of rash action are strongly correlated with risky behaviors, but research has shown little overlap *between* these two types of measures. A meta-analysis conducted by Cyders and Coskunpinar (48) found that effect sizes for the relationship between self-report and behavioral task measures of rash action are small, ranging from $r = 0.097$ to 0.134, suggesting that at least 99% of the variance between these types of measures is unshared. This indicates that self-report and behavioral measures of rash action assess complementary, but separate, constructs. In some ways, this lack of overlap is not surprising, as these different task domains assess separate aspects of rash action. Self-report measures likely represent stable tendencies toward general behaviors (trait-like impulsivity) reflecting predominately emotional/motivational mechanisms of rash action, whereas behavioral tasks are more likely snapshots of behavior (state-like impulsivity) in response to stimuli, reflecting predominately cognitive mechanisms of rash action (9).

Self-report measurement of negative urgency has important strengths in the context of psychopathology. First, it has content and ecological validity as it reflects the individuals' subjective experience of patterns of thoughts, emotions, and behaviors in daily life, which can easily be generalized to the real world (50). Second, it has strong face validity, in that questions and results can be easily interpreted without making assumptions since they are based on direct and clear questions to the respondents (29, 48). Finally, it is inexpensive and easy to administer to a large group of people (48). However, this type of assessment has some limitations that make it less ideal in designing or testing the efficacy of treatments. Self-report measurement is limited by self-awareness, openness, and social desirability (48, 51), making the assessment only as good as what a person knows and is willing to report about the self. For example, in a clinical trial, individuals might not report on less socially desirable aspects of the self, and thus baseline levels might be underestimates of the true level of negative urgency, making measuring change over the trial more difficult. Relatedly, measuring negative urgency repeatedly in short succession might lead to participant fatigue or might influence an individual's responses in undue ways, further contributing to error in the measurement. For example, in a clinical trial, individuals might report a reduction in negative urgency after treatment, because they assume such a reduction is expected and not due to any true changes in the trait in response to treatment. Additionally, because the UPPS-P evaluates general tendencies, changes that do occur in shorter time frames might not be accurately assessed *via* this measure (i.e., it is not designed to assess shorter fluctuations in behavior). Finally, self-report measures are difficult to translate into animal models. Behavioral tasks designed to measure the behavioral expression of negative urgency in lab settings would be an excellent complementary approach to address these limitations and to better design and assess treatment effectiveness.

## ANIMAL MODELS OF NEGATIVE URGENCY

The use of animal models would greatly enhance the capability to deconstruct possible underlying neural mechanisms of negative urgency and allow for greater manipulation of testing variables to determine new therapeutic targets. There are numerous papers describing external validity, including the specific criteria animal models must meet and how different facets of external validity simulate conditions, neurobiology, and behavior seen in clinical populations (e.g., 52–55). The earliest characterization of these criteria included the requirement for animal models to demonstrate the same etiology, symptoms, response to treatment, and biochemistry seen in human populations (54). These criteria were the foundation for decades of work establishing a well-defined framework for animal models. The traditional framework, proposed by Willner (55), included three types of validity: *predictive validity* (i.e., the model predicts some criterion of interest), *face validity* (i.e., the model looks similar to the human condition), and *construct validity* (i.e., the animal model measures what is intended to measure) (55). Expansions and modifications of these criteria provide a more granular method for establishing reliable, translatable animal models, taking into account several factors that represent critical points for similarity. Geyer and Markou (53) emphasized the additional importance of *etiological validity* (i.e., the model has the same etiology as human condition) and *convergent/discriminant validity* (i.e., the model is associated with other related models but unrelated to models that are disparate with the underlying condition). Belzung and Lemoine (52) further emphasized *induction validity* (i.e., etiological effects on observable behaviors in animals have similar effects in humans) and *remission validity* (i.e., similarity in response to treatment across animal and human conditions).

Any animal model of negative urgency must fulfill these validity requirements; we evaluate existing and potential models in terms of these criteria (**Table 1**). For the sake of simplicity, we have not included every measure, but rather those we believe most strictly comply to a model of negative urgency. We also highlight the types of validity each model satisfies, where applicable, which aids in determining translatability.

At present, studies investigating negative urgency in animals are sparse. One proposed method for generating negative urgency (utilized in both animal and human models) involves unexpected reward omission (56–58). In one study, humans or rats were trained to perform an operant task (button pressing or lever pressing, respectively) and were rewarded with either money or a food pellet, respectively (56). Increases in response rates and decreases in response latencies were dependent variables constituting measures of negative urgency. This task has many strengths, including that it can and has been applied across human and animal models and that it appears to have adequate predictive and face validity for the emotional change. The task is especially analogous in clinical and preclinical administration (56); however, this task lacks the "rash action" component necessary to accurately assess negative urgency. For the model to have good external validity, there must be some procedure in place to assess the effect of this induced negative urgency on impulsive behavior. In short, this model does not provide any negative consequences of impulsive behavior generated through negative affect. Therefore, although this task shows some promise, further research is required for better, more representative models.

## SUGGESTIONS FOR OBJECTIVE TRANSLATIONAL MODELS OF NEGATIVE URGENCY

### Affective State

Clinical designs for incitement of negative affect in humans include the International Affective Picture System (IAPS), the Paced Auditory Serial Addition Test (PASAT), and social rejection, although there are no analogous methods in animal models (59, 60). The IAPS involves presentation of positive, neutral, or negative images (61). Numerous studies have shown that the administration of the IAPS is effective in producing transient negative emotion with resultant changes in brain activity or behavior (62–66). However, none of these studies has demonstrated increased impulsive, rash behavior associated with that negative affect. The PASAT is a procedure in which subjects must serially add a quickly vocalized list of numbers and is a demonstrated lab-induced stressor (67). Implementation of a social rejection protocol has generated changes in response inhibition during a Go/No-Go task (64, 68), thus linking negative affect with rash action. A meta-analysis by Westerman (69) outlines numerous other mood induction paradigms (including video clips, writing, etc). and describes the strengths and drawbacks of each. For example, the Imagination mood induction procedure requires the subject to imagine an emotion-laden experience from their past, and the Velten mood induction procedure requires the participants to make negative self-references (69). Unfortunately, these methods are not conducive to reproduction with animal models.

Although these findings suggest usefulness of these methods in humans, translatability to animals is questionable at best. There is no comparable method to many of these procedures (IAPS, PASAT, Imagination, Velten) in preclinical studies. While social isolation models in rodents can elicit behavioral modifications, these are typically utilized to produce depressive states and may instigate neurobiological alterations that have little connection to impulsivity and may hinder the ability to interpret results (54, 70, 71). For greatest translatability, the methods by which negative urgency are elicited should be as similar as possible in human and animal subjects.

**TABLE 1 |** Methods for induction of negative affect and measurement of impulsive responding. This table lists several possible suggestions for induction of negative affect in animals and humans and impulsivity assessment. It also outlines which types of validity (which describes translatability) are fulfilled with each task. NEO-PI-R: NEO Personality Inventory, revised; IAPS: International Affective Picture System; na: no available data.

| TASK | APPLICABLE IN HUMANS | APPLICABLE IN ANIMALS | TYPES OF VALIDITY | | | | | |
|---|---|---|---|---|---|---|---|---|
| | | | FACE | CONSTRUCT | ETIOLOGICAL | CONVERGENT | INDUCTION | REMISSION |
| **INDUCTION OF NEGATIVE AFFFECT** | | | | | | | | |
| REWARD OMMISSION TASK | + | + | + | + | + | + | + | na |
| IAPS | + | | | | | | | |
| Paced Auditory Serial Addition Test | + | | | | | | | |
| IMAGINATION Mood Induction Procedure | + | | | | | | | |
| VELTEN Mood Induction Procedure | + | | | | | | | |
| SOCIAL REJECTION (humans) | + | | | | | | | |
| SOCIAL ISOLATION (animals) | | + | | + | | | + | na |
| FOOT SHOCK | | + | | + | | | | na |
| FOOD DEPRIVATION | | + | | + | | | + | na |
| ACUTE RESTRAINT STRESS | | + | | + | | | + | na |
| **MEASURES OF IMPULSIVITY** | | | | | | | | |
| DELAY DISCOUNTING | + | + | + | + | + | + | + | + |
| GO/NO-GO | + | + | + | + | + | + | + | + |
| STOP SIGNAL | + | + | + | + | + | + | + | na |
| CONTINUOUS PERFORMANCE TASK | + | + | + | + | + | + | + | na |
| BALLOON ANALOGUE RISK TASK | + | | | + | | | | na |
| ERIKSEN FLANKER TASK | + | | | | | | | |
| **SELF-REPORT MEASURES** | | | | | | | | |
| UPPS-P | + | | | | | + | | |
| NEO-PI-R (Impulsiveness facet) | + | | | | | + | | |

Currently, there are several animal models capable of inducing stress, anxiety, and depression, such as restraint stress, foot shock, and the forced swim test (72–75). Many of these suffer from limited translatability to clinical models, due to ethical or feasibility restraints. Additionally, these models typically result in long-term effects (including downstream effects on neurotransmitter systems), in addition to immediate, negative states. For an animal model to have good face and etiological validity, there must be some instigating event that engenders a transitory negative state without conferring semi-permanent or permanent change. Given the effects of corticosterone on numerous brain regions, including the hippocampus (76, 77), the task should avoid chronic stressors and focus on events that primarily lead to depressive-like states. Additionally, it is important to limit exposure to the negative stimulus to avoid creation of a disposition to depression often seen after repeated administration (78). This distinction permits researchers to narrow investigations to discrete elicited state-like behavior rather than long term, trait-like behavior.

## Impulsive Choice

Delay discounting is based on the premise that reinforcer influence on behavior decreases as a function of the delay to its delivery (79). In one version of this task, the adjusting amounts version, subjects complete several trials in which they must choose between a small, immediate reward and a larger, delayed reward and every choice of the immediate reinforcer decreases the amount of reinforcer available upon choice of the immediate reinforcer on the next trial (80, 81). In this manner, repeated choice of the immediate reinforcer results in overall suboptimal levels of reinforcer across the session. Although delay discounting is typically thought to assess levels of cognitive impulsivity (82), the design of the task is such that impulsive-like responding is rewarded immediately (immediate reinforcer) and is then consequently paired with decrease in immediate reinforcer volume. Through manipulation of the length of the delay to the larger reward and the use of the hyperbolic discounting equation, we are able to generate a "discounting curve" that describes the steepness or "impulsivity" of each individual. This curve can be thought of as a measure of how long the subject is willing to wait for a specific reward, a measure of "cognitive impulsivity."

Previous work has demonstrated the translatability of delay discounting. The delay discounting model has considerable face validity (52). The basic premise is identical in both human and animal models, particularly in the Experiential Discounting Task for humans, which requires the participant to experience the delay during the task, rather than afterwards, eliminating the need for the subject to "imagine" the delay while continuing to respond (83). In the animal version, subjects are also required to experience the delay during the session. Furthermore, one of the proposed mechanisms of external validity is the requirement that the task must measure the same changes in behavior upon treatment (remission validity) (52). Although this version of delay discounting most closely resembles the version administered in animals, there are possible limitations in test–retest reliability and conflating the delay and probability of receiving reward (84). A more common administration (the adjusting amounts version) involves presenting a delayed choice that will be accessible at some point in the future rather than implementing the delay during the task itself. The adjusting amounts version is also efficient at generating discounting curves and there is no demonstrable difference in effect between delayed rewards during the task and those imagined in the future (85). The animal version of delay discounting described here is accurate enough to detect the same decreases in impulsivity after stimulant (methamphetamine/amphetamine) administration observed in clinical applications (86–91). Given the demonstrated ability of the delay discounting task to evaluate changes in impulsive, rash behavior, and the translatability of those results, it may provide a valid mechanism to analyze behavior motivated by a negative emotional state.

### Impulsive Action

In the Go/No-Go task, the subject is required to respond on a specified manipulandum upon presentation of some stimulus during "Go" trials and must inhibit that response upon presentation of some stimulus during "No-Go" trials (92, 93). This method is used to measure action restraint in a number of animal models of disease, including alcohol use disorder (94). A meta-analysis found a significant correlation between results on clinical applications of the task with self-report measures of negative urgency (48). A recent study examining the association between induced negative urgency and performance on the Go/No-Go task revealed that greater activation in brain regions involved in inhibitory processes was correlated with higher levels of urgency (64–66, 68). An investigation into the effects of social rejection on impulsivity found that subjects reporting higher levels of negative affect completed significantly fewer successful No-Go trials (95). There is also evidence that responding in the Go/No-Go task predicts relapse rates in abstinent alcoholics (96). Administration of this task in an animal model of negative urgency could pave the way toward understanding what neural correlates underlie this association.

### Conclusions on Translational Tasks

In conclusion, although the literature on animal models of negative urgency is sparse, there are some interesting and promising attempts to model negative urgency preclinically. The very nature of negative urgency centers upon behavioral reactions to emotional states, suggesting an internalizing primary aspect of the trait that is integrated with an externalizing behavioral outcome. Therefore, any reliable, translatable model of negative urgency must include a method for inducing negative affect in addition to the demonstration of an externalizing behavior of some interest. Unfortunately, the design of preclinical models of internalizing affective disorders is inherently problematic. Emotional states, such as depression, are not easily represented in non-human subjects, which limits the ability to devise translational, behavioral measures (52, 78, 97–99). Any animal model seeking to evaluate affectivity must demonstrate the capacity not only to induce a specific emotional state, but also to effectively identify alterations in that state under manipulation. Since evaluating the subjective experiences of animals is difficult, this is a challenging prospect; however, the translatability of the model is necessary for the generation of meaningful results (52).

Ideally, the behavior evoked by the induction of negative affect should be immediately reinforcing, yet ultimately yield suboptimal results. Cyders and Smith (100) proposed that rash or ill-advised actions during times of negative arousal, such as consuming alcohol upon receipt of bad news, provide immediate relief, reinforcing the behavior (100). Alternatively, more adaptive coping mechanisms are not implemented, limiting the reinforcement of these responses. For example, then, engagement in repeated alcohol intake to alleviate negative affectivity is reinforced and the behavior becomes more frequent, despite being detrimental in the long term. The key in an animal model is to devise a task that provides an opportunity to access a preferred reward (food, sucrose, mating), paired with loss of a highly valued resource or punishment, such as excessive lever pressing, resulting in smaller amounts of reward over time.

## NEURAL AND GENETIC CORRELATES OF NEGATIVE URGENCY AND POTENTIAL TREATMENT TARGETS

There are numerous excellent reviews outlining human brain structures and systems believed to contribute to the experience of negative urgency (2, 101) and other emotion-related constructs (9, 102–104). Given the implicit obstacles associated with neuroimaging in rodents and the lack of definitive homologous prefrontal regions in rodent brains, there has been limited information gleaned from animal neuroimaging studies.

### Human Neuroimaging

Research concerning the neurobiology underlying negative urgency follows two primary tracts: structures and systems that represent bottom-up processing and structures and systems that are associated with top-down regulatory control. Regions representing bottom-up processing, such as the amygdala, have connections to regions regulating top-down control, including the orbitofrontal cortex (OFC), the ventral medial prefrontal cortex (vmPFC), and the dorsolateral PFC (dlPFC).

These connections constitute a reciprocal system by which both systems integrate to detect negative affect, determine the salience of that affect, and initiate or inhibit behavior in reaction (2). For instance, the amygdala is greatly involved with the experience of negative emotions (105) and projects to, and receives back projections from, the OFC (106). The OFC and its medial sector, the vmPFC, play a role in modulating emotion-based behavior and reactivity (105) and can inhibit behavior that is emotion-based (107). The ability of top-down regulatory systems to control emotion-based behavior is essential for preservation of long-term goals. There is emerging evidence that negative urgency relates to variations in neural activity in these and other subcortical [ventral striatum (VST) and caudate nucleus (CAU)] and frontal (dlPFC) brain regions (57, 64, 68, 108, 109).

There is a wealth of information concerning the function of these brain regions from neuroimaging studies, implicating the association of various structures in negative-urgency-mediated ill-advised behaviors, particularly in alcohol use disorder populations and social drinkers. The insula (INS), which plays a role in emotional processing, shows greater activation during negative urgency in adolescent binge drinkers (110). The caudate (CAU) demonstrates greater activation in response to alcohol cues in social drinkers (64, 68). The mOFC/vmOFC, primarily engaged in evaluation of rewarding stimuli to determine action, is activated more strongly to alcohol odor cues, while activation of the lOFC, which evaluates punishing stimuli, was related to negative urgency in social drinkers (63). The PFC, particularly the dlPFC, is heavily recruited during cognitive tasks in subjects high in negative urgency (111, 112). Finally, the amygdala, which is specifically involved in processing negative emotions (113) and is an important hub in negative urgency (101), shows greater activation in response to negative mood images and during negative mood evaluation in cocaine users with personality disorders (114, 115). Taken together, these findings imply a dysregulation in this interconnected system of regions associated with emotional processing and emotion-based behavioral control, which is likely contributing to maladaptive actions in pathological populations.

Emerging evidence from functional connectivity studies indicates that these structures interact to direct emotional lability and drive behavior. Dysfunction in the vmPFC impacts its association with the amygdala, resulting in potentiated response to emotional cues (116). Non-treatment-seeking alcoholics have aberrant anterior insular cortex connectivity, a region associated with assignment of emotional states to interoceptive bodily stimuli (117). There is evidence of increased cortico-limbic connectivity in cocaine-dependent subjects, associated with emotion-based impulsivity (118). A model-free, resting-state study of alcohol-dependent subjects found increased within-network connectivity in salience, orbitofrontal, and default mode networks and increased between-network connectivity associated with higher self-reported ratings of negative urgency (119). These findings indicate interconnected, functionally coupled sets of brain regions associated with emotional activation and responding, which must be better understood to further development of more targeted treatment strategies. There are numerous avenues for further exploration using connectivity tools, which would immeasurably enhance insight into underlying mechanisms of behavior. Unfortunately, neuroimaging techniques are inherently difficult to conduct in animal models and may be confounded by agents used to anesthetize subjects, limiting investigations at the preclinical level.

## Human Neurotransmitter Systems

Function in many of the above brain regions is largely mediated by dopamine (DA) and serotonin (5HT) transmitter systems. These systems interact to influence emotion-based decision-making. Researchers have reported that low levels of 5HT are associated with greater incidences of rash or maladaptive behavior involving risk and increases in negative affect (120–125). Conversely, subjects with lower mono-amino oxidase, responsible for the breakdown of 5HT, display higher levels of aggression and negative urgency (126), which suggests that it may be the dysregulation of serotonin that influences emotional lability rather than simply a depletion. Interestingly, high 5HT levels in the PFC are correlated with socially adept behavior in monkeys (127), while low levels of 5HT in the anterior cingulate cortex are correlated with inhibited emotional regulation (124). It is important to note that these associations are receptor-dependent. The 5HT system is composed of several types of receptors and transporters, which may infer opposite effects upon activation. For instance, a reduction in 5HT available at $5HT_{2c}$ and $5HT_{1a}$ receptor sites increases likelihood of impulsive, rash behavior, while low 5HT at $5HT_{2a}$ receptor sites reduces risky behavior (128, 129). This dichotomy in receptor effects is important when determining possible pharmacological treatments. Although $5HT_{2c}$ and $5HT_{1a}$ receptors are more common, any prospective treatment targeting this system would be better served to attempt pharmacological effects specified for these receptors.

Alternatively, greater levels of DA activity are associated with a higher tendency to act (130), greater behavioral disinhibition (131), and greater reward-seeking and risk-taking behaviors (132, 133). DA is highly influential in the OFC–amygdala circuit (considered to be the "reward" circuit), particularly at D2 and D4 receptor sites, and it is theorized that DA effects on rash action may stem from D2 activation decreasing the value of delayed rewards (134). A recent study evaluating DA availability using positron emission tomography (PET) found that increased levels of DA in the putamen were associated with greater levels of impulsivity on the delay discounting task (135). The DA system in the OFC–amygdala circuit is modulated by serotonergic input through both direct and indirect mechanisms (136, 137). 5HT systems that subsume information processing influence DA pathways that underlie approach behavior (120, 138); therefore, decreased 5HT levels would result in diminished suppression of rash, ill-advised behavior.

## Human Genetics

Overall, it is well-established that behavior consistent with negative urgency is associated with depleted 5HT levels in the PFC and overactive DA in the OFC–amygdala circuit. There are a number of genetic polymorphisms possibly contributing to the imbalances observed in populations endorsing elevated negative urgency. Certain alleles of the serotonin transporter gene (5HTTLPR) and DA receptor genes (DRD2, DRD3, and DRD4) have all been associated with fluctuations in 5HT and DA levels and, thus, frequency of emotion-based rash behaviors (139–144). Associations between DA and 5HT are also present in an animal model of negative urgency. Yates et al. found that increased DA transporter function in the nucleus accumbens and greater 5HT transporter function in the OFC are mediated by higher exhibited negative urgency in a reward omission task (57). This neurobiological similarity highlights the usefulness of animal models to further elucidate the correlation between negative urgency and risky behavior, such as alcohol consumption.

There is limited information regarding the association between these neurotransmitter systems and negative urgency in alcohol use disorder populations. There are numerous lines of evidence indicating that decreased levels of 5HT are strongly associated with increased alcohol consumption and risk for future alcohol problems (145–147). One recent study reported that negative urgency (as measured by UPPS-P) mediated the relationship between alcohol abuse and genetically driven decreases in 5HT availability (148). In this study, higher polygenic 5HT scores (indicating lower 5HT function) were positively correlated with higher self-reported negative urgency and greater levels of alcohol consumption. At this time, there are no preclinical investigations evaluating the relationship between these transmitter systems, alcohol overconsumption, and negative urgency, although one study did report an increase in negative affect during cocaine withdrawal in rats in the reward omission task (58).

In addition to the influence of the DA and 5HT systems, there is evidence that polymorphisms of the GABRA2 gene, which codes for the $GABA_A$a2 receptor, are also associated with both alcoholism risk and negative urgency (149). Villafuerte (150) identified an association between impulsiveness and alcoholism with genetic variants of the GABRA2 gene in a family strongly endorsing alcoholism (150). This same study reported that this association was mediated by activation during reward or loss. Further research uncovered that impulsiveness, particularly negative urgency, mediates the association between the GABRA2 gene and alcoholism (151). In addition, lower levels of gamma-Aminobutyric acid (GABA) in the dlPFC are correlated with greater reports of negative urgency (152). This region is implicated in the effortful control of behavior and is heavily activated during behavioral inhibition tasks in subjects high in negative urgency. Lack of GABA in this brain region may inhibit function, decreasing the ability of the dlPFC to efficiently regulate behavior.

## Implications for Treatment

Taken together, these findings provide excellent opportunities for translation to animal models, with the ultimate goal of improving clinical treatment. Translation of negative urgency to preclinical models would improve treatment in three main ways.

First, it allows for more precise identification of the neural correlates of negative urgency in human neuroimaging studies. Examining these regions translationally allows for more precision in the identified regions, circuits, and neurotransmitter systems. For example, identified neural substrates mediating negative urgency may be manipulated in animal models, and support of those hypotheses would provide data suggesting potential mechanisms through which those substrates may be manipulated to aid in treatment. Thus, this would help determine if these brain correlates are simply associated with negative urgency or are a causal mechanism in these maladaptive behaviors. This could lead to novel neurological and physiological targets.

Relatedly, animal models provide a unique opportunity to further elucidate neural underpinnings of behavior through manipulation of genetic predispositions. There are several lines of mice and rats selectively bred to prefer alcohol, including alcohol-preferring rats, high alcohol-drinking rats, and high alcohol-preferring mice (153, 154). Behavioral models can be used to compare responding to negative urgency in these subjects to responding observed in low alcohol-preferring subjects. These methods have demonstrated the ability to identify behavioral characteristics inherited alongside the predilection to prefer and consume alcohol, including impulsive-like responding in a delay discounting task (81, 155). Furthermore, they increase understanding of contributions of specific brain regions, networks, and neurotransmitter systems on alcohol consumption and associated risky behavior (156–160). Manipulation of brain region function in selectively bred animals through lesion studies, or neurotransmitter systems through pharmacological agents, grants researchers the ability to assess how each component affects behavior and determine what modifications may be employed to alter that behavior. Importantly, upon development of an animal model of negative urgency, researchers can better understand the relationship of negative affect and alcohol consumption. Although research implies that trait negative urgency contributes to the progression of alcohol use disorder, is it possible that prolonged heavy alcohol use increases the influence of negative affect? As noted above, research in humans suggests that the immediate relief from negative emotions provided by alcohol consumption increases the likelihood of repeated pairings. Animals that are selectively bred to prefer alcohol grant researchers the ability to evaluate this premise and manipulate factors, such as neurotransmitter systems, which facilitate this association. The use of selectively bred animals is recommended when investigating the interaction of two traits (alcohol preference and negative urgency).

Second, it enables the testing of novel compounds and their ability to reduce negative urgency-like behaviors, which, if successful, could then be applied and tested in clinical models. This treatment may be pharmacological, as in a drug purported to reduce anxiety (targeting the affective aspect), or behavioral, such as training the subject to reduce excessive lever pressing in times of stress (targeting the rash behavior aspect). Examining these treatments in animals first allows for testing of initial feasibility, safety, and effectiveness prior to implementing such interventions in humans. These treatments may produce objective, quantifiable outcomes that can then be administered in a clinical setting. Given the demonstrated influence of negative urgency on increased alcohol consumption in alcohol use disorder populations and the increased elucidation of neural mechanisms underlying this association, developing novel therapeutic targets through animal models should constitute the next step toward more efficacious treatment options. Upon design of a translational, externally valid animal model, there are numerous possible targets of investigation. In particular, administration of agents designed to boost 5HT availability, specifically in the PFC, could generate a cascading effect downstream in the DA system of the OFC–amygdala circuit. Alternatively, increasing levels of GABA in the dlPFC may heighten the ability of this region to function efficiently, alleviating the heavy cognitive load required by subjects with high negative urgency to inhibit behavior.

Translation to animal models in this way has provided greater understanding of neural correlates of behavior in several domains. For instance, the symptoms of bipolar disorder are often alleviated through lithium administration, which also serves to decrease incidents of suicidal behavior (161–163). Valproate, an alternate method for bipolar disorder treatment, is also efficacious in relieving symptoms, but has no effect on suicidal behavior (164). A study evaluating the effects of these drugs on impulsivity using the delay discounting task revealed that lithium was more effective at reducing impulsive behavior in that paradigm, which may underlie the decrease in suicide attempts in that population (165). Models of Parkinson's and Alzheimer's disease have provided valuable information on the neural deterioration or malfunctioning that accompany the symptoms of those disorders (166–170). Animal models of depression have helped identify brain network and neurotransmitter systems associated with negative affect (171–174). One of the most useful tools of the animal model is to administer pharmacological therapies to attempt to identify what neurobiological mechanisms underlie symptoms and behavior.

Third, it allows for the manipulation of negative urgency in human studies and how changing the immediate expression of the trait can be clinically applied. Such studies would help test the viability of potential interventions in changing negative urgency in the human laboratory. It would also allow the use of a behavioral task of negative urgency as an objective marker of change for clinical trials of negative-urgency-based interventions, avoiding limitations related to self-report, as described above. Therefore, it is clear that the use of objective translational paradigms of negative urgency would be conducive to advancing research concerning the treatment of addictive disorders, as well as other comorbid disorders related to negative urgency.

## CONCLUSIONS, LIMITATIONS, AND SUGGESTIONS FOR FUTURE WORK

We propose two important gaps in research on negative urgency that should be filled as next steps in the long-term goal of intervening on negative urgency. First, existing translational approaches for negative urgency only assess negative affect or impulsive behavior, but not both. We suggest that only by combining these two aspects of negative urgency into one model can we increase the validity of the model in both animal and human subjects. There is still some work to do to figure out the most valid way to create such a translational model. In devising a translatable method to accurately evaluate negative urgency, and more importantly to develop a model that is sensitive enough to detect changes in behavior, investigators should seek to preserve as many aspects of validity as possible (**Table 1**). Of course, other potential methods could be developed, but should meet minimal validity criteria. Importantly, many of the methods of inducing negative emotions in humans have limited translatability, hindering the design of a truly translational task. The reward omission task may be a prime place to start to induce negative emotion across human and animal models. However, other approaches to induce negative affect translationally may need to be species specific. For example, food restriction might be effective and useful in animal models, but these methods have feasibility and ethical restraints in human work. In an animal model, acute restraint stress, food deprivation, and foot shock are demonstrably effective at inciting negative affect; however, these methods may lead to increased corticotrophin levels or persistent depressive-like symptoms, so exposure should be minimal. Any combination of these methods should be thoroughly vetted and rigorously tested to establish both construct and predictive validity. In contrast, several of the impulsivity methods are highly translatable (**Table 1**) and serve as good starting points in designing a new model. Of these impulsivity tasks, the delay discounting task would be the most effective for use of cognitive impulsivity inquiries, while the Go/No-Go task would be most informative for measures of motor impulsivity.

One limitation of investigations of negative urgency is the difficulty in parsing specific emotional reactions for evaluation. There is inherently a great deal of overlap in experience of emotion; anger, fear, and sadness often co-occur and the neural underpinnings of singular emotions are highly interconnected. An excellent review from Price (175) on the neurocircuitry of mood disorders describes this phenomenon very succinctly, identifying several structures, including the primary structures of the limbic system and hippocampal regions, which contribute to various emotions and how those structures interconnect. Although the ability to efficiently unravel such closely related emotions (sadness, stress, etc). would be ideal, it has not yet been successfully accomplished and negative urgency has been shown and theorized to relate to multiple different negative emotions, including sadness, stress, and anger. Unfortunately, the inability to untangle specific emotions may hinder the ability of animal research to completely model the human experience.

Another important caveat of developing a translational model of negative urgency is the distinction between state and trait behavior, which show little overlap (46). This might limit the feasibility of developing a translational model. Current self-report evaluations of negative urgency in humans are effective at assessing trait levels of negative urgency; a similar trait-like construct may be modeled in animals through selective breeding. For example, the high alcohol-preferring mouse lines have demonstrated higher impulsive behavior in the delay discounting task (76), making them an ideal model for investigations of trait impulsivity. State behavior is successfully measured in both human and animal models, allowing for the potential of strong concordance between these groups. Although state and trait approaches do not overlap strongly, researchers propose that increased overlap would likely occur through increased specificity in the measures (46). For example, performing a behavioral task under a negative emotional state would theoretically lead to larger correlations between the state measure and the trait of negative urgency.

Second, research has yet to examine identified human neural and genetic correlates of negative affect in animal models. There are numerous avenues for exploration that are well supported in the field and should be manipulated in animal models to test their potential treatment value. Abundant research implicates dysfunction of the serotonin and dopamine systems in regulation of the OFC–amygdala circuit may contribute to behavioral disinhibition during negative emotional states. There is also evidence of the contribution of GABA unavailability in the PFC, which may account for the excessive activation during response inhibition in subjects high in negative urgency. Identifying agents that efficiently reduce impulsive behavior during negative urgency in an animal model provides a basis for potential applications in a clinical setting. Future work should aim to further elucidate the influence of the OFC–amygdala circuit (emotional processing) and regions of the prefrontal cortex (behavioral control) in negative urgency. Novel pharmacological treatments can be discovered through manipulation strategies only available in animal models, which can then be applied in a clinical setting. It should be noted that although several lines of research have identified rodent brain regions as homologous to the human prefrontal cortex regions, there is no definitive nomenclature that accurately confirms these regions (169), which may limit translatability of neural data across preclinical and clinical models, although this type of work has been successful in related disorders (for review, see Ref. 93).

In conclusion, we suggest that future studies should seek to devise and test a valid translational model of negative urgency that is easily administered in both animals and human subjects. We hope that our review not only answers some questions about how to do this, but also creates new questions that can improve and advance this work more in the future. The long-term goal of such work will be to bring together basic research on negative urgency and clinical practice of addiction medicine, for more effective prevention, treatment, and rehabilitation of addictive disorders. We suggest that development of this model will allow for determination of prime neurological and physiological treatment targets, the testing of treatment effectiveness in the preclinical and the clinical laboratory, and, ultimately, improvement in negative-urgency-related treatment response and effectiveness. Given that negative urgency is a transdiagnostic risk factor that impedes treatment success, the impact of this work could be large in reducing client suffering and societal costs.

## AUTHOR CONTRIBUTIONS

All authors contributed to the overall direction and goals of this review. The original concept was generated and broadened by MC, who was also responsible for edits and comments. EA wrote the introduction to urgency, outlined research in clinical subjects using the UPPS self-report measure, and contributed to editing and comments. MH wrote the bulk of the paper, including sections on animal models and possible neural correlates for investigation and contributed to overall edits and comments.

## REFERENCES

1. Whiteside SP, Lynam DR. The five factor model and impulsivity: using a structural model of personality to understand impulsivity. *Psychol Bull* (2001) 30(4):669–89. doi: 10.1016/S0191-8869(00)00064-7
2. Cyders MA, Smith GT. Emotion-based dispositions to rash action: positive and negative urgency. *Psychol Bull* (2008) 134(6):807–28. doi: 10.1037/a0013341
3. Coskunpinar A, Dir AL, Cyders MA, E. Multidimensionality in impulsivity and alcohol use: a meta-analysis using the UPPS model of impulsivity. *Alcohol Clin Exp Res* (2013) 37(9):1441–50. doi: 10.1111/acer.12131
4. Hershberger A, Connors M, Um M. et al. *Int J Ment Health Addiction* (2018) 16:366. doi: 10.1007/s11469-017-9783-6
5. Berg JM, Latzman RD, Bliwise NG, Lilienfeld SO. Parsing the heterogeneity of impulsivity: a meta-analytic review of the behavioral implications of the UPPS for psychopathology. *Psychol Assess* (2015) 27(4):1129–46. doi: 10.1037/pas0000111
6. Dalley JW, Robbins TW. Fractionating impulsivity: neuropsychiatric implications. *Nat Rev Neurosci* (2017) 18:158. doi: 10.1038/nrn.2017.8
7. Khadka S, Stevens MC, Aslanzadeh F, Narayanan B, Hawkins KA, Austad CS, et al. Composite impulsivity-related domains in college students. *J Psychiatr Res* (2017) 90:118–25. doi: 10.1016/j.jpsychires.2017.02.016
8. Cyders MA, Coskunpinar A. Is urgency emotionality? Separating urgent behaviors from effects of emotional experiences. *Pers Individ Dif* (2010) 48(7):839–44. doi: 10.1016/j.paid.2010.02.009
9. Sharma L, Markon KE, Clark LA. Toward a theory of distinct types of 'impulsive' behaviors: a meta-analysis of self-report and behavioral measures. *Psychol Bull* (2014) 140(2):374–408. doi: 10.1037/a0034418
10. Segerstrom SC, Smith GT. Personality and coping: individual differences in responses to emotion. *Annu Rev Psychol* (2019) 70(1):651–71. doi: 10.1146/annurev-psych-010418-102917
11. Costa PT, McCrae RR. Four ways five factors are basic. *Personality and Individual Differences* (1992) 13(6):653–65.
12. Digman JM. Higher-order factors of the Big Five. *J Pers Soc Psychol* (1997) 73(6):1246–56. doi: 10.1037//0022-3514.73.6.1246
13. Markon KE, Krueger RF, Watson D. Delineating the structure of normal and abnormal personality: an integrative hierarchical approach. *J Pers Soc Psychol* (2005) 88(1):139–57. doi: 10.1037/0022-3514.88.1.139
14. Gross JJ. The emerging field of emotion regulation: an integrative review. *Rev Gen Psychol* (1998) 2(3):271–99. doi: 10.1037//1089-2680.2.3.271
15. Gratz K, Roemer L. Multidimensional assessment of emotion regulation and dysregulation: development, factor structure, and initial validation of the difficulties in emotion regulation scale. *J Psychopathol Behav Assess* (2004) 26(1):41–54. doi: 10.1023/B:JOBA.0000007455.08539.94
16. Fossati A, Gratz KL, Maffei C, Borroni S. Impulsivity dimensions, emotion dysregulation, and borderline personality disorder features among Italian nonclinical adolescents. *Borderline Pers Disord Emotion dysregulation* (2014) 1:5–26. doi: 10.1186/2051-6673-1-5
17. Fischer S, Smith GT, Cyders MA. Another look at impulsivity: a meta-analytic review comparing specific dispositions to rash action in their relationship to bulimic symptoms. *Clin Psychol Rev* (2008) 28(8):1413–25. doi: 10.1016/j.cpr.2008.09.001
18. Settles RE, Fischer S, Cyders MA, Combs JL, Gunn RL, Smith GT. Negative urgency: a personality predictor of externalizing behavior characterized by neuroticism, low conscientiousness, and disagreeableness. *J Abnorm Psychol* (2012) 121(1):160. doi: 10.1037/a0024948
19. Spillane NS, Smith GT, Kahler CW. Impulsivity-like traits and smoking behavior in college students. *Addict Behav* (2010) 35(7):700–5. doi: 10.1016/j.addbeh.2010.03.008
20. Pang RD, Hom MS, Geary BA, Doran N, Spillane NS, Guillot CR, et al. Relationships between trait urgency, smoking reinforcement expectancies, and nicotine dependence. *J Addict Dis* (2014) 33(2):83–93. doi: 10.1080/10550887.2014.909695
21. Lee DC, Peters JR, Adams ZW, Milich R, Lynam DR. Specific dimensions of impulsivity are differentially associated with daily and non-daily cigarette smoking in young adults. *Addict Behav* (2015) 46:82–5. doi: 10.1016/j.addbeh.2015.03.009

22. Dvorak RD, Day AM. Marijuana and self-regulation: examining likelihood and intensity of use and problems. *Addict Behav* (2014) 39(3):709–12. doi: 10.1016/j.addbeh.2013.11.001
23. Wardell JD, Strang NM, Hendershot CS. Negative urgency mediates the relationship between childhood maltreatment and problems with alcohol and cannabis in late adolescence. *Addict Behav* (2016) 56:1–7. doi: 10.1016/j.addbeh.2016.01.003
24. Wolitzky-Taylor K, McBeth J, Guillot CR, Stone MD, Kirkpatrick MG, Zvolensky M, et al. Transdiagnostic processes linking anxiety symptoms and substance use problems among adolescents. *J Addict Dis* (2016) 35(4):266–77. doi: 10.1080/10550887.2016.1207969
25. Guller L, Zapolski TC, Smith GT. Personality measured in elementary school predicts middle school addictive behavior involvement. *J Psychopathol* (2015) 37(3): 523–32. doi: 10.1007/s10862-014-9474-6
26. Littlefield AK, Stevens AK, Cunningham S, Jones RE, King KM, Schumacher JA, et al. Stability and change in multi-method measures of impulsivity across residential addictions treatment. *Addict Behav* (2015) 42:126–9. doi: 10.1016/j.addbeh.2014.11.002
27. Littlefield AK, Sher KJ, Wood PK. Is "maturing out" of problematic alcohol involvement related to personality change? *J Abnorm Psychol* (2009) 118(2):360. doi: 10.1037/a0015125
28. Cyders MA, Coskunpinar A, VanderVeen JD. Urgency: a common transdiagnostic endophenotype for maladaptive risk taking. In Zeigler-Hill V, Marcus DK (Eds.), *The dark side of personality: Science and practice in social, personality, and clinical psychology*. Washington, DC, US: American Psychological Association (2016). p. 157–88. doi: 10.1037/14854-009
29. Um M, Hershberger AR, Whitt ZT, Cyders MA, e. dysregulation. Recommendations for applying a multi-dimensional model of impulsive personality to diagnosis and treatment. *Borderline Personal Disord Emot Dysregul* (2018) 5(1):6. doi: 10.1186/s40479-018-0084-x
30. Hershberger AR, Um M, Cyders MA. The relationship between the UPPS-P impulsive personality traits and substance use psychotherapy outcomes: a meta-analysis. *Drug Alcohol Depend* (2017) 178:408–16. doi: 10.1016/j.drugalcdep.2017.05.032
31. Zapolski TC, Settles RE, Cyders MA, Smith GT. Borderline personality disorder, bulimia nervosa, antisocial personality disorder, ADHD, substance use: common threads, common treatment needs, and the nature of impulsivity. *Indep Pract* (2010) 30(1):20.
32. Kiluk BD, Nich C, Babuscio T, Carroll KM. Quality versus quantity: acquisition of coping skills following computerized cognitive–behavioral therapy for substance use disorders. *Addiction* (2010) 105(12):2120–7. doi: 10.1111/j.1360-0443.2010.03076.x
33. Magill M, Kiluk BD, McCrady BS, Tonigan JS, Longabaugh R. Research E. Active ingredients of treatment and client mechanisms of change in behavioral treatments for alcohol use disorders: progress 10 years later. *Alcohol Clin Exp Res* (2015) 39(10):1852–62. doi: 10.1111/acer.12848
34. Adams ZW, Kaiser AJ, Lynam DR, Charnigo RJ, Milich R. Drinking motives as mediators of the impulsivity-substance use relation: pathways for negative urgency, lack of premeditation, and sensation seeking. *Addict Behav* (2012) 37(7):848–55. doi: 10.1016/j.addbeh.2012.03.016
35. Caspi A, Roberts BW. Personality development across the life course: The argument for change and continuity. *Psychol Inq* (2001) 12(2):49–66. doi: 10.1207/S15327965PLI1202_01
36. Zapolski TC, Smith GT. Pilot study: implementing a brief DBT skills program in schools to reduce health risk behaviors among early adolescents. *J Sch Nurs* (2017) 33(3):198–204. doi: 10.1177/1059840516673188
37. Margolin A, Schuman-Olivier Z, Beitel M, Arnold RM, Fulwiler CE, Avants SK. A preliminary study of spiritual self-schema (3-S+) therapy for reducing impulsivity in HIV-positive drug users. *J Clin Psychol* (2007) 63(10):979–99. doi: 10.1002/jclp.20407
38. Axelrod SR, Perepletchikova F, Holtzman K, Sinha R. Emotion regulation and substance use frequency in women with substance dependence and borderline personality disorder receiving dialectical behavior therapy. *Am J Drug Alcohol Abuse* (2011) 37(1):37–42. doi: 10.3109/00952990.2010.535582
39. Weiss NH, Tull MT, Davis LT, Searcy J, Williams I, Gratz KL. A preliminary experimental investigation of emotion dysregulation and impulsivity in risky behaviours. *Behav Change* (2015) 32(2):127–42. doi: 10.1017/bec.2015.5
40. Santos-Ruiz A, Robles-Ortega H, Pérez-García M, Peralta-Ramírez MI. Effects of the cognitive–behavioral therapy for stress management on executive function components. *Spanish J Psychology* (2017) 20:E11–9. doi: 10.1017/sjp.2017.10
41. Rinne T, van den Brink W, Wouters L, van Dyck R. SSRI treatment of borderline personality disorder: a randomized, placebo-controlled clinical trial for female patients with borderline personality disorder. *Am J Psychiatry* (2002) 159(12):2048–54. doi: 10.1176/appi.ajp.159.12.2048
42. Amaro H, Magno-Gatmaytan C, Meléndez M, Cortés DE, Arevalo S, Margolin A. Addiction treatment intervention: an uncontrolled prospective pilot study of spiritual self-schema therapy with Latina women. *Subst Abus* (2010) 31(2): 117–25. doi: 10.1080/08897071003641602
43. Cyders MA, Smith GT, Spillane NS, Fischer S, Annus AM, Peterson C. Integration of impulsivity and positive mood to predict risky behavior: development and validation of a measure of positive urgency. *Psychol Assess* (2007) 19(1):107–18. doi: 10.1037/1040-3590.19.1.107
44. Lynam D, Smith G, Cyders M, Fischer S, Whiteside S. The UPPS-P: a multidimensional measure of risk for impulsive behaviour (2007).
45. Argyriou E, Um M, Wu W, Cyders MA. Measurement invariance of the UPPS-P impulsive behavior scale across age and sex across the adult life span. *Assessment* 0(0):1073191119832660.
46. Zapolski TC, Cyders MA, Smith GT. Positive urgency predicts illegal drug use and risky sexual behaviour. *Psychol Addict Behav* (2009) 23(2):348. doi: 10.1037/a0014684
47. Cyders MA. Impulsivity and the sexes: measurement and structural invariance of the UPPS-P Impulsive Behavior Scale. *Assessment* (2013) 20(1):86–97. doi: 10.1177/1073191111428762
48. Cyders MA, Coskunpinar A. Measurement of constructs using self-report and behavioral lab tasks: is there overlap in nomothetic span and construct representation for impulsivity? *Clinical Psychol Rev* (2011) 31(6):965–82. doi: 10.1016/j.cpr.2011.06.001
49. Cyders MA, Coskunpinar A. The relationship between self-report and lab task conceptualizations of impulsivity. *J Res Pers* (2012) 46(1):121–4. doi: 10.1016/j.jrp.2011.11.005
50. Sperry SH, Lynam DR, Walsh MA, Horton LE, Kwapil TR. Examining the multidimensional structure of impulsivity in daily life. *Pers Individ Dif* (2016) 94:153–8. doi: 10.1016/j.paid.2016.01.018
51. Holtgraves T. Social desirability and self-reports: testing models of socially desirable responding. *Pers Soc Psychol Bull* (2004) 30(2):161–72. doi: 10.1177/0146167203259930
52. Belzung C, Lemoine M. Criteria of validity for animal models of psychiatric disorders: focus on anxiety disorders and depression. *Biol Mood Anxiety Disord* (2011) 1(1):9–23. doi: 10.1186/2045-5380-1-9
53. Geyer MA, Markou A. Animal models of psychiatric disorders. *Psychopharmacology: the fourth generation of progress* (1995) 787–98.
54. McKinney WT, Bunney WE. Animal model of depression: i. Review of evidence: implications for research. *Arch Gen Psychiatry* (1969) 21(2):240–8. doi: 10.1001/archpsyc.1969.01740200112015
55. Willner PJP. The validity of animal models of depression. *Psychopharmacology* (1984) 83(1):1–16. doi: 10.1007/BF00427414
56. Gipson CD, Beckmann JS, Adams ZW, Marusich JA, Nesland TO, Yates JR, et al. A translational behavioral model of mood-based impulsivity: implications for substance abuse. *Drug Alcohol Depend* (2012) 122(1–2):93–9. doi: 10.1016/j.drugalcdep.2011.09.014
57. Yates JR, Darna M, Gipson CD, Dwoskin LP, Bardo MT. Dissociable roles of dopamine and serotonin transporter function in a rat model of negative urgency. *Behav Brain Res* (2015) 291:201–8. doi: 10.1016/j.bbr.2015.05.023
58. Barker AT, Rebec GV. Cocaine withdrawal alters the reward omission effect and enhances traits of negative urgency in rats across multiple days of testing. *Drug Alcohol Depend* (2016) 163:S19–S24. doi: 10.1016/j.drugalcdep.2015.11.040
59. Holdwick DJ, Jr., Wingenfeld SA. The subjective experience of PASAT testing: does the PASAT induce negative mood? *Arch Clin Neuropsychol* (1999) 14(3):273–84. doi: 10.1093/arclin/14.3.273
60. Tombaugh TN. A comprehensive review of the Paced Auditory Serial Addition Test (PASAT). *Arch Clin Neuropsychol* (2006) 21(1):53–76. doi: 10.1016/j.acn.2005.07.006
61. Lang P, Bradley M, Cuthbert B. *International affective picture system (IAPS):*

*Technical manual and affective ratings 1997*. Gainesville, FL: NIMH Center for the Study of Emotion and Attention, University of Florida (2009).

62. Craig AR, Maxfield AD, Stein JS, Renda CR, Madden GJ. Do the adjusting-delay and increasing-delay tasks measure the same construct: delay discounting? *Behav Pharmacol* (2014) 25(4):306–15. doi: 10.1097/FBP.0000000000000055
63. Cyders MA, Dzemidzic M, Eiler WJ, Coskunpinar A, Karyadi K, Kareken DA. Negative urgency and ventromedial prefrontal cortex responses to alcohol cues: fMRI evidence of emotion-based impulsivity. *Alcohol Clin Exp Res* (2014) 38(2):409–17. doi: 10.1111/acer.12266
64. Chester DS, Lynam DR, Milich R, DeWall CN. Craving versus control: negative urgency and neural correlates of alcohol cue reactivity. *Drug Alcohol Depend* (2016) 163:S25–S28. doi: 10.1016/j.drugalcdep.2015.10.036
65. Cohen-Gilbert JE, Nickerson LD, Sneider JT, Oot EN, Seraikas AM, Rohan ML, et al. College binge drinking associated with decreased frontal activation to negative emotional distractors during inhibitory control. *Front Psychol* (2017) 8:1650. doi: 10.3389/fpsyg.2017.01650
66. Savulich G, Riccelli R, Passamonti L, Correia M, Deakin J, Elliott R, et al. Effects of naltrexone are influenced by childhood adversity during negative emotional processing in addiction recovery. *Transl Psychiatry* (2017) 7(3):e1054. doi: 10.1038/tp.2017.34
67. Lejuez CW, Kahler CW, Brown RA. A modified computer version of the Paced Auditory Serial Addition Task (PASAT) as a laboratory-based stressor. *Behavior Therapist* (2003) 26(4):290–3.
68. Chester DS, Lynam DR, Milich R, Powell DK, Andersen AH, DeWall CN. How do negative emotions impair self-control? A neural model of negative urgency. *Neuroimage* (2016) 132:43–50. doi: 10.1016/j.neuroimage.2016.02.024
69. Westermann R, Spies K, Stahl G, Hesse FW. Relative effectiveness and validity of mood induction procedures: a meta- analysis. *Eur J Social Psychology* (1996) 26(4):557–80.
70. Shetty RA, Sadananda M. Brief social isolation in the adolescent Wistar-Kyoto rat model of endogenous depression alters corticosterone and regional monoamine concentrations. *Neurochem Res* (2017) 42(5):1470–7. doi: 10.1007/s11064-017-2203-2
71. Doherty FD, O'Mahony SM, Peterson VL, O'Sullivan O, Crispie F, Cotter PD, et al. Post-weaning social isolation of rats leads to long-term disruption of the gut microbiota-immune-brain axis. *Brain Behav Immun* (2018) 68:261–73. doi: 10.1016/j.bbi.2017.10.024
72. Ohi K, Mikuni M, Takahashi K. Stress adaptation and hypersensitivity in 5-HT neuronal systems after repeated foot shock. *Pharmacol Biochem Behav* (1989) 34(3):603–8. doi: 10.1016/0091-3057(89)90566-2
73. West AP. Neurobehavioral studies of forced swimming: the role of learning and memory in the forced swim test. *Prog Neuropsychopharmacol Biol Psychiatry* (1990) 14(6):863–IN864. doi: 10.1016/0278-5846(90)90073-P
74. Conrad CD, Magariños AM, LeDoux JE, McEwen BS. Repeated restraint stress facilitates fear conditioning independently of causing hippocampal CA3 dendritic atrophy. *Behav Neurosci* (1999) 113(5):902–13. doi: 10.1037//0735-7044.113.5.902
75. Conrad CD, Grote KA, Hobbs RJ, Ferayorni A. Sex differences in spatial and non-spatial Y-maze performance after chronic stress. *Neurobiol Learn Mem* (2003) 79(1):32–40. doi: 10.1016/S1074-7427(02)00018-7
76. Bodnoff SR, Humphreys AG, Lehman JC, Diamond DM, Rose GM, Meaney MJ. Enduring effects of chronic corticosterone treatment on spatial learning, synaptic plasticity, and hippocampal neuropathology in young and mid-aged rats. *J Neurosci* (1995) 15(1 Pt 1):61–9. doi: 10.1523/JNEUROSCI.15-01-00061.1995
77. Schaaf MJM, De Kloet ER, Vreugdenhil E. Corticosterone effects on BDNF expression in the hippocampus implications for memory formation. *Stress* (2000) 3(3):201–8. doi: 10.3109/10253890009001124
78. Willner P, Mitchell PJ. The validity of animal models of predisposition to depression. *Behav Pharmacol* (2002) 13(3):169–88. doi: 10.1097/00008877-200205000-00001
79. Ainslie G, Herrnstein RJ. Preference reversal and delayed reinforcement. *Anim Learn Behav* (1981) 9(4):476–82. doi: 10.3758/BF03209777
80. Mazur JE. An adjusting procedure for studying delayed reinforcement. Commons ML; Mazur JE; Nevin JA. *Quantitative Analyses of Behavior*, Hillsdale, New Jersey: Lawrence Erlbaum Associates, Inc. (1987) Volume 4, p. 55–72.
81. Oberlin BG, Grahame NJ. High-alcohol preferring mice are more impulsive than low-alcohol preferring mice as measured in the delay discounting task. *Alcohol Clin Exp Res* (2009) 33(7):1294–303. doi: 10.1111/j.1530-0277.2009.00955.x
82. Bickel WK, Marsch LA. Toward a behavioral economic understanding of drug dependence: delay discounting processes. *Addiction* (2001) 96(1):73–86. doi: 10.1046/j.1360-0443.2001.961736.x
83. Reynolds B, Schiffbauer R. Measuring state changes in human delay discounting: an experiential discounting task. *Behav Processes* (2004) 67(3):343–56. doi: 10.1016/j.beproc.2004.06.003
84. Smits RR, Stein JS, Johnson PS, Odum AL, Madden GJ. Test–retest reliability and construct validity of the Experiential Discounting Task. *Exp Clin Psychopharmacol* (2013) 21(2):155–63. doi: 10.1037/a0031725
85. Madden GJ, Begotka AM, Raiff BR, Kastern LL. Delay discounting of real and hypothetical rewards. *Exp Clin Psychopharmacol* (2003) 11(2):139–45. doi: 10.1037/1064-1297.11.2.139
86. Wade TR, de Wit H, Richards JB. Effects of dopaminergic drugs on delayed reward as a measure of impulsive behavior in rats. *Psychopharmacology* (2000) 150(1):90–101. doi: 10.1007/s002130000402
87. De Wit H, Enggasser JL, Richards JB. Acute administration of d-amphetamine decreases impulsivity in healthy volunteers. *Neuropsychopharmacology* (2002) 27(5):813–25. doi: 10.1016/S0893-133X(02)00343-3
88. Pietras CJ, Cherek DR, Lane SD, Tcheremissine OV, Steinberg JL. Effects of methylphenidate on impulsive choice in adult humans. *Psychopharmacology* (2003) 170(4):390–8. doi: 10.1007/s00213-003-1547-2
89. Perry JL, Stairs DJ, Bardo MT. Impulsive choice and environmental enrichment: effects of d-amphetamine and methylphenidate. *Behav Brain Res* (2008) 193(1):48–54. doi: 10.1016/j.bbr.2008.04.019
90. Shiels K, Hawk LW, Jr., Reynolds B, Mazzullo RJ, Rhodes JD, Pelham WE, Jr., et al. Effects of methylphenidate on discounting of delayed rewards in attention deficit/hyperactivity disorder. *Exp Clin Psychopharmacol* (2009) 17(5):291. doi: 10.1037/a0017259
91. Oberlin BG, Bristow RE, Heighton ME, Grahame NJ. Pharmacologic dissociation between impulsivity and alcohol drinking in high alcohol preferring mice. *Alcohol Clin Exp Res* (2010) 34(8):1363–75. doi: 10.1111/j.1530-0277.2010.01220.x
92. Nosek BA, Banaji MR. The go/no-go association task. *Soc Cogn* (2001) 19(6):625–66. doi: 10.1521/soco.19.6.625.20886
93. Simmonds DJ, Pekar JJ, Mostofsky SH. Meta-analysis of Go/No-go tasks demonstrating that fMRI activation associated with response inhibition is task-dependent. *Neuropsychologia* (2008) 46(1):224–32. doi: 10.1016/j.neuropsychologia.2007.07.015
94. Olmstead MC. Animal models of drug addiction: where do we go from here? *Q J Exp Psychol (Hove)* (2006) 59(4):625–53. doi: 10.1080/17470210500356308
95. Chester DS, Lynam DR, Milich R, DeWall CN. Social rejection magnifies impulsive behavior among individuals with greater negative urgency: an experimental test of urgency theory. *J Exp Psychol Gen* (2017) 146(7):962. doi: 10.1037/xge0000308
96. Reyes-Huerta HE, dos Santos C, Martínez K. Impulsive mechanisms influencing relapse in alcohol drinking. *Med Hypotheses* (2018) 112:27–9. doi: 10.1016/j.mehy.2018.01.007
97. Belzung C. Innovative drugs to treat depression: did animal models fail to be predictive or did clinical trials fail to detect effects? *Neuropsychopharmacology* (2014) 39(5):1041–51. doi: 10.1038/npp.2013.342
98. Stewart AM, Kalueff AV. Developing better and more valid animal models of brain disorders. *Behav Brain Res* (2015) 276:28–31. doi: 10.1016/j.bbr.2013.12.024
99. Czéh B, Fuchs E, Wiborg O, Simon M. Animal models of major depression and their clinical implications. *Prog Neuropsychopharmacol Biol Psychiatry* (2016) 64:293–310. doi: 10.1016/j.pnpbp.2015.04.004
100. Cyders MA, Flory K, Rainer S, Smith GT. The role of personality dispositions to risky behavior in predicting first-year college drinking. *Addiction* (2009) 104(2):193–202. doi: 10.1111/j.1360-0443.2008.02434.x
101. Smith GT, Cyders MA. Integrating affect and impulsivity: the role of positive and negative urgency in substance use risk. *Drug Alcohol Depend* (2016) 163:S3–S12. doi: 10.1016/j.drugalcdep.2015.08.038
102. Carver CS, Johnson SL, Joormann J. Serotonergic function, two-mode models of self-regulation, and vulnerability to depression: what depression has in common with impulsive aggression. *Psychol Bull* (2008) 134(6):912–43. doi: 10.1037/a0013740
103. Phillips ML, Ladouceur CD, Drevets WC. A neural model of voluntary and automatic emotion regulation: implications for understanding the pathophysiology and neurodevelopment of bipolar disorder. *Mol Psychiatry* (2008) 13:833. doi: 10.1038/mp.2008.65

104. Wilcox CE, Pommy JM, Adinoff B,. Neural circuitry of impaired emotion regulation in substance use disorders. *Am J Psychiatry* (2016) 173(4):344–61. doi: 10.1176/appi.ajp.2015.15060710
105. Davidson RJ. Affective neuroscience and psychophysiology: toward a synthesis. *Psychophysiology* (2003) 40(5):655–65. doi: 10.1111/1469-8986.00067
106. Lewis MD. Bridging emotion theory and neurobiology through dynamic systems modeling. *Behavioral and Brain Sciences* (2005) 28(2):169–94.
107. Lewis MD, Todd RM, Honsberger MJ. Event-related potential measures of emotion regulation in early childhood. *Neuroreport* (2007) 18(1):61–5. doi: 10.1097/WNR.0b013e328010a216
108. Clark L, Stokes PR, Wu K, Michalczuk R, Benecke A, Watson BJ, et al. Striatal dopamine D2/D3 receptor binding in pathological gambling is correlated with mood-related impulsivity. *NeuroImage* (2012) 63(1):40–6. doi: 10.1016/j.neuroimage.2012.06.067
109. Albein-Urios N, Verdejo-Román J, Asensio S, Soriano-Mas C, Martínez-González JM, Verdejo-García A. Re-appraisal of negative emotions in cocaine dependence: dysfunctional corticolimbic activation and connectivity. *Addict Biol* (2014) 19(3):415–26. doi: 10.1111/j.1369-1600.2012.00497.x
110. Xiao L, Bechara A, Gong Q, Huang X, Li X, Xue G, et al. Abnormal affective decision making revealed in adolescent binge drinkers using a functional magnetic resonance imaging study. *Psychol Addict Behav* (2013) 27(2):443–54. doi: 10.1037/a0027892
111. Albein-Urios N, Martinez-González JM, Lozano Ó, Clark L, Verdejo-García A. Comparison of impulsivity and working memory in cocaine addiction and pathological gambling: implications for cocaine-induced neurotoxicity. *Drug Alcohol Depend* (2012) 126(1):1–6. doi: 10.1016/j.drugalcdep.2012.03.008
112. Barkley-Levenson E, Xue F, Droutman V, Miller LC, Smith BJ, Jeong D, et al. Prefrontal cortical activity during the Stroop task: new insights into the why and the who of real-world risky sexual behavior. *Ann Behav Med* (2018) 52(5):367–79. doi: 10.1093/abm/kax019
113. Phan KL, Wager T, Taylor SF, Liberzon I. Functional neuroanatomy of emotion: a meta-analysis of emotion activation studies in PET and fMRI. *Neuroimage* (2002) 16(2):331–48. doi: 10.1006/nimg.2002.1087
114. Albein-Urios N, Martinez-Gonzalez JM, Lozano Ó, Moreno-López L, Soriano-Mas C, Verdejo-Garcia A. Negative urgency, disinhibition and reduced temporal pole gray matter characterize the comorbidity of cocaine dependence and personality disorders. *Drug Alcohol Depend* (2013) 132(1):231–7. doi: 10.1016/j.drugalcdep.2013.02.008
115. Cyders MA, Dzemidzic M, Eiler WJ, Coskunpinar A, Karyadi KA, Kareken DA. Negative urgency mediates the relationship between amygdala and orbitofrontal cortex activation to negative emotional stimuli and general risk-taking. *Cereb Cortex* (2015) 25(11):4094–102. doi: 10.1093/cercor/bhu123
116. Motzkin JC, Philippi CL, Wolf RC, Baskaya MK, Koenigs M. Ventromedial prefrontal cortex is critical for the regulation of amygdala activity in humans. *Biol Psychiatry* (2015) 77(3):276–84. doi: 10.1016/j.biopsych.2014.02.014
117. Halcomb ME, Chumin EJ, Goñi J, Dzemidzic M, Yoder KK. Aberrations of anterior insular cortex functional connectivity in nontreatment-seeking alcoholics. *Psychiat Res-Neuroim* (2019) 284:21–8. doi: 10.1016/j.pscychresns.2018.12.016
118. Contreras-Rodríguez O, Albein-Urios N, Vilar-López R, Perales JC, Martínez-Gonzalez JM, Fernández-Serrano MJ, et al. Increased corticolimbic connectivity in cocaine dependence versus pathological gambling is associated with drug severity and emotion-related impulsivity. *Addict Biol* (2016) 21(3):709–18. doi: 10.1111/adb.12242
119. Zhu X, Cortes CR, Mathur K, Tomasi D, Momenan R. Model-free functional connectivity and impulsivity correlates of alcohol dependence: a resting-state study. *Addict Biol* (2017) 22(1):206–17. doi: 10.1111/adb.12272
120. Spoont MR. Modulatory role of serotonin in neural information processing: implications for human psychopathology. *Psychol Bull* (1992) 112(2):330–50. doi: 10.1037//0033-2909.112.2.330
121. Depue RA, Collins PF. Neurobiology of the structure of personality: dopamine, facilitation of incentive motivation, and extraversion. *Behavioral and Brain Sciences* (1999) 22:491–517. doi: 10.1017/S0140525X99002046
122. Menahem Krakowski. Violence and serotonin: influence of impulse control, affect regulation, and social functioning. *J Neuropsychiatry Clin Neurosci* (2003) 15(3):294–305. doi: 10.1176/appi.neuropsych.15.3.294
123. Cools R, Blackwell A, Clark L, Menzies L, Cox S, Robbins TW. Tryptophan depletion disrupts the motivational guidance of goal-directed behavior as a function of trait impulsivity. *Neuropsychopharmacology* (2005) 30(7):1362–73. doi: 10.1038/sj.npp.1300704
124. Frankle WG, Lombardo I, New AS, Goodman M, Talbot PS, Huang Y, et al. Brain serotonin transporter distribution in subjects with impulsive aggressivity: a positron emission study with [11C]McN 5652. *Am J Psychiatry* (2005) 162(5):915–23. doi: 10.1176/appi.ajp.162.5.915
125. Winstanley CA, Eagle DM, Robbins TW. Behavioral models of impulsivity in relation to ADHD: translation between clinical and preclinical studies. *Clinical Psychol Rev* (2006) 26(4):379–95. doi: 10.1016/j.cpr.2006.01.001
126. Chester DS, DeWall CN, Derefinko KJ, Estus S, Peters JR, Lynam DR, et al. Monoamine oxidase A (MAOA) genotype predicts greater aggression through impulsive reactivity to negative affect. *Behav Brain Res* (2015) 283:97–101. doi: 10.1016/j.bbr.2015.01.034
127. Raleigh MJ, Brammer GL. Individual differences in serotonin-2 receptors and social behavior in monkeys. *Soc Neurosci Abst* (1993).
128. Winstanley CA, Theobald DE, Dalley JW, Glennon JC, Robbins TW. 5-HT2A and 5-HT2C receptor antagonists have opposing effects on a measure of impulsivity: interactions with global 5-HT depletion. *Psychopharmacology (Berl)* (2004) 176(3-4):376–85. doi: 10.1007/s00213-004-1884-9
129. Carli M, Baviera M, Invernizzi RW, Balducci C. Dissociable contribution of 5-HT1A and 5-HT2A receptors in the medial prefrontal cortex to different aspects of executive control such as impulsivity and compulsive perseveration in rats. *Neuropsychopharmacology* (2006) 31(4):757–67. doi: 10.1038/sj.npp.1300893
130. Depue RA, Luciana M, Arbisi P, Collins P, Leon A. Dopamine and the structure of personality: relation of agonist-induced dopamine activity to positive emotionality. *J Pers Soc Psychol* (1994) 67(3):485–98. doi: 10.1037/0022-3514.67.3.485
131. Cardinal RN, Winstanley CA, Robbins TW, Everitt BJ. Limbic corticostriatal systems and delayed reinforcement. *Ann NY Acad Sci* (2004) 1021(1):33–50. doi: 10.1196/annals.1308.004
132. Spear LP. Neurobehavioral changes in adolescence. *Curr Dir Psychol Sci* (2000) 9(4):111–4. doi: 10.1111/1467-8721.00072
133. Spear LP. Rewards, aversions and affect in adolescence: emerging convergences across laboratory animal and human data. *Dev Cogn Neurosci* (2011) 1(4):390–403. doi: 10.1016/j.dcn.2011.08.001
134. Limosin F, Loze JY, Dubertret C, Gouya L, Ades J, Rouillon F, et al. Impulsiveness as the intermediate link between the dopamine receptor D2 gene and alcohol dependence. *Psychiatr Genet* (2003) 13(2):127–29. doi: 10.1097/01.ypg.0000066963.66429.00
135. Smith CT, Wallace DL, Dang LC, Aarts E, Jagust WJ, D'Esposito M, et al. Modulation of impulsivity and reward sensitivity in intertemporal choice by striatal and midbrain dopamine synthesis in healthy adults. *J Neurophysiol* (2016) 115(3): 1146–56. doi: 10.1152/jn.00261.2015
136. Howell LL, Czoty PW, Byrd LD. Pharmacological interactions between serotonin and dopamine on behavior in the squirrel monkey. *Psychopharmacology* (1997) 131(1): 40–8. doi: 10.1007/s002130050263
137. Fink KB, Gothert M. 5-HT receptor regulation of neurotransmitter release. *Pharmacol Rev* (2007) 59(4):360–417. doi: 10.1124/pr.107.07103
138. Patterson CM, Newman JP. Reflectivity and learning from aversive events: Toward a psychological mechanism for the syndromes of disinhibition. *Psychol Rev* (1993) 100(4):716–36. doi: 10.1037//0033-295X.100.4.716
139. Auerbach JG, Faroy M, Ebstein R, Kahana M, Levine J. The association of the dopamine D4 receptor gene (DRD4) and the serotonin transporter promoter gene (5-HTTLPR) with temperament in 12-month-old infants. *J Child Psychol Psychiatry* (2001) 42(6):777–83. doi: 10.1111/1469-7610.00774
140. Lakatos K, Nemoda Z, Birkas E, Ronai Z, Kovacs E, Ney K, et al. Association of D4 dopamine receptor gene and serotonin transporter promoter polymorphisms with infants' response to novelty. *Mol Psychiatry* (2003) 8(1):90–7. doi: 10.1038/sj.mp.4001212
141. Munafo MR, Clark TG, Moore LR, Payne E, Walton R, Flint J. Genetic polymorphisms and personality in healthy adults: a systematic review and meta-analysis. *Mol Psychiatry* (2003) 8(5):471–84. doi: 10.1038/sj.mp.4001326
142. Hu X, Oroszi G, Chun J, Smith TL, Goldman D, Schuckit MA. An expanded evaluation of the relationship of four alleles to the level of response to alcohol and the alcoholism risk. *Alcohol Clin Exp Res* (2005) 29(1):8–16. doi: 10.1097/01.ALC.0000150008.68473.62
143. Beitchman JH, Baldassarra L, Mik H, De Luca V, King N, Bender D, et al. Serotonin transporter polymorphisms and persistent, pervasive childhood aggression. *Am J Psychiatry* (2006) 163(6):1103–5. doi: 10.1176/ajp.2006.163.6.1103
144. Hu XZ, Lipsky RH, Zhu G, Akhtar LA, Taubman J, Greenberg BD, et al. Serotonin transporter promoter gain-of-function genotypes are linked to

obsessive-compulsive disorder. *Am J Hum Genet* (2006) 78(5):815–26. doi: 10.1086/503850

145. Ballenger JC, Goodwin FK, Major LF, Brown GL. Alcohol and central serotonin metabolism in man. *Arch Gen Psychiatry* (1979) 36(2):224–7. doi: 10.1001/archpsyc.1979.01780020114013
146. LeMarquand D, Pihl RO, Benkelfat C. Serotonin and alcohol intake, abuse, and dependence: clinical evidence. *Biol Psychiatry* (1994) 36(5):326–37. doi: 10.1016/0006-3223(94)90630-0
147. Farren CK, Tipton KF. Trait markers for alcoholism: clinical utility. *Alcohol Alcohol* (1999) 34(5):649–65. doi: 10.1093/alcalc/34.5.649
148. Wang FL, Chassin L. Negative urgency mediates the relation between genetically influenced serotonin functioning and alcohol problems. *Clin Psychol Sci* (2018) 6(1):106–22. doi: 10.1177/2167702617733817
149. Edenberg HJ, Dick DM, Xuei X, Tian H, Almasy L, Bauer LO, et al. Variations in GABRA2, encoding the α2 subunit of the GABAA receptor, are associated with alcohol dependence and with brain oscillations. *Am J Hum Genet* (2004) 74(4):705–14. doi: 10.1086/383283
150. Villafuerte S, Heitzeg MM, Foley S, Wendy Yau WY, Majczenko K, Zubieta JK, et al. Impulsiveness and insula activation during reward anticipation are associated with genetic variants in GABRA2 in a family sample enriched for alcoholism. *Mol Psychiatry* (2011) 17:511. doi: 10.1038/mp.2011.33
151. Villafuerte S, Strumba V, Stoltenberg SF, Zucker RA, Burmeister M. Impulsiveness mediates the association between GABRA2 SNPs and lifetime alcohol problems. *Genes Brain Behav* (2013) 12(5):525–31. doi: 10.1111/gbb.12039
152. Boy F, Evans CJ, Edden RAE, Lawrence AD, Singh KD, Husain M, et al. Dorsolateral prefrontal γ-aminobutyric acid in men predicts individual differences in rash impulsivity. *Biol Psychiatry* (2011) 70(9):866–72. doi: 10.1016/j.biopsych.2011.05.030
153. Grahame NJ, Li T-K, Lumeng L. Selective breeding for high and low alcohol preference in mice. *Behav Genet* (1999) 29(1):47–57. doi: 10.1023/A:1021489922751
154. McBride WJ, Rodd ZA, Bell RL, Lumeng L, Li TK. The alcohol-preferring (P) and high-alcohol-drinking (HAD) rats—Animal models of alcoholism. *Alcohol* (2014) 48(3):209–15. doi: 10.1016/j.alcohol.2013.09.044
155. Wilhelm CJ, Mitchell SH. Rats bred for high alcohol drinking are more sensitive to delayed and probabilistic outcomes. *Genes Brain Behav* (2008) 7(7):705–13. doi: 10.1111/j.1601-183X.2008.00406.x
156. Murphy JM, McBride WJ, Lumeng L, Li TK. Contents of monoamines in forebrain regions of alcohol-preferring (P) and -nonpreferring (NP) lines of rats. *Pharmacol Biochem Behav* (1987) 26(2):389–92. doi: 10.1016/0091-3057(87)90134-1
157. McBride WJ, Murphy JM, Lumeng L, Li TK. Serotonin, dopamine and GABA involvement in alcohol drinking of selectively bred rats. *Alcohol* (1990) 7(3):199–205. doi: 10.1016/0741-8329(90)90005-W
158. Schulte T, Oberlin BG, Kareken DA, Marinkovic K, Müller-Oehring EM, Meyerhoff DJ, et al. How acute and chronic alcohol consumption affects brain networks: insights from multimodal neuroimaging. *Alcohol Clin Exp Res* (2012) 36(12):2017–27. doi: 10.1111/j.1530-0277.2012.01831.x
159. Giuliano C, Peña-Oliver Y, Goodlett CR, Cardinal RN, Robbins TW, Bullmore ET, et al. Evidence for a long-lasting compulsive alcohol seeking phenotype in rats. *Neuropsychopharmacology* (2017) 43:728. doi: 10.1038/npp.2017.105
160. Winkler MC, Greager EM, Stafford J, Bachtell RK. Methamphetamine self-administration reduces alcohol consumption and preference in alcohol-preferring P rats. *Addict Biol* (2018) 23(1):90–101. doi: 10.1111/adb.12476
161. Cipriani A, Pretty H, Hawton K, Geddes JR. Lithium in the prevention of suicidal behavior and all-cause mortality in patients with mood disorders: a systematic review of randomized trials. *Am J Psychiatry* (2005) 162(10):1805–19. doi: 10.1176/appi.ajp.162.10.1805
162. Baldessarini RJ, Tondo L, Davis P, Pompili M, Goodwin FK, Hennen J. Decreased risk of suicides and attempts during long-term lithium treatment: a meta-analytic review. *Bipolar Disord* (2006) 8(5p2):625–39. doi: 10.1111/j.1399-5618.2006.00344.x
163. Crane CA, Godleski SA, Przybyla SM, Schlauch RC, Testa M. The proximal effects of acute alcohol consumption on male-to-female aggression: a meta-analytic review of the experimental literature. *Trauma Violence Abuse* (2016) 17(5):520–31. doi: 10.1177/1524838015584374
164. Patorno E, Bohn RL, Wahl PM, Avorn J, Patrick AR, Liu J, et al. Anticonvulsant medications and the risk of suicide, attempted suicide, or violent death. *JAMA* (2010) 303(14):1401–9. doi: 10.1001/jama.2010.410
165. Halcomb ME, Gould TD, Grahame NJ. Lithium, but not valproate, reduces impulsive choice in the delay-discounting task in mice. *Neuropsychopharmacology* (2013) 38(10):1937. doi: 10.1038/npp.2013.89
166. Nitta A, Itoh A, Hasegawa T, Nabeshima T. β-Amyloid protein-induced Alzheimer's disease animal model. *Neurosci Lett* (1994) 170(1):63–6. doi: 10.1016/0304-3940(94)90239-9
167. Di Marzo V, Hill MP, Bisogno T, Crossman AR, Brotchie JM. Enhanced levels of endogenous cannabinoids in the globus pallidus are associated with a reduction in movement in an animal model of Parkinson's disease. *FASEB J* (2000) 14(10):1432–8. doi: 10.1096/fasebj.14.10.1432
168. Bories C, Arsenault D, Lemire M, Tremblay C, De Koninck Y, Calon F. Transgenic autoinhibition of p21-activated kinase exacerbates synaptic impairments and fronto-dependent behavioral deficits in an animal model of Alzheimer's disease. *Aging (Albany NY)* (2017) 9(5):1386. doi: 10.18632/aging.101239
169. Nascimento G, Bortolanza M, Bariotto K, Leite-Panissi C, Del Bel E. Effects of L-DOPA and doxicycline administration on nociceptive responses in an animal model of Parkinson's disease. *J Cereb Blood Flow Metab* (2017), Sage Publications Inc 2455 Teller Rd, Thousand Oaks, CA 91320 USA.
170. Rizzi N, Brunialti E, Cerri S, Cermisoni G, Levandis G, Cesari N, et al. In vivo imaging of early signs of dopaminergic neuronal death in an animal model of Parkinson's disease. *Neurobiol Dis* (2018) 114:74–84. doi: 10.1016/j.nbd.2018.02.005
171. Kennett GA, Chaouloff F, Marcou M, Curzon G. Female rats are more vulnerable than males in an animal model of depression: the possible role of serotonin. *Brain Res* (1986) 382(2):416–21. doi: 10.1016/0006-8993(86)91355-7
172. Dremencov E, Gispan-Herman I, Rosenstein M, Mendelman A, Overstreet DH, Zohar J, et al. The serotonin–dopamine interaction is critical for fast-onset action of antidepressant treatment: in vivo studies in an animal model of depression. *Prog Neuropsychopharmacol Biol Psychiatry* (2004) 28(1):141–7. doi: 10.1016/j.pnpbp.2003.09.030
173. Liu X-C, Erhardt S, Goiny M, Engberg G, Mathé AA. Decreased levels of kynurenic acid in prefrontal cortex in a genetic animal model of depression. *Acta Neuropsychiatr* (2017) 29(1):54–8. doi: 10.1017/neu.2016.31
174. Qiao H, An S-C, Xu C, Ma X-M. Role of proBDNF and BDNF in dendritic spine plasticity and depressive-like behaviors induced by an animal model of depression. *Brain Res* (2017) 1663:29–37. doi: 10.1016/j.brainres.2017.02.020
175. Price JL, Drevets WC. Neurocircuitry of Mood Disorders. *Neuropsychopharmacology* (2009) 35:192–216.
176. Laubach M, Amarante LM, Swanson K, White SR. What, if anything, is rodent prefrontal cortex? *Cognition and Behavior* (2018) 5:5–28. doi: 10.31234/osf.io/c2a79

9

# Resonance-Paced Breathing Alters Neural Response to Visual Cues: Proof-of-Concept for a Neuroscience-Informed Adjunct to Addiction Treatments

***Marsha E. Bates[1,2]*, Laura M. Lesnewich[2,3], Sarah Grace Uhouse[2,3], Suril Gohel[4] and Jennifer F. Buckman[1,2]***

*[1] Cardiac Neuroscience Laboratory, Department of Kinesiology and Health, Rutgers University-New Brunswick, Piscataway, NJ, United States, [2] Center of Alcohol Studies, Rutgers University-New Brunswick, Piscataway, NJ, United States, [3] Cardiac Neuroscience Laboratory, Department of Psychology, Rutgers University-New Brunswick, Piscataway, NJ, United States, [4] Department of Health Informatics, School of Health Professions, Rutgers University-Newark, Newark, NJ, United States*

****Correspondence:***
*Marsha E. Bates*
*mebates@smithers.rutgers.edu*

Conscious attempts to regulate alcohol and drug use are often undermined by automatic attention and arousal processes that are activated in the context of salient cues. Response to these cues involves body and brain signals that are linked via dynamic feedback loops, yet no studies have targeted the cardiovascular system as a potential conduit to alter automatic neural processes that maintain cue salience. This proof-of-concept study examined within-person changes in neural response to parallel but unique sets of visual alcohol-related cues at two points in time: prior to versus following a brief behavioral intervention. The active intervention was resonance breathing, a rhythmical breathing task paced at 0.1 Hz (6 breaths per minute) that helps normalize neurocardiac feedback. The control intervention was a low-demand cognitive task. Functional magnetic resonance imaging (fMRI) was used to assess changes in brain response to the cues presented before (A1) and after (A2) the intervention in 41 emerging adult men and women with varying drinking behaviors. The resonance breathing group exhibited significantly less activation to A2 cues compared with A1 cues in left inferior and superior lateral occipital cortices, right inferior lateral occipital cortex, bilateral occipital pole, and temporal occipital fusiform cortices. This group also showed significantly greater activation to A2 cues compared with A1 cues in medial prefrontal, anterior and posterior cingulate, and precuneus cortices, paracingulate, and lingual gyri. The control group showed no significant changes. Thus, following resonance breathing, activation in brain regions involved in visual processing of cues was reduced, while activation in brain areas implicated in behavioral control, internally directed cognition, and brain–body integration was increased. These findings provide preliminary evidence that manipulation of the cardiovascular system with resonance breathing alters neural activation in a manner theoretically consistent with a dampening of automatic sensory input and strengthening of higher-level cognitive processing.

**Keywords: alcohol, biofeedback, cardiovascular, neural reactivity, functional magnetic resonance imaging, heart rate variability, respiration, resonance breathing**

## INTRODUCTION

Moment-to-moment changes in internal states (e.g., cognition, emotion, visceral processes, moods) and environments (e.g., cues, persons) influence decisions to use alcohol and other drugs (1). These dynamic, intra-individual change processes derive from the body's ability to collect and relay information to the brain about the environment (afferent neural traffic), as well as from the brain's ability to integrate this information and generate a behavioral response (efferent neural traffic). In other words, behavior is influenced by both body and brain signals that are linked via reflexive and predictive bidirectional feedback (2, 3).

In the case of the cardiovascular system, this feedback loop (**Figure 1**) has been extensively documented in terms of its neurophysiology and functional anatomy in rodent and primate models [e.g., (4, 5)]; parallel functional anatomy emerged in a meta-analysis of human neuroimaging studies (6). The loop maintains signaling between the brain and heart via the vagus and sympathetic nerves, baroreceptors located on the aortic arch, carotid artery, and other vessel walls, and a network of brain regions referred to as the central autonomic network (4). These bodies of literature reveal how the brain elicits cardiovascular signals that promote arousal (e.g., increasing heart rate and blood pressure) that, in turn, prepare the organism for goal-directed behavior to respond to in-the-moment demands. Through this loop, feedback from the heart and vasculature is integrated with other autonomic information and relayed to forebrain structures that mediate cognitive and emotional experience

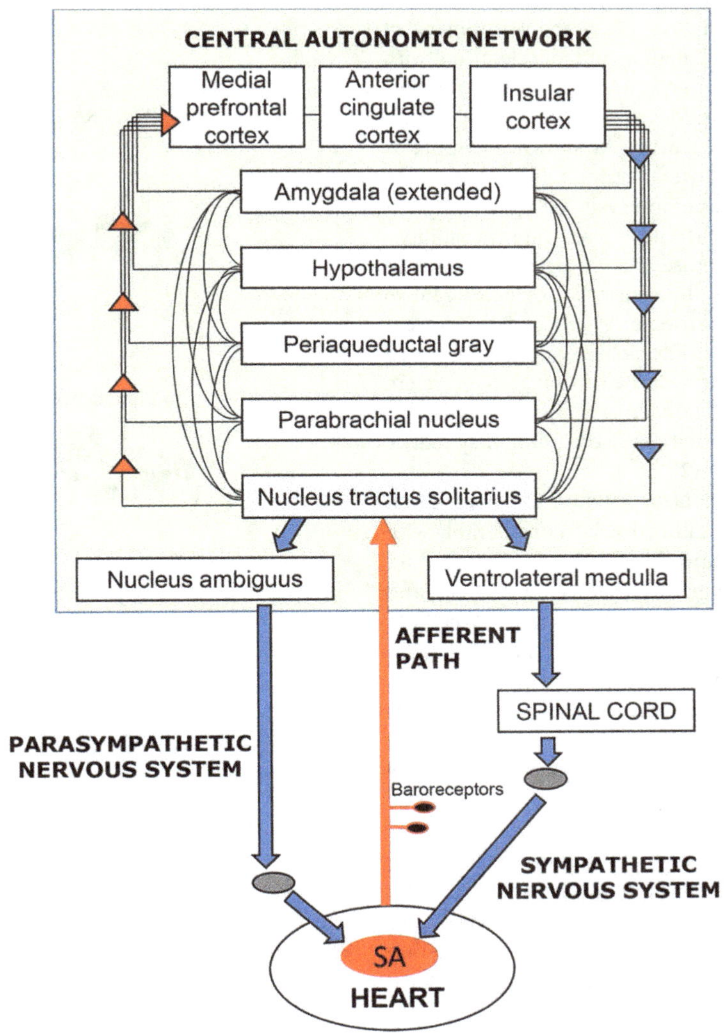


**FIGURE 1** | Schematic overview of the neurocardiac feedback loop. Efferent information (blue arrows) emanates from cortical, subcortical, and brain stem structures of the central-autonomic network and flows to the sinoatrial (SA) node of the heart via the sympathetic and parasympathetic branches of the autonomic nervous system. Afferent information (red arrows) from the heart and blood vessels is conveyed back to the brain via baroreceptors located mainly in the walls of the aortic and carotid arteries. Afferent signals enter the brain (shaded in green) via the nucleus tractus solitarius in the brain stem and are integrated with other sensory, cognitive, and affective information as it ascends to cortical regions, including the medial frontal, cingulate, and insular cortices.

(7–9). Consideration of cardiovascular processes as embedded components of affect and cognition implies that these processes contribute to motivated human behavior, including behavioral flexibility toward alcohol and other drugs (10–12). This is important because several non-invasive, low-cost behavioral interventions that help normalize cardiovascular functioning have demonstrated efficacy across various mental and physical health conditions (13–20).

Two compelling qualities of the neurocardiac feedback loop for intervention development are its plasticity and responsivity to relatively simple behavioral interventions. Afferent stream activation of the neurocardiac feedback loop can be accomplished by manipulating peripheral functions, such as respiration and muscle flexion (21–24). Breathing paced at 6 breaths per minute (0.1 Hz) is slower and more rhythmical than typical breathing (12–20 breaths per minute). It creates resonance within the cardiovascular system by synchronizing cardiac oscillations driven by respiratory sinus arrhythmia (i.e., the phenomena of heart rate acceleration with inhalation and deceleration with exhalation) with cardiac oscillations driven by the baroreflex, which links heart rate acceleration/deceleration to corresponding changes in the blood pressure (21, 25). As shown in **Figure 2**, breathing at this frequency lowers systolic blood pressure, increases variability in the time intervals between R-spikes of the electrocardiogram (ECG) (i.e., heart rate variability), generates large oscillations in pulse transit time (i.e., vascular tone variability), and increases the sensitivity of heart rate to changes in blood pressure (i.e., baroreflex gain) (12, 21). A recent meta-analysis found that clinical interventions involving paced breathing at a resonance frequency of the cardiovascular system resulted in large effect size reductions in anxiety and stress (26). Preliminary evidence also suggested paced breathing may reduce craving for appetitive substances (27).

The brain structures of the central autonomic network that participate in cardiovascular signaling overlap considerably with those that process reward, emotion, and habit formation (28), including medial prefrontal, cingulate, and insular cortices, and amygdala. These structures also figure prominently in current translational models of putative addiction neurocircuitry (29–31), with the brain stem serving as the first point of neural integration of afferent autonomic and somatic signals from the body. Psychophysiological evidence suggests that the neurocardiac feedback loop may participate in substance use behaviors through its contribution to attention capture by stimulating cues, affective modulation, and relay of visceral reactivity to the brain [e.g., (32–36)], but little research has extended these findings to the neural structures that comprise the central autonomic network. Nonetheless, converging lines of evidence suggest that ineffective or maladaptive functioning of this feedback loop can set into motion a cascade of biological events that alter one's ability to adaptively modulate affect, arousal, and stress response (2, 37, 38).

Neural cue reactivity studies, wherein brain activation is measured while participants are exposed to salient alcohol- or drug-related cues, have received significant attention in the neuroscience and psychology of addiction literatures (39, 40). Cue reactivity studies typically compare within-person differences in

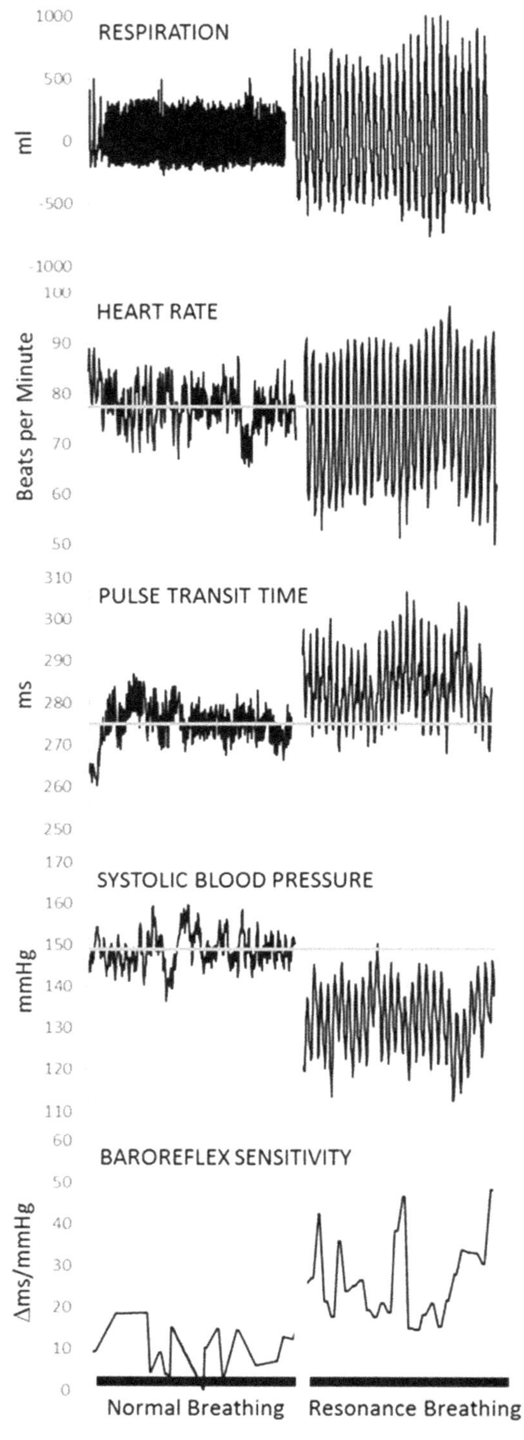


**FIGURE 2** | Physiological data from one representative individual collected during a 5-min baseline task (normal breathing) and a 5-min resonance breathing task. Resonance breathing elicited instantaneous changes in respiration, heart rate, pulse transit time (i.e., vascular tone), systolic arterial pressure, and baroreflex sensitivity such that oscillations were magnified and more rhythmic across all measures. In addition, resonance breathing decreased systolic pressure, improved vascular tone, and increased the sensitivity of the neurocardiac feedback loop (i.e., baroreflex). Adapted from (12). Used with permission.

brain activation to alcohol or drug cues versus control cues (40). There is substantial evidence that elevated alcohol and drug cue neural reactivity is found in individuals with substance use disorders (40–42). Increased neural (43) and cardiac (44) cue reactivity also has been associated with increased drug craving (2, 37, 38). Experimental evidence suggests that heightened neural (45) and cardiovascular (46) reactivity to alcohol and drug cues is related to high risk substance use in non-clinical populations. Thus, altered reactivity to affective and appetitive stimuli appears to increase the likelihood that individuals will be susceptible to contextual influences on substance use, even following extended periods of abstinence (47, 48). This raises the question of whether behavioral interventions that enhance the efficiency of neurocardiac signaling might be used to alter neurocardiac activation to contextual challenges that promote substance use and relapse (49, 50).

This proof-of-concept study examined whether stimulating the afferent stream of the neurocardiac feedback loop with a 5-min course of resonance breathing can affect subsequent neural activation to visual alcohol cues. In contrast to cue reactivity paradigms that compare neural activation to alcohol versus control cues, this study examined within-person changes in neural response to alcohol cues at two points in time. We compared neural activation with unique sets of alcohol cues viewed prior to versus following the breathing task. Because this is the first study of its kind, there is no empirical literature to guide predictions about brain activation changes when participants are exposed to visual cues following resonance breathing. Based on the anatomy of the central autonomic network (4, 5) and drug cue salience networks (28, 40), we hypothesized that significant changes in activation may be observed in brainstem, medial prefrontal, cingulate, and insular cortices, as well as in the amygdala. We further allowed for the possibility of spreading activation, wherein structures within the central autonomic network that share additional network circuitry with regions outside the central autonomic network (e.g., the mesocorticolimbic circuit, ventral striatum) may exhibit activation changes as well. Significant changes in neural response were not anticipated in the group that viewed alcohol cues before and after completing a low-demand cognitive task.

# METHODS

## Participants

Forty-nine men and women, ages 18 to 25 years, were recruited at a large, northeast U.S. university and in the surrounding community through advertisements targeting alcohol drinkers. Initial inclusion criteria for all participants assessed via self-report were fluency in English, right-handedness, near 20/20 vision (corrected), and alcohol consumption at least once per month. Exclusion criteria assessed via self-report included: MRI contraindications (e.g., permanent metal in the body, claustrophobia), abnormal hearing, any serious medical condition (e.g., epilepsy, diabetes), cardiovascular problems (e.g., hypertension, heart murmur), current learning disability or attention difficulties, loss of consciousness for longer than 30 min, and, for women, pregnancy. To reduce heterogeneity related to psychiatric comorbidities and poly-substance use, lifetime diagnosis of a bipolar disorder or psychosis (e.g., schizophrenia, schizoaffective disorder), past year psychiatric/psychological treatment, past year cannabis use exceeding four times per month in the past year, other past year illicit drug use more than twice per month, past or current substance use treatment (including Alcoholics Anonymous/Narcotics Anonymous), and substance use during pregnancy on the part of the biological mother also were exclusionary.

Half of the participants were recruited based on meeting the National Institute on Alcohol Abuse and Alcoholism (NIAAA) "low risk" drinking criteria [i.e., no more than 5 drinks per day for men (4 drinks per day for women), no more than 14 drinks per week for men (7 drinks per week for women)], as well as an additional criterion of not binge drinking more than once in the past 6 months. The other half met DSM-IV-TR criteria (51) for alcohol dependence. This proof-of-concept examination of resonance breathing as a neurally active intervention included all participants with the exception that data from eight participants were excluded due to excessive motion in the scanner. The final sample (n = 41) had a mean age of 21.4 (SD = 1.9) years and was racially and ethnically diverse (27% Asian, 27% black/African American, 29% white, 17% other/multiple race; 11% Latino/a); 46% of the participants identified as female.

## Procedures

Potential participants who gave verbal consent completed a telephone screening interview to determine initial eligibility. Eligible participants were asked to abstain from alcohol and drug use (except caffeine and nicotine) for 24 h prior to the experimental session. After screening, they were randomized into the active intervention (i.e., resonance breathing) or the control intervention (i.e., vanilla task), with drinking profiles being approximately equally distributed in both groups.

Upon arrival at the imaging center, participants provided written informed consent, supplied a breath sample to verify zero blood alcohol concentration, and completed a MRI safety screener and self-report questionnaires regarding alcohol use, mood state (Positive and Negative Affect Scale) (52), and stress (Perceived Stress Scale) (53). Basic physiological measures (e.g., temperature, blood pressure, weight) and a urine sample were collected; participants with a positive urine screen for cocaine, methamphetamine, opiates, and/or benzodiazepines (One Step Multi-Drug Screen Test Panel) were excluded. Participants with a positive urine screen for marijuana were asked additional follow-up questions about their drug use, and those with marijuana use exceeding four times per month were excluded. Women were screened for pregnancy using a standard urine dipstick. All participants were trained to use an MRI-compatible response box and to perform their assigned intervention task. Task training lasted approximately 2 min. Participants then were fitted with ECG sensors and a respiration belt and positioned in the scanner.

The overall paradigm (**Figure 3A**) involved four 5-min tasks: 1) viewing a set of nature picture cues, 2) viewing a set

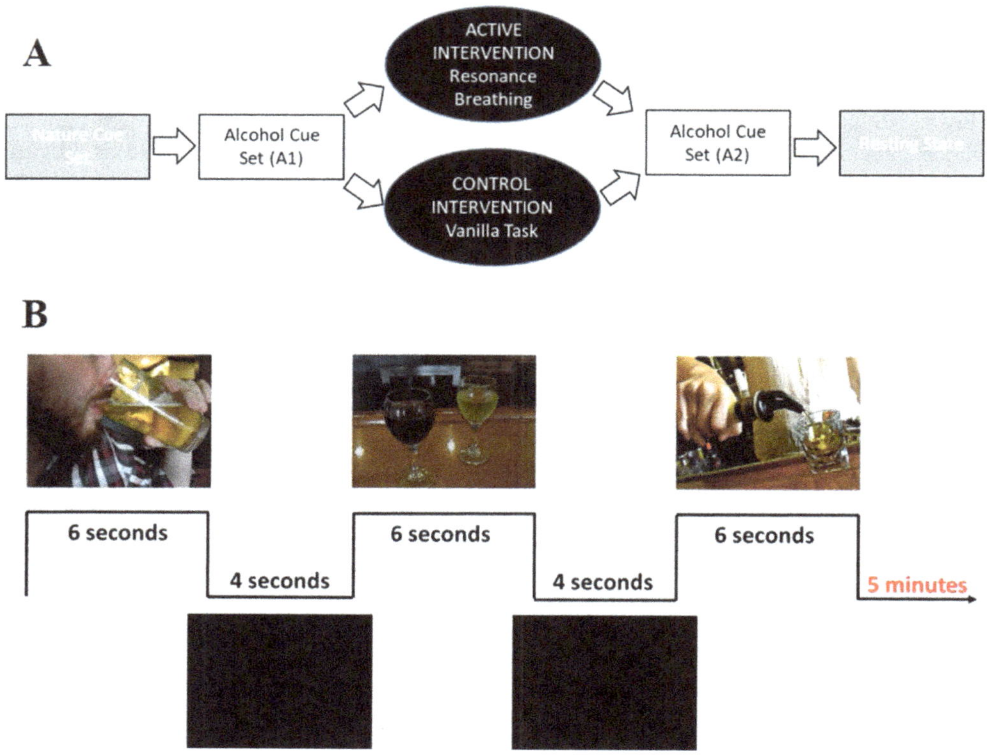


**FIGURE 3 |** Visual depiction of the study and cue task design. Panel **(A)** shows the complete study design. Participants first viewed a set of nature picture cues (data not shown). Participants then viewed a set of alcohol picture cues (A1), followed by a 5-min intervention task (active condition: resonance breathing; control condition: vanilla task). They then immediately viewed a second, distinct set of alcohol picture cues (A2). The study ended with a 6-min resting state task (data not shown). Panel **(B)** shows representative images from the alcohol cue tasks, both of which involved viewing 30 unique images that were presented for 6 s, with 4-s inter-stimulus intervals.

of alcohol picture cues (A1), 3) performing the intervention task, 4) viewing a second, distinct set of alcohol picture cues (A2); a 6-min resting state task was then performed. After each task, participants responded to the question, "How much are you currently craving alcohol right now?" using a track ball on a visual analogue scale (VAS, 43) anchored from "not at all" (0) to "extremely" (100). Stimulus cues were presented using E-Prime software (Psychology Software Tools Inc.). Images were projected onto a screen positioned at the rear of the scanner bore and viewed through a mirror attached to the head coil. A trigger pulse synchronized the start of each task with the E-Prime software. Total scan time was approximately 45 min.

Data from the two alcohol cue tasks (A1, A2) were analyzed in the present study. Each task included 30 unique images that were presented for 6 s with 4-s inter-stimulus intervals (**Figure 3B**), a design driven by the larger study's broader goal of characterizing the relationship between cardiovascular and neural reactivity. The alcohol cues were drawn from prior studies in our and others' laboratories (34, 54, 55). Each participant's self-reported preferred beverage (i.e., beer, wine, "straight" liquor, or mixed drinks) made up approximately 50% of the images to which they were exposed. Participants were instructed to pay attention to the images and to press a response box button when they saw an image that contained their preferred drink.

Between the A1 and A2 cue sets, participants in the active intervention (resonance breathing) synchronized their breathing with a visual pacer at the rate of 0.1 Hz (i.e., 6 breaths per minute). Compliance to the breathing task was verified via analysis of the respiratory signal. Time series respiratory frequency data were Fourier transformed, and the shape of the spectrum was visually inspected; all participants showed a respiratory peak at 0.1 Hz and spectral characteristics consistent with resonance breathing. Participants in the control intervention group completed a low-demand cognitive "vanilla" task wherein different colored rectangles were presented for 10 s each; they were instructed to silently count the number of blue rectangles (56).

After exiting the scanner, participants were compensated for their time. Those who met the criteria for alcohol dependence were given an informational brochure on alcohol use disorders and treatment options. This study was approved by the university's institutional review board for the protection of human subjects involved in research.

## Imaging Parameters and Pre-Processing

Imaging data were collected using a 3T Siemens Trio scanner and 12-channel head coil. Standard localizer, anatomical, scout, and field map scans were collected. High-resolution anatomical images were acquired using a T1-weighted MPRAGE protocol with parameters: repetition time (TR) = 1,900 ms, echo time (TE) = 2.51 ms, matrix = 256 × 256 voxels, field-of-view (FOV) = 256 mm, voxel size = 1 × 1 × 1 mm, 176 1-mm sagittal slices (.5 mm gap). Functional blood oxygen level-dependent (BOLD) data were acquired using single-shot gradient echo-planar imaging (EPI) sequences with parameters: TR = 2,000 ms, TE = 25 ms, flip, angle = 90°, matrix = 64 × 64 voxels, FOV = 192 mm, voxel size = 3 × 3 × 3 mm, 35 contiguous 3-mm sagittal slices (1 mm gap). ECG and respiration data were collected using a MRI-compatible BIOPAC acquisition system (Biopac Systems, Goleta, CA) as part of the larger study.

FSL 5.0.9 software was used to conduct image preprocessing and data analysis (FMIRB's Software Library, https://fsl.fmrib.ox.ac.uk). Non-brain tissue was removed from all anatomical and BOLD images using FSL's Brain Extraction Tool (BET, 57) by estimating each image's center of gravity and manually adjusting BET parameters as necessary until an optimal result was obtained. BOLD data were motion-corrected using FSL's MCFLIRT (58), and the output was reviewed to identify participants with excessive motion during the resting-state scan. Excessive motion was defined conservatively as mean absolute and/or relative displacement greater than .5 mm. A paired t-test was performed to compare mean framewise displacement between the randomized intervention groups. No significant differences were observed in motion between the groups ($p > 0.05$). BOLD images were segmented into gray matter, white matter (WM), and cerebral spinal fluid (CSF) using FSL's FAST (59). Probability maps of CSF and WM were derived, and time-series data for these signals were extracted from each participant. These nuisance parameters (i.e., WM, CSF) along with extended head motion parameters were used as covariates in the linear regression models implemented in FSL to decrease the effects of signals-of-no-interest. BOLD data were registered to standard space with a two-step process using FMRIB's Linear Image Registration Tool (FLIRT) (60). The data were first registered to the T1-weighted anatomical image and then to MNI-152 standard space using 9 degrees-of-freedom and SINC interpolation. All data were visually inspected for gross errors in registration. A high pass temporal filter was set to 50 s, and spatial smoothing was set to a 6-mm full-width at half-maximum Gaussian kernel.

## Statistical Analyses

Analyses of the BOLD data from the A1 and A2 cue reactivity tasks were performed using a two-step process. Subject-level effects were calculated using first-level analyses in FSL's FEAT, and group effects were determined using higher-level analyses. In the first-level analysis, each alcohol image event was modeled and convolved with a double-gamma hemodynamic response function (HRF), and the mean task activation for A1 and A2 was calculated for each participant. In the higher-level analysis stage, two sets of analyses were performed using Randomise, the non-parametric permutation-testing tool implemented in FSL (61). First, one-sample $t$-tests were conducted to characterize neural activation in each intervention group before (A1) and after (A2) the intervention. Next, to examine intervention effects on neural activation to visual stimuli, paired $t$-tests with two contrasts were conducted on each intervention group (i.e., resonance breathing, control) separately (61). For each contrast, 5,000 permutations were calculated. One contrast (A1 > A2) was designed to determine brain areas that demonstrated greater activation pre- compared to post-intervention task, and the second contrast (A2 > A1) was designed to determine brain areas that demonstrated greater activation post-intervention compared to pre-intervention task. Threshold-free cluster enhancement was employed (62), and activation was considered significant at $p < 0.05$ (corrected for multiple comparisons using FSL Randomise).

A repeated-measures mixed model was used to assess the effect of resonance breathing on VAS craving scores. Craving data for one participant was missing due to equipment failure; thus, data from 40 participants were available for analysis. A between-subjects factor of intervention group (resonance breathing, control) and a within-subjects factor of craving scores following A1 and A2, as well as their interaction, were modeled. To examine the relationship between VAS craving scores and brain regions that exhibited significant pre-intervention to post-intervention changes, regions-of-interest (ROIs) were defined by creating 6-mm spheres around the peak voxel of each significant cluster of activation for the A1 > A2 and A2 > A1 contrasts. Mean activation values of these ROIs were extracted for each participant from the subject-level A1 and A2 cope images. Pearson correlations were then used to test the associations between ROI activation and VAS craving scores at A1 and A2. Point biserial correlations were used to examine the relationship of binary drinking status (low-risk = 0, alcohol dependent = 1) to ROI activation at A2 in the resonance breathing group. These analyses were performed using SAS 9.4 software (SAS Institute, Cary, NC, USA).

# RESULTS

## Neuroimaging

Both intervention groups exhibited widespread neural activity in response to the visual alcohol cues, including in bilateral posterior parahippocampal gyri, temporal occipital fusiform cortices, lateral occipital cortices (inferior and superior divisions), postcentral gyri, and cerebellum at A1 and A2. The resonance breathing group (n = 22) additionally showed significant activation in bilateral inferior frontal gyri, left insula, left pallidum, left putamen, left amygdala, and left thalamus (A1, A2), and left precentral gyrus (A1). The control group (n = 19) additionally showed significant activation in the right thalamus (A1) and left precentral gyrus (A2). These results are shown in **Figure 4**.

Participants in the resonance breathing group demonstrated greater activation in response to alcohol cues pre-breathing compared with post-breathing (A1>A2) in left inferior and superior lateral occipital cortices and right inferior lateral occipital cortex, as well as bilateral occipital pole and temporal occipital fusiform cortices. They also demonstrated greater activation post-breathing compared with pre-breathing (A2 > A1) in

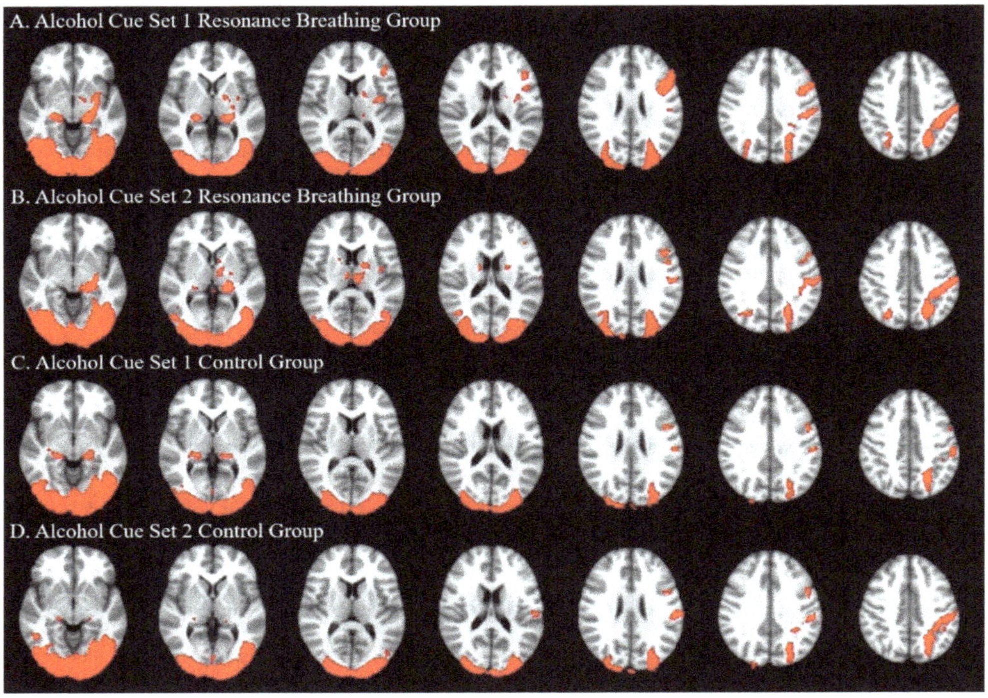


**FIGURE 4 |** Significant Neural Activation to Visual Alcohol Cue Sets. One-sample *t*-tests were used to identify areas of significant neural activation during alcohol cue set viewing. The neural responses of the active intervention (resonance breathing) group are shown in Panels **(A)** (A1 task, cues viewed prior to the intervention) and **(B)** (A2 task, cues viewed after the intervention). The neural responses of the control intervention (vanilla task) group are shown in Panels **(C)** (A1 task, cues viewed prior to the intervention) and **(D)** (A2 task, cues viewed after the intervention). Axial slices are shown in MNI standard space at z = −6 (first slice) and every fourth subsequent slice. Images are oriented using radiological convention. Areas of significant activation are shown in red.

voxels spanning precuneus cortex, posterior cingulate gyrus, and bilateral lingual gyri, as well as in medial prefrontal cortex (MPFC), paracingulate gyrus, and anterior cingulate cortex (ACC). These results are shown in **Table 1** and **Figure 5**.

The control group analysis yielded no significant activation in either the A1 > A2 or A2 > A1 contrasts, indicating that there were no statistically significant changes in brain activation in response to visual alcohol cues in the group that performed the control task.

## Self-Report

Surveys administered prior to the neuroimaging session revealed that the sample as a whole had low-moderate perceived stress (mean ± standard deviation = 17 ± 6), and positive (mean ± standard deviation = 30.7±9.7) and negative (mean ± standard deviation = 13.9 ± 6.2) affect scores that were similar to those reported from the original general adult normative sample (52). There were no differences in affect or stress between the intervention groups nor between the drinking groups (all $p > .05$).

Craving was measured in the scanner after exposure to each cue block. The results of a repeated-measures (A1, A2) mixed model indicated that there was a significant main effect of group on craving, but no main effect of task (i.e., from pre- to post-intervention). Participants randomized to the resonance breathing intervention group reported lower levels

**TABLE 1 |** Anatomical location at peak voxel coordinates in significant clusters of activation in resonance breathing group.

| A1>A2 Contrast | | | | | |
|---|---|---|---|---|---|
| | | MNI Coordinates | | | |
| **Cluster Size** | **Z** | **x** | **y** | **z** | **Peak Voxel Anatomical Location** |
| 2,433 | 6.80 | −30 | −96 | 10 | Occipital pole (L) |
| 1,339 | 6.95 | 28 | −90 | 4 | Occipital pole (R) |
| 10 | 4.74 | 28 | −38 | −24 | Temporal fusiform cortex (R) |
| **A2>A1 Contrast** | | | | | |
| | | MNI Coordinates | | | |
| **Cluster Size** | **Z** | **x** | **y** | **z** | **Peak Voxel Anatomical Location** |
| 2,141 | 7.81 | 2 | −78 | 42 | Precuneus Cortex |
| 283 | 5.89 | −2 | 50 | 0 | Paracingulate Gyrus/ Medial Prefrontal Cortex |
| 150 | 4.74 | −16 | −50 | −2 | Lingual Gyrus (L) |
| 16 | 5.35 | 6 | −24 | 40 | Posterior Cingulate Cortex |
| 15 | 4.44 | 2 | −22 | 32 | Posterior Cingulate Cortex |
| 2 | 3.81 | 0 | −56 | 10 | Precuneus Cortex |
| 1 | 6.87 | −2 | −6 | 36 | Anterior Cingulate Cortex |

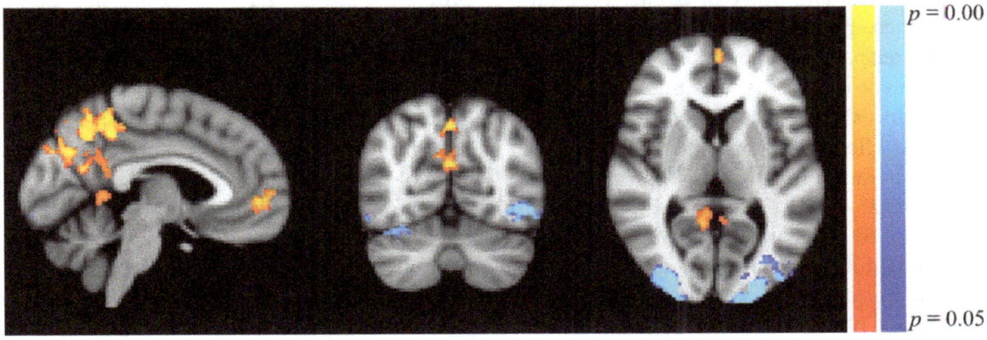


**FIGURE 5 |** Significant Clusters of Activation in Resonance Breathing Group. Blue-cyan clusters represent regions with greater activation during A1 compared to A2 (A1 > A2), and red-yellow clusters represent regions with greater activation during A2 compared with A1 (A2 > A1). Voxels were thresholded at $p < 0.05$. Image is shown in MNI standard space at x = −4, y = −66, z = 6, and oriented using radiological convention.

of in-the-moment craving compared to those randomized to the control intervention group [$F(76,1) = 5.76$, $p = 0.0188$; least square mean ± standard error of resonance breathing group = 28.1 ± 4.5 and of control group = 43.7 ± 4.7]. The group–task interaction was not statistically significant, suggesting that changes in subjective reports of craving pre- to post-intervention did not significantly differ between the two groups.

No significant correlations were observed at A1 between VAS craving scores and the ten cluster activation scores in the full sample ($r$ range, −0.24 to 0.09, all $p > .05$). In addition, there were no significant correlations at A2 between craving scores and the ten cluster activation scores within either group (resonance breathing group $r$ range, −0.32 to 0.28, all $p > .05$; control group $r$ range, −0.42 to 0.44, all $p > .05$). Lastly, there were no significant correlations at A2 between drinking status (AUD vs. low risk) and the ten-cluster activation scores in the resonance breathing group ($r$ range, −0.27 to 0.28, all $p > .05$).

## DISCUSSION

Evidence that visceral afferent signaling influences stimulus processing argues for intervention development aimed at manipulating cardiovascular signals to alter detection and neural processing of affective stimuli (63). The results of the present study provide the first proof-of-concept evidence that a brief behavioral intervention of resonance breathing can significantly alter drinkers' neural activation to visual alcohol cues. The observed changes in brain activity included both decreases and increases in the activation of distinct brain regions.

In the group that performed resonance breathing between the visual cue tasks, but not in the control group, there was reduced activation in occipital regions from the first set of alcohol cues to the second, different set of alcohol cues. This pattern of results suggests that the breathing intervention prompted a subsequent decrease in visual cortex activation when individuals were confronted with alcohol-related visual stimuli. The specificity of these changes to alcohol-related content is unclear as this proof-of-concept study did not include a cue set of non-alcohol–related images presented before and after the intervention. Indeed, visual cortex activation to many types of images, including faces, is modulated by their emotional and social significance (64–66). Multiple lines of evidence also support the involvement of the visual cortex in appetitive cue processing. Several meta-analyses found that drug users consistently showed increased activation in occipital regions in response to drug-related cues compared to controls, even when non-visual drug-related stimuli were presented (41, 67–69). Increased visual cortex activation has been observed in individuals with behavioral addictions, such as pathological gambling, as well (70–72). Thus, although the literature suggests that the role of the visual cortex in alcohol and drug cue reactivity is not specific, decreased activation in the lateral occipital cortices following resonance breathing would be consistent with decreased perception, representation, and recognition of the images (73) and/or may potentially reflect less attention being directed toward the cues by the amygdala (66) or higher cortical areas (74).

In parallel with reduced visual processing of the cues, we observed increased activation in bilateral medial prefrontal, anterior and posterior cingulate, and precuneus cortices during the second alcohol cue task, only in the resonance breathing group. The ACC and MPFC, as regions of the central autonomic network, bi-directionally influence, and are influenced by, afferent cardiovascular signaling. Resonance breathing increases cardiovascular input to the brain via activation of brainstem nuclei that share connectivity with the ACC and MPFC (4) and are thought to give rise to the visceral experience of emotion (75). Functionally, the ACC is a part of the mesocorticolimbic circuit, which is thought to be involved in conflict monitoring and the regulation of cognitive and emotional processing by integrating input and modulating processing in other regions (76, 77). The MPFC is considered to be part of a cognitive control system in the brain that promotes goal-directed behaviors (78) by using incoming information to predict the most adaptive response based on past experience (79).

Hypothetically, increased activation of MPFC and ACC in response to alcohol cues following the breathing intervention would be consistent with heightened internal monitoring of cognitive-emotional state and enhanced cognitive control. At the same time, some studies have identified these regions as sites of heightened reactivity to alcohol and other drug cues (42), and heightened reactivity in these regions has been related to post-treatment drinking and relapse, although the results in this area have not been consistent (80). Thus, it is unclear whether or under what circumstances these and other brain regions accentuate or restrain cue-elicited craving and substance use behaviors. Evidence for individual differences in brain areas most reactive to appetitive cues (42) and inconsistencies in replication add further complication to interpretation. More nuanced examination of intra-individual changes in neural activation across brain areas, and perhaps also across simultaneously operating psychological and physiological systems involved in motivated behavior, are needed.

The posterior cingulate cortex (PCC) and the precuneus showed increased activation to visual alcohol cues following the breathing intervention, but not the control task. Both of these regions are considered core nodes of the default mode network, a functional brain network involved in self-referential thought and mind-wandering (81) that shows preserved connectivity during cognitive load (82). The lingual gyrus, a brain region involved in visual encoding and higher-order analysis of complex visual stimuli (83), also showed increased activation only in the resonance breathing group. This gyrus has been implicated in spontaneous thought and often co-activates with the default mode network (84). Whether increased activation in these regions potentially plays a role in promoting self-regulation in response to alcohol or other affectively valenced cues is unknown, but warrants further investigation. One possibility is that following resonance breathing the brain reverts to its "baseline" resting state (85) for some amount of time despite activation by salient cues, rather than transitioning to a heightened state of arousal.

We did not observe acute changes in self-reported craving levels in the resonance breathing group following the second presentation of alcohol cues (absence of significant cue task by group interaction), nor were craving levels related to brain clusters of activation in response to cues at A1 or A2. Several factors likely contributed to these null findings. Randomization into resonance breathing and control groups in the present study did not result in equivalent mean craving rating scores; the resonance breathing group reported significantly lower craving levels throughout the study. Failures of randomization in small samples are common (86), and future studies may benefit from selecting participants with high levels of self-reported craving and/or matching on craving levels across intervention groups. It may also be that the brief 5-min duration of resonance breathing did not affect conscious self-estimates of craving in the present sample, or that resonance breathing works in a way that affects a different pathway, such as the operation of cue salience (50), rather than consciously experienced craving levels. The present data are limited in not speaking to these alternative speculations.

## Implications for Clinical Translation

If replicated and extended, the current findings that a brief, 5-min bout of resonance breathing changed neural activation in brain areas implicated in affective and appetitive stimulus processing could have clinical implications for individuals who show elevated neural reactivity in response to appetitive cues (44). Resonance breathing is the active mechanism of heart rate variability biofeedback, an empirically supported behavioral intervention for disorders with core features of affective and emotional dysregulation (13, 14, 17, 26) including alcohol use disorders (44, 87, 88). Emerging evidence suggests that heart rate variability biofeedback and paced breathing interventions reduce self-reported craving for alcohol and other appetitive stimuli, such as food (27, 89). While standard heart rate variability biofeedback delivery protocols include five to ten 1-h sessions and home practice (90, 91), resonance breathing itself produces immediate physiological effects (see **Figure 2**). This proof-of-concept study was novel in examining whether resonance breathing also elicits immediate neural effects. The findings provide an initial step in validating resonance breathing as an in-the-moment behavioral tool that potentially could be used ad lib in the natural environment to alter neural activation, both before and during contexts of heightened risk for substance use. Accessible smart phone applications are available to self-administer resonance breathing and HRV biofeedback, suggesting promise for a scalable intervention tool if future research is successful in demonstrating that such effects are linked to reduced alcohol and drug use behaviors.

## Limitations and Directions for Future Research

As a proof-of-concept study, these findings should be interpreted with caution and used for the generation of future hypotheses regarding the effects of resonance breathing on neural activation to alcohol-related visual stimuli, behavioral correlates of alcohol use such as in-the-moment craving, and actual use behaviors. Importantly, the changes observed in neural activation to the cues following the resonance breathing intervention should not be considered specific to alcohol-cue reactivity, as this study did not include a comparison condition of matched, non-alcohol cues presented before and after the intervention. This study also was limited in not being sufficiently powered to examine sensitively the relation of individual differences in alcohol use behaviors to changes in neural activation following resonance breathing. We note that the cue presentation paradigm of the present study was designed in line with the goal of better understanding afferent cardiovascular input to neural reactivity and thus was not typical of those used in many other fMRI studies of cue reactivity. A recent meta-analysis found that cue paradigm and type did not significantly influence neural response patterns associated with cue reactivity however (28), suggesting the fMRI assessment of neural activation is robust to multiple cue presentation approaches. Future studies should include larger samples to link current and chronic substance use behaviors to cue reactivity, and a design that counterbalances and compares neural response to alcohol-related and non-alcoholic beverage cues. Specificity may be addressed also by comparisons to non-alcohol or drug-related, yet positive or negative affectively valenced, visual cue sets.

## Conclusion

In summary, this study presents preliminary evidence that individuals ranging in drinking behaviors from low-risk to alcohol-dependent may be less visually engaged by alcohol cues and initiate greater top-down cognitive processing of cues following resonance breathing. This is consistent with the broader literature on resonance breathing that shows it normalizes neurocardiac feedback and improves autonomic nervous system regulation (25). Moreover, it points to a potential neural foundation for the effects of resonance breathing and adds to the scientific premise for the use of heart rate variability biofeedback as an intervention for brain-based mental and physical health conditions. More highly powered studies are needed to replicate and extend these neural activation results. Critical next steps are to understand how the cardiovascular and neural changes elicited by resonance breathing are linked to changes in the subjective experience of craving and alcohol use behaviors.

## AUTHOR CONTRIBUTIONS

MB and JB designed the study. MB and LL wrote the first draft of the article. All authors contributed to writing sections of the manuscript. LL and SU collected all data. LL and SU post-processed the imaging data. LL, SU, and SG performed the data analyses. All authors read and approved the final manuscript.

## ACKNOWLEDGMENTS

We acknowledge Dr. Evgeny Vaschillo, an originator of heart rate variability biofeedback and the study of cardiovascular resonance. We also thank the staff and students of the Cardiac Neuroscience Laboratory for their assistance in screening and testing participants.

## REFERENCES


1. Shiffman S, Stone AA, Hufford MR. Ecological momentary assessment. *AnnRev Clin Psychol* (2008) 4:1–32. doi: 10.1146/annurev.clinpsy.3.022806.091415
2. Tracey KJ. Reflex control of immunity. *Nat Rev Immunol* (2009) 9:418–28. doi: 10.1038/nri2566
3. Gianaros PJ, Jennings JR. Host in the machine: a neurobiological perspective on psychological stress and cardiovascular disease. *Am Psychol* (2018) 73:1031–44. doi: 10.1037/amp0000232
4. Benarroch EE. The central autonomic network. In: Low PA, editor. *Clinical Autonomic Disorders*. 2nd ed Lippincott-Raven (1997). p. 17–23.
5. Goldstein DS. *The autonomic nervous system in health and disease*. New York: Marcel Dekker, Inc. (2001).
6. Beissner F, Meissner K, Bar KJ, Napadow V. The autonomic brain: an activation likelihood estimation meta-analysis for central processing of autonomic function. *J Neurosci* (2013) 33:10503–11. doi: 10.1523/JNEUROSCI.1103-13.2013
7. Lacey BC, Lacey JI. Some autonomic-central nervous system interrelationships. In: Blank P, editor. *Physiological Correlations of Emotion*. Academic Press (1970). p. 205–27. doi: 10.1016/B978-0-12-102850-3.50016-5
8. Iversen S, Iversen L, Saper CB. The autonomic nervous system and the hypothalamus. In: Kandel ER, Schwartz CE, Jessell TM, editors. *Principle of Neural Science*. McGraw-Hill (2000). p. 960–81.
9. Critchley HD. Neural mechanisms of autonomic, affective, and cognitive integration. *J Compar Neurol* (2005) 493:154–66. doi: 10.1002/cne.20749
10. Bates ME, Buckman JF. Emotional dysregulation in the moment: why some college students may not mature out of hazardous alcohol and drug use. In: White HR, Rabiner DL, editors. *College drinking and drug use*. The Guilford Press (2011). p. 83–101.
11. Bates ME, Buckman JF. Integrating body and brain systems in addiction neuroscience. In: Miller P, editor. *Biological Research on Addiction: Comprehensive Addictive Behaviors and Disorders*. Elsevier (2013). doi: 10.1016/B978-0-12-398335-0.00020-0
12. Buckman JF, Vaschillo EG, Fonoberova M, Mezic I, Bates ME. The translational value of psychophysiology methods and mechanisms: multilevel, dynamic, personalized. *J Stud Alcohol Drugs* (2018) 79:229–38. doi: 10.15288/jsad.2018.79.229
13. Hassett AL, Radvanski DC, Vaschillo E, Vaschillo B, Sigal LH, Karavidas MK, et al. A pilot study of the efficacy of heart rate variability (HRV) biofeedback in patients with fibromyalgia. *Appl Psychophysiol Biofeedback* (2007) 32:1–10. doi: 10.1007/s10484-006-9028-0
14. Karavidas MK, Lehrer PM, Vaschillo E, Vaschillo B, Marin H, Buyske S, et al. Preliminary results of an open label study of heart rate variability biofeedback for the treatment of major depression. *Appl Psychophysiol Biofeedback* (2007) 32:19–30. doi: 10.1007/s10484-006-9029-z
15. Windhorst U. Muscle proprioceptive feedback and spinal networks. *Brain Res Bull* (2007) 73:155–202. doi: 10.1016/j.brainresbull.2007.03.010
16. Reiner R. Integrating a portable biofeedback device into clinical practice for patients with anxiety disorders: results of a pilot study. *Appl Psychophysiol Biofeedback* (2008) 33:55–61. doi: 10.1007/s10484-007-9046-6
17. Siepmann M, Aykac V, Unterdorfer J, Petrowski K, Mueck-Weymann M. A pilot study on the effects of heart rate variability biofeedback in patients with depression and in healthy subjects. *Appl Psychophysiol Biofeedback* (2008) 33:195–201. doi: 10.1007/s10484-008-9064-z
18. Zucker TL, Samuelson KW, Muench F, Greenberg MA, Gevirtz RN. The effects of respiratory sinus arrhythmia biofeedback on heart rate variability and posttraumatic stress disorder symptoms: a pilot study. *Appl Psychophysiol Biofeedback* (2009) 34:135–43. doi: 10.1007/s10484-009-9085-2
19. Sutarto AP, Wahab MN, Zin NM. Resonant breathing biofeedback training for stress reduction among manufacturing operators. *Int J Occup Saf Ergon* (2012) 18:549–61. doi: 10.1080/10803548.2012.11076959
20. Eddie D, Kim C, Bates ME, Lehrer P, Deneke E. A pilot study of brief heart rate variability biofeedback to reduce craving in young adult men receiving inpatient treatment for substance use disorders. *Appl Psychophysiol Biofeedback* (2014) 39:181–92. doi: 10.1007/s10484-014-9251-z
21. Lehrer PM, Vaschillo E, Vaschillo B, Lu SE, Eckberg DL, Edelberg R, et al. Heart rate variability biofeedback increases baroreflex gain and peak expiratory flow. *Psychosomatic Med* (2003) 65:796–805. doi: 10.1097/01.PSY.0000089200.81962.19
22. Vaschillo E, Vaschillo B, Lehrer P. Heartbeat synchronizes with respiratory rhythm only under specific circumstances. *Chest* (2004) 126:1385–6. doi: 10.1016/S0012-3692(15)31329-5
23. Lehrer P, Vaschillo E, Trost Z, France CR. Effects of rhythmical muscle tension at 0.1Hz on cardiovascular resonance and the baroreflex. *Biol Psychol* (2009) 81:24–30. doi: 10.1016/j.biopsycho.2009.01.003
24. Vaschillo EG, Vaschillo B, Pandina RJ, Bates ME. Resonances in the cardiovascular system caused by rhythmical muscle tension. *Psychophysiology* (2010) 48:927–36. doi: 10.1111/j.1469-8986.2010.01156.x
25. Vaschillo EG, Vaschillo B, Buckman JF, Pandina RJ, Bates ME. The investigation and clinical significance of resonance in the heart rate and vascular tone baroreflexes. In: Fred A, Filipe J, Gamboa H, editors. *Biomedical Engineering Systems and Technologies: Communications in Computer and Information Science* Springer (2011). p. 224–37. doi: 10.1007/978-3-642-18472-7_18
26. Goessl VC, Curtiss JE, Hofmann SG. The effect of heart rate variability biofeedback training on stress and anxiety: a meta-analysis. *Psychol Med* (2017) 47:2578–86. doi: 10.1017/S0033291717001003

27. Alayan N, Eller L, Bates ME, Carmody DP. Current evidence on heart rate variability biofeedback as a complementary anticraving intervention. *J Altern Complement Med* (2018) 24:1039–50. doi: 10.1089/acm.2018.0019
28. Noori HR, Cosa Linan A, Spanagel R. Largely overlapping neuronal substrates of reactivity to drug, gambling, food and sexual cues: a comprehensive meta-analysis. *Eur Neuropsychopharmacol* (2016) 26:1419–30. doi: 10.1016/j.euroneuro.2016.06.013
29. Kelley AE, Berridge KC. The neuroscience of natural rewards: relevance to addictive drugs. *J Neurosci* (2002) 22:3306–11. doi: 10.1523/JNEUROSCI.22-09-03306.2002
30. Naqvi NH, Bechara A. The hidden island of addiction: the insula. *Trends Neurosci* (2009) 32:56–67. doi: 10.1016/j.tins.2008.09.009
31. Koob GF, Volkow ND. Neurocircuitry of addiction. *Neuropsychopharmacology* (2010) 35:217–38. doi: 10.1038/npp.2009.110
32. Sinha R, Fuse T, Aubin LR, O'malley SS. Psychological stress, drug-related cues and cocaine craving. *Psychopharmacology (Berl)* (2000) 152:140–8. doi: 10.1007/s002130000499
33. Thayer JF, Lane RD. A model of neurovisceral integration in emotion regulation and dysregulation. *J Affect Disord* (2000) 61:201–16. doi: 10.1016/S0165-0327(00)00338-4
34. Vaschillo EG, Bates ME, Vaschillo B, Lehrer P, Udo T, Mun EY, et al. Heart rate variability response to alcohol, placebo, and emotional picture cue challenges: effects of 0.1-Hz stimulation. *Psychophysiology* (2008) 45:847–58. doi: 10.1111/j.1469-8986.2008.00673.x
35. Garland EL, Carter K, Ropes K, Howard MO. Thought suppression, impaired regulation of urges, and Addiction-Stroop predict affect-modulated cue-reactivity among alcohol dependent adults. *Biol Psychol* (2012a) 89:87–93. doi: 10.1016/j.biopsycho.2011.09.010
36. Garland EL, Franken IH, Sheetz JJ, Howard MO. Alcohol attentional bias is associated with autonomic indices of stress-primed alcohol cue-reactivity in alcohol-dependent patients. *Exp Clin Psychopharmacol* (2012b) 20:225–35. doi: 10.1037/a0027199
37. Porges SW, Doussard-Roosevelt JA, Maita AK. Vagal tone and the physiological regulation of emotion. *Monogr Soc Res Child Dev* (1994) 59(167–186):250–83. doi: 10.2307/1166144
38. Hugdahl K. Cognitive influences on human autonomic nervous system function. *Curr Opin Neurobiol* (1996) 6:252–8. doi: 10.1016/S0959-4388(96)80080-8
39. Kuhn S, Gallinat J. Common biology of craving across legal and illegal drugs—a quantitative meta-analysis of cue-reactivity brain response. *Eur J Neurosci* (2011) 33:1318–26. doi: 10.1111/j.1460-9568.2010.07590.x
40. Jasinska AJ, Stein EA, Kaiser J, Naumer MJ, Yalachkov Y. Factors modulating neural reactivity to drug cues in addiction: a survey of human neuroimaging studies. *Neurosci Biobehav Rev* (2014) 38:1–16. doi: 10.1016/j.neubiorev.2013.10.013
41. Schacht JP, Anton RF, Myrick H. Functional neuroimaging studies of alcohol cue reactivity: a quantitative meta-analysis and systematic review. *Addict Biol* (2013) 18:121–33. doi: 10.1111/j.1369-1600.2012.00464.x
42. Hanlon CA, Dowdle LT, Gibson NB, Li X, Hamilton S, Canterberry M, et al. Cortical substrates of cue-reactivity in multiple substance dependent populations: transdiagnostic relevance of the medial prefrontal cortex. *Transl Psychiatry* (2018) 8:186. doi: 10.1038/s41398-018-0220-9
43. Myrick H, Anton RF, Li X, Henderson S, Drobes D, Voronin K, et al. Differential brain activity in alcoholics and social drinkers to alcohol cues: relationship to craving. *Neuropsychopharmacology* (2004) 29:393–402. doi: 10.1038/sj.npp.1300295
44. Witteman J, Post H, Tarvainen M, De Bruijn A, Perna Ede S, Ramaekers JG, et al. Cue reactivity and its relation to craving and relapse in alcohol dependence: a combined laboratory and field study. *Psychopharmacology (Berl)* (2015) 232:3685–96. doi: 10.1007/s00213-015-4027-6
45. Dager AD, Anderson BM, Stevens MC, Pulido C, Rosen R, Jiantonio-Kelly RE, et al. Influence of alcohol use and family history of alcoholism on neural response to alcohol cues in college drinkers. *Alcohol Clin Exp Res* (2013) 37 Suppl 1:E161–171. doi: 10.1111/j.1530-0277.2012.01879.x
46. Mun EY, Von Eye A, Bates ME, Vaschillo EG. Finding groups using model-based cluster analysis: heterogeneous emotional self-regulatory processes and heavy alcohol use risk. *Dev Psychol* (2008) 44:481–95. doi: 10.1037/0012-1649.44.2.481
47. Tiffany ST. The role of cognitive factors in reactivity to drug cues. In: Drummond DC, Tiffany ST, editors. *Addictive Behaviour: Cue Exposure Theory and Practice*. Wiley (1995).
48. Robinson TE, Berridge KC. Review. The incentive sensitization theory of addiction: some current issues. *Philos Trans R Soc London— B: Biol Sci* (2008) 363:3137–46. doi: 10.1098/rstb.2008.0093
49. Marlatt GA. Section I. theoretical perspectives on relapse: taxonomy of high-risk situations for alcohol relapse: evolution and development of a cognitive-behavioral model. *Addiction* (1996) 91:S37–49. doi: 10.1111/j.1360-0443.1996.tb02326.x
50. Grusser SM, Wrase J, Klein S, Hermann D, Smolka MN, Ruf M, etal. Cue-induced activation of the striatum and medial prefrontal cortex is associated with subsequent relapse in abstinent alcoholics. *Psychopharmacology* (2004) 175:296–302. doi: 10.1007/s00213-004-1828-4
51. American Psychiatric Association. *Diagnostic and statistical manual of mental disorders*. Washington, DC: American Psychiatric Association (2000).
52. Crawford JR, Henry JD. The Positive and Negative Affect Schedule (PANAS): construct validity, measurement properties and normative data in a large non-clinical sample. *Br J Clin Psychol* (2004) 43:245–65. doi: 10.1348/0144665031752934
53. Cohen S, Karmarck T, Mermelstein R. A global measure of perceived stress. *J Health Soc Behav* (1983) 24:385–96. doi: 10.2307/2136404
54. Tapert SF, Cheung EH, Brown GG, Frank LR, Paulus MP, Schweinsburg AD, et al. Neural response to alcohol stimuli in adolescents with alcohol use disorder. *Arch Gen Psychiatry* (2003) 60:727–35. doi: 10.1001/archpsyc.60.7.727
55. Ray S, Hanson C, Hanson SJ, Bates ME. fMRI BOLD response in high-risk college students (Part 1): during exposure to alcohol, marijuana, polydrug and emotional picture cues. *Alcohol Alcohol* (2010) 45:437–43. doi: 10.1093/alcalc/agq042
56. Jennings JR, Kamarck T, Stewart C, Eddy M, Johnson P. Alternate cardiovascular baseline assessment techniques: vanilla or resting baseline. *Psychophysiology* (1992) 29, 742-50. doi: 10.1111/j.1469-8986.1992.tb02052.x
57. Smith SM. Fast robust automated brain extraction. *Hum Brain Mapp* (2002) 17:143–55. doi: 10.1002/hbm.10062
58. Jenkinson M, Bannister P, Brady M, Smith SA. Improved optimization for the robust and accurate linear registration and motion correction of brain images. *Neuroimage* (2002) 17:825–41. doi: 10.1006/nimg.2002.1132
59. Zhang Y, Brady MS, Smith S. Segmentation of brain MR images through a hidden Markov random field model and the expectation-maximization algorithm. *IEEE Transact Med Imaging* (2001) 20:45–57:S. doi: 10.1109/42.906424
60. Jenkinson M, Smith S. A global optimisation method for robust affine registration of brain images. *Med Image Anal* (2001) 5:143–56. doi: 10.1016/S1361-8415(01)00036-6
61. Winkler AM, Ridgway GR, Webster MA, Smith SM, Nichols TE. Permutation inference for the general linear model. *Neuroimage* (2014) 92:381–97. doi: 10.1016/j.neuroimage.2014.01.060
62. Smith SM, Nichols TE. Threshold-free cluster enhancement: addressing problems of smoothing, threshold dependence and localisation in cluster inference. *Neuroimage* (2009) 44:83–98. doi: 10.1016/j.neuroimage.2008.03.061
63. Critchley HD, Garfinkel SN. Interactions between visceral afferent signaling and stimulus processing. *Front Neurosci* (2015) 9:286. doi: 10.3389/fnins.2015.00286
64. Adolphs R. Neural systems for recognizing emotion. *Curr Opin Neurobiol* (2002) 12:169–77. doi: 10.1016/S0959-4388(02)00301-X
65. Schupp HT, Junghoefer M, Weike AI, Hamm AO. Emotional facilitation of sensory processing in the visual cortex. *Psychol Sci* (2003) 14:7–13. doi: 10.1111/1467-9280.01411
66. Vuilleumier P, Pourtois G. Distributed and interactive brain mechanisms during emotion face perception: evidence from functional neuroimaging. *Neuropsychologia* (2007) 45:174–94. doi: 10.1016/j.neuropsychologia.2006.06.003
67. Chase HW, Eickhoff SB, Laird AR, Hogarth L. The neural basis of drug stimulus processing and craving: an activation likelihood estimation meta-analysis. *Biol Psychiatry* (2011) 70:785–93. doi: 10.1016/j.biopsych.2011.05.025
68. Engelmann JM, Versace F, Robinson JD, Minnix JA, Lam CY, Cui Y, et al. Neural substrates of smoking cue reactivity: a meta-analysis of fMRI studies. *Neuroimage* (2012) 60:252–62. doi: 10.1016/j.neuroimage.2011.12.024

69. Hanlon CA, Dowdle LT, Naselaris T, Canterberry M, Cortese BM. Visual cortex activation to drug cues: a meta-analysis of functional neuroimaging papers in addiction and substance abuse literature. *Drug Alcohol Depend* (2014) 143:206–12. doi: 10.1016/j.drugalcdep.2014.07.028
70. Potenza MN, Steinberg MA, Skudlarski P, Fulbright RK, Lacadie CM, Wilber MK, et al. Gambling urges in pathological gambling: a functional magnetic resonance imaging study. *Arch Gen Psychiatry* (2003) 60:828–36. doi: 10.1001/archpsyc.60.8.828
71. Crockford DN, Goodyear B, Edwards J, Quickfall J, El-Guebaly N. Cue-induced brain activity in pathological gamblers. *Biol Psychiatry* (2005) 58:787–95. doi: 10.1016/j.biopsych.2005.04.037
72. Goudriaan AE, De Ruiter MB, Van Den Brink W, Oosterlaan J, Veltman DJ. Brain activation patterns associated with cue reactivity and craving in abstinent problem gamblers, heavy smokers and healthy controls: an fMRI study. *Addict Biol* (2010) 15:491–503. doi: 10.1111/j.1369-1600.2010.00242.x
73. Grill-Spector K, Kourtzi Z, Kanwisher N. The lateral occipital complex and its role in object recognition. *Vision Res* (2001) 41:1409–22. doi: 10.1016/S0042-6989(01)00073-6
74. Kanwisher N, Wojciulik E. Visual attention: insights from brain imaging. *Nat Rev Neurosci* (2000) 1:91–100. doi: 10.1038/35039043
75. Venkatraman A, Edlow BL, Immordino-Yang MH. The Brainstem in Emotion: A Review. *Front Neuroanat* (2017) 11:15. doi: 10.3389/fnana.2017.00015
76. Bush G, Luu P, Posner MI. Cognitive and emotional influences in anterior cingulate cortex. *Trends Cogn Sci* (2000) 4:215–22. doi: 10.1016/S1364-6613(00)01483-2
77. Botvinick MM, Cohen JD, Carter CS. Conflict monitoring and anterior cingulate cortex: an update. *Trends Cogn Sci* (2004) 8:539–46. doi: 10.1016/j.tics.2004.10.003
78. Ridderinkhof KR, Ullsperger M, Crone EA, Nieuwenhuis S. The role of the medial frontal cortex in cognitive control. *Science* (2004) 306:443–7. doi: 10.1126/science.1100301
79. Euston DR, Gruber AJ, Mcnaughton BL. The role of medial prefrontal cortex in memory and decision making. *Neuron* (2012) 76:1057–70. doi: 10.1016/j.neuron.2012.12.002
80. Courtney KE, Schacht JP, Hutchison K, Roche DJ, Ray LA. Neural substrates of cue reactivity: association with treatment outcomes and relapse. *Addict Biol* (2016) 21:3–22. doi: 10.1111/adb.12314
81. Buckner RL, Andrews-Hanna JR, Schacter DL. The brain's default network: anatomy, function, and relevance to disease. *Ann N Y Acad Sci* (2008) 1124:1–38. doi: 10.1196/annals.1440.011
82. Fransson P, Marrelec G. The precuneus/posterior cingulate cortex plays a pivotal role in the default mode network: evidence from a partial correlation network analysis. *Neuroimage* (2008) 42:1178–84. doi: 10.1016/j.neuroimage.2008.05.059
83. Machielsen WC, Rombouts SA, Barkhof F, Scheltens P, Witter MP. FMRI of visual encoding: reproducibility of activation. *Hum Brain Mapp* (2000) 9:156–64. doi: 10.1002/(SICI)1097-0193(200003)9:3<156::AID-HBM4>3.0.CO;2-Q
84. Fox KC, Spreng RN, Ellamil M, Andrews-Hanna JR, Christoff K. The wandering brain: meta-analysis of functional neuroimaging studies of mind-wandering and related spontaneous thought processes. *Neuroimage* (2015) 111:611–21. doi: 10.1016/j.neuroimage.2015.02.039
85. Gusnard DA, Raichle ME, Raichle ME. Searching for a baseline: functional imaging and the resting human brain. *Nat Rev Neurosci* (2001) 2:685–94. doi: 10.1038/35094500
86. Kang M, Ragan BG, Park JH. Issues in outcomes research: an overview of randomization techniques for clinical trials. *J Athl Train* (2008) 43:215–21. doi: 10.4085/1062-6050-43.2.215
87. Penzlin AI, Siepmann T, Illigens BM, Weidner K, Siepmann M. Heart rate variability biofeedback in patients with alcohol dependence: a randomized controlled study. *Neuropsychiatr Dis Treat* (2015) 11:2619–27. doi: 10.2147/NDT.S84798
88. Penzlin AI, Barlinn K, Illigens BM, Weidner K, Siepmann M, Siepmann T. Effect of short-term heart rate variability biofeedback on long-term abstinence in alcohol dependent patients—a one-year follow-up. *BMC Psychiatry* (2017) 17:325. doi: 10.1186/s12888-017-1480-2
89. Eddie D, Conway FN, Alayan N, Buckman J, Bates ME. Assessing heart rate variability biofeedback as an adjunct to college recovery housing programs. *J Subst Abuse Treat* (2018) 92:70–6. doi: 10.1016/j.jsat.2018.06.014
90. Lehrer PM, Vaschillo E, Vaschillo B. Resonant frequency biofeedback training to increase cardiac variability: rationale and manual for training. *Appl Psychophysiol Biofeedback* (2000) 25:177–91. doi: 10.1023/A:1009554825745
91. Lehrer P, Vaschillo B, Zucker T, Graves J, Katsamanis M, Aviles M, et al. Protocol for Heart Rate Variability Biofeedback Training. *Biofeedback* (2013) 41:98–109 doi: 10.5298/1081-5937-41.3.08.

10

# Impact of Substance use Disorder Pharmacotherapy on Executive Function

*Kevin Butler*[1] *and Bernard Le Foll*[1,2,3,4,5,6,7*]

[1] *Translational Addiction Research Laboratory, Centre for Addiction and Mental Health, University of Toronto, Toronto, ON, Canada,* [2] *Alcohol Research and Treatment Clinic, Acute Care Program, Centre for Addiction and Mental Health, Toronto, ON, Canada,* [3] *Campbell Family Mental Health Research Institute, Centre for Addiction and Mental Health, Toronto, ON, Canada,* [4] *Department of Family and Community Medicine, University of Toronto, Toronto, ON, Canada,* [5] *Department of Pharmacology and Toxicology, University of Toronto, Toronto, ON, Canada,* [6] *Division of Brain and Therapeutics, Department of Psychiatry, University of Toronto, Toronto, ON, Canada,* [7] *Institute of Medical Sciences, University of Toronto, Toronto, ON, Canada*

***Correspondence:***
*Bernard Le Foll*
*bernard.lefoll@camh.ca*

Substance use disorders are chronic, relapsing, and harmful conditions characterized by executive dysfunction. While there are currently no approved pharmacotherapy options for stimulant and cannabis use disorders, there are several evidence-based options available to help reduce symptoms during detoxification and aid long-term cessation for those with tobacco, alcohol and opioid use disorders. While these medication options have shown clinical efficacy, less is known regarding their potential to enhance executive function. This narrative review aims to provide a brief overview of research that has investigated whether commonly used pharmacotherapies for these substance use disorders (nicotine, bupropion, varenicline, disulfiram, acamprosate, nalmefene, naltrexone, methadone, buprenorphine, and lofexidine) effect three core executive function components (working memory, inhibitory control and cognitive flexibility). While pharmacotherapy-induced enhancement of executive function may improve cessation outcomes in dependent populations, there are limited and inconsistent findings regarding the effects of these medications on executive function. We discuss possible reasons for the mixed findings and suggest some future avenues of work that may enhance the understanding of addiction pharmacotherapy and cognitive training interventions and lead to improved patient outcomes.

**Keywords: addiction, cognitive enhancement, cognitive flexibility, executive function, inhibitory control, pharmacotherapy, substance use disorder, working memory**

## INTRODUCTION

Substance use disorders are chronic, relapsing conditions (1) with huge costs to the individual and to society. For example, using data from 2015, Peacock et al. (2) estimate global prevalence of past 30 day heavy alcohol use, daily smoking and past year opioid use at 18.4, 15.2, and 0.37%, respectively and they estimate disease burden with the number of disability-adjusted life years (the number of years lost due to ill-health, disability, or early death) as 170.9 million, 85.0 million and 27.8 million for tobacco smoking, alcohol, and illicit drug use, respectively. Indeed, alcohol, heroin, and tobacco have previously been rated amongst the most harmful misused drugs when considering harms to both the individual and to others (3).

There are several psychological/behavioral treatments available for substance use disorders [for a brief overview see McGovern and carroll (4)]. While there are no approved pharmacotherapies for stimulant and cannabis use disorders, evidence-based pharmacological agents are available for tobacco, alcohol and opioid use disorders (TUD, AUD, and OUD, respectively). Medications currently approved for these disorders include nicotine replacement therapy, bupropion, varenicline (for TUD), disulfiram, acamprosate, naltrexone, nalmefene (for AUD), methadone, buprenorphine, naltrexone, and lofexidine (for OUD). While previous research has found these drugs to be efficacious, relapse in drug dependence is 40–60% (5) suggesting efficacy is limited and that there is room for improvement in the management of addictions.

Cognitive processes may be important targets for the treatment of substance use disorders (6, 7). In particular, executive dysfunction is considered a hallmark of addiction (8, 9) and may represent a good transdiagnostic target across addictive disorders. Impairments in executive function may contribute to the initiation and maintenance of problematic drug use. For instance, executive function at an early age predicts subsequent substance use (10) and performance comparisons across drug users, non-addicted family members and healthy controls suggest that deficits in executive function may be a cognitive endophenotype associated with drug dependence vulnerability (11, 12). Executive function deficits are also related to relapse, worse clinical outcomes and poor treatment adherence (13–19) with exacerbation of executive function impairments observed during early abstinence which may contribute to relapse (20–22).

While the clinical efficacy of approved pharmacotherapy for TUD, AUD, and OUD is recognized, there has been far less research conducted on the cognitive effects of these medications (23) despite potential cognitive enhancement effects contributing to clinical efficacy. Therefore, the goal of this review is to provide a brief and selective, narrative summary of the evidence examining the impact of nicotine, bupropion, varenicline, disulfiram, acamprosate, nalmefene, naltrexone, methadone, buprenorphine, and lofexidine on executive function. We do not include medications used off-label to treat substance use disorders due to the wide-range of off-label prescribing practices, limited, or inconsistent evidence for clinical efficacy and because we cannot be certain which of these medications will continue to look effective as the evidence base for them increases. This review complements the recent systematic review that investigated general cognitive effects of pharmacotherapy for substance use disorders (23). While this earlier review provides a good overview of the cognitive impact of substance use disorder medication, its discussion of the impact on executive function could be considered limited by the general approach to cognition that has been taken. The current review fractionates executive function and focuses on working memory, inhibitory control, and cognitive flexibility as there is general agreement that these are the three core executive function components and that other higher-order executive functions such as decision-making, planning, problem-solving, and reasoning may require these basic components (24, 25). Additionally, the current review also takes a translational approach by including relevant findings from research with non-human animals where human research is scarce or it adds to an understanding of drug effects.

## PHARMACOTHERAPIES FOR TOBACCO USE DISORDER

### Nicotine

The nicotinic acetylcholine receptor agonist nicotine is used in those with TUD as a replacement therapy where it can be delivered in many forms including chewing gum and adhesive skin patches. When used as an aid to quit smoking or chewing tobacco, nicotine replacement therapy helps to manage withdrawal symptoms associated with cessation and can increase the rate of quitting by up to 50–70% (26). Both $\alpha_4\beta_2$ and $\alpha_7$ nicotinic receptor subtypes have been implicated in cognitive enhancement (27). Indeed, a considerable amount of evidence exists regarding the cognitive enhancing effects of nicotine. For instance, nicotine can improve some abstinence associated cognitive impairments (28). Additionally, a 2010 meta-analysis suggests that fine motor, alerting attention-accuracy and response time, orienting attention reaction time, short-term episodic memory accuracy, and working memory reaction time are particularly sensitive to enhancement following administration of nicotine (29). Furthermore, because the studies included in this meta-analysis used non-smokers or non-/minimally deprived smokers the cognitive enhancement is unlikely to be driven by relief from withdrawal but, instead, represents true cognitive enhancement.

However, reported effects of nicotine on working memory are far from consistent. Animal work suggests that working memory (radial-arm maze) performance is improved by nicotine administration (30) and that methamphetamine or ketamine-induced impairments in working memory (radial-arm maze, odor span task) can be improved by nicotine (31, 32). On the other hand, no effect on working memory (digit recall, serial addition/subtraction, n-back task, digit span, spatial span, letter-number sequencing, odor span task) has been seen in human studies that have administered 2 and 4 mg nicotine gum relative to placebo in healthy non-smoking participants (33–35). Another study found that 15 mg nicotine patches improved working memory (n-back task reaction time) in deprived smokers relative to placebo while they had no benefit in healthy non-smokers but instead impaired performance with significantly fewer hits, more misses and false alarms and a trend toward longer reaction times (36). Taken together this suggests that nicotine may improve working memory when there is impaired baseline performance present but has no effect or impairs performance when baseline performance is higher (37).

Nicotine administration has also been found to improve inhibitory control (antisaccade task, errors of commission on a continuous performance task) deficits that are induced by overnight smoking abstinence (38). However, 7 mg nicotine patches do not improve inhibitory control (stop-signal task, go/nogo task, antisaccade task) in healthy non-smokers (39, 40). In contrast to the findings of these studies, several nicotine administration studies in animals have shown that nicotine can induce disinhibition with increased impulsive responding evident across a range of behavioral tasks (41–47). Similarly, acute cigarette smoking may bias responding to more impulsive action and impulsive choices (48, 49). As with the effect of nicotine on working memory, the mixed findings with nicotine apparently able to improve, impair or have no effect on inhibitory control may be due to baseline differences in performance and several previous studies support this idea. For example, nicotine enhances inhibitory control (fewer errors of commission on a continuous performance task) in non-smokers that have low levels of attention but not in those with high levels of attention (50) while in another study, nicotine enhanced inhibitory control (fewer errors of commission on a continuous performance task) in those with a diagnosis of schizophrenia but not in healthy controls (51). Finally, the effect of chronic nicotine exposure on impulsivity in rats may be influenced by baseline levels of impulsivity with nicotine inducing greater impulsive choice in those with lower trait impulsivity (52, 53).

Few studies have examined the effects of nicotine on cognitive flexibility and those which have reveal mixed findings, much as studies assessing working memory and inhibitory control have. Acute cigarette smoking has been shown to impair cognitive flexibility (more intra-dimensional set-shifting errors on an intra-extra dimensional set-shifting task) in high but not low dependent smokers (54) and (greater difficulty integrating reinforcement history on a reversal learning task) relative to never and former smokers (55). Cognitive flexibility has also been shown to be impaired (poorer learning of strategies to complete the task in the Wisconsin Card Sorting test) by 7 mg nicotine patch administration relative to placebo in non-smokers with high but not low levels of attention (50). Nicotine administration at high (18 mg/Kg/day × 4 weeks) but not low dose (6.3 mg/Kg/day × 4 weeks) also impaired cognitive flexibility (increased perseverative responding to previously non-reinforced stimuli in a reversal learning task) in mice (56). Conversely, improvements in cognitive flexibility (attentional set-shifting task) and reversal of nicotine withdrawal-induced impairment in cognitive flexibility (reversal learning task) have both been reported in rats (57, 58). While in another human study, cognitive flexibility (attentional switching on the flexibility of attention test) was not changed by nicotine (59). As with working memory and inhibitory control, mixed findings like these suggest that baseline performance levels may be influential in determining cognitive effects of nicotine. As nicotine can induce dopamine release (60), as smoking does in humans (61), a more biological explanation for the mixed findings reported throughout this section might be that performance and dopamine levels are related such that at optimal dopamine levels executive function performance is at its peak i.e., the inverted "U" curve theory (62, 63). Release of dopamine by nicotine could therefore improve or impair performance depending on initial dopamine levels.

## Bupropion

Used clinically for depression as well as a smoking cessation aid, bupropion is a norepinephrine-dopamine reuptake inhibitor and a nicotinic acetylcholine receptor antagonist. Bupropion reduces the severity of nicotine craving and withdrawal symptoms, its clinical effectiveness as a smoking cessation aid is comparable to nicotine replacement therapy and is independent of its antidepressant effect (64, 65). Symptoms that improve in depressed patients that respond to bupropion include those reflecting cognitive disturbance (66). Indeed, one study in patients with major depressive disorder has shown that while serotonin selective reuptake inhibitor-treated patients show cognitive impairments including worse cognitive flexibility relative to matched healthy controls, bupropion-treated patients had normalized cognitive performance with better cognitive flexibility but with no significant mean difference compared to controls (67). Further, another study in those with major depressive disorder found that 8 weeks of bupropion treatment lead to improvements on tasks requiring cognitive flexibility (Trail Making B), working memory and reasoning [A not B Task; (68)].

Few studies have investigated the effects of bupropion on executive function in smokers and the findings of existing studies have been equivocal. One study in 24 smokers with high interest in quitting reported that working memory (correct response times on an N-Back task) was improved by bupropion compared to placebo on the first day of a quit attempt (69). In contrast, another study in 58 smokers (36 male, 22 female) found that bupropion enhanced working memory (Digit Span task) in females but not males whereas it enhanced inhibitory control (inhibiting choice of immediate rewards over a larger, delayed reward) in males but not females during early abstinence (70). A final study in smokers investigated effects of both abstinence and bupropion on cognitive function in adults with schizophrenia. However, in this study 1 week of abstinence was not associated with deficits in working memory (Digit Span task) and controlling for abstinence status, bupropion wasn't associated with better working memory performance (71). Similar null findings have been observed in healthy participants where working memory (Digit Span task) was not improved by either a single dose (150mg) or 2 weeks repeated administration (150 mg x 6days followed by 300 mg x 8days) of bupropion (72). However, in an animal study there were positive effects of bupropion on inhibitory control. In this study, rats were perinatally exposed to polychlorinated biphenyls thought to decrease medial prefrontal cortical dopamine levels and cause subsequent inhibitory control deficits assessed with a differential reinforcement of low rates of responding (DRL) task. This study showed that bupropion improved inhibitory control performance on the DRL task (73).

## Varenicline

As a partial agonist at $\alpha_4\beta_2$ nicotinic acetylcholine receptors, varenicline has been found to reduce craving and the pleasurable effects of tobacco and is more effective for smoking cessation than both nicotine replacement therapy and bupropion (74). Varenicline can reverse withdrawal-associated working memory impairment (75). Patterson et al. (75) showed that in abstinent smokers varenicline, vs. placebo, improved reaction times on correct N-back trials with no significant effects on task accuracy. Interestingly, slower correct responses on the N-Back task predict more rapid resumption of smoking during a short period of abstinence in smokers receiving placebo but not varenicline (76). Beyond simply improving withdrawal-associated impairment, varenicline (0.5 mg/day × 3days followed by 1 mg/day × 4days) administered to non-smokers has been shown to also improve working memory performance (77) with a significant positive association found between plasma varenicline levels and visual-spatial working memory in another non-smoker study (78). There are mixed findings regarding working memory performance in studies with other populations for instance varenicline (1 mg/day × 3 days) attenuated withdrawal-associated working memory impairments in smokers with schizophrenia (79) but did not improve working memory in smokers with schizophrenia who are not treatment-seeking and could continue to smoke (80, 81). Mixed working memory findings have also been found with varenicline in human studies with populations that have other substance abuse problems. For example, varenicline has been shown to improve working memory in heavy drinkers; with larger improvements predicting less alcohol-primed *ad libitum* drinking (82), but not in non-treatment seeking methamphetamine dependent participants (83). While an animal study found that varenicline improves working memory in cocaine-experienced monkeys (84). These mixed findings for other substances of abuse and across different species make it difficult to draw firm conclusions regarding varenicline's cognitive impact. However, as described above evidence suggests that there is some cognitive benefit for certain types of abstinent smoker (75).

Studies regarding varenicline effects on inhibitory control are also mixed. For instance, animal studies indicate that varenicline increases premature responding (failure to inhibit a response during a wait period) on a 5-Choice Serial Reaction Time task (85) however, using a similar 3-Choice task, Ohmura et al. (86) demonstrate that this pro-impulsive effect is evident for nicotine-naïve but not nicotine-exposed or nicotine-abstinent animals. In human studies there was no significant effect of varenicline, compared to placebo, on inhibitory control assessed with a stop-signal task in treatment-seeking smokers (87). In contrast, impulsive responding was increased on a stop-signal task by cigarette smoking and by varenicline [albeit to a smaller degree than smoking; (48)]. However, Austin et al. (48) also found that varenicline attenuated smoking-induced impulsive responding. Varenicline has also been found to reduce antisaccadic error rate (an oculomotor measure of disinhibition) in those with schizophrenia/schizoaffective disorder regardless of smoking status (80).

Fewer studies have reported effects of varenicline on cognitive flexibility. Animal studies have provided mixed findings with Gould et al. (84) finding no effect of varenicline on reversal learning (at doses that give maximum improvement in working memory) in rhesus monkeys. However, varenicline reduced ketamine-induced impairments in reversal learning (accuracy and perseverative responding) and improved working memory (accuracy at long delays on a delay match to sample task) in rhesus and pigtail monkeys (88). In studies related more specifically to smoking, varenicline reversed nicotine withdrawal-induced deficits in the number of reversals on a probabilistic reversal learning task administered to rats (58). While in a human study comparing 24 abstinent smokers with 20 non-smokers, impairments on a reversal learning task (increased response shifting with decisions less sensitive to available evidence) found in abstinent smokers were attenuated by varenicline. In addition, decreased mesocorticolimbic activity associated with shifting in abstinent smokers was increased to the level of non-smokers by varenicline (89). It should be noted that as with nicotine, varenicline produces elevation of dopamine (90).

## PHARMACOTHERAPIES FOR ALCOHOL USE DISORDER

### Disulfiram

By inhibiting the enzyme aldehyde dehydrogenase, disulfiram administration leads to acetaldehyde accumulation when alcohol is consumed. This results in an unpleasant reaction consisting of tachycardia, flushing, nausea, and vomiting. This aversion therapy creates the expectancy of negative consequences that are thought to deter alcohol use. Disulfiram is an efficacious treatment in supervised and high compliance open label studies but not blinded studies suggesting that expectancy may be a requirement of clinical effectiveness [for a review and meta-analysis of efficacy see Skinner et al. (91)]. There is evidence that anti-addictive effects may be mediated by an additional mechanism of action. For example, in rats disulfiram reduces drug-induced reinstatement of cocaine seeking via dopamine β-hydroxylase inhibition (92). Similarly reductions in chocolate self-administration and reinstatement of chocolate seeking have also been observed in rats treated with disulfiram (93) and there are reports that it may have potential for treatment of pathological gambling (94, 95) and cocaine dependence (96).

Few studies have investigated disulfiram's cognitive effects (see Pujol et al. (23) for an overview). In terms of executive function, there were no effects of disulfiram on working memory assessed with the Digit Span Test (97). Similarly, Gilman et al. (98) found no group differences on an extensive test battery, including tasks assessing executive function, when comparing 11 alcoholic patients receiving disulfiram and 37 alcoholic patients not receiving the drug. In contrast, disulfiram administration has been shown to improve inhibitory control (by inhibiting preference for immediate gain at the expense of reduced net gain) in rats that were making suboptimal choices but not those whose choices were already optimal (94).

### Acamprosate

Although the precise mechanism of action is not fully understood, acamprosate is thought to correct imbalance in inhibitory and excitatory neurotransmission induced by chronic alcohol exposure (99). Acamprosate has been found to be a safe and efficacious anti-craving and anti-relapse agent (100). There have been limited studies examining acamprosate effects on executive function. The drugs proposed mechanism of action at NMDA receptors suggests acamprosate would have negative effects on learning and memory, indeed previous cognitive work in healthy participants indicates an acamprosate-induced impairment in delayed free recall. However, working memory was unaffected by acamprosate in the same participants (101). Similarly, there was no significant effect of acamprosate on working memory performance of rats in a three-panel runway task. Although, performance (both errors and latency) was better in acamprosate and scopolamine-treated rats compared to when they were administered the muscarinic acetylcholine receptor antagonist alone (102). There have been mixed findings with studies investigating cognitive flexibility. While Ralevski et al. (103) found no significant effects of acamprosate in 23 alcohol-dependent schizophrenic patients on the Wisconsin Card Sorting Test, animal studies suggest that acamprosate reverses chronic alcohol-induced impairments in attentional set-shifting including reducing task perseveration (104). More recent evidence suggests that these cognitive effects may be related to acamprosate's calcium moiety as a sodium salt version of the drug failed to reverse chronic alcohol-induced deficits in cognition (105).

### Nalmefene

Approved in Europe but not in America, nalmefene is an antagonist at μ-opioid and δ-opioid receptors as well as a partial agonist at κ-opioid receptors thus reducing the positive, rewarding effects of acute alcohol consumption. Nalmefene has greater affinity for κ-opioid receptors than naltrexone does (106). Nalmefene also differs from naltrexone in having a longer half-life, greater bioavailability and no observed dose-dependent liver toxicity [see review by Niciu and Arias (107)]. To the best of our knowledge, there has not been any published research investigating the effects of nalmefene on executive function. However, the κ-opioid receptor agonists nalfurafine and U50,488 produce deficits in inhibitory control (DRL, delay-discounting and stop-signal tasks) in mice and rats (108, 109). U50,488 also produces deficits in cognitive flexibility (modified water maze task) in mice that are reversed by the κ-opioid receptor antagonist nor-binaltorphimine (110). Another κ-opioid receptor agonist U69,593 enhances, while nor-binaltorphimine disrupts working memory (Y-maze) in mice (111). Future studies with nalmefene are warranted because these animal studies suggest that modulation of κ-opioid receptors effects executive function which may be beneficial in disorders characterized by executive dysfunction, such as addiction. Studies examining general cognitive effects of nalmefene are also scarce with one report suggesting increases in subjective alertness but no effect on a choice reaction time task (112).

## PHARMACOTHERAPIES FOR ALCOHOL AND OPIOID USE DISORDERS

### Naltrexone

Pharmacologically, naltrexone has greatest affinity for the μ-opioid receptor but is an antagonist at all opioid receptors and it reduces the rewarding effects as well as craving and desire for alcohol and opiates (113, 114). Indeed, mice lacking the μ-opioid receptor do not self-administer alcohol (115). There have been a small number of human and animal studies examining the effects of naltrexone on executive function. After 8 weeks of administration, Hatsukami et al. (116) found no significant differences in working memory (digit span backwards) in overweight men who were administered either naltrexone (300 mg/day) or placebo. In contrast, animal research suggests naltrexone in rats improves working memory performance (radial arm maze) compared to saline administration (117) and that naltrexone reverses deficits in working memory (radial arm maze) that have been induced by exposure to microwaves (118). However, one study did find the opposite with microwave exposure failing to induce deficits in radial arm maze performance and naltrexone treated rats taking longer to complete the task relative to saline treated animals (119).

In animal studies examining the effects of naltrexone on inhibitory control, naltrexone had no significant effect on delay discounting (inhibiting choice of immediate reward over a larger, delayed reward) when administered alone in rats and mice (120, 121). In contrast, naltrexone has been shown to improve inhibitory control in a rat gambling task (by inhibiting preference for immediate gain at the expense of reduced net gain) in animals that made more suboptimal choices at baseline (122). Additionally, naltrexone pre-treatment improved morphine-induced decrements in impulsive choice (120). Similarly, naloxone (a drug which is used clinically for acute opioid overdose and is a non-selective opioid antagonist which, like naltrexone, blocks μ-opioid receptors with greatest affinity) attenuates drug-induced inhibitory control deficits (five-choice serial reaction time task) in rats (123). In humans, the acute effect of naltrexone (50 mg) on inhibitory control (inhibiting choice of immediate reward over a larger, delayed reward) has been investigated in abstinent alcoholics and healthy controls. Naltrexone did not improve impulsive choice reliably across abstinent alcoholic participants, but performance was instead dependent on personality. Across both abstinent alcoholics and healthy controls, those with greater external locus of control made fewer impulsive choices on naltrexone and the opposite was true for individuals with greater internal locus of control (124). As perceptions of control may be influenced by tonic frontal dopamine (125) and frontal dopaminergic tone may account for individual differences in impulsive choice (126) it is interesting to note here that previous evidence suggests that the opioid system appears to have a role in modulating dopamine tone (127).

Research regarding the effect of naltrexone on cognitive flexibility has been mixed. A study in rats suggests that aged relative to young rats have impaired flexibility on an attentional set-shifting task (extradimensional shifting) and that this age-related impairment was reversed by naltrexone while there was no effect of naltrexone on the performance of younger rats (128). In humans, no significant difference in cognitive flexibility (Color Trails task) was found between abstinent heroin abusers receiving naltrexone therapy and healthy controls whereas buprenorphine-maintained patients showed impairments in cognitive flexibility (129) while, an earlier study in overweight men suggested there was no significant effect of receiving high dose naltrexone (300 mg/day) on cognitive flexibility (Trails B) after 8 weeks of treatment compared to placebo (116).

## PHARMACOTHERAPIES FOR OPIOID USE DISORDER

### Methadone

As a μ-opioid receptor agonist that also has antagonist properties at the glutamatergic NMDA receptor, methadone is used clinically as an analgesic and is used in OUD where it may be used in long-term maintenance therapy or to manage withdrawal during detoxification (130). Several studies have investigated executive function in patients receiving methadone maintenance therapy. Studies tend to differ in terms of the methadone dose and duration of treatment as well as by comparator i.e., healthy controls with no history of substance abuse, former opioid abusers not in methadone maintenance therapy, or within subject comparisons such as pre-/during therapy and peak/trough concentration following dosing (for studies comparing methadone maintenance therapy with buprenorphine see next section). These differences may account for some equivocal findings described below.

Studies have shown that methadone maintenance therapy is associated with poorer working memory. For instance, those who had been on short-term (at least 30 days) or long-term (at least 6 months) methadone maintenance scored in the lower portion of the normal range for working memory (letter-digit ordering) based on normative test data (131). Working memory (letter number sequencing) was also worse in those in methadone maintenance therapy (mean duration of treatment: 38.66 months; mean dose of methadone: 83.82 mg/day) compared to abstinent heroin abusers although this difference only approached significance (132). Methadone users (mean duration of treatment: 41.48 months) also had significantly worse working memory (2-back task) compared to healthy controls (133). While in another study using a within-subject design working memory (n-back task and modified Sternberg task) was assessed in methadone-maintained patients (mean duration of treatment: 48.9 months; mean dose of methadone: 97.5 mg/day) at approximately 120 min and 26 h after dosing (to coincide with peak and trough methadone concentrations). While there were no differences on the modified Sternberg task, *n*-back performance was slower when testing time coincided with peak methadone concentration. In addition, higher doses of methadone were associated with decreased n-back hit rate (134). However, some studies have found no significant differences in working memory when comparing methadone-maintained patients with healthy controls with no history of substance abuse (135) or with abstinent former opioid abusers (136). The average doses of methadone used in these two studies was 15.14 and 67.2 mg/day, respectively. Taken together it appears that methadone may impair working memory on certain tasks and when higher doses are taken. However, more studies are needed that take into account baseline cognitive performance levels.

Two studies (described above) assessed the effects of methadone maintenance therapy on inhibitory control (132, 133). These studies found that methadone maintenance was associated with poorer inhibitory control (five-digit test) compared to abstinent heroin abusers (132) and poorer inhibitory control (stop-signal task) when compared to healthy controls (133). In another study however, no correlations between dose or duration of methadone maintenance therapy were found in patients where the mean duration of treatment was 8.6 years and the mean dose was 124.2 mg/day (137). Perhaps the longer duration of treatment lead to tolerance of cognitive effects in some participants. Surprisingly, opposite findings have been observed with better inhibitory control (stop-signal task) found in methadone maintenance therapy compared to abstinent opiate dependent participants (138). In their study, Liao et al. (138) found that stop-signal reaction time was significantly shorter in methadone-maintained participants compared to abstinent participants and was no different when compared to healthy controls. Another study comparing methadone-maintained patients and healthy controls stratified patients by duration of treatment (short term: <12 months or long term: ≥12 months) and by dose (low dose: <80 mg/day or high dose: ≥80 mg/day). This study found that healthy participants made more inhibitory errors (errors of commission) on a continuous performance task compared to short term and low dose methadone-maintained patients (139). However, short term and low dose methadone-maintained patients also had the slowest reaction times on the task and the methadone group tended to have poorer sustained attention than healthy controls assessed on the same task. Therefore, the lower number of inhibitory errors found in short term and low dose methadone-treated patients could be due to general task disengagement in this group.

Most studies investigating the effects of methadone maintenance therapy on cognitive flexibility have demonstrated that treatment is associated with impaired flexibility. Those who had been on short-term (at least 30 days) or long-term (at least 6 months) methadone maintenance scored in the lower portion of the normal range for cognitive flexibility (trail making test) based on normative test data (131). In addition, worse cognitive flexibility assessed using a range of cognitive flexibility tasks (trail making test, oral trails, Wisconsin Card Sorting test, switching of attention task) has been reported in methadone-maintained patients compared to abstinent opioid abusers (132, 136) and healthy controls (135, 140, 141). One study found no improvement in cognitive flexibility (trail making test) when comparing opiate dependent participants at baseline and again following 2 months on methadone maintenance therapy (142) and surprisingly, in one study improved flexibility (trail making test) was found as methadone dose increased (134). A further study compared former opiate dependent participants that had been medication free for 10 years with those whom had been on methadone maintenance for the past 10 years (143). This study demonstrated that methadone maintenance was associated with a selective flexibility deficit. While both groups were able to acquire and reverse information about positive and negative outcomes under neutral conditions, Levy-Gigi et al. (143) found that the methadone-maintained group were impaired at reversing positive outcomes when these were presented in a drug-related context.

## Buprenorphine

As a non-selective, mixed agonist-antagonist at opioid receptors (partial agonist at μ-opioid receptor, antagonist at κ- and δ-opioid receptors as well as weak partial agonist at nociception receptors) buprenorphine is used as an analgesic as well as to help manage withdrawal symptoms during opioid detoxification. During detoxification, buprenorphine may be used as short or long-term opioid replacement therapy (for longer-term use it is often combined with the pure opioid antagonist naloxone) and it appears to have similar clinical effectiveness to methadone at managing opioid withdrawal (144).

Few studies have investigated the effects of buprenorphine on executive function. One study investigating the impact of different doses on working memory administered buprenorphine/naloxone to opioid dependent patients at a starting dose of 8 mg/2 mg going up to 16 mg/4 mg and then 32 mg/8 mg with 7–10 days at each dose. This study found that there was no impairment in working memory (N-back task) as the dose increased four-fold (145). However, poorer working memory (Letter-Number Sequencing task, Paced Auditory Serial Addition task) has previously been found in opioid-dependent patients treated with buprenorphine/naloxone compared to healthy controls (146, 147). Rapeli et al. (147) also compare buprenorphine/naloxone treated patients with methadone-maintained patients at several time points (1. 2months, 2. 6–9months and 3. 12–17months after starting substitution therapy) and show that for one of the working memory tasks (Letter-Number Sequencing task) the buprenorphine/naloxone treated group improved between the second and third time points while the methadone treated groups performance remained stable across time. Working memory (digit span backwards) was however not found to be significantly different between patients on either buprenorphine (mean dose: 10.6 mg/day) or methadone (mean dose: 82.7 mg/day) maintenance therapy (mean duration of treatment 48 months across both maintenance therapies) or between these patients (combined in to one group) and healthy controls in a study from another group (148).

Very few studies have assessed the effect of buprenorphine on inhibitory control. One study already mentioned in this section above (148) found that opiate-dependent patients on either buprenorphine and methadone maintenance therapy didn't differ in inhibitory control (Haylings Sentence Completion test) but that when compared to healthy controls these patients (combined in to one group) performed significantly worse. However, another study comparing buprenorphine-maintained opioid dependent patients (mean duration of therapy: 5.4 years; mean dose: 9 mg/day) with both methadone-maintained patients (mean duration of therapy: 8.3 years; mean dose: 66 mg/day) and healthy non-opiate dependent controls found that the buprenorphine treated group performed better than the methadone treated group and no different from controls on the Iowa gambling task (149). The Iowa gambling task is traditionally considered a decision-making task but to perform well on the task it requires the ability to inhibit selection of decks that provide higher immediate gains but long-term losses (150). While, Haylings Sentence Completion test involves inhibition of sensible words that could be used to complete sentences (151). While inhibition is required by both tasks the Iowa gambling task is less semantic and the differing task demands and neural underpinnings may account for the differing findings from these studies.

Several studies have assessed the effect of buprenorphine on cognitive flexibility. Two studies already mentioned in this section above also included an assessment of cognitive flexibility (145, 149). One of these studies did not find impairments in cognitive flexibility (trail making task) with a four-fold increase in the dose of buprenorphine/naloxone given to opioid dependent patients (145). However, in the other study mentioned buprenorphine-maintained patients made fewer perseverative errors on the Wisconsin Card Sorting task compared to methadone-maintained patients with their performance falling somewhere between the group treated with methadone and healthy controls (149). In other studies, a within-subject design found that intravenous infusion of 0.6 mg of buprenorphine to healthy males over 150 min resulted in a significant deterioration in cognitive flexibility (trail making test) compared to a drug-free baseline assessment (152). Studies comparing opioid dependent patients on buprenorphine to healthy controls assessing cognitive flexibility (trail making test, color trails task) have tended to find that the treated patients perform less well than healthy control (129, 153). However, in tasks comparing the cognitive flexibility of buprenorphine and methadone-treated opioid dependent patients two studies failed to find a significant difference in cognitive flexibility in direct contrast to Pirastu et al. (149) (154, 155). While maintenance therapy doses and durations of treatment across these studies were similar, these two latter studies used the trail making test while the Wisconsin Card Sorting task was used by Pirastu et al. (149). The different cognitive demands of these tasks may help explain the differences seen across these studies. In the trail making test participants are required to shift backwards and forwards between numbers and letters in a predictable manner (156). While in contrast, in the Wisconsin Card Sorting task participants are unaware of what shifts will be required when task rules change and must work these out for themselves using feedback (157).

## Lofexidine

Approved for the management of acute opioid detoxification in the United Kingdom in 1994 and more recently by the Food and Drug Administration in the United States in 2018, lofexidine is an $\alpha_{2A}$ adrenergic receptor agonist that has historically been used to reduce blood pressure and is now used to alleviate opioid withdrawal symptoms (158). To the best of our knowledge, there has not been any published research investigating lofexidine's effects on executive function. Studies examining general cognitive effects of lofexidine are also scarce. However, one report in 14 opioid dependent participants, suggests there may be a dose-related deterioration in simple reaction time, continuous performance, procedural memory, and mathematical processing when lofexidine is added to methadone maintenance therapy (159). Nevertheless, other $\alpha_{2A}$ adrenergic receptor agonists have been shown to selectively improve prefrontal cortex mediated cognitive functions (160).

## DISCUSSION

The aim of this review was to provide a brief narrative overview of the evidence for effects of some of the most commonly approved and prescribed pharmacotherapies for TUD, AUD, and OUD on the three core executive functions (working memory, inhibitory control and cognitive flexibility). Enhancement of executive function is likely to be an important target for the treatment of substance use disorders and may contribute to clinical efficacy of existing medications since executive dysfunction is thought to contribute to poor treatment adherence, worse clinical outcomes and relapse (13–19). However, for most of the approved pharmacotherapies reviewed it was difficult to draw firm conclusions regarding effects on executive function. This is due to a surprising lack of well-powered empirical research evaluating the effects of pharmacotherapy on executive function, and because of the extent of contradictory findings. A similar conclusion was made by a recent systematic review of the general cognitive effects of existing pharmacotherapy (23).

Both hypo- and hyperdopaminergic states have been postulated to account for various addiction phenomenon in the absence and presence of drug cues (161). Positron-emission tomography (PET) studies in substance abusing populations suggest that there are decreases in both dopamine release and dopamine $D_2$ receptors (162, 163). Indeed, the dopamine hypothesis of drug addiction (164) implicates a long-lasting hypodopaminergic state throughout the addiction cycle including persistence of this state in withdrawal. For example, PET imaging with a high affinity dopamine $D_{2/3}$ receptor radioligand has established that there is a smaller amphetamine-induced dopamine release in the cortex and midbrain of abstinent alcoholics than in healthy controls (165). Many of the pharmacotherapies reviewed here have direct or indirect effects on dopamine levels. In line with the inverted "U" shaped dose response curve for dopamine effects on executive function (62) drugs that enhance dopamine levels in individuals with a low baseline level of dopamine would be expected to enhance executive function while potentially impairing the performance of individuals with a higher dopaminergic starting point. Mixed findings in the current review may be attributable to differing dopaminergic baselines. In this regard, medicated substance dependent patients with lower baseline dopamine and greater cognitive impairments may receive greater cognitive benefit than less cognitively impaired patients with a higher dopaminergic baseline. While it may be more difficult to demonstrate cognitive improvements in healthy participants or there may be paradoxical impairment in performance.

Substance use disorder pharmacotherapies have been shown to be efficacious however they do not work for everyone. Identifying for whom they do, and do not, work is an important unmet clinical need. While it is evident that executive dysfunction is observed during early abstinence which may contribute to relapse (20–22) much more work is required in order to determine whether a drugs positive effects on executive function are predictive of positive cessation outcomes. Previous PET imaging studies with a high affinity dopamine $D_{2/3}$ receptor radioligand have suggested that the extent to which methylphenidate induces increases in dopamine are predictive of relapse and response to behavioral and psychological treatments in methamphetamine and cocaine abusers (166, 167). Future research should investigate whether clinical effectiveness of pharmacotherapy (i.e., sustained cessation) is related to individual differences in the ability of the drugs to improve cognitive function and whether this is associated with baseline differences or changes in dopamine levels.

Existing and novel cognitive enhancers may be beneficial for substance abuse disorders and studies investigating effects of cognitive enhancers are on-going (7). Whether it is existing pharmacotherapies being evaluated for their effects on cognition, or novel cognitive enhancers being evaluated for the potential to improve executive function and clinical outcomes in substance dependent populations, it is important to consider how cognition will be assessed. The current narrative review illustrates that even when the number of studies assessing different components of executive function are small, a wide variety of tasks and outcome measures are used which can make cross-study comparisons difficult. Future studies should carefully consider which tasks are best suited to assess relevant cognitive functions. Future work should also consider the potential cognitive enhancers mechanism of action and abuse potential. For example, modafinil is a promising cognitive enhancer but it's addictive potential has been illustrated in studies examining effects on behavioral sensitization and conditioned place preference (168).

An alternative approach to try and improve executive function in addiction has been with cognitive training most notably working memory training and inhibitory control training. Training of working memory has been found to improve working memory performance and reduce subsequent drug use in methadone-maintained patients and problem drinkers compared to control conditions (169, 170). Similarly, inhibitory control training using an alcohol-related Go/NoGo task has previously been found to reduce post-training alcohol consumption as effectively as a Brief Alcohol Intervention (171). Reduced drug use post-training suggests that interventions based on these types of training procedure may improve clinical outcomes and further supports the targeting of executive function in addiction. However, future studies should consider whether pharmacotherapy could compliment and even facilitate such training. Inhibitory control training, for example, may work via the devaluation of reward-related stimuli (172) and given that some of the drugs reviewed here e.g., varenicline, disulfiram, nalmefene, and naltrexone may devalue substances of abuse (either by reducing the positive rewarding effects of substances or by pairing them with an unpleasant reaction) it would be interesting to see whether these drugs are able to facilitate inhibitory control training and improve dependent populations control over substance use in real-world settings.

In this review we have examined the evidence for executive function enhancement by commonly prescribed, labeled pharmacotherapy for TUD, AUD, and OUD as any such enhancement may contribute to clinical efficacy. However, it should be noted that the act of detoxification might itself be expected to improve executive function. Future studies should include appropriate controls or take this variable in to account when estimating the cognitive effects of medications used to assist detoxification maintenance. While a potential strength of this review is that it has evaluated the cognitive impact of only those medications with a high degree of evidence for efficacy in treating TUD, AUD, and OUD this does mean that we may have missed important trends in findings with those medications that are used off-label to treat these disorders (e.g., topiramate). In addition, this review excluded off-label pharmacotherapy for other substance use disorders such as the stimulants cocaine and methamphetamine. These disorders are persistent public health problems for which there are no approved pharmacotherapy options (173, 174). While the relative lack of evidence for consistent and positive pharmacotherapy effects, coupled with a wide-range of off-label prescribing practices lead us to exclude such research this too may have led to missing important trends in findings and consequently limited our discussion.

## CONCLUSIONS

There are several efficacious pharmacotherapy options available for TUD, AUD, and OUD. Evidence is limited and conflicting regarding whether they can improve executive function in dependent populations. It should be noted that baseline differences in dopamine and performance may contribute to an explanation for why inconsistent findings exist. So far, strategies aimed at enhancing cognition to help with improving cessation rates in dependent populations have not been successfully implemented in the clinic. However, there has been limited research conducted in this area and cognitive enhancement remains a potential strategy that is worth exploring further. The issue of abuse liability of drugs that can be cognitive enhancers needs to be taken in to consideration when designing such studies. Moreover, studies should now move beyond simply assessing cognitive effects in order to establish whether an improved cognitive response is related to clinical efficacy and if this is also associated with baseline or changes in dopamine. This approach may assist future personalized medicine strategies.

## AUTHOR CONTRIBUTIONS

All authors contributed to conception of this review, KB drafted the manuscript and all authors contributed to manuscript revision, read and approved the submitted version.

## REFERENCES


1. Leshner AI. Addiction is a brain disease, and it matters. *Science*. (1997) 278:45–7. doi: 10.1126/science.278.5335.45
2. Peacock A, Leung J, Larney S, Colledge S, Hickman M, Rehm J, et al. Global statistics on alcohol, tobacco and illicit drug use: 2017 status report. *Addiction*. (2018) 113:1905–26. doi: 10.1111/add.14234
3. Nutt DJ, King LA, Phillips LD. Drug harms in the UK: a multicriteria decision analysis. *Lancet*. (2010) 376:1558–65. doi: 10.1016/S0140-6736(10)61462-6
4. McGovern MP, Carroll KM. Evidence-based practices for substance use disorders. *Psychiatr Clin North Am*. (2003) 26:991–1010. doi: 10.1016/S0193-953X(03)00073-X
5. McLellan AT, Lewis DC, O'Brien CP, Kleber HD. Drug dependence, a chronic medical illness: implications for treatment, insurance, and outcomes evaluation. *JAMA*. (2000) 284:1689–95. doi: 10.1001/jama.284.13.1689
6. Brady KT, Gray KM, Tolliver BK. Cognitive enhancers in the treatment of substance use disorders: clinical evidence. *Pharmacol Biochem Behav*. (2011) 99:285–94. doi: 10.1016/j.pbb.2011.04.017
7. Sofuoglu M, DeVito EE, Waters AJ, Carroll KM. Cognitive enhancement as a treatment for drug addictions. *Neuropharmacology*. (2013) 64:452–63. doi: 10.1016/j.neuropharm.2012.06.021
8. Verdejo-Garcia, A. (2017). Chapter 16 - executive dysfunction in addiction. In: Goldberg E, editor. *Executive Functions in Health and Disease*. San Diego, CA: Academic Press (2017). p. 395–403.
9. Verdejo-Garcia A, Bechara A, Recknor EC, Perez-Garcia M. Executive dysfunction in substance dependent individuals during drug use and abstinence: an examination of the behavioral, cognitive and emotional correlates of addiction. *J Int Neuropsychol Soc*. (2006) 12:405–15. doi: 10.1017/S1355617706060486
10. Aytaclar S, Tarter RE, Kirisci L, Lu S. Association between hyperactivity and executive cognitive functioning in childhood and substance use in early adolescence. *J Am Acad Child Adolesc Psychiatry*. (1999) 38:172–8. doi: 10.1097/00004583-199902000-00016
11. Ersche KD, Turton AJ, Chamberlain SR, Muller U, Bullmore ET, Robbins TW. Cognitive dysfunction and anxious-impulsive personality traits are endophenotypes for drug dependence. *Am J Psychiatry*. (2012) 169:926–36. doi: 10.1176/appi.ajp.2012.11091421
12. Gierski F, Hubsch B, Stefaniak N, Benzerouk F, Cuervo-Lombard C, Bera-Potelle C, et al. Executive functions in adult offspring of alcohol-dependent probands: toward a cognitive endophenotype? *Alcohol Clin Exp Res*. (2013) 37(Suppl. 1):E356–63. doi: 10.1111/j.1530-0277.2012.01903.x
13. Albein-Urios N, Pilatti A, Lozano O, Martinez-Gonzalez JM, Verdejo-Garcia A. The value of impulsivity to define subgroups of addicted individuals differing in personality dysfunction, craving, psychosocial adjustment, and wellbeing: a latent class analysis. *Arch Clin Neuropsychol*. (2014) 29:38–46. doi: 10.1093/arclin/act072
14. Bates ME, Pawlak AP, Tonigan JS, Buckman JF. Cognitive impairment influences drinking outcome by altering therapeutic mechanisms of change. *Psychol Addict Behav*. (2006) 20:241–53. doi: 10.1037/0893-164X.20.3.241
15. Blume AW, Marlatt GA. The role of executive cognitive functions in changing substance use: what we know and what we need to know. *Ann Behav Med*. (2009) 37:117–25. doi: 10.1007/s12160-009-9093-8
16. Dominguez-Salas S, Diaz-Batanero C, Lozano-Rojas OM, Verdejo-Garcia A. Impact of general cognition and executive function deficits on addiction treatment outcomes: systematic review and discussion of neurocognitive pathways. *Neurosci Biobehav Rev*. (2016) 71:772–801. doi: 10.1016/j.neubiorev.2016.09.030
17. Goncalves PD, Ometto M, Malbergier A, Martins P, Beraldo L, Santos B, et al. Executive functioning and outpatient treatment adherence after intensive inpatient care in cocaine dependence: a six-month follow-up study. *Drug and Alcohol Depend*. (2017) 171:e75. doi: 10.1016/j.drugalcdep.2016.08.214
18. Loughead J, Wileyto EP, Ruparel K, Falcone M, Hopson R, Gur R, et al. Working memory-related neural activity predicts future smoking relapse. *Neuropsychopharmacology*. (2015) 40:1311–20. doi: 10.1038/npp.2014.318
19. Miller L. Predicting relapse and recovery in alcoholism and addiction: neuropsychology, personality, and cognitive style. *J Subst Abuse Treat*. (1991) 8:277–91. doi: 10.1016/0740-5472(91)90051-B

20. Ashare RL, Falcone M, Lerman C. Cognitive function during nicotine withdrawal: Implications for nicotine dependence treatment. *Neuropharmacology.* (2014) 76(PtB):581–91. doi: 10.1016/j.neuropharm.2013.04.034
21. Rapeli P, Kivisaari R, Autti T, Kahkonen S, Puuskari V, Jokela O, et al. Cognitive function during early abstinence from opioid dependence: a comparison to age, gender, and verbal intelligence matched controls. *BMC Psychiatry.* (2006) 6:9. doi: 10.1186/1471-244X-6-9
22. Zinn S, Stein R, Swartzwelder HS. Executive functioning early in abstinence from alcohol. *Alcohol Clin Exp Res.* (2004) 28:1338–46. doi: 10.1097/01.ALC.0000139814.81811.62
23. Pujol CN, Paasche C, Laprevote V, Trojak B, Vidailhet P, Bacon E, et al. Cognitive effects of labeled addictolytic medications. *Prog Neuropsychopharmacol Biol Psychiatry.* (2018) 81:306–32. doi: 10.1016/j.pnpbp.2017.09.008
24. Diamond A. Executive functions. *Annu Rev Psychol.* (2013) 64:135–68. doi: 10.1146/annurev-psych-113011-143750
25. Miyake A, Friedman NP, Emerson MJ, Witzki AH, Howerter A, Wager TD. The unity and diversity of executive functions and their contributions to complex "Frontal Lobe" tasks: a latent variable analysis. *Cogn Psychol.* (2000) 41:49–100. doi: 10.1006/cogp.1999.0734
26. Stead LF, Perera R, Bullen C, Mant D, Hartmann-Boyce J, Cahill K, et al. Nicotine replacement therapy for smoking cessation. *Cochrane Database Syst Rev.* (2012) 11:Cd000146. doi: 10.1002/14651858.CD000146.pub4
27. Levin ED, Bradley A, Addy N, Sigurani N. Hippocampal alpha 7 and alpha 4 beta 2 nicotinic receptors and working memory. *Neuroscience.* (2002) 109:757–65. doi: 10.1016/S0306-4522(01)00538-3
28. Atzori G, Lemmonds CA, Kotler ML, Durcan MJ, Boyle J. Efficacy of a nicotine (4 mg)-containing lozenge on the cognitive impairment of nicotine withdrawal. *J Clin Psychopharmacol.* (2008) 28:667–74. doi: 10.1097/JCP.0b013e31818c9bb8
29. Heishman SJ, Kleykamp BA, Singleton EG. Meta-analysis of the acute effects of nicotine and smoking on human performance. *Psychopharmacology.* (2010) 210:453–69. doi: 10.1007/s00213-010-1848-1
30. Levin ED, Briggs SJ, Christopher NC, Rose JE. Chronic nicotinic stimulation and blockade effects on working memory. *Behav Pharmacol.* (1993) 4:179–82. doi: 10.1097/00008877-199304000-00010
31. Mizoguchi H, Ibi D, Takase F, Nagai T, Kamei H, Toth E, et al. Nicotine ameliorates impairment of working memory in methamphetamine-treated rats. *Behav Brain Res.* (2011) 220:159–63. doi: 10.1016/j.bbr.2011.01.036
32. Rushforth SL, Steckler T, Shoaib M. Nicotine improves working memory span capacity in rats following sub-chronic ketamine exposure. *Neuropsychopharmacology.* (2011) 36:2774–81. doi: 10.1038/npp.2011.224
33. Heishman SJ, Snyder FR, Henningfield JE. Performance, subjective, and physiological effects of nicotine in non-smokers. *Drug Alcohol Depend.* (1993) 34:11–8. doi: 10.1016/0376-8716(93)90041-N
34. Kleykamp BA, Jennings JM, Blank MD, Eissenberg T. The effects of nicotine on attention and working memory in never-smokers. *Psychol Addict Behav.* (2005) 19:433–8. doi: 10.1037/0893-164X.19.4.433
35. MacQueen DA, Drobes DJ. Validation of the human odor span task: effects of nicotine. *Psychopharmacology.* (2017) 234:2871–82. doi: 10.1007/s00213-017-4680-z
36. Grundey J, Amu R, Ambrus GG, Batsikadze G, Paulus W, Nitsche MA. Double dissociation of working memory and attentional processes in smokers and non-smokers with and without nicotine. *Psychopharmacology.* (2015) 232:2491–501. doi: 10.1007/s00213-015-3880-7
37. Niemegeers P, Dumont GJ, Quisenaerts C, Morrens M, Boonzaier J, Fransen E, et al. The effects of nicotine on cognition are dependent on baseline performance. *Eur Neuropsychopharmacol.* (2014) 24:1015–23. doi: 10.1016/j.euroneuro.2014.03.011
38. Dawkins L, Powell JH, West R, Powell J, Pickering A. A double-blind placebo-controlled experimental study of nicotine: II–effects on response inhibition and executive functioning. *Psychopharmacology.* (2007) 190:457–67. doi: 10.1007/s00213-006-0634-6
39. Ettinger U, Faiola E, Kasparbauer AM, Petrovsky N, Chan RC, Liepelt R, et al. Effects of nicotine on response inhibition and interference control. *Psychopharmacology.* (2017) 234:1093–111. doi: 10.1007/s00213-017-4542-8
40. Wignall ND, de Wit H. Effects of nicotine on attention and inhibitory control in healthy nonsmokers. *Exp Clin Psychopharmacol.* (2011) 19:183–91. doi: 10.1037/a0023292
41. Blondel A, Sanger DJ, Moser PC. Characterisation of the effects of nicotine in the five-choice serial reaction time task in rats: antagonist studies. *Psychopharmacology.* (2000) 149:293–305. doi: 10.1007/s002130000378
42. Dallery J, Locey ML. Effects of acute and chronic nicotine on impulsive choice in rats. *Behav Pharmacol.* (2005) 16:15–23. doi: 10.1097/00008877-200502000-00002
43. Kelsey JE, Niraula A. Effects of acute and sub-chronic nicotine on impulsive choice in rats in a probabilistic delay-discounting task. *Psychopharmacology.* (2013) 227:385–92. doi: 10.1007/s00213-013-2984-1
44. Kirshenbaum AP, Jackson ER, Brown SJ, Fuchs JR, Miltner BC, Doughty AH. Nicotine-induced impulsive action: sensitization and attenuation by mecamylamine. *Behav Pharmacol.* (2011) 22:207–21. doi: 10.1097/FBP.0b013e328345ca1c
45. Kolokotroni KZ, Rodgers RJ, Harrison AA. Acute nicotine increases both impulsive choice and behavioural disinhibition in rats. *Psychopharmacology.* (2011) 217:455–73. doi: 10.1007/s00213-011-2296-2
46. Mazur GJ, Wood-Isenberg G, Watterson E, Sanabria F. Detrimental effects of acute nicotine on the response-withholding performance of spontaneously hypertensive and Wistar Kyoto rats. *Psychopharmacology.* (2014) 231:2471–82. doi: 10.1007/s00213-013-3412-2
47. Tsutsui-Kimura I, Ohmura Y, Izumi T, Yamaguchi T, Yoshida T, Yoshioka M. Nicotine provokes impulsive-like action by stimulating alpha4beta2 nicotinic acetylcholine receptors in the infralimbic, but not in the prelimbic cortex. *Psychopharmacology.* (2010) 209:351–9. doi: 10.1007/s00213-010-1804-0
48. Austin AJ, Duka T, Rusted J, Jackson A. Effect of varenicline on aspects of inhibitory control in smokers. *Psychopharmacology.* (2014) 231:3771–85. doi: 10.1007/s00213-014-3512-7
49. Hogarth L, Stillwell DJ, Tunney RJ. BIS impulsivity and acute nicotine exposure are associated with discounting global consequences in the Harvard game. *Hum Psychopharmacol.* (2013) 28:72–9. doi: 10.1002/hup.2285
50. Poltavski DV, Petros T. Effects of transdermal nicotine on attention in adult non-smokers with and without attentional deficits. *Physiol Behav.* (2006) 87:614–24. doi: 10.1016/j.physbeh.2005.12.011
51. Barr RS, Culhane MA, Jubelt LE, Mufti RS, Dyer MA, Weiss AP, et al. The effects of transdermal nicotine on cognition in nonsmokers with schizophrenia and nonpsychiatric controls. *Neuropsychopharmacology.* (2008) 33:480–90. doi: 10.1038/sj.npp.1301423
52. Kayir H, Semenova S, Markou A. Baseline impulsive choice predicts the effects of nicotine and nicotine withdrawal on impulsivity in rats. *Prog Neuropsychopharmacol Biol Psychiatry.* (2014) 48:6–13. doi: 10.1016/j.pnpbp.2013.09.007
53. Kolokotroni KZ, Rodgers RJ, Harrison AA. Trait differences in response to chronic nicotine and nicotine withdrawal in rats. *Psychopharmacology.* (2014) 231:567–80. doi: 10.1007/s00213-013-3270-y
54. Nesic J, Rusted J, Duka T, Jackson A. Degree of dependence influences the effect of smoking on cognitive flexibility. *Pharmacol Biochem Behav.* (2011) 98:376–84. doi: 10.1016/j.pbb.2011.01.015
55. Butler K, Rusted J, Gard P, Jackson A. Performance monitoring in nicotine dependence: considering integration of recent reinforcement history. *Pharmacol Biochem Behav.* (2017) 156:63–70. doi: 10.1016/j.pbb.2017.04.004
56. Ortega LA, Tracy BA, Gould TJ, Parikh V. Effects of chronic low- and high-dose nicotine on cognitive flexibility in C57BL/6J mice. *Behav Brain Res.* (2013) 238:134–45. doi: 10.1016/j.bbr.2012.10.032
57. Allison C, Shoaib M. Nicotine improves performance in an attentional set shifting task in rats. *Neuropharmacology.* (2013) 64:314–20. doi: 10.1016/j.neuropharm.2012.06.055
58. Jackson A, Silk S, Buhidma Y, Shoaib M. Varenicline, the clinically effective smoking cessation agent, restores probabilistic response reversal performance during withdrawal from nicotine. *Addict Biol.* (2017) 22:1316–28. doi: 10.1111/adb.12423
59. Mancuso G, Warburton DM, Melen M, Sherwood N, Tirelli E. Selective effects of nicotine on attentional processes. *Psychopharmacology.* (1999) 146:199–204. doi: 10.1007/s002130051107
60. Cumming P, Rosa-Neto P, Watanabe H, Smith D, Bender D, Clarke PB, et al. Effects of acute nicotine on hemodynamics and binding of [11C]raclopride

to dopamine D2,3 receptors in pig brain. *Neuroimage*. (2003) 19:1127–36. doi: 10.1016/S1053-8119(03)00079-X

61. Le Foll B, Guranda M, Wilson AA, Houle S, Rusjan PM, Wing VC, et al. Elevation of dopamine induced by cigarette smoking: novel insights from a [11C]-+-PHNO PET study in humans. *Neuropsychopharmacology*. (2014) 39:415–24. doi: 10.1038/npp.2013.209
62. Cools R, D'Esposito M. Inverted-U-shaped dopamine actions on human working memory and cognitive control. *Biol Psychiatry*. (2011) 69:e113–125. doi: 10.1016/j.biopsych.2011.03.028
63. Luijten M, Veltman DJ, Hester R, Smits M, Nijs IM, Pepplinkhuizen L, et al. The role of dopamine in inhibitory control in smokers and non-smokers: a pharmacological fMRI study. *Eur Neuropsychopharmacol*. (2013) 23:1247–56. doi: 10.1016/j.euroneuro.2012.10.017
64. Hughes JR, Stead LF, Hartmann-Boyce J, Cahill K, Lancaster T. Antidepressants for smoking cessation. *Cochrane Database Syst Rev*. (2014) 8:Cd000031. doi: 10.1002/14651858.CD000031.pub4
65. Wu P, Wilson K, Dimoulas P, Mills EJ. Effectiveness of smoking cessation therapies: a systematic review and meta-analysis. *BMC Public Health*. (2006) 6:300. doi: 10.1186/1471-2458-6-300
66. Fabre LF, Brodie HK, Garver D, Zung WW. A multicenter evaluation of bupropion versus placebo in hospitalized depressed patients. *J Clin Psychiatry*. (1983) 44:88–94.
67. Gualtieri CT, Johnson LG. Bupropion normalizes cognitive performance in patients with depression. *MedGenMed*. (2007) 9:22. Available online at: https://www.medscape.com/viewarticle/550429
68. Gorlyn M, Keilp J, Burke A, Oquendo M, Mann JJ, Grunebaum M. Treatment-related improvement in neuropsychological functioning in suicidal depressed patients: paroxetine vs. *bupropion Psychiatry Res*. (2015) 225:407–12. doi: 10.1016/j.psychres.2014.12.004
69. Perkins KA, Karelitz JL, Jao NC, Gur RC, Lerman C. Effects of bupropion on cognitive performance during initial tobacco abstinence. *Drug Alcohol Depend*. (2013) 133:283–6. doi: 10.1016/j.drugalcdep.2013.05.003
70. Ashare RL, McKee SA. Effects of varenicline and bupropion on cognitive processes among nicotine-deprived smokers. *Exp Clin Psychopharmacol*. (2012) 20:63–70. doi: 10.1037/a0025594
71. Evins AE, Deckersbach T, Cather C, Freudenreich O, Culhane MA, Henderson DC, et al. Independent effects of tobacco abstinence and bupropion on cognitive function in schizophrenia. *J Clin Psychiatry*. (2005) 66:1184–90. doi: 10.4088/JCP.v66n0915
72. Chevassus H, Farret A, Gagnol JP, Poncon CA, Costa F, Roux C, et al. Psychological and physiological effects of bupropion compared to methylphenidate after prolonged administration in healthy volunteers (NCT00285155). *Eur J Clin Pharmacol*. (2013) 69:779–87. doi: 10.1007/s00228-012-1418-z
73. Meyer AE, Miller MM, Nelms Sprowles JL, Levine LR, Sable HJ. A comparison of presynaptic and postsynaptic dopaminergic agonists on inhibitory control performance in rats perinatally exposed to PCBs. *Neurotoxicol Teratol*. (2015) 50:11–22. doi: 10.1016/j.ntt.2015.05.009
74. Mills EJ, Wu P, Spurden D, Ebbert JO, Wilson K. Efficacy of pharmacotherapies for short-term smoking abstinance: a systematic review and meta-analysis. *Harm Reduct J*. (2009) 6:25. doi: 10.1186/1477-7517-6-25
75. Patterson F, Jepson C, Strasser AA, Loughead J, Perkins KA, Gur RC, et al. Varenicline improves mood and cognition during smoking abstinence. *Biol Psychiatry*. (2009) 65:144–9. doi: 10.1016/j.biopsych.2008.08.028
76. Patterson F, Jepson C, Loughead J, Perkins K, Strasser AA, Siegel S, et al. Working memory deficits predict short-term smoking resumption following brief abstinence. *Drug Alcohol Depend*. (2010) 106:61–4. doi: 10.1016/j.drugalcdep.2009.07.020
77. Mocking RJ, Patrick Pflanz C, Pringle A, Parsons E, McTavish SF, Cowen PJ, et al. Effects of short-term varenicline administration on emotional and cognitive processing in healthy, non-smoking adults: a randomized, double-blind, study. *Neuropsychopharmacology*. (2013) 38:476–84. doi: 10.1038/npp.2012.205
78. Kozak K, Dermody SS, Rabin RA, Zack M, Barr MS, Tyndale RF, et al. Effects of varenicline on cognitive function in non-smokers with schizophrenia. *Schizophr Res*. (2017) 197:562–563. doi: 10.1016/j.schres.2017.03.023
79. Wing VC, Wass CE, Bacher I, Rabin RA, George TP. Varenicline modulates spatial working memory deficits in smokers with schizophrenia. *Schizophr Res*. (2013) 149:190–1. doi: 10.1016/j.schres.2013.06.032
80. Hong LE, Thaker GK, McMahon RP, Summerfelt A, Rachbeisel J, Fuller RL, et al. Effects of moderate-dose treatment with varenicline on neurobiological and cognitive biomarkers in smokers and nonsmokers with schizophrenia or schizoaffective disorder. *Arch Gen Psychiatry*. (2011) 68:1195–206. doi: 10.1001/archgenpsychiatry.2011.83
81. Smith RC, Amiaz R, Si TM, Maayan L, Jin H, Boules S, et al. Varenicline effects on smoking, cognition, and psychiatric symptoms in schizophrenia: a double-blind randomized trial. *PLoS ONE*. (2016) 11:e0143490. doi: 10.1371/journal.pone.0143490
82. Roberts W, McKee SA. Effects of varenicline on cognitive performance in heavy drinkers: dose-response effects and associations with drinking outcomes. *Exp Clin Psychopharmacol*. (2018) 26:49–57. doi: 10.1037/pha0000161
83. Kalechstein AD, Mahoney JJ, Verrico CD, De La Garza R. Short-term, low-dose varenicline administration enhances information processing speed in methamphetamine-dependent users. *Neuropharmacology*. (2014) 85:493–8. doi: 10.1016/j.neuropharm.2014.05.045
84. Gould RW, Garg PK, Garg S, Nader MA. Effects of nicotinic acetylcholine receptor agonists on cognition in rhesus monkeys with a chronic cocaine self-administration history. *Neuropharmacology*. (2013) 64:479–88. doi: 10.1016/j.neuropharm.2012.08.004
85. Wouda JA, Riga D, De Vries W, Stegeman M, van Mourik Y, Schetters D, et al. Varenicline attenuates cue-induced relapse to alcohol, but not nicotine seeking, while reducing inhibitory response control. *Psychopharmacology*. (2011) 216:267–77. doi: 10.1007/s00213-011-2213-8
86. Ohmura Y, Sasamori H, Tsutsui-Kimura I, Izumi T, Yoshida T, Yoshioka M. Varenicline provokes impulsive action by stimulating alpha4beta2 nicotinic acetylcholine receptors in the infralimbic cortex in a nicotine exposure status-dependent manner. *Pharmacol Biochem Behav*. (2017) 154:1–10. doi: 10.1016/j.pbb.2017.01.002
87. Rhodes JD, Hawk LW Jr, Ashare RL, Schlienz NJ, Mahoney MC. The effects of varenicline on attention and inhibitory control among treatment-seeking smokers. *Psychopharmacology* (2012) 223:131–8. doi: 10.1007/s00213-012-2700-6
88. Terry AV Jr, Plagenhoef M, Callahan PM. Effects of the nicotinic agonist varenicline on the performance of tasks of cognition in aged and middle-aged rhesus and pigtail monkeys. *Psychopharmacology* (2016) 233:761–71. doi: 10.1007/s00213-015-4154-0
89. Lesage E, Aronson SE, Sutherland MT, Ross TJ, Salmeron BJ, Stein EA. Neural signatures of cognitive flexibility and reward sensitivity following nicotinic receptor stimulation in dependent smokers: a randomized trial. *JAMA Psychiatry* (2017) 74:632–40. doi: 10.1001/jamapsychiatry.2017.0400
90. Di Ciano P, Guranda M, Lagzdins D, Tyndale RF, Gamaleddin I, Selby P, et al. Varenicline-induced elevation of dopamine in smokers: a preliminary [(11)C]-(+)-PHNO PET Study. *Neuropsychopharmacology* (2016) 41:1513–20. doi: 10.1038/npp.2015.305
91. Skinner MD, Lahmek P, Pham H, Aubin HJ. Disulfiram efficacy in the treatment of alcohol dependence: a meta-analysis. *PLoS ONE* (2014) 9:e87366. doi: 10.1371/journal.pone.0087366
92. Schroeder JP, Cooper DA, Schank JR, Lyle MA, Gaval-Cruz M, Ogbonmwan YE, et al. Disulfiram attenuates drug-primed reinstatement of cocaine seeking via inhibition of dopamine beta-hydroxylase. *Neuropsychopharmacology* (2010) 35:2440–9. doi: 10.1038/npp.2010.127
93. Zaru A, Maccioni P, Colombo G, Gessa GL. Disulfiram inhibits chocolate self-administration and reinstatement to chocolate seeking in rats. *Pharmacol Biochem Behav*. (2016) 148:119–27. doi: 10.1016/j.pbb.2016.04.008
94. Di Ciano P, Manvich DF, Pushparaj A, Gappasov A, Hess EJ, Weinshenker D, et al. Effects of disulfiram on choice behavior in a rodent gambling task: association with catecholamine levels. *Psychopharmacology* (2018) 235:23–35. doi: 10.1007/s00213-017-4744-0
95. Mutschler J, Buhler M, Grosshans M, Diehl A, Mann K, Kiefer F. Disulfiram, an option for the treatment of pathological gambling? *Alcohol Alcohol*. (2010) 45:214–6. doi: 10.1093/alcalc/agp093

96. Gaval-Cruz M, Weinshenker D. Mechanisms of disulfiram-induced cocaine abstinence: antabuse and cocaine relapse. *Mol Interv.* (2009) 9:175–87. doi: 10.1124/mi.9.4.6
97. Peeke SC, Prael AR, Herning RI, Rogers W, Benowitz NL, Jones RT. Effect of disulfiram on cognition, subjective response, and cortical-event-related potentials in nonalcoholic subjects. *Alcohol Clin Exp Res.* (1979) 3:223–9. doi: 10.1111/j.1530-0277.1979.tb05304.x
98. Gilman S, Adams KM, Johnson-Greene D, Koeppe RA, Junck L, Kluin KJ, et al. Effects of disulfiram on positron emission tomography and neuropsychological studies in severe chronic alcoholism. *Alcohol Clin Exp Res.* (1996) 20:1456–61. doi: 10.1111/j.1530-0277.1996.tb01149.x
99. Scott LJ, Figgitt DP, Keam SJ, Waugh J. Acamprosate: a review of its use in the maintenance of abstinence in patients with alcohol dependence. *CNS Drugs* (2005) 19:445–64. doi: 10.2165/00023210-200519050-00006
100. Plosker GL. Acamprosate: a review of its use in alcohol dependence. *Drugs* (2015) 75:1255–68. doi: 10.1007/s40265-015-0423-9
101. Schneider U, Wohlfarth K, Schulze-Bonhage A, Haacker T, Muller-Vahl KR, Zedler M, et al. Effects of acamprosate on memory in healthy young subjects. *J Stud Alcohol* (1999) 60:172–5. doi: 10.15288/jsa.1999.60.172
102. Okulicz-Kozaryn I, Midolajczak P, Szczawinska K, Kaminska E, Kus K. Effects of acamprosate and scopolamine on the working memory of rats in a three-panel runway task. *J Basic Clin Physiol Pharmacol.* (2001) 12:197–216. doi: 10.1515/JBCPP.2001.12.3.197
103. Ralevski E, O'Brien E, Jane JS, Dean E, Dwan R, Petrakis I. Effects of acamprosate on cognition in a treatment study of patients with schizophrenia spectrum disorders and comorbid alcohol dependence. *J Nerv Ment Dis.* (2011) 199:499–505. doi: 10.1097/NMD.0b013e3182214297
104. Hu W, Morris B, Carrasco A, Kroener S. Effects of acamprosate on attentional set-shifting and cellular function in the prefrontal cortex of chronic alcohol-exposed mice. *Alcohol Clin Exp Res.* (2015) 39:953–61. doi: 10.1111/acer.12722
105. Pradhan G, Melugin PR, Wu F, Fang HM, Weber R, Kroener S. Calcium chloride mimics the effects of acamprosate on cognitive deficits in chronic alcohol-exposed mice. *Psychopharmacology* (2018) 235:2027–40. doi: 10.1007/s00213-018-4900-1
106. Michel ME, Bolger G, Weissman BA. Binding of a new opiate antagonist, nalmefene, to rat brain membranes. *Methods Find Exp Clin Pharmacol.* (1985) 7:175–7.
107. Niciu MJ, Arias AJ. Targeted opioid receptor antagonists in the treatment of alcohol use disorders. *CNS Drugs* (2013) 27:777–87. doi: 10.1007/s40263-013-0096-4
108. Abraham AD, Fontaine HM, Song AJ, Andrews MM, Baird MA, Kieffer BL, et al. kappa-opioid receptor activation in dopamine neurons disrupts behavioral inhibition. *Neuropsychopharmacology* (2018) 43:362–72. doi: 10.1038/npp.2017.133
109. Walker BM, Kissler JL. Dissociable effects of kappa-opioid receptor activation on impulsive phenotypes in wistar rats. *Neuropsychopharmacology* (2013) 38:2278–85. doi: 10.1038/npp.2013.129
110. Daumas S, Betourne A, Halley H, Wolfer DP, Lipp HP, Lassalle JM, et al. Transient activation of the CA3 Kappa opioid system in the dorsal hippocampus modulates complex memory processing in mice. *Neurobiol Learn Mem.* (2007) 88:94–103. doi: 10.1016/j.nlm.2007.02.001
111. Wall PM, Messier C. U-69,593 microinjection in the infralimbic cortex reduces anxiety and enhances spontaneous alternation memory in mice. *Brain Res.* (2000) 856:259–80. doi: 10.1016/S0006-8993(99)01990-3
112. Yeomans MR, Wright P, Macleod HA, Critchley JA. Effects of nalmefene on feeding in humans. dissociation of hunger and palatability *Psychopharmacology* (1990) 100:426–32. doi: 10.1007/BF02244618
113. Johansson BA, Berglund M, Lindgren A. Efficacy of maintenance treatment with naltrexone for opioid dependence: a meta-analytical review. *Addiction* (2006) 101:491–503. doi: 10.1111/j.1360-0443.2006.01369.x
114. Rosner S, Hackl-Herrwerth A, Leucht S, Vecchi S, Srisurapanont M, Soyka M. Opioid antagonists for alcohol dependence. *Cochrane Database Syst Rev.* (2010) 8:Cd001867. doi: 10.1002/14651858.CD001867.pub3
115. Roberts AJ, McDonald JS, Heyser CJ, Kieffer BL, Matthes HW, Koob GF, et al. mu-Opioid receptor knockout mice do not self-administer alcohol. *J Pharmacol Exp Ther.* (2000) 293:1002–8. Available online at: http://jpet.aspetjournals.org/content/293/3/1002
116. Hatsukami DK, Mitchell JE, Morley JE, Morgan SF, Levine AS. Effect of naltrexone on mood and cognitive functioning among overweight men. *Biol Psychiatry* (1986) 21:293–300. doi: 10.1016/0006-3223(86)90050-8
117. Canli T, Cook RG, Miczek KA. Opiate antagonists enhance the working memory of rats in the radial maze. *Pharmacol Biochem Behav.* (1990) 36:521–5. doi: 10.1016/0091-3057(90)90250-L
118. Lai H, Horita A, Guy AW. Microwave irradiation affects radial-arm maze performance in the rat. *Bioelectromagnetics* (1994) 15:95–104. doi: 10.1002/bem.2250150202
119. Cobb BL, Jauchem JR, Adair ER. Radial arm maze performance of rats following repeated low level microwave radiation exposure. *Bioelectromagnetics* (2004) 25:49–57. doi: 10.1002/bem.10148
120. Kieres AK, Hausknecht KA, Farrar AM, Acheson A, de Wit H, Richards JB. Effects of morphine and naltrexone on impulsive decision making in rats. *Psychopharmacology* (2004) 173:167–74. doi: 10.1007/s00213-003-1697-2
121. Oberlin BG, Bristow RE, Heighton ME, Grahame NJ. Pharmacologic dissociation between impulsivity and alcohol drinking in high alcohol preferring mice. *Alcohol Clin Exp Res.* (2010) 34:1363–75. doi: 10.1111/j.1530-0277.2010.01220.x
122. Di Ciano P, Le Foll B. Evaluating the impact of naltrexone on the rat gambling task to test its predictive validity for gambling disorder. *PLoS ONE* (2016) 11:e0155604. doi: 10.1371/journal.pone.0155604
123. Wiskerke J, Schetters D, van Es IE, van Mourik Y, den Hollander BR, Schoffelmeer AN, et al. mu-Opioid receptors in the nucleus accumbens shell region mediate the effects of amphetamine on inhibitory control but not impulsive choice. *J Neurosci.* (2011) 31:262–72. doi: 10.1523/JNEUROSCI.4794-10.2011
124. Mitchell JM, Tavares VC, Fields HL, D'Esposito M, Boettiger CA. Endogenous opioid blockade and impulsive responding in alcoholics and healthy controls. *Neuropsychopharmacology* (2007) 32:439–49. doi: 10.1038/sj.npp.1301226
125. Declerck CH, Boone C, De Brabander B. On feeling in control: a biological theory for individual differences in control perception. *Brain Cogn.* (2006) 62:143–76. doi: 10.1016/j.bandc.2006.04.004
126. Kelm MK, Boettiger CA. Effects of acute dopamine precusor depletion on immediate reward selection bias and working memory depend on catechol-O-methyltransferase genotype. *J Cogn Neurosci.* (2013) 25:2061–71. doi: 10.1162/jocn_a_00464
127. Spanagel R, Herz A, Shippenberg TS. Opposing tonically active endogenous opioid systems modulate the mesolimbic dopaminergic pathway. *Proc Natl Acad Sci USA.* (1992) 89:2046–50. doi: 10.1073/pnas.89.6.2046
128. Rodefer JS, Nguyen TN. Naltrexone reverses age-induced cognitive deficits in rats. *Neurobiol Aging* (2008) 29:309–13. doi: 10.1016/j.neurobiolaging.2006.10.005
129. Messinis L, Lyros E, Andrian V, Katsakiori P, Panagis G, Georgiou V, et al. Neuropsychological functioning in buprenorphine maintained patients versus abstinent heroin abusers on naltrexone hydrochloride therapy. *Hum Psychopharmacol.* (2009) 24:524–31. doi: 10.1002/hup.1050
130. Mattick RP, Breen C, Kimber J, Davoli M. Methadone maintenance therapy versus no opioid replacement therapy for opioid dependence. *Cochrane Database Syst Rev.* (2009) 8:Cd002209. doi: 10.1002/14651858.CD002209.pub2
131. Soyka M, Zingg C, Koller G, Hennig-Fast K. Cognitive function in short- and long-term substitution treatment: are there differences? *World J Biol Psychiatry* (2010) 11:400–8. doi: 10.3109/15622970902995604
132. Verdejo A, Toribio I, Orozco C, Puente KL, Perez-Garcia M. Neuropsychological functioning in methadone maintenance patients versus abstinent heroin abusers. *Drug Alcohol Depend* (2005) 78:283–8. doi: 10.1016/j.drugalcdep.2004.11.006
133. Zeng H, Su D, Jiang X, Zhu L, Ye H. The similarities and differences in impulsivity and cognitive ability among ketamine, methadone, and non-drug users. *Psychiatry Res.* (2016) 243:109–14. doi: 10.1016/j.psychres.2016.04.095
134. Rass O, Kleykamp BA, Vandrey RG, Bigelow GE, Leoutsakos JM, Stitzer ML, et al. Cognitive performance in methadone maintenance patients: effects of time relative to dosing and maintenance dose level. *Exp Clin Psychopharmacol.* (2014) 22:248–56. doi: 10.1037/a0035712

135. Mazhari S, Keshvari Z, Sabahi A, Mottaghian S. Assessment of cognitive functions in methadone maintenance patients. *Addict Health* (2015) 7: 109–16. Available online at: http://ahj.kmu.ac.ir/index.php/ahj/article/view/298/262
136. Mintzer MZ, Copersino ML, Stitzer ML. Opioid abuse and cognitive performance. *Drug Alcohol Depend* (2005) 78:225–30. doi: 10.1016/j.drugalcdep.2004.10.008
137. Elkana O, Adelson M, Doniger GM, Sason A, Peles E. Cognitive function is largely intact in methadone maintenance treatment patients. *World J Biol Psychiatry* (2017) 1–11. doi: 10.1080/15622975.2017.1342047
138. Liao DL, Huang CY, Hu S, Fang SC, Wu CS, Chen WT, et al. Cognitive control in opioid dependence and methadone maintenance treatment. *PLoS ONE* (2014) 9:e94589. doi: 10.1371/journal.pone.0094589
139. Bracken BK, Trksak GH, Penetar DM, Tartarini WL, Maywalt MA, Dorsey CM, et al. Response inhibition and psychomotor speed during methadone maintenance: impact of treatment duration, dose, and sleep deprivation. *Drug Alcohol Depend* (2012) 125:132–9. doi: 10.1016/j.drugalcdep.2012.04.004
140. Darke S, Sims J, McDonald S, Wickes W. Cognitive impairment among methadone maintenance patients. *Addiction* (2000) 95:687–95. doi: 10.1046/j.1360-0443.2000.9556874.x
141. Wang GY, Wouldes TA, Kydd R, Jensen M, Russell BR. Neuropsychological performance of methadone-maintained opiate users. *J Psychopharmacol.* (2014) 28:789–99. doi: 10.1177/0269881114538541
142. Gruber SA, Tzilos GK, Silveri MM, Pollack M, Renshaw PF, Kaufman MJ, et al. Methadone maintenance improves cognitive performance after two months of treatment. *Exp Clin Psychopharmacol.* (2006) 14:157–64. doi: 10.1037/1064-1297.14.2.157
143. Levy-Gigi E, Keri S, Shapiro AR, Sason A, Adelson M, Peles E. Methadone maintenance patients show a selective deficit to reverse positive outcomes in drug-related conditions compared to medication free prolonged opiate abstinence. *Drug Alcohol Depend* (2014) 144:111–8. doi: 10.1016/j.drugalcdep.2014.08.016
144. Gowing L, Ali R, White JM, Mbewe D. Buprenorphine for managing opioid withdrawal. *Cochrane Database Syst Rev.* (2017) 2:Cd002025. doi: 10.1002/14651858.CD002025.pub5
145. Mintzer MZ, Correia CJ, Strain EC. A dose-effect study of repeated administration of buprenorphine/naloxone on performance in opioid-dependent volunteers. *Drug Alcohol Depend* (2004) 74:205–9. doi: 10.1016/j.drugalcdep.2003.12.008
146. Rapeli P, Fabritius C, Alho H, Salaspuro M, Wahlbeck K, Kalska H. Methadone vs. buprenorphine/naloxone during early opioid substitution treatment: a naturalistic comparison of cognitive performance relative to healthy controls *BMC Clin Pharmacol.* (2007) 7:5. doi: 10.1186/1472-6904-7-5
147. Rapeli P, Fabritius C, Kalska H, Alho H. Cognitive functioning in opioid-dependent patients treated with buprenorphine, methadone, and other psychoactive medications: stability and correlates. *BMC Clin Pharmacol.* (2011) 11:13. doi: 10.1186/1472-6904-11-13
148. Darke S, McDonald S, Kaye S, Torok M. Comparative patterns of cognitive performance amongst opioid maintenance patients, abstinent opioid users and non-opioid users. *Drug Alcohol Depend* (2012) 126:309–15. doi: 10.1016/j.drugalcdep.2012.05.032
149. Pirastu R, Fais R, Messina M, Bini V, Spiga S, Falconieri D, et al. Impaired decision-making in opiate-dependent subjects: effect of pharmacological therapies. *Drug Alcohol Depend* (2006) 83:163–8. doi: 10.1016/j.drugalcdep.2005.11.008
150. Bechara A, Damasio AR, Damasio H, Anderson SW. Insensitivity to future consequences following damage to human prefrontal cortex. *Cognition* (1994) 50:7–15. doi: 10.1016/0010-0277(94)90018-3
151. Chan RCK, Shum D, Toulopoulou T, Chen EYH. Assessment of executive functions: Review of instruments and identification of critical issues. *Arch Clin Neuropsychol.* (2008) 23:201–16. doi: 10.1016/j.acn.2007.08.010
152. Jensen ML, Sjogren P, Upton RN, Foster DJ, Bonde P, Graae C, et al. Pharmacokinetic-pharmacodynamic relationships of cognitive and psychomotor effects of intravenous buprenorphine infusion in human volunteers. *Basic Clin Pharmacol Toxicol.* (2008) 103:94–101. doi: 10.1111/j.1742-7843.2008.00250.x
153. Soyka M, Lieb M, Kagerer S, Zingg C, Koller G, Lehnert P, et al. Cognitive functioning during methadone and buprenorphine treatment: results of a randomized clinical trial. *J Clin Psychopharmacol.* (2008) 28:699–703. doi: 10.1097/JCP.0b013e31818a6d38
154. Giacomuzzi S, Thill C, Riemer Y, Garber K, Ertl M. Buprenorphine- and methadone maintenance treatment: influence on aspects of cognitive and memory performance. *Open Addict J.* (2008) 1:5–6. doi: 10.2174/1874941000801010005
155. Loeber S, Kniest A, Diehl A, Mann K, Croissant B. Neuropsychological functioning of opiate-dependent patients: a nonrandomized comparison of patients preferring either buprenorphine or methadone maintenance treatment. *Am J Drug Alcohol Abuse.* (2008) 34:584–93. doi: 10.1080/00952990802308239
156. Bowie CR, Harvey PD. Administration and interpretation of the Trail Making Test. *Nat Protoc.* (2006) 1:2277–81. doi: 10.1038/nprot.2006.390
157. Grant DA, Berg EA. A behavioral analysis of degree of reinforcement and ease of shifting to new responses in a Weigl-type card-sorting problem. *J Exp Psychol.* (1948) 38:404–11. doi: 10.1037/h0059831
158. Gish EC, Miller JL, Honey BL, Johnson PN. Lofexidine, an {alpha}2-receptor agonist for opioid detoxification. *Ann Pharmacother.* (2010) 44:343–51. doi: 10.1345/aph.1M347
159. Schroeder JR, Schmittner J, Bleiberg J, Epstein DH, Krantz MJ, Preston KL. Hemodynamic and cognitive effects of lofexidine and methadone coadministration: a pilot study. *Pharmacotherapy* (2007) 27:1111–9. doi: 10.1592/phco.27.8.1111
160. Ramos BP, Arnsten AF. Adrenergic pharmacology and cognition: focus on the prefrontal cortex. *Pharmacol Ther.* (2007) 113:523–36. doi: 10.1016/j.pharmthera.2006.11.006
161. Leyton M, Vezina P. Dopamine ups and downs in vulnerability to addictions: a neurodevelopmental model. *Trends Pharmacol Sci.* (2014) 35:268–76. doi: 10.1016/j.tips.2014.04.002
162. Thiruchselvam T, Malik S, Le Foll B. A review of positron emission tomography studies exploring the dopaminergic system in substance use with a focus on tobacco as a co-variate. *Am J Drug Alcohol Abuse* (2017) 43:197–214. doi: 10.1080/00952990.2016.1257633
163. Volkow ND, Fowler JS, Wang GJ, Baler R, Telang F. Imaging dopamine's role in drug abuse and addiction. *Neuropharmacology* (2009) 56(Suppl. 1):3–8. doi: 10.1016/j.neuropharm.2008.05.022
164. Melis M, Spiga S, Diana M. The dopamine hypothesis of drug addiction: hypodopaminergic state. *Int Rev Neurobiol.* (2005) 63:101–54. doi: 10.1016/S0074-7742(05)63005-X
165. Narendran R, Mason NS, Paris J, Himes ML, Douaihy AB, Frankle WG. Decreased prefrontal cortical dopamine transmission in alcoholism. *Am J Psychiatry* (2014) 171:881–8. doi: 10.1176/appi.ajp.2014.13121581
166. Martinez D, Carpenter KM, Liu F, Slifstein M, Broft A, Friedman AC, et al. Imaging dopamine transmission in cocaine dependence: link between neurochemistry and response to treatment. *Am J Psychiatry* (2011) 168:634–41. doi: 10.1176/appi.ajp.2010.10050748
167. Wang GJ, Smith L, Volkow ND, Telang F, Logan J, Tomasi D, et al. Decreased dopamine activity predicts relapse in methamphetamine abusers. *Mol Psychiatry* (2012) 17:918–25. doi: 10.1038/mp.2011.86
168. Wuo-Silva R, Fukushiro DF, Borcoi AR, Fernandes HA, Procopio-Souza R, Hollais AW, et al. Addictive potential of modafinil and cross-sensitization with cocaine: a pre-clinical study. *Addict Biol.* (2011) 16:565–79. doi: 10.1111/j.1369-1600.2011.00341.x
169. Houben K, Wiers RW, Jansen A. Getting a grip on drinking behavior: training working memory to reduce alcohol abuse. *Psychol Sci.* (2011) 22:968–75. doi: 10.1177/0956797611412392
170. Rass O, Schacht RL, Buckheit K, Johnson MW, Strain EC, Mintzer MZ. A randomized controlled trial of the effects of working memory training in methadone maintenance patients. *Drug Alcohol Depend* (2015) 156:38–46. doi: 10.1016/j.drugalcdep.2015.08.012

171. Bowley C, Faricy C, Hegarty B, Johnstone SJ, Smith LJ, Kelly PJ, et al. The effects of inhibitory control training on alcohol consumption, implicit alcohol-related cognitions and brain electrical activity. *Int J Psychophysiol.* (2013) 89:342–8. doi: 10.1016/j.ijpsycho.2013.04.011

172. Wessel JR, O'Doherty JP, Berkebile MM, Linderman D, Aron AR. Stimulus devaluation induced by stopping action. *J Exp Psychol Gen.* (2014) 143:2316–29. doi: 10.1037/xge0000022

173. Czoty PW, Stoops WW, Rush CR. Evaluation of the "Pipeline" for development of medications for cocaine use disorder: a review of translational preclinical, human laboratory, and clinical trial research. *Pharmacol Rev.* (2016) 68:533–62. doi: 10.1124/pr.115.011668

174. Lee NK, Jenner L, Harney A, Cameron J. Pharmacotherapy for amphetamine dependence: a systematic review. *Drug Alcohol Depend* (2018) 191:309–37. doi: 10.1016/j.drugalcdep.2018.06.038

# 11

# A Novel Hierarchical LATER Process Model: Evaluating Latent Sources of Variation in Reaction Times of Adult Daily Smokers

*Nicole J. Roberts*[1]*, *Zita Oravecz*[1,2], *Briana N. Sprague*[1] *and Charles F. Geier*[1]*

[1] *Department of Human Development and Family Studies, The Pennsylvania State University, University Park, PA, United States,* [2] *Institute for CyberScience, The Pennsylvania State University, University Park, PA, United States*

***Correspondence:**
*Nicole J. Roberts*
*njr175@psu.edu*
*Charles Geier*
*cfg2@psu.edu*

Reaction time data from cognitive tasks continue to be a key way to assess decision-making in various contexts to better understand addiction. The goal of this paper is twofold: to introduce a nuanced modeling approach for reaction time data and to demonstrate the novel insights it can provide into the decision processes of nicotine-dependent individuals in different contexts. We focus on the Linear Approach to Threshold with Ergodic Rate (LATER) model, which is a cognitive process model that describes reaction time data in terms of two distinct aspects of cognitive functioning: speed of information accumulation ("accretion") and threshold amount of information needed prior to execution ("caution"). We introduce a novel hierarchical extension to the LATER model to simultaneously account for differences across persons and experimental conditions, both in the accretion and caution parameters. This approach allows for the inclusion of person-specific predictor variables to explain between-person variation in terms of accretion and caution together with condition-specific predictors to model experimental condition manipulations. To highlight the usefulness of this model, we analyze reaction time data from a study on adult daily cigarette smokers. Participants performed a monetary incentivized Go/No-Go task during two testing sessions, once while following their typical smoking patterns and again following 12 h of verified smoking abstinence. Our main results suggest that regardless of trial type, smokers in a period of abstinence have faster accretion rates, and lower caution thresholds relative to smoking as usual.

**Keywords: smoking, cognition, cognitive model, abstinence, Go/NoGo task**

## INTRODUCTION

A fundamental goal of psychiatry and neuroscience research is to understand how and why humans make decisions and behave as they do across various contexts. In particular, work aimed at understanding how exposure to addictive substances like nicotine impacts and alters decision-making is of considerable interest. The examination of reaction time data acquired from cognitive tasks continues to be a major way to assess decision-making, yet traditional analysis of such data (e.g., evaluation of group-level means and variances) limits the extent to which we can assess or estimate latent (psychological) processes that may be underlying the decision/behavior. To address these limitations, *cognitive process models* were developed, which use theoretically derived model parameters that represent latent psychological constructs to better account for individual differences in the complex processes underlying human decisions and behavior; see, for example, Stout et al. (1), Yechiam et al. (2), Cohen et al. (3), and Hauser et al. (4) for a variety of models and applications.

In this paper, we focus on one particular process model, the Linear Approach to Threshold with Ergodic Rate (LATER) model, which was developed to capture individual differences in the underlying mechanisms of decision-making using data from reaction time tasks (5, 6). We extend the basic LATER model hierarchically in order to assess sources of both individual and experimental condition specific differences in reaction times. Moreover, we cast the hierarchical LATER model in the Bayesian framework, which provides a convenient approach for simultaneous estimation of person-specific LATER process parameters and regression coefficients related to person-specific (e.g., age) and condition-specific (e.g., experimental manipulation of reward, smoking status) effects. Additionally, casting the model in the Bayesian framework allows for inference in terms of statements about posterior probabilities. We assert that coalescing advanced process models with experimental manipulations (e.g., abstinence vs. smoking to satiety in smokers) can help us better understand how drug exposure (e.g., nicotine) affects the underlying mental processes guiding decision-making and behavior, and may provide insights for a better understanding of addiction, particularly at the individual level.

In the sections that follow, we first describe the use of process models and specify the LATER model we hierarchically extended and employed. We then apply this novel model to reaction time data obtained from a sample of adult daily smokers to demonstrate its potential utility in addiction research.

## Modeling Reaction Times With the LATER Model

The time interval between stimulus presentation and initiation of a behavioral response is defined as the reaction time, or latency, and includes multiple underlying physiological processes occurring on varying time scales. For example, relatively rapid processes, on the order of tens of milliseconds, include transduction of the external stimulus energy to a neural response, signal propagation time from the periphery to the central nervous system and back, and muscle activation, among others. More temporally extended processes comprising reaction time include brain network-level computations (on the order of hundreds of milliseconds) related to making a decision, that is, forming and maintaining internal representations of the stimuli, then planning and executing a goal-directed motor plan. It is believed that these central, network-level computations comprise a majority of the reaction time (7, 8). As fast sensory and motor times are relatively fixed, reaction time variability is therefore a useful approximation of *decision time* (9). In other words, reaction time largely reflects the time needed to decide.

Researchers utilize tailored tasks that attempt to delineate the cognitive processes underlying reaction times in order to gain insight into decision processes and factors that influence them. However, reaction times are typically evaluated in terms of average performance across groups and/or study conditions. This approach disregards the potential variability in the processes underlying latency values, i.e., intraindividual variability across trials in a task. Indeed, in experimental paradigms, reaction time can vary significantly between one trial to the next, even if the same experimental conditions are maintained (9).

Capturing variability in reaction times with process models can provide additional information about the underlying mechanisms of decisions. One major theoretical framework for understanding decision-making holds that the brain accumulates relevant information until the resultant probability reaches a threshold that warrants action (10). The length of time in which it takes to reach this threshold depends on the dynamics of the rise-to-threshold (10). The LATER model describes the latency distributions of observed reaction times by characterizing the decision-making process in terms of two cognitive variables. The first is *caution*, or the amount of information needed to exceed a threshold to respond. The caution parameter represents the attitude toward partial prior information in a similar manner as a loss function represents the attitude toward risk (11). The second variable is *accretion*, or the rate (speed) of information accumulation. Bickel and colleagues (11) argue that caution can be seen as assigning an operational definition to the degree of conservatism toward ambiguity, and accretion rate as the assimilating capacity.

Utilizing the LATER model to describe reaction time data based on accretion rates and caution thresholds better reflects the actual shape of reaction time data relative to traditional averaging approaches. One of the most salient properties of the stochastic distribution of reaction times is that they are generally positive skewed; the distributions rise rapidly and then fall off slowly with a long, right-tailed skew. This is a near universal finding, regardless of stimulus type (e.g., visual, auditory), response (e.g., manual, oculomotor), or species [see Ref. (12)]. Interestingly, when plotted, this skewed distribution does not fit any of the traditional mathematical distributions like Gaussian or Poisson particularly well [e.g., Refs. (9, 12, 13)]. However, if one wants to examine the underlying mechanisms for the variability, rather than its effect (14, 15), then the *reciprocal* of the reaction time should be examined. If reciprocal latencies are plotted cumulatively (a reciprobit plot), a straight line will be obtained. This represents the *rate* at which the decision reaches completion, and follows a normal, Gaussian distribution (see below). Accordingly, the LATER model explains this general feature of reaction time distribution by appropriately modeling the rate of rise for each trial, varying in a Gaussian fashion, which explains the observed shape of latency distributions [see Ref. (12) for review].

This results in describing reaction time distributions by utilizing a model with a decision signal starting point, which then rises at a constant rate until it reaches a threshold value, at which point a response is initiated. Accordingly, the LATER model is a sequential-sampling model, which assumes that during the course of a trial, information is accumulated sequentially until a threshold amount of information is reached and a response is executed. Indeed, the LATER model explains the observed features of reaction time distributions by assuming that a stimulus triggers a neuronal decision signal to rise linearly until it reaches a threshold value in which a response is then executed. This rate of rise for each trial varies in a Gaussian fashion, explaining the observed shape of latency distributions. Modeling reaction time with the LATER model has provided novel insight into the cognitive components (accretion, caution) underlying reaction times in healthy individuals [see Ref. (12) for review and additional details on the original LATER model].

We argue that the LATER model can benefit from being cast in a hierarchical/multilevel framework (16, 17). Oravecz et al. (18) described a hierarchical extension to the LATER model that allowed for a person-specific accretion rate. We extend this approach by allowing for individual differences in both accretion *and* caution parameters. The multilevel extension enables us to model the individual-level repeated measures of reaction times with the LATER process and pool information across the resulting latent, person-specific accretion and caution parameters *via* joint population (group-level) distributions. The multilevel framework also provides us with a statistically principled way to add person-level predictors on these two latent parameters (e.g., to test if the number of cigarettes smoked per day is related to slower information accumulation). In our proposed model, all latent person-specific parameters and corresponding regression coefficients are estimated simultaneously, as opposed to first obtaining point estimates of caution and accretion for each person and then regressing those on predictors, which can lead to bias in the regression coefficient estimates [see Ref. (19)]. Importantly, we will also introduce condition-specific predictors to capture how accretion and caution differ as a function of experimental manipulation (e.g., smoking as usual vs. abstinence). The estimation of condition and person-specific effects is again simultaneous. The ability to have different groups and experimental manipulations within the same model also allows for direct statistical comparisons between the conditions/groups.

## Specification of the Hierarchical LATER Model

Next we introduce the model specification for the hierarchical LATER model. We start with describing the LATER model as originally outlined [see Ref. (5); for reviews see Refs. (9, 12)], but with multilevel extensions to both caution and accretion parameters. Then we describe how the single-step regression is formulated on the person-specific caution (threshold) and accretion rate (information accumulation), and we finish with showing how condition-specific effects can be incorporated in the same model.

Data will be denoted as $y_{p,i}$ for person $p$ and trial $i$. We allow each subject $p$ to have their own accretion ($v_p$) and caution ($\theta_p$) parameters. On a trial $i$, a trial and person-specific realization of the accretion rate, $z_{p,i}$ is modeled through a normal (Gaussian) distribution with the following specification:

$$Z_{p,i} \sim N(v_p, 1) \tag{1}$$

We can get the predicted response time (or latency) at trial $i$ for person $p$ ($y_{p,i}$) by dividing the person-specific caution by the person-specific accretion rate on trial $i$:

$$y_{p,i} = \frac{\theta_p}{Z_{p,i}},$$

which can be rearranged to yield:

$$\frac{z_{p,i}}{\theta_p} = \frac{1}{y_{p,i}}$$

To get the distribution of $\frac{z_{p,i}}{\theta_p}$, we divide the distribution of $z_{p,i}$ specified in Equation 1 by $\theta_p$:

$$\frac{z_{p,i}}{\theta_p} = \frac{1}{y_{p,i}} \sim N\left(\frac{v_p}{\theta_p}, \frac{1}{\theta_p^2}\right)$$

To summarize, the LATER model assumes sequential sampling; it assumes that over the course of a trial, information is accumulated sequentially until a threshold amount of information is reached, at which time a response is executed. This resulting accretion process (i.e., information accumulation) is assumed to be linear and eventually reaches a fixed threshold, with a rate that is random from trial to trial, as shown in **Figure 1**. Importantly, this trial-to-trial random rate is one of the key motivations to model reaction time with the LATER model approach.

To model similarities across individuals in terms of accretion and caution, we will assume that all person-specific LATER process parameters come from joint group-level (or level-2 or population) distributions. These group-level distributions also provide for a straightforward manner to regress these parameters on relevant person predictors (e.g., cigarettes smoked per day) to further improve the model. Therefore, in our application, the means of the population distributions of caution and accretion are made into the function of person predictors. Assume that $K$ person covariates are measured and $x_{p,k}$ denotes the score of person $p$ on covariate $k$ ($k = 1, \ldots, K$). For example, in our application we considered that age, gender, cigarettes smoked per day, and nicotine dependence level (as assessed by the Fagerström Test for Nicotine Dependence; FTND) could be possible sources of individual differences among persons; therefore, we included them as person predictors. All person-specific covariate scores are collected into a vector, with the length $K$+1, denoted as $\mathbf{x}_p = (1, x_{p1}, x_{p2}, \ldots, x_{pK})^T$, where the first element is an intercept. The group-level distribution of the person-specific accretion parameters $v_p$ is then formulated as

$$v_p = \mathbf{x}_p \beta v + \varepsilon_{p,v}$$

where vector $\boldsymbol{\beta}_v$, of dimension $1 \times (K+1)$, contains the regression weights for the person predictors (e.g., association between FTND and accretion) and $\varepsilon_{p,v}$ is normally distributed with

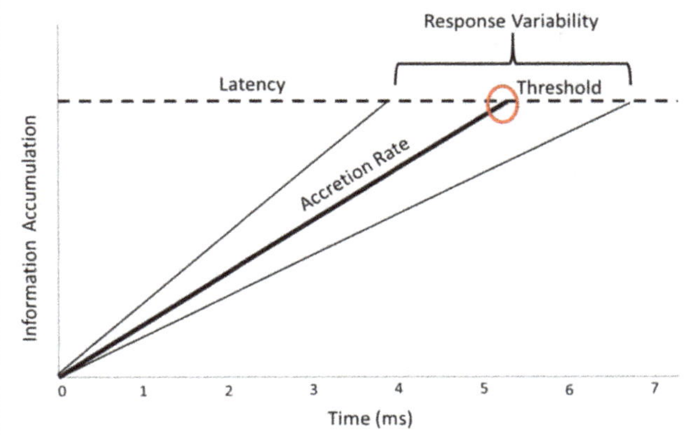


**FIGURE 1 |** Visual representation of the cognitive processes (accretion rate and caution threshold) examined in the Linear Approach to Threshold with Ergodic Rate (LATER) model.

mean 0 and variance $\sigma_v^2$, quantifying residual unexplained inter-individual differences (random effects). Following similar logic, the group-level distribution of the person-specific caution parameters was modeled similarly: $\theta_p = \mathbf{x}_p \beta_\theta + \varepsilon_{p,\theta.}$ Besides person-specific differences, covariates capturing experimental conditions can also be included in the model. In our application (described below), smokers completed the task under two conditions, smoking as usual vs. abstinent. Abstinence was operationalized as abstaining from smoking for a minimum of 12 h. Baseline measures of exhaled CO were taken during a screening procedure, allowing for verification of an abstinence state. The task was composed of two trial types, reward vs. neutral. The design was completely crossed; all participants completed both conditions and trial types (smoking as usual-reward trials, smoking as usual-neutral trials, abstinent-reward trials, abstinent-neutral trials). We selected smoking as usual and neutral as the baseline, and dummy coded the neutral–abstinent, reward–abstinent, and reward–smoking as usual conditions. The regression coefficients corresponding to these dummy-coded condition-specific variables represent the deviations of a condition from the baseline (i.e., smoking as usual-neutral reward).

We denote these covariates for every data point as $g_{n,c}$ where $n = (1, 2, \ldots, N)$, with $N$ representing the total number of reaction times in the experiment and $c = (1, 2, \ldots, C)$, and $C$ representing the number of dummy-coded conditions minus 1 (baseline). Corresponding regression coefficients are denoted as $\delta_{v,c}$ for accretion and $\delta_{\theta,c}$ for the caution threshold. **Table 1** shows the conditions (reward vs. neutral and smoking as usual vs. abstinent) with corresponding regression terms for further clarification of the design. To formulate the LATER model with these experimental condition effects, we introduce a more general notation than that of Equation 1 for data $y_{p,i}$: we stack all trials for the persons $p$ under each other, resulting in a long vector of reaction time scores, where $n$ stands for a single trial (up to $N$), and then we rewrite the model as:

**TABLE 1 |** Describes the design matrix of the current study; the two conditions (Smoke as Usual, Abstinent) and two trial types (reward, neutral) with corresponding regression terms are shown here for the person-specific pater parameters.

| | Smoke as Usual | Abstinent |
|---|---|---|
| Neutral | $\delta_{v,1}, \delta_{\theta,1}$ | Baselines |
| Reward | $\delta_{v,3}, \delta_{\theta,3}$ | $\delta_{v,2}, \delta_{\theta,2}$ |

$$y_n \sim N\left(\frac{v_n}{\theta_n}, \frac{1}{\theta_n^2}\right)$$

For example, with the three conditions we introduced, the accretion is then modeled as:

$$v_n = v_p + g_{n,1}\delta_{v,1} + g_{n,2}\delta_{v,2} + g_{n,3}\delta_{v,3}$$

which can be written in a more general form:

$$v_n = v_p + \mathbf{g}\delta_v$$

Similar formulation applies to the caution parameter:

$$\theta_n = \theta_{p\,+}\mathbf{g}\delta_\theta$$

This formulation allows us to model the effect of the experimental manipulation in terms of meaningful process model parameters while also capturing individual differences in these parameters.

## Modeling in the Hierarchical Bayesian Framework

The hierarchically extended LATER model was cast in the Bayesian framework. In this framework, both data and model parameters are defined as random variables and the Bayesian model specifies their joint probability distribution (20). With this approach, statistical inference is focused on the posterior probability distribution of the parameters, which is derived by combining the likelihood and prior distribution on the model parameters based on Bayes' rule. The prior distributions are integral parts of the model; the mean of the prior suggests the likely parameter value, and the variance of the prior distribution reflects the level of uncertainty about the possible values of the parameter of interest. This analysis is the mathematically normative way to reallocate credibility across parameter values as new data arrive (21).

In the Bayesian framework, inferences about parameters are based on the posterior probability distributions of the parameters. The posterior distribution is stochastically approximated by taking a large number of samples from it, and then calculating posterior point estimates, posterior standard deviations (similar to that of the standard error), and posterior credible intervals for each parameter. One of the key strengths in fitting a hierarchical model with a Bayesian statistical approach is that these algorithms are able to fit increasingly complex models to the data (22). This is especially useful for our model as we can estimate all person-specific parameters, group-level variances, and regression coefficients corresponding to person and condition effects simultaneously. Parameter estimation was implemented in Stan (23); software code for the model is provided in **Appendix A**. The utilized data and accompanying R script are also provided as an **Online Supplement** on the project's Open Science Framework (OSF) page: https://osf.io/5h8m4/?view_only=f6c1e50dcfa04244bba428d6cf259d36

## Model Application—Smokers

We fit the hierarchical LATER model to data from "go" trials from a Go/No-Go task performed by a group of adult daily smokers to gain further insight into cognitive changes associated with smoking abstinence. While the Go/No-Go task is a paradigm typically used to investigate inhibitory control (no-go trials), it can also be a highly informative task in terms of assessing what cognitive mechanisms support "go" decisions (12, 24). Notably, go trials in this task far outnumber the number of no-go trials, increasing power and adding an additional dimension of rich data to analyze from this classic task. Prior studies have utilized the Go/No-Go behavioral paradigm to study the effect of nicotine use on cognitive systems using reaction times [e.g., Refs. (25–27)]; these studies manipulate the task environment in various ways, such as smoking status (e.g., daily smoker vs. non-smoker) and session type (e.g., smoking to satiety vs. abstinent). However, findings from these studies thus far have only demonstrated differences in reaction times (and error rates) between these various manipulations. While these studies have been informative in highlighting the fact that nicotine impacts task performance under particular task manipulations, they fail to explain how. That is, what are the underlying mechanisms of reaction times (i.e., components of decision-making) that nicotine affects?

Given widespread effects of nicotine on cognitive brain systems [e.g., Refs. (25, 26, 28–35)], we hypothesize that nicotine will affect psychological (cognitive) processes important for decision-making, including caution threshold and accretion rates. Furthermore, given that nicotine is known to alter (decrease) responsiveness to non-drug (e.g., money), particularly during periods of smoking abstinence [e.g., Refs. (33, 36–38)], we hypothesize that the availability of rewards may differentially impact caution and accretion depending on smoking status, as these likely interact with reward processes during incentivized decision-making [e.g., Ref. (29)]. We suggest that these effects may be masked or confounded when analyzing latencies via traditional average mean scores. In addition, traditional analysis is often based on averaging task performance across individuals per experimental condition, disregarding possible intraindividual differences that may be present. Failure to account for such differences may contribute to inconsistent results found in previous work [see Ref. (39)]. By utilizing the LATER process modeling approach instead of relying on statistical summaries of raw reaction times, substantively meaningful latent model parameters (accretion and threshold) are calculated and updated in a trial-by-trial manner, better capturing intraindividual processes. Moreover, by allowing individual differences in the latent process model parameters, this ensures that condition-specific differences are not biased by an averaging artifact. To this end, our proposed modeling approach was employed in an attempt to elucidate the effects of nicotine exposure (smoke as usual vs. abstinence) on cognitive functioning and potential moderating effects of rewards on Go/No-Go task performance.

The current dataset has previously been explored via the traditional frequentist approach to examine the effects of reward and smoking conditions on the latency and accuracy of task performance (see Ref. 40). However, it is not well understood which cognitive parameters nicotine affects. As a result, it remains unknown if non-drug rewards affect particular components of cognitive functioning in smokers. One goal in extending the LATER model was to explore intraindividual differences among daily cigarette smokers in their information accumulation and caution cognitive processes. In addition, we also wanted to study the difference in these two processes across experimental conditions (i.e., reward/neutral condition; smoke as usual/abstinence).

# METHODS

## Participants

After Institutional Review Board approval, 23 smokers were recruited *via* community advertisements. Inclusion criteria were the following: a) ≥18 years old, b) smoked at least four cigarettes/day for the past 12 months, c) inhale while smoking, and d) no intention to quit smoking in the next 1 month. Exclusion criteria were the following: a) women who were pregnant or lactating, or who planned to become pregnant or breastfeed during the study, and b) other tobacco use within the past 12 months. Participants who dropped out before completing the study ($n$ = 5) were excluded, leaving a final sample of 17 (5 females). While this is a relatively low sample size, each person has a high number of trials (750), which facilitate the estimation of the person-specific process parameters. Fewer trials would certainly result in more uncertainty (higher posterior standard deviation) in the parameter estimates; however, via hierarchical modeling, we pool information across participants to improve parameter estimation. Moreover, a large number of trials in fact are not uncommon in the Go/NoGo literature, as it helps build a prepotent response. In addition, as we take a multilevel modeling approach, we pool information across persons, which helps handle outlier effects and reduces the risk of model over-fitting. The mean age of these participants was 31.06 ($SD$ = 13.82). Participants identified as Caucasian, (66.7%), Asian (27.8%), and mixed race (5.6%). Participants reported smoking an average of 11.08 cigarettes per day. The sample exhibited low nicotine dependence on the Fagerström Test of Nicotine Dependence (FTND), with a mean score of 2.61 ($SD$ = 2.35).

## Procedure

Participants attended a baseline session. A coVita|Bedfont Micro Smokerlyzer® was used to monitor CO levels. The Beck Depression Inventory–II (41) and the Center for Epidemiologic Studies Depression Scale–Revised (42) were used to screen for current depression. A screening for dependence on drugs other than nicotine was also administered. Participants then completed the FTND (43). Participants then attended two counterbalanced sessions—smoke as usual and abstinent. For the abstinent session, participants were instructed not to smoke for at least 12 h before the session. For the smoke as usual session, participants were instructed to continue their regular smoking habits.

Participants began the experimental sessions by providing a CO sample to ensure abstinence or smoke as usual conditions. Abstinence was determined by a CO level of at least one half of the participant's CO level at their baseline session. Individuals then completed a recent nicotine, alcohol, and substance use measure, and the Questionnaire of Smoking Urges–Brief (QSU) (44). Participants reporting the use of alcohol or other substances within 24 h before experimental sessions were asked to return at a later date when they had refrained from substance use. Investigators then administered a measure of nicotine withdrawal, followed by an antisaccade (inhibitory control) and a working memory task (not reported here), as well as a monetary incentivized Go/No-Go task. Each session lasted approximately 2 h. Results of questionnaires utilized in the current analyses and additional demographics can be found in **Table 2**.

## Go/No-Go Task

An incentivized version of the Go/No-Go task was administered *via* a computer with a 17-in. monitor presented in E-Prime (Psychology Software Tools, Inc., Pittsburgh, PA). The task consisted of three trial types: frequent-Go (FGO; 75%), infrequent-Go (IFGO; 12.5%), and NoGo trials (12.5%) (45). Only data from the FGO trials are analyzed in this study as a main aim of the current modeling approach was to examine inter-individual variability in reaction times. Including IFGO trials would introduce additional sources of variability, confounding the findings. The participants were required to press the space bar on a computer keyboard using the index finger of their dominant hand. Each trial consisted of the presentation of a colored square for 400 ms followed by the presentation of a fixation cross for 400 ms. Responses were collected during this 800-ms period. Participants were instructed to respond as quickly and as accurately as possible. Trials with reactions times <150 ms were excluded from analyses to avoid the inclusion of potentially premature responses. This was a threshold that we set in order to ensure that the response was in fact a reaction to the stimulus. If reaction times are too fast, they are not a reaction to the stimulus; rather they reflect general responding. Utilizing a threshold is well documented in the reaction time literature [see, e.g., Ref. (40)] (46). The trial types were presented pseudo-randomly. Participants completed 10 runs, and each run was composed of 100 trials. Five runs were preceded by a ring of dollar signs ($), indicating the availability of monetary reward depending on run performance. Five runs were preceded by a ring of pound signs (#), indicating that no monetary reward was available. The order of runs was randomized. Participants were instructed that they could earn up to $5.00 in addition to their participation earnings, and that faster and more accurate performance on rewarded blocks would result in a greater reward amount. Participants were instructed that they would receive the earned rewards once they had completed the study and the investigators analyzed their data. At the end of the trials, the participants were told that they were getting the full reward amount.

**TABLE 2** | Participant characteristics.

| | Mean | SD |
|---|---|---|
| Age | 34.15 | 18.31 |
| Age of first use | 19.63 | 5.34 |
| FTND | 2.63 | 11.32 |
| Avg. cigarettes per day | 2.29 | 11.00 |

*FTND, Fagerström test for nicotine dependence.*

## Bayesian Data Analysis

In the present application of the model, we used weakly informative prior distributions, specified in **Appendix A**. As we had no prior knowledge, we chose weakly informative priors so that the prior distributions would have very little impact on the results. Parameters were estimated by running six chains with 2,000 iterations each, discarding the first 1,000 samples as burn-in. Convergence of the six chains was tested by the $\hat{R}$ statistic (the Gelman–Rubin convergence statistic, used to test the degree of convergence of a random Markov Chain; see Ref. 47). $\hat{R}$ is calculated by taking the ratio of variance within and between chains. $\hat{R}$ was lower than 1.01 for all parameters (conventional criterion being $\hat{R}$ <1.1), indicating no problems with convergence. The full R script and accompanying data that allow for replicating the analysis can be found on the Open Science Framework website of the project[1].

# RESULTS

## Individual Differences in the Decisions on Go Trials

We estimated an accretion and a caution threshold parameter for each person. Results show individual differences in accretion rate and caution threshold (**Figure 2**). Caution parameter estimates ranged between 2 and 6, while accretion rate was between 0.7 and 1.6. To relate these two scales, a person, for example, with caution parameter 4 and accretion rate 1 would need ¼ s (250 ms) to give a response. Alternatively, the same reaction time can arise from a faster accretion rate (e.g., 1.5) but also higher caution (e.g., 6). As can be seen in **Figure 2**, various combinations of accretion rates and caution parameters can result in very similar reaction times.

[1] https://osf.io/5h8m4/?view_only=f6c1e50dcfa04244bba428d6cf259d36

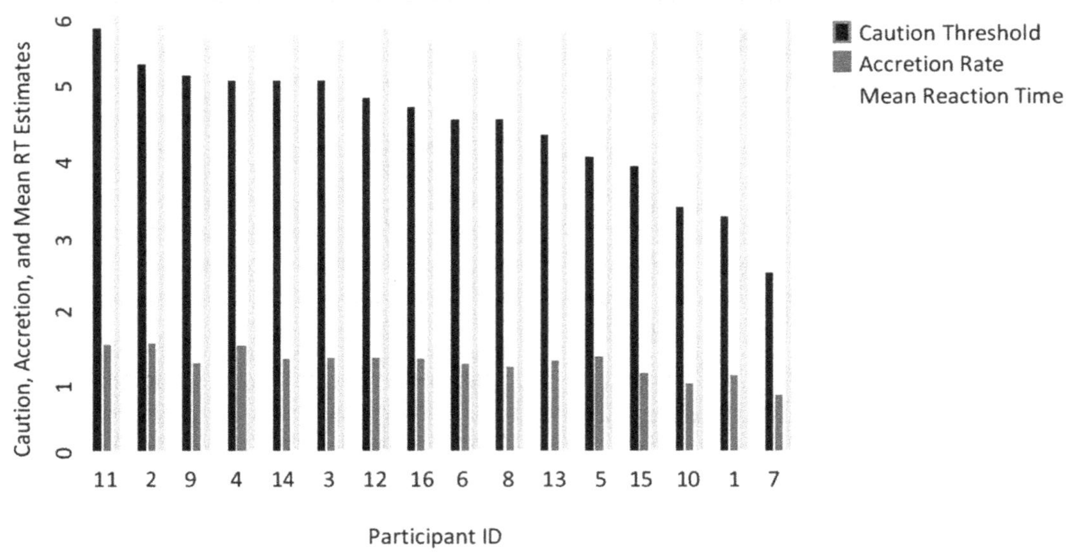


**FIGURE 2 |** Individual differences in participants' accretion, caution, and mean reaction time (RT) estimates. *Note.* Mean RT is log transformed. Mean reaction times were included in the figure to demonstrate the different combinations of caution and accretion, which could result in similar RTs.

We included person-level predictors (chronological age, age of smoking initiation, FTND score, average number of cigarettes smoked per day) to predict individual differences in accretion or caution, but no predictors explained differences in either parameter. Regression coefficients estimates and corresponding 95% credible intervals are reported in **Appendix B**.

## Condition-Specific Differences in the Decisions on the Go Trials

We were interested in capturing differences in the decisions on the Go trials in periods when smokers abstained from smoking (vs. smoking as usual) and when a reward was offered depending on their performance (vs. neutral condition with no reward). These conditions were crossed for each person for a two-by-two design. We chose the neutral trials in the smoke as usual session as our baseline, and modeled the differences in the neutral and abstained from smoking, and the abstinent and smoking as usual reward conditions in terms of accretion and caution. Results are reported in **Table 3**. All accretion parameters had posterior distributions that had posterior mass largely concentrated away from zero, indicating support for a difference in these conditions on accretion, compared to the baseline (neutral trial, smoke as usual) condition. The $\delta_{v,1}$ and $\delta_{v,3}$ accretion parameters reveal that regardless of trial condition (neutral vs. reward), abstaining from smoking was associated with faster information accumulation compared to smoking as usual. The $\delta_{v,2}$ accretion estimate indicated that when smoking as usual, smokers had slower accretion rates relative to reward trials.

Compared to the baseline condition, regardless of trial condition, smokers had a lower caution threshold when in a period of abstinence, relative to the baseline condition ($\delta_{\theta,1}$,$\delta_{\theta,3}$)

**TABLE 3 |** Summary of the regression weights where response speed was modeled with the LATER model.

| Condition | Posterior mean | Posterior SD | 95% CrI |
|---|---|---|---|
| Neutral, abstinent | −0.3638 | 0.0552 | (−0.4763, −0.2613) |
| Reward, smoke as usual | 0.1231 | 0.0565 | (0.0153 , 0.2360) |
| Reward, abstinent | −0.2494 | 0.0556 | (−0.3573, −0.1384) |
| Neutral, abstinent | −0.0655 | 0.0145 | (−0.0938, −0.0376) |
| Reward, smoke as usual | 0.0835 | 0.0150 | (0.0537, 0.1120) |
| Reward, abstinent | −0.0068 | 0.0147 | (−0.0352 , 0.0222) |

*Negative Posterior Means indicate faster accretion rates and lower caution thresholds; positive values indicate slower accretion rates and higher caution thresholds. Mean and SD are posterior mean and standard deviation. "Neutral" refers to a neutral trial; "Reward" refers to a reward trial. CrI, credibility interval; SD, standard deviation.*

The $\delta_{\theta,3}$ parameter had a 95% confidence interval containing 0, indicating less confidence for a meaningful difference between this parameter (abstinent, reward) to the baseline (smoke as usual, reward). The $\delta_{\theta,2}$ parameter indicates a larger caution threshold in the reward trials relative to the neutral trials in the smoke as usual session, suggesting that participants are integrating reward information into their cognitive appraisals of whether or not to execute a "go" response.

## Model Fit

In addition to overall model convergence, we tested how well the LATER model fit the actual observed data through posterior predictive checks (PPCs). For this, we generated 100 new data sets from the posterior distributions of the LATER model parameters. **Figure 3** shows smoothed blue curves of these generated datasets overlaying the experimental data

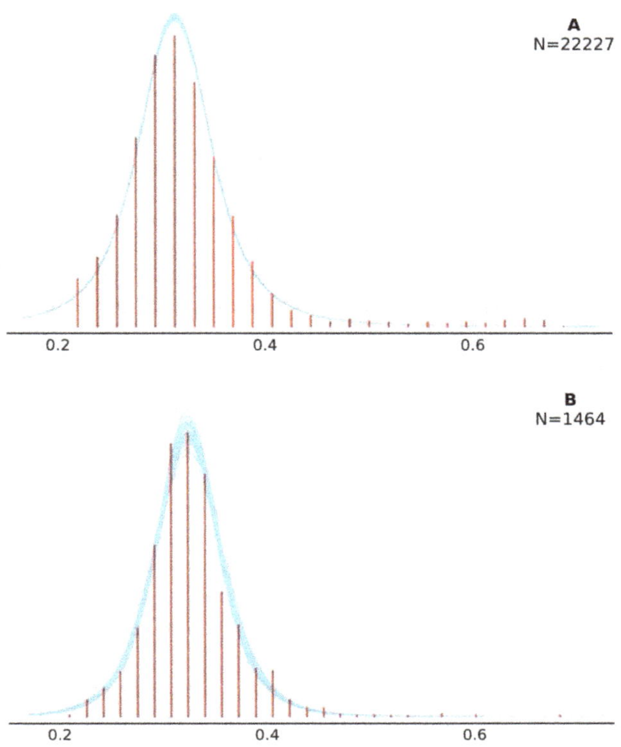


**FIGURE 3 |** Visual summary of the posterior predictive checks. Checks were completed with 100 generated data sets. Smoothed histograms of these generated datasets are depicted by the blue curves. The distribution of the experimental data is shown with the red bars. Plot **(A)** shows these checks on the level of the full data set, while Plot **(B)** shows it for a randomly selected participant.

(red histogram). Plot A depicts the full data PPC results, and Plot B displays a randomly selected participant's data. Overall, the LATER model adequately fit the experimental data well, demonstrated by generated data sets, which nicely overlay the real experimental data (i.e., the blue curves follow the same pattern of the red histogram). The results were analyzed in the Bayesian framework, which does not utilize traditional indices to show goodness of fit (e.g., CFI) but relies on PPCs. This entails "simulating replicated data under the fitted model and then comparing these to the observed data" (48, p. 158). Systematic discrepancies within these graphical checks are indicative of poor model fit. Here, our graphical PPCs shown in **Figure 3** do not reveal any systematic misfit.

## DISCUSSION

In this paper, we articulated model implementation of a novel hierarchically extended LATER model, which parses reaction time into two distinct aspects of cognitive functioning: accretion rate and caution threshold. This model extension enables researchers to account for and compare differences in sources of variation related to experimental conditions and person-specific differences in accretion and threshold. We demonstrated the applicability and benefits of this model by applying it to reaction time data from a group of adult daily smokers, identifying condition and trial level effects. We aimed to place emphasis on both modeling and the nuanced substantive findings that this modeling makes possible. That is, we presented a novel hierarchical extension to the LATER model in order to account for differences across persons and experimental conditions simultaneously. We showcase the strength of this approach by demonstrating what researchers can learn about smoking status and the influence of rewards utilizing this modeling approach.

In the original analyses of the data, Lydon et al., (40) reported that task performance was more accurate (in regards to error processing) on rewarded trials relative to the neutral trials, but only in the smoke as usual session. There were no differences between reward and neutral trials during the abstinent session. And importantly, there were no significant differences in mean reaction times between the abstinent and smoke as usual sessions, regardless of the trial type. Here, our findings demonstrate differences in both cognitive parameters underlying reaction times.

In the current analyses, in the accretion parameter, the baseline (or comparative) condition was smoke as usual, neutral trials. Our results demonstrated the following: Relative to our baseline condition, when smokers were in an abstinent state, they had faster accretion rates in both reward and neutral trials. When smokers were smoking as usual, they had slower accretion rates when a reward was at stake relative to neutral trials. In regards to the caution threshold, again the baseline was smoke as usual, neutral trials. Relative to this baseline condition, when a participant was in a period of abstinence, regardless of the trial type (reward, neutral), s/he utilized a lower caution threshold. Compared to the baseline smoke as usual neutral condition, when a reward was at stake (still smoking as usual condition), smokers utilized a larger caution threshold.

Our study is the first to combine advanced process models with experimental manipulations to examine the effects of smoking on behavior. Understanding how rewards affect decisions is critical as contingency management treatment programs encourage continued abstinence by increasing the value associated with continued abstinence (49). Our findings demonstrate differences in both accretion and caution parameters when smokers were abstinent relative to smoking as usual: faster accretion rates and lower caution thresholds when participants were in a period of abstinence, regardless of trial type. This overall main finding falls in line with other studies demonstrating abstinence-related reward-insensitivities (28, 33, 36), with important implications for contingency management programs. If incentives used in smoking interventions are not overcoming cognitive deficits produced by acute nicotine withdrawal, incentives may fail to change the value associated with continued smoking abstinence, undermining the allocations of cognitive resources needed in attempts to remain abstinent. Future work should focus on examining the generalizability of reward/reward insensitivity, particularly in an abstinence state, to other types of motivating incentives (e.g., food, social praise) in order to investigate if alternative incentives can impact cognitive performance in deprived smokers in order to inform the development of effective interventions.

Interestingly, when smokers were smoking as usual, rewarded trials produced slower accretion rates and increased caution thresholds. This finding suggests that when participants were smoking as usual, they seemed to be more careful in their decision time, perhaps a speed-accuracy tradeoff. Indeed, Lydon et al. (40) reported fewer errors when examining the no/go trials of this task in rewarded vs. neutral trials when participants were smoking as usual. Additionally, additional processing demands/time could have been needed in order to integrate information about the reward into the decision process.

To our knowledge, a LATER process model has never been applied to cigarette smokers to examine the underlying mechanisms of reaction or decision times. However, our findings fall in line with other research groups attempting to examine differences in underlying mechanisms of decision-making based on smoking state. Zack et al. (50) found that adolescent heavy smokers made more errors on a rapid information processing task relative to when they were smoking as usual, in line with the current results. These results support the notion that that accretion rate, the speed of information accumulation, is affected by abstinence. In a resting state magnetic resonance imaging study, Lerman and colleagues (30) reported that weaker inter-network connectivity (salience and default) predicted less suppression of default mode activity during performance of a working memory task. They argue that alterations in the coupling of these networks, and the inability to disengage from the default mode network, may be critical in cognitive alterations that underlie dependence. In our study, the trial type (reward vs. neutral) did not make a difference when smokers were in a period of abstinence. This could be due to alterations in the coupling of these networks as found in the study by Lerman and colleagues.

There are notable limitations in the current study. We implemented our model in the Bayesian statistical framework, which allowed us to fit a complex model to reaction time data in a single step. However, there are limitations to utilizing a Bayesian framework, namely in the computation power needed to implement such approaches. The current analysis was carried out using parallel computations [six cores running six Markov chain Monte Carlo (MCMC) chains] and took about 25 min. However, due to recent advances in statistical software, computational difficulty is becoming less of an issue. In addition, we had a limited sample size and unbalanced gender. However, as described in our Methods section, our implementation of a process model that utilizes a sequential sampling method and hierarchical modeling handles small sample sizes better than traditional approaches. We have made our scripts and data available to facilitate researchers utilizing this approach, hopefully with larger samples and more balanced samples to overcome this limitation in future work.

Taken together, our hierarchical extension of the LATER process model is able to separate the reaction time of the go trials into two cognitive processes, accretion and caution, while simultaneously accounting for differences in groups/session (smoke as usual vs. abstinent) and experimental condition (reward vs. neutral trials). Combing these approaches provides additional nuanced insight into nicotine's effects on behavior.

Our model examines differences across individuals together with condition specific differences. This is an important extension of the model as it is critical for researchers to have the ability to test both between- and within-person differences in experimental conditions. Continual use of marrying cognitive process models with experimental condition manipulations will help elucidate factors that may impact decision-making in smokers, and can be extended to additional types of addiction. This modeling approach can and should be used in future research; by combining this approach with other tasks, group conditions, etc., researchers can better understand the cognitive processes underlying decision-making within particular groups. These cognitive factors have the potential to inform the development and improvement of intervention programs by understanding which cognitive mechanisms need to be targeted by interventions. Although we did not find an association between individual level predictors and accretion/caution parameters, our novel extension to the LATER model puts us in a position to assess this in the future with larger sample sizes, more diverse samples (e.g., varying levels of nicotine dependence), and other types of addiction.

## AUTHOR CONTRIBUTIONS

NR contributed to data acquisition, analysis, interpretation, drafting the manuscript, and study conception and design. BS contributed to data analysis and drafting the manuscript. ZO and CG contributed to study conception and design, data analysis, interpretation, and drafting the manuscript.

## REFERENCES

1. Stout JC, Busemeyer JR, Lin A, Grant SJ, Bonson KR. Cognitive modelling analysis of decision-making processes in cocaine abusers. *Psychon Bull Rev* (2004) 11(4):742–7. doi: 10.3758/BF03196629
2. Yechiam E, Busemeyer JR, Stout JC, Bechara A. Using cognitive models to map relations between neuropsychological disorders and human decision-making deficits. *Psychol Sci* (2005) 16(12):973–8. doi: 10.1111/j.1467-9280.2005.01646.x
3. Cohen JR, Asarnow RF, Sabb FW, Bilder RM, Bookheimer SY, Knowlton BJ, et al. A unique adolescent response to reward prediction errors. *Nat Neurosci* (2010) 13(6):669. doi: 10.1038/nn.2558
4. Hauser TU, Iannaccone R, Walitza S, Brandeis D, Brem S. Cognitive flexibility in adolescence: neural and behavioral mechanisms of reward prediction error processing in adaptive decision making during development. *Neuroimage* (2015) 104:347–54. doi: 10.1016/j.neuroimage.2014.09.018
5. Reddi BAJ, Carpenter RH. The influence of urgency on decision time. *Nat Neurosci* (2000) 3(8):827. doi: 10.1038/77739
6. Ratcliff R. Putting noise into neurophysiological models of simple decision making. *Nat Neurosci* (2001) 4(4):336. doi: 10.1038/85956
7. Brenner E, Smeets JB. How people achieve their amazing temporal precision in interception. *J Vis* (2015) 15(3):8–8. doi: 10.1167/15.3.8
8. Rubinstein A. Response time and decision making: an experimental study. *Judgm Decis Mak* (2013) 8(5):540–51.
9. Noorani I. LATER models of neural decision behavior in choice tasks. *Front Integr Neurosci* (2014) 8:67. doi: 10.3389/fnint.2014.00067
10. Noorani I, Carpenter RHS. Re-starting a neural race: anti-saccade correction. *Eur J Neurosci* (2014) 39(1):159–64. doi: 10.1111/ejn.12396
11. Bickel WK, Jarmolowicz DP, Mueller ET, Gatchalian KM, McClure SM. Are

executive function and impulsivity antipodes? A conceptual reconstruction with special reference to addiction. *Psychopharmacology* (2012) 221(3):361–87. doi: 10.1007/s00213-012-2689-x

12. Noorani I, Carpenter RHS. The LATER model of reaction time and decision. *Neurosci Biobehav Rev* (2016) 64:229–51. doi: 10.1016/j.neubiorev.2016.02.018
13. Whelan R. Effective analysis of reaction time data. *Psychol Rec* (2008) 58(3):475–82. doi: 10.1007/BF03395630
14. Carpenter RHS, Reddi BAJ, Anderson AJ. A simple two-stage model predicts response time distributions. *J Physiol* (2009) 587(16):4051–62. doi: 10.1113/jphysiol.2009.173955
15. Carpenter RHS. Contrast, probability, and saccadic latency: evidence for independence of detection and decision. *Curr Biol* (2004) 14(17):1576–80. doi: 10.1016/j.cub.2004.08.058
16. Bryk AS, Raudenbush SW. Application of hierarchical linear models to assessing change. *Psychol Bull* (1987) 101(1):147. doi: 10.1037//0033-2909.101.1.147
17. Raudenbush SW, Bryk AS. Hierarchical linear models: applications and data analysis methods. *Sage* (2002) 1.
18. Oravecz Z, Huentelman M, Vandekerckhove J. Sequential Bayesian updating for big data. In: *Big Data in Cognitive Science*. London and New York: Routledge Taylor & Francis Group. (2016). p. 13–33.
19. Pagan A. Econometric issues in the analysis of regressions with generated regressors. *Int Econ Rev* (1984) 25:221–47. doi: 10.2307/2648877
20. Gelman A, Carlin JB, Stern HS, Dunson DB, Vehtari A, Rubin DB. *Bayesian Data Analysis* Vol. 2. Boca Raton, FL: CRC Press (2014).
21. Kruschke JK, Aguinis H, Joo H. The time has come: Bayesian methods for data analysis in the organizational sciences. *Organ Res Methods* (2012) 15(4):722–52. doi: 10.1177/1094428112457829
22. Turner RM, Jackson D, Wei Y, Thompson SG, Higgins JP. Predictive distributions for between-study heterogeneity and simple methods for their application in Bayesian meta-analysis. *Stat Med* (2015) 34(6):984–98. doi: 10.1002/sim.6381
23. STAN Development team. Stan Modeling Language: User's Guide and Reference Manual. Version 2.11.0. http://mc-stan.org.
24. Noorani I, Gao MJ, Pearson BC, Carpenter RHS. Predicting the timing of wrong decisions with LATER. *Exp Brain Res* (2011) 209(4):587–98. doi: 10.1007/s00221-011-2587-1
25. Spinella M. Correlations between orbitofrontal dysfunction and tobacco smoking. *Addict Biol* (2002) 7(4):381–4. doi: 10.1080/1355621021000005964
26. Dinn WM, Aycicegi A, Harris CL. Cigarette smoking in a student sample: neurocognitive and clinical correlates. *Addict Behav* (2004) 29(1):107–26. doi: 10.1016/j.addbeh.2003.07.001
27. Reynolds B, Patak M, Shroff P, Penfold RB, Melanko S, Duhig AM. Laboratory and self-report assessments of impulsive behavior in adolescent daily smokers and nonsmokers. *Exp Clin Psychopharmacol* (2007) 15(3):264. doi: 10.1037/1064-1297.15.3.264
28. Dawkins L, Acaster S, Powell JH. The effects of smoking and abstinence on experience of happiness and sadness in response to positively valenced, negatively valenced, and neutral film clips. *Addict Behav* (2007) 32(2):425–31. doi: 10.1016/j.addbeh.2006.05.010
29. Geier CF, Sweitzer M, Denlinger R, Sparacino G, Donny E. Abstinent adult daily smokers show reduced anticipatory but elevated saccade-related brain responses during a rewarded antisaccade task. *Psychiat Res Neuroim* (2014) 223(2):140–7. doi: 10.1016/j.pscychresns.2014.04.007
30. Lerman C, Gu H, Loughead J, Ruparel K, Yang Y, Stein EA. Large-scale brain network coupling predicts acute nicotine abstinence effects on craving and cognitive function. *JAMA Psychiatry* (2014) 71(5):523–30. doi: 10.1001/jamapsychiatry.2013.4091
31. Perkins KA, Lerman C, Coddington SB, Jetton C, Karelitz JL, Scott JA, et al. Initial nicotine sensitivity in humans as a function of impulsivity. *Psychopharmacology* (2008) 200(4):529–44. doi: 10.1007/s00213-008-1231-7
32. Sweitzer MM, Donny EC, Dierker LC, Flory JD, Manuck SB. Delay discounting and smoking: association with the Fagerström test for nicotine dependence but not cigarettes smoked per day. *Nicotine Tob Res* (2008) 10(10):1571–5. doi: 10.1080/14622200802323274
33. Sweitzer MM, Geier CF, Joel DL, McGurrin P, Denlinger RL, Forbes EE, et al. Dissociated effects of anticipating smoking versus monetary reward in the caudate as a function of smoking abstinence. *Biol Psychiatry* (2014) 76(9):681–8. doi: 10.1016/j.biopsych.2013.11.013
34. Wilson SJ, Sayette MA. Neuroimaging craving: urge intensity matters. *Addiction* (2015) 110(2):195–203. doi: 10.1111/add.12676
35. Zelle SL, Gates KM, Fiez JA, Sayette MA, Wilson SJ. The first day is always the hardest: functional connectivity during cue exposure and the ability to resist smoking in the initial hours of a quit attempt. *NeuroImage* (2017) 151:24–32. doi: 10.1016/j.neuroimage.2016.03.015
36. Dawkins L, Powell JH, West R, Powell J, Pickering A. A double-blind placebo controlled experimental study of nicotine: I—effects on incentive motivation. *Psychopharmacology* (2006) 189(3):355–67. doi: 10.1007/s00213-006-0588-8
37. Powell J, Tait S, Lessiter J. Cigarette smoking and attention to signals of reward and threat in the Stroop paradigm. *Addiction* (2002) 97(9):1163–70. doi: 10.1046/j.1360-0443.2002.00117.x
38. Peters J, Bromberg U, Schneider S, Brassen S, Menz M, Banaschewski T, et al. Lower ventral striatal activation during reward anticipation in adolescent smokers. *Am J Psychiatry* (2011) 168(5):540–9. doi: 10.1176/appi.ajp.2010.10071024
39. Lee MD. How cognitive modeling can benefit from hierarchical Bayesian models. *J Math Psychol* (2011) 55(1):1–7. doi: 10.1016/j.jmp.2010.08.013
40. Lydon DM, Roberts NJ, Geier CF. Reduced influence of monetary incentives on Go/NoGo performance during smoking abstinence. *Nicotine Tob Res* (2014) 17(9):1178–81. doi: 10.1093/ntr/ntu283
41. Beck AT, Steer RA, Brown GK. Beck depression inventory–II. *San Antonio* (1996) 78(2):490–8. doi: 10.1037/t00742-000
42. Eaton WW, Smith C, Ybarra M, Muntaner C, Tien A. Center for Epidemiologic studies depression scale: review and revision (CESD and CESD-R). (2004). doi: 10.1037/t29280-000
43. Heatherton TF, Kozlowski LT, Frecker RC, Fagerstrom KO. The Fagerström test for nicotine dependence: a revision of the Fagerström tolerance questionnaire. *Br J Addict* (1991) 86(9):1119–27. doi: 10.1111/j.1360-0443.1991.tb01879.x
44. Cox LS, Tiffany ST, Christen AG. Evaluation of the brief questionnaire of smoking urges (QSU-brief) in laboratory and clinical settings. *Nicotine Tob Res* (2001) 3(1):7–16. doi: 10.1080/14622200020032051
45. Chikazoe J, Jimura K, Hirose S, Yamashita KI, Miyashita Y, Konishi S. Preparation to inhibit a response complements response inhibition during performance of a stop-signal task. *J Neurosci* (2009) 29(50):15870–7. doi: 10.1523/JNEUROSCI.3645-09.2009
46. Hallett PE. Primary and secondary saccades to goals defined by instructions. *Vision research*, 18(10) (1978) 1279–96.
47. Gelman A, Rubin DB. Inference from iterative simulation using multiple sequences (with Discussion). *Statistical Science* (1992) 7:457–511.
48. Gelman A, Hill J. Data analysis using regression and multilevel/hierarchical models. Cambridge University Press (2006).
49. Prendergast M, Podus D, Finney J, Greenwell L, Roll J. Contingency management for treatment of substance use disorders: a meta-analysis. *Addiction* (2006) 101(11):1546–60.
50. Zack M, Belsito L, Scher R, Eissenberg T, Corrigall WA. Effects of abstinence and smoking on information processing in adolescent smokers. *Psychopharmacology* (2001) 153(2):249–57. doi: 10.1007/s002130000552

# 12

# Molecular Imaging of Opioid and Dopamine Systems: Insights into the Pharmacogenetics of Opioid use Disorders

*Jamie A. Burns[1], Danielle S. Kroll[1], Dana E. Feldman[1], Christopher Kure Liu[1], Peter Manza[1], Corinde E. Wiers[1], Nora D. Volkow[1,2] and Gene-Jack Wang[1]**

*[1] National Institute on Alcohol Abuse and Alcoholism, Bethesda, MD, United States, [2] National Institute on Drug Abuse, Bethesda, MD, United States*

***Correspondence:***
*Gene-Jack Wang*
*gene-jack.wang@nih.gov*

Opioid use in the United States has steadily risen since the 1990s, along with staggering increases in addiction and overdose fatalities. With this surge in prescription and illicit opioid abuse, it is paramount to understand the genetic risk factors and neuropsychological effects of opioid use disorder (OUD). Polymorphisms disrupting the opioid and dopamine systems have been associated with increased risk for developing substance use disorders. Molecular imaging studies have revealed how these polymorphisms impact the brain and contribute to cognitive and behavioral differences across individuals. Here, we review the current molecular imaging literature to assess how genetic variations in the opioid and dopamine systems affect function in the brain's reward, cognition, and stress pathways, potentially resulting in vulnerabilities to OUD. Continued research of the functional consequences of genetic variants and corresponding alterations in neural mechanisms will inform prevention and treatment of OUD.

**Keywords: opioid use disorder, neuroimaging, genetics, positron emission tomography, PET, polymorphism, opioid receptors, dopamine receptors**

## INTRODUCTION

Opioid use in the United States has steadily risen since the late 1990s, along with staggering increases in overdose fatalities (1). The use of illicit opioids such as heroin and fentanyl has increased dramatically, contributing to opioid-related morbidity and mortality (2). With approximately 115 Americans dying each day from an opioid overdose, this epidemic is now considered a public health emergency (3). The surge in prescription and illicit opioid abuse necessitates further investigation into the genetic risk factors and neuropsychological effects of opioid use disorder (OUD).

The roles of the opioid and dopamine (DA) systems in substance use disorders (SUDs) are well recognized (4). Drug reward and incentive salience develop during the acute effects of drug-taking and correspond to changes in opioid and DA signaling in the basal ganglia (5). Incentive salience is defined by the association of previously neutral stimuli with drug use, which promotes compulsive drug-seeking (4). Stress responses associated with withdrawal involve decreased DA signaling along reward pathways, increased dynorphin-mediated kappa opioid (KOP) receptor signaling, and increased corticotropin-releasing factor (CRF) signaling in the amygdala (4). These same principles apply to OUD. For example, Wang et al. (6) used positron-emission tomography (PET) imaging with

[$^{11}$C]raclopride to demonstrate lower dopamine receptor 2 (D2R) and 3 (D3R) availability in the striatum of opioid-dependent patients compared to controls. Another [$^{11}$C]raclopride PET study found low striatal D2/3 receptor availability and low presynaptic DA in OUD patients compared to controls (7), which has also been found for other SUDs including cocaine, alcohol, methamphetamine, and cannabis [reviewed in Refs. (8, 9)]. Low D2R levels have also been associated with sleep deprivation (10–12) and lower socioeconomic status (13, 14). These factors may contribute to lower D2R availability found in SUDs, particularly since SUDs and sleep deprivation are highly comorbid (15). Other preclinical studies have found dynorphin-mediated KOP receptor signaling inhibits dopaminergic signaling and modulates aversive emotional states that maintain drug dependence (16–18). Based on these studies, both the opioid and DA signaling systems are implicated in OUD.

However, there are opposing views on these systems' involvement in addiction. For example, there are studies that report no disruption of D2R in OUD, including no difference in baseline D2R availability in methadone-maintained OUD patients compared to controls (19). Moreover, PET studies of opioid-dependent patients on medications for OUD (MOUD) found no increase in striatal DA release in response to opioid administration (19, 20). Studies of other SUDs also present slight inconsistencies in their effects on the dopamine system. Imaging studies in individuals with alcohol use disorder (AUD) have reported marked reductions in dopamine release and in striatal D2R, and most preclinical studies have documented significant reductions in dopamine neuronal firing and tonic dopamine release (9, 21–27). However, studies in rodents have also reported dynamic changes in dopamine release with increases and decreases in accumbens at various days post alcohol withdrawal (28). The discrepancies in the preclinical studies are likely to reflect in part time at which the measurements were made (early versus late withdrawal) as well as the alcohol models used (active versus passive administration). Thus, further research is required to understand the complex relationship between opioid and DA systems in SUDs.

While it has long been postulated that genetics influence an individual's susceptibility to addiction, there has been little success in pinpointing genes with well-defined, causal roles in SUDs (29). Nevertheless, OUD is highly heritable, with an estimated 50% genetic contribution (30–32). The use of candidate gene studies and genome-wide association studies has revealed several polymorphisms that reliably associate with SUDs; however, addiction is a polygenic disease with complex genetic interactions and therefore individual polymorphisms will likely only account for a fraction of the total genetic risk for OUD (33–35). Polymorphisms in the opioid signaling system have been associated with addiction, as well as addiction treatment response (29). For example, several studies have identified a single nucleotide polymorphism (SNP) in the *OPRM1* gene that associates with improved response to naltrexone treatment in individuals with AUD (36–39). Other *OPRM1* SNPs may also play a role in nicotine dependence and treatment response (40–42). Additionally, genetic variations in the DA system have been linked to various SUDs as DA modulates reward and aversion pathways central to addiction (29, 43). For example, polymorphisms in the genes coding for dopamine 1 receptor (D1R) and D2R are associated with OUD, cocaine use disorder (CUD), and AUD (6, 22, 44). In addition, polymorphisms in the gene *DAT1*, which codes for dopamine transporters (DAT), have been associated with CUD and AUD (45–47). In line with this, reduced striatal DAT availability has been associated with OUD (48–53) and DAT availability has been associated with various other SUDs (51, 54–62).

In this review, we compiled findings related to the genetics of the opioid and DA systems and corresponding changes in brain and behavior as evidenced by PET neuroimaging. Functional and structural magnetic resonance imaging (MRI) is another useful tool in examining altered neural circuits in individuals with SUDs, as well as in polymorphism carriers. However, we will limit the scope to molecular imaging as the literature on MRI in OUD was recently reviewed (63–66). Integrating genetics with regional changes in receptor binding may help uncover circuits relevant for the pathophysiology of OUD, and thereby inform precision-based prevention and treatment.

## THE OPIOID RECEPTOR SYSTEM

## OPRM1

### *OPRM1* Background

The *OPRM1* gene codes for the MOP receptor, an inhibitory G-protein coupled receptor (GPCR) that binds endogenous opioid peptides such as β-endorphin and enkephalins as well as exogenous opioids such as morphine and heroin (67). MOP receptors are required to establish morphine place preference and physical dependence (68). MOP receptors are expressed throughout the brain's reward pathways including the mesocorticolimbic network as illustrated in **Figure 1**; their proposed mechanism for positive reinforcement in OUD is through disinhibition of DA neurons that trigger drug reward upon DA release (69, 70). Originally it was thought that MOP receptor agonists hyperpolarize GABAergic interneurons of the ventral tegmental area (VTA), reducing GABA-mediated inhibitory input to DA neurons and thereby increasing DA signaling by disinhibition (69). However, most evidence now suggests that the rostromedial tegmental nucleus mediates opioid-induced disinhibition of DA neurons (71–73). There is preclinical evidence of DA-independent opioid-induced reward, but the mechanism is not well understood (74, 75).

The effects of prolonged opioid exposure on MOP receptors, whether in the context of chronic pain management or substance abuse, are not fully understood. Bolger et al. (76) demonstrated an upregulation in MOP receptor in rat brain after chronic heroin administration. However, several other studies have demonstrated that both morphine and buprenorphine administration downregulate MOP receptors in rat brain (76, 77) including striatum (78). Clinically, prolonged exposure to opioids results in tolerance and increased opioid dose requirements; several proposed mechanisms may explain this phenomenon, including phosphorylation and arrestin-driven uncoupling of the GPCR and receptor internalization and degradation

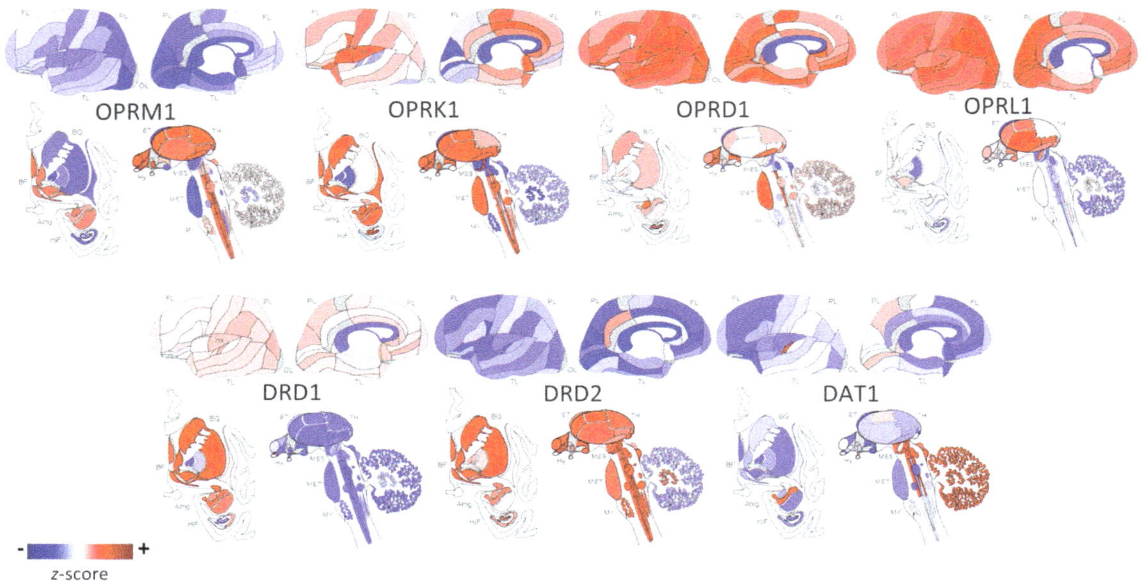


**FIGURE 1 |** Regional distribution of receptor types in the human brain. Opioid and dopamine receptor gene expression in the human brain [Opioid Receptor Mu 1 (OPRM1), Opioid Receptor Kappa 1 (OPRK1), Opioid Receptor Delta 1 (OPRD1), Opioid Related Nociceptin Receptor 1 (OPRL1), Dopamine Receptor D1 (DRD1), Dopamine Receptor D2 (DRD2), Dopamine Active Transporter 1 (DAT1)]. Images constructed using Allen Human Brain Atlas. Data displayed are from one donor: H0351.2002, 39 years, M, Black or African American. The color bar displays expression values using *z*-score normalization. Color scale was altered to highlight regional differences in gene expression per receptor type; therefore, the absolute scale differs across each of the receptor subtypes. For quantitative results from all six postmortem donor brains, visit http://human.brain-map.org/static/brainexplorer.

(79–82). However, several studies cloned MOP receptors in human embryonic kidney cells and found that morphine does not promote MOP receptor endocytosis (80, 83–85), which results in protracted desensitization that could contribute to tolerance (86). Yet, several opioids including methadone, etorphine, and [D-Ala2, N-MePhe4, Gly-ol]-enkephalin (DAMGO) induced the expected receptor sequestration in cell line models (79, 80, 87, 88). A study in rats also showed MOP receptor internalization in the striatum and habenula after acute etorphine, but not morphine administration (80). These findings were replicated in the rat's locus coeruleus where neurons showed MOP receptor internalization in response to DAMGO and methadone, but not morphine (89). Downregulation of MOP receptors is agent-specific as some opioids are more effective at activating the G-protein response than others (87). The concept of biased agonism explains differential activation patterns and intracellular signaling cascades based on ligand structure and GPCR conformations (90, 91). In the case of MOP receptors, ligands may preferentially activate G-protein coupling or β-arrestin recruitment (92). Schmid et al. (92) reported that fentanyl promotes bias toward β-arrestin recruitment, while morphine is relatively unbiased in mouse models and cell lines. Given that β-arrestin drives MOP receptor internalization and is associated with respiratory suppression and tolerance, these findings have clinical significance and may explain the differences in ligand-mediated MOP receptor internalization (92–95). Specifically, the increased lethality of fentanyl and structurally related synthetic opioids may not be due solely to greater potency, but also due to the preferential activation of an intracellular pathway that promotes respiratory depression (92, 96).

## *OPRM1* Polymorphisms

Genetic variations of *OPRM1,* the gene encoding for MOP, have been studied in the context of vulnerabilities to SUDs, treatment response, and relapse. Whole genome sequencing has identified 3,324 *OPRM1* polymorphisms, the most commonly studied of which, rs1799971 (A118G), has a global minor allele frequency of 19% (97). Located on exon 1 of *OPRM1*, this SNP results in an asparagine replaced by an aspartate at position 40, which is in the amino-terminus of the receptor (98, 99). In preclinical studies, the G allele was associated with lower MOP receptor expression in transfected cell lines (100–103). In [$^{11}$C]carfentanil PET scans, the G allele was also associated with lower global MOP receptor expression (104) and lower expression in anterior cingulate cortex (ACC), nucleus accumbens (NAc), and thalamus compared to the common genotype (105). One proposed mechanism suggests that the amino acid substitution removes an extracellular glycosylation site, potentially interfering with the protein's folding or incorporation into the cell membrane (101). Other studies found that the G allele results in reduced levels of MOP receptor mRNA expression, although the underlying mechanism remains unknown (103). For example, a post-mortem study of heterozygotes for A118G found the wild-type A allele had twice the mRNA expression than the G variant in cortical and pons tissue samples (103). An *in vitro* study of G allele-transfected cells also showed reduced mRNA and lower receptor protein levels when compared to the wild-type allele (103). Oertel et al. (106) propose that rs1799971 creates a novel methylation site that suppresses transcription of *OPRM1*.

Interestingly, an initial *in vitro* study reported increased binding affinity of β-endorphin to the variant receptor (107); though subsequent *in vitro* studies were unable to replicate this finding (100, 108).

## Genetic Association Studies: *OPRM1* and OUD

Several studies have investigated the effects of genetic variations in *OPRM1* on susceptibility to SUDs, including OUD. A systematic review and meta-analysis of 13 studies of the A118G polymorphism in OUD found significant associations of the G allele with CUD and OUD in Asian populations, but not in African American, Caucasian, or Hispanic populations (109). However, a behavioral study linked the G allele with increased addiction severity in Caucasian males with OUD (110). This could be attributable to the varying prevalence of the rs1799971 minor allele across ethnicities; for example, the G allele frequency is greater in Asian populations than in Caucasians (30–40% and 11–15%, respectively), and it is less than 5% in African American populations (107, 111, 112). Another study examined four low-frequency SNPs of *OPRM1* in a cohort of European Americans and African Americans; only one polymorphism, rs62638690, was associated with both cocaine and heroin addiction in European Americans; however, it did not withstand correction for multiple testing (113). This may suggest that while *OPRM1* polymorphisms alter vulnerability to OUD, the effects are race- and/or ethnicity-dependent. Finally, an intron 2 polymorphism, rs9479757, was not associated with OUD in a Chinese population, but OUD patients with the minor allele were found to consume higher levels of opioids (114). Further, Xu et al. (115) found the rs9479757 minor allele associated with addiction severity among Chinese OUD patients (115). These findings are outlined in **Table 1**.

Additionally, the A118G polymorphism may have relevance for OUD treatment. In a mouse model of A118G, the analgesic, anxiolytic, and hyperlocomotor effects of buprenorphine were attenuated in carriers of the minor G allele (162). In a study of opioid-dependent chronic pain patients, carriers of the minor G allele required higher morphine equivalent daily doses than AA homozygotes (163). This may be attributed to reduced MOP receptor functioning in carriers of the G allele that results in an increased opioid requirement for pain management (163, 164). However, a meta-analysis of the association between rs1799971 and methadone treatment response among OUD patients was inconclusive (165).

Several studies have examined associations between *OPRM1* polymorphisms and stress response, as MOP receptors help regulate stress levels *via* tonic inhibition of the hypothalamic–pituitary–adrenal (HPA) axis (166). Naloxone is an opioid receptor antagonist with highest affinity for MOP receptors, thus eliciting an HPA axis stress response upon binding (167). Several studies demonstrate that healthy heterozygotes of A118G have increased stress response to naloxone compared to non-G allele carriers (168–170). Given the role of stress dysregulation in vulnerability to SUDs, this provides a potential mechanism for this SNP as a risk factor for OUD (167).

The A118G SNP has also been associated with personality traits relevant to SUDs (171). Several studies assessed participants with the five-factor NEO, a personality inventory that scores in domains of "Openness to Experience, Conscientiousness, Extraversion, Agreeableness, and Neuroticism" (172). High Neuroticism, low Conscientiousness, and low Agreeableness scores are associated with SUDs (173–176). Specifically, higher scores on Neuroticism and lower scores on Conscientiousness, Agreeableness, and Extraversion have been associated with OUD (177, 178). Compared to A118 homozygotes, carriers of the G allele scored lower on the Conscientiousness factor (170), which is associated with task organization and execution, and reflects control over impulsivity (179). Moreover, Pecina et al. (105) found that G carriers had higher Neuroticism scores than non-carriers, which negatively correlated with baseline MOP receptor availability in the anterior insula and subgenual ACC as assessed with [$^{11}$C]carfentanil PET. However, Hernandez-Avila et al. (180) found no association between A118G and NEO personality dimensions in healthy and substance-dependent volunteers; thus, the role of this polymorphism in moderating personality is uncertain. Love et al. (181) used [$^{11}$C]carfentanil PET in a study of healthy volunteers and assessed participants with the Revised NEO Personality Inventory, which includes domains "Impulsiveness" and "Deliberation," that have been associated with negative risk-taking, including drug use (182, 183). Participants with high Impulsivity and low Deliberation scores showed higher baseline MOP receptor availability in several brain regions including the ACC and amygdala (181). Further, in response to a pain stress challenge, subjects with high Impulsivity/low Deliberation scores demonstrated a larger reduction in MOP receptor availability from baseline compared to low Impulsivity/high Deliberation scores in regions including the orbitofrontal cortex and amygdala (181). This suggests a possible mechanism for the role of personality traits in shaping vulnerabilities to SUDs.

## Molecular Imaging: MOP Receptor and OUD

Several studies have used PET imaging to investigate MOP receptor availability in OUD patients receiving MOUD. The radioligand [$^{11}$C]carfentanil is widely used in PET studies as it is a highly potent MOP-selective receptor agonist (184). [$^{18}$F]cyclofoxy is less frequently used as it is both a MOP receptor and KOP receptor agonist, with some preliminary evidence of MOP receptor preference (185–188).

A number of studies have examined the effects of buprenorphine, a high-affinity MOP receptor partial agonist and KOP and delta opioid (DOP) receptor antagonist (189–191) in the treatment of OUD. Using [$^{11}$C]carfentanil PET imaging, Greenwald et al. (192) investigated the duration of binding of buprenorphine at MOP receptor and the corresponding effects on withdrawal in 10 OUD patients. They found that 50–60% MOP receptor occupancy by buprenorphine was required for withdrawal suppression (192). At 28 h after buprenorphine, 46% of whole-brain MOP receptors were

**TABLE 1** | Polymorphisms associated with OUD in the opioid system and molecular imaging correlates.

| Gene | Polymorphism | Location | Finding | Author | Year | n | Ethnicity | Imaging Correlates |
|---|---|---|---|---|---|---|---|---|
| ***OPRM1*** | **rs1799971** | Exon 1 | Risk factor for OUD | Kumar et al. (116) | 2012 | 330 | Indian | -Lower baseline MOP receptor binding potential in NAc and amygdala of tobacco smokers (117–119) -Greater DA release in the right caudate and ventral pallidum in response to smoking (120) |
| | | | | Kapur et al. (121) | 2007 | 282 | Indian | |
| | | | | Deb et al. (122) | 2010 | 169 | Indian | |
| | | | | Tan et al. (123) | 2003 | 137 | Indian | |
| | | | | Nagaya et al. (124) | 2012 | 160 | Malaysian males | |
| | | | | Szeto et al. (111) | 2001 | 296 | Chinese | |
| | | | | Bart et al. (125) | 2004 | 309 | Caucasian | |
| | | | | Drakenberg et al. (126) | 2006 | 65 | Caucasian | |
| | | | No significant association with OUD | Bond et al. (107) | 1998 | 31 | African American | |
| | | | | Luo et al. (127) | 2003 | 100 | African American | |
| | | | | Gelernter et al. (112) | 1999 | 288 | African American | |
| | | | | Crowley et al. (128) | 2003 | 195 | African American | |
| | | | | Zhang et al. (40) | 2006 | 600 | Caucasian | |
| | | | | Bond et al. (107) | 1998 | 52 | Caucasian | |
| | | | | Gelernter et al. (112) | 1999 | 492 | Caucasian | |
| | | | | Franke et al. (129) | 2001 | 652 | Caucasian | |
| | | | | Luo et al. (127) | 2003 | 231 | Caucasian | |
| | | | | Crowley et al. (128) | 2003 | 229 | Caucasian | |
| | | | | Levran et al. (130) | 2008 | 596 | Caucasian | |
| | | | | Nikolov et al. (131) | 2011 | 3,283 | Caucasian | |
| | | | | Bond et al. (107) | 1998 | 67 | Hispanic | |
| | | | | Gelernter et al. (112) | 1999 | 94 | Hispanic | |
| | | | | Li et al. (132) | 2000 | 434 | Chinese | |
| | | | | Zhang et al. (133) | 2007 | 332 | Chinese | |
| | | | | Shi et al. (114) | 2002 | 145 | Chinese | |
| | | | | Tan et al. (123) | 2003 | 208 | Chinese | |
| | | | | Tan et al. (123) | 2003 | 156 | Malay | |
| | | | No significant association with methadone dose | Crettol et al. (134) | 2008 | 238 | Caucasian | |
| | | | Prolonged abstinence without agonist therapy | Levran et al. (135) | 2017 | 596 | Caucasian | |
| | **rs62638690** | Exon 2 | Protective against OUD | *Clarke et al. (113) | 2013 | 1,377 | European American | |
| | **rs510769** | Intron 1 | Risk factor for OUD | *Levran et al. (130) | 2008 | 596 | Caucasian | |
| | **rs3778151** | Intron 1 | Risk factor for OUD | *Levran et al. (130) | 2008 | 596 | Caucasian | |
| | **rs9479757** | Intron 2 | Higher opioid consumption | Shi et al. (114) | 2002 | 145 | Chinese | |
| | | | Addiction severity | Xu et al. (115) | 2014 | 332 | Male Chinese | |
| ***OPRD1*** | **rs569356** | Promoter | Risk factor for OUD | *Zhang et al. (136) | 2008 | 1,063 | European American | |
| | | | No significant association with OUD | Nelson et al. (137) | 2014 | 2,954 | Australian | |
| | **rs4654327** | 3' UTR | Risk factor for OUD | Gao et al. (138) | 2017 | 774 | Chinese | |
| | | | No significant association with OUD | Nelson et al. (137) | 2014 | 2,954 | Australian | |
| | **rs1042114** | Exon 1 | Risk factor for OUD | Nagaya et al. (139) | 2018 | 1,002 | Malay males | |
| | | | | Zhang et al. (136) | 2008 | 1,063 | European American | |
| | | | | Crist et al. (140) | 2013 | 566 | Caucasian males | |
| | | | No significant association with OUD | Nelson et al. (137) | 2014 | 2,954 | Australian | |
| | **rs2234918** | Exon 3 | Risk factor for OUD | Huang et al. (141) | 2018 | 1,331 | Chinese | |
| | | | | Mayer et al. (142) | 1997 | 218 | Caucasian | |
| | | | No significant association with OUD | Xu et al. (143) | 2002 | 754 | Chinese | |
| | | | | Levran et al. (130) | 2008 | 596 | Caucasian | |
| | | | | Zhang et al. (136) | 2008 | 1,063 | European American | |
| | | | | Franke et al. (144) | 1999 | 406 | Caucasian | |
| | | | | Crist et al. (140) | 2013 | 2,502 | Mixed | |
| | | | No significant association with methadone dose | Crettol et al. (134) | 2008 | 455 | Caucasian | |
| | **rs508448** | Intron 1 | Earlier onset OUD | Gao et al. (138) | 2017 | 774 | Chinese | |
| | | | No significant association with OUD | Nelson et al. (137) | 2014 | 2,954 | Australian | |
| | **rs581111** | Intron 1 | Risk factor for OUD | Crist et al. (140) | 2013 | 1,006 | African American | |
| | | | Higher relapse rates on buprenorphine | Clarke et al. (145) | 2014 | 582 | Caucasian females | |
| | | | No significant association with OUD | Nelson et al. (137) | 2014 | 2,954 | Australian | |

*(Continued)*

**TABLE 1** | Continued

| Gene | Polymorphism | Location | Finding | Author | Year | n | Ethnicity | Imaging Correlates |
|---|---|---|---|---|---|---|---|---|
| | **rs678849** | Intron 1 | Risk factor for OUD | Sharafshah et al. (146) | 2017 | 404 | Iranian | |
| | | | Abstinence-induced withdrawal severity | *Jones et al. (147) | 2016 | 19 | Mixed | |
| | | | Higher relapse rates on buprenorphine | Crist et al. (148) | 2013 | 77 | African American | |
| | | | | Crist et al. (149) | 2018 | 55 | African American | |
| | | | Lower relapse rates on methadone | Crist et al. (148) | 2013 | 77 | African American | |
| | | | No significant association with relapse rates on methadone | Crist et al. (149) | 2018 | 55 | African American | |
| | | | No significant association with OUD | Nelson et al. (137) | 2014 | 2,954 | Australian | |
| | | | | Zhang et al. (136) | 2008 | 1,063 | European American | |
| | **rs2236857** | Intron 1 | Risk factor for OUD | Sharafshah et al. (146) | 2017 | 404 | Iranian | |
| | | | | Nelson et al. (137) | 2014 | 2,954 | Australian | |
| | | | | *Levran et al. (130) | 2008 | 596 | Caucasian | |
| | | | No significant association with OUD | Zhang et al. (136) | 2008 | 1,063 | European American | |
| | | | Protective against stress response in OUD | Huang et al. (141) | 2018 | 1,331 | Chinese | |
| | **rs2236857+ rs581111 haplotype†** | Intron 1 | Risk factor for OUD | Nelson et al. (137) | 2014 | 2,954 | Australian | |
| | **rs2236855** | Intron 1 | Risk factor for OUD | Sharafshah et al. (146) | 2017 | 404 | Iranian | |
| | | | | Nelson et al. (137) | 2014 | 2954 | Australian | |
| | | | No significant association with OUD | Zhang et al. (136) | 2008 | 1,063 | European American | |
| | | | | Crist et al. (140) | 2013 | 566 | Caucasian males | |
| | **rs760589** | Intron 1 | Risk factor for OUD | Sharafshah et al. (146) | 2017 | 404 | Iranian | |
| | | | | *Nelson et al. (137) | 2014 | 2,954 | Australian | |
| | **rs2236861** | Intron 1 | Risk factor for OUD | Beer et al. (150) | 2013 | 284 | Western European | |
| | | | | *Levran et al. (130) | 2008 | 596 | Caucasian | |
| | | | | *Nelson et al. (137) | 2014 | 2,954 | Australian | |
| | **rs529520** | Intron 1 | Higher methadone requirement | Luo et al. (151) | 2017 | 257 | Chinese | |
| | | | Higher relapse rates on buprenorphine | Clarke et al. (145) | 2014 | 582 | Caucasian females | |
| | | | Risk factor for OUD | *Nelson et al. (137) | 2014 | 2,954 | Australian | |
| | | | No significant association with OUD | Zhang et al. (136) | 2008 | 1,063 | European American | |
| | **rs10753331** | Intron 1 | Abstinence-induced withdrawal severity | Jones et al. (147) | 2016 | 19 | Mixed | |
| | | | Risk factor for OUD | Crist et al. (140) | 2013 | 566 | Caucasian | |
| | **rs3766951** | Intron 1 | Risk factor for OUD | Nelson et al. (137) | 2014 | 2,954 | Australian | |
| | | | | *Levran et al. (130) | 2008 | 596 | Caucasian | |
| | **rs2298897** | Intron 1 | Risk factor for OUD | Nelson et al. (137) | 2014 | 2,954 | Australian | |
| **OPRK1** | **rs1051660** | Exon 2 | Risk factor for OUD | Yuferov et al. (152) | 2004 | 291 | Mixed | |
| | | | | Gerra et al. (153) | 2007 | 176 | Caucasian Italian | |
| | **rs702764** | Exon 4 | No significant association with OUD | Nagaya et al. (139) | 2018 | 1,002 | Malay males | |
| | | | | Zhang et al. (136) | 2008 | 1,063 | European American | |
| | **rs997917** | Intron 2 | Risk factor for OUD | Albonaim et al. (154) | 2017 | 404 | Iranian | |
| | | | No significant association with OUD | Zhang et al. (136) | 2008 | 1,063 | European American | |
| | **rs6985606** | Intron 2 | Risk factor for OUD | Albonaim et al. (154) | 2017 | 404 | Iranian | |
| | | | No significant association with OUD | Zhang et al. (136) | 2008 | 1,063 | European American | |
| | **rs6473797** | Intron 2 | Protective against OUD | *Levran et al. (130) | 2008 | 596 | Caucasian | |
| | | | Naloxone-precipitated withdrawal severity | Jones et al. (147) | 2016 | 29 | Mixed | |
| | | | No significant association with OUD | Albonaim et al. (154) | 2017 | 404 | Iranian | |

*(Continued)*

**TABLE 1** | Continued

| Gene | Polymorphism | Location | Finding | Author | Year | n | Ethnicity | Imaging Correlates |
|---|---|---|---|---|---|---|---|---|
| ***PDYN*** | **rs35286281 H allele** | Promoter | Risk factor for OUD | Yuanyuan et al. (155) | 2018 | 1,107 | Chinese | |
| | | | | Wei et al. (156) | 2011 | 604 | Chinese | |
| | | | No significant association with OUD | Hashemi et al. (157) | 2018 | 435 | Iranian | |
| | **rs1997794** | Promoter | Risk factor for OUD | Clarke et al. (158) | 2012 | 2,618 | European American females | |
| | | | | Clarke et al. (159) | 2009 | 858 | Chinese females | |
| | | | No significant association with OUD | Nagaya et al. (139) | 2018 | 1,002 | Malaysian males | |
| | **rs2281285** | Intron 2 | No significant association with OUD | Hashemi et al. (157) | 2018 | 435 | Iranian | |
| | **rs910080** | 3' UTR | Risk factor for OUD | Nagaya et al. (139) | 2018 | 1,002 | Malaysian males | |
| | | | | Clarke et al. (158) | 2012 | 2,618 | European American females | |
| | | | | Wei et al. (156) | 2011 | 604 | Chinese | |
| | | | | Hashemi et al. (157) | 2018 | 435 | Iranian | |
| | | | No significant association with OUD | Clarke et al. (158) | 2012 | 2,618 | European American males | |
| | **rs1022563** | 3' UTR | Risk factor for OUD | Clarke et al. (158) | 2012 | 2,618 | European American females | |
| | | | | Clarke et al. (159) | 2009 | 858 | Chinese females | |
| | | | | Wei et al. (156) | 2011 | 604 | Chinese | |
| | | | No significant association with OUD | Nagaya et al. (139) | 2018 | 1,002 | Malaysian males | |
| | **rs2235749** | 3' UTR | Risk factor for OUD | Wei et al. (156) | 2011 | 604 | Chinese | |
| | | | No significant association with OUD | Hashemi et al. (157) | 2018 | 435 | Iranian | |
| ***OPRL1*** | **rs6512305** | Intron 1 | Risk factor for OUD | *Xuei et al. (160) | 2008 | 1,923 | European American | |
| | **rs6090043** | Intron 1 | Risk factor for OUD | *Xuei et al. (160) | 2008 | 1,923 | European American | |
| | | | No significant association with OUD | Briant et al. (161) | 2010 | 447 | African American | |
| | **rs6090041** | Intron 1 | Risk factor for OUD | Briant et al. (161) | 2010 | 447 | Caucasian | |
| | | | No significant association with OUD | Briant et al. (161) | 2010 | 447 | African American | |
| | | | | Xuei et al. (160) | 2008 | 1,923 | European American | |
| | **rs6090043+ rs6090041 haplotype‡1** | Intron 1 | Risk factor for OUD | Briant et al. (161) | 2010 | 447 | Mixed | |
| | **rs6090043+ rs6090041 haplotype‡2** | Intron 1 | Risk factor for OUD | Briant et al. (161) | 2010 | 447 | Caucasian | |
| | | | No significant association with OUD | Briant et al. (161) | 2010 | 447 | African American | |

*SNP associations refer to the minor allele.*
**Nominal significance.*
*† rs2236857 + rs581111 GA haplotype (coupled minor alleles).*
*‡[1] rs6090043 + rs6090041 AT haplotype.*
*‡[2] rs6090043 + rs6090041 GC haplotype.*

occupied, indicating inadequate withdrawal suppression (192). This may reflect the half-life of oral buprenorphine, which ranges from 28 to 37 h (193). Plasma concentrations of buprenorphine were time-dependent and correlated with levels of MOP receptor occupancy in brain (192, 194). Considering the minor allele of rs1799971 may lower MOP receptor expression, it stands to reason that this SNP may influence the dose of buprenorphine required to achieve adequate withdrawal suppression.

In two studies, heroin-dependent patients maintained on varying doses of buprenorphine underwent several [$^{11}$C]carfentanil PET scans (194, 195). Buprenorphine was shown to reduce MOP receptor availability in a dose-dependent manner, and decreased MOP receptor availability correlated with decreased heroin craving and withdrawal symptoms (194, 195). After detoxification from buprenorphine, OUD participants demonstrated higher regional binding potential of MOP receptor particularly in the inferior frontal and anterior cingulate cortex compared to healthy controls (195). Yet, an animal study found buprenorphine maintenance down-regulates MOP receptor in rat brains (77). The higher MOP receptor binding potential among OUD participants found by Zubieta et al. (195) could reflect opioid or buprenorphine induced downregulation of enkephalins and β-endorphins in brain with a consequent reduced competition for [$^{11}$C]carfentanil binding to MOP.

Another study used [$^{18}$F]cyclofoxy PET scans in 14 methadone-maintained patients and 14 healthy controls (185).

The methadone-maintained patients demonstrated 19–32% lower cyclofoxy binding than the controls in thalamus, caudate, anterior cingulate cortex, middle temporal cortex, and the middle frontal cortex (185). The lower [$^{18}$F]cyclofoxy binding in the brain of OUD participants correlated with plasma methadone levels, likely reflecting the steady-state methadone occupancy of MOP receptors (185). These findings contrast with those obtained in OUD patients treated with buprenorphine who showed much greater levels of MOP occupancy consistent with the partial agonist effects of buprenorphine as compared to the full agonist effects of methadone (192). This discrepancy could also reflect less receptor internalization associated with a partial agonist and, therefore, greater levels of receptor occupancy by the radioligand.

PET studies have also investigated the effects of A118G on MOP receptor availability in individuals with SUDs. For example, the G allele has been associated with lower baseline MOP receptor binding potential in NAc and amygdala of smokers (146–148). Thus, A118G may shape predispositions to substance abuse by affecting MOP receptor availability, which could contribute to aberrant dopaminergic signaling. A [$^{11}$C]raclopride PET study of tobacco smokers found that the G allele associated with greater DA release in the right caudate and ventral pallidum in response to smoking compared to the A allele (120). This is further evidence of the association between A118G and drug reward, which may increase vulnerability to SUDs (120). Longitudinal studies are needed to clarify the link between opioid receptor availability and SUDs.

## OPRK1

### *OPRK1* Background

*OPRK1* codes for the KOP receptor, an inhibitory GPCR that is implicated in the brain's stress or anti-reward system (196). KOP receptors are the most abundant opioid receptors in the human brain and are highly expressed in key brain regions of the stress axis such as the prefrontal cortex and amygdala (197) as well as in reward-related regions including the VTA, NAc core, dorsal striatum, and substantia nigra as seen in **Figure 1** (187, 198–201). KOP receptors are coupled with calcium channels and are localized in presynaptic terminals of dopaminergic cells; activation of KOP receptors inhibits adenylyl cyclase and calcium currents, thereby inhibiting DA release (199, 202–204). Prodynorphin (*PDYN*) codes for the precursor to the dynorphin peptide, which is the endogenous ligand to the KOP receptor. Using a phospho-selective antibody against KOP receptors, Land et al. (16) demonstrated that both stress paradigms and CRF injections elicit dynorphin-dependent KOP receptor activation in the basolateral amygdala, NAc, and hippocampus of mice. This indicates the key role KOP receptor signaling plays in stress and dysphoria. In general, KOP receptor agonists have anxiogenic properties in humans (205, 206) while KOR antagonists demonstrate anxiolytic properties in animal models (207, 208). However, there is evidence of dose-dependent effects; in a mouse study, KOP receptor agonist, U50,488H, was anxiolytic at high doses but anxiogenic in low doses (209). KOP receptor signaling may also influence stress responses associated with relapse; for example, heroin-dependent rats treated with KOP receptor antagonists show reduced anxiety- and stress-induced reinstatement of drug-seeking behavior (210, 211).

KOP receptor signaling is also involved in an array of physiological functions such as mood modulation, pain perception, learning and memory, and behavioral response to drugs of abuse (212, 213). Within the NAc, dynorphin signaling inhibits DA release, which leads to aversive effects on mood (214). In individuals with SUDs, KOP receptor-mediated dynorphin signaling drives negative affective states during drug withdrawal (215). One [$^{11}$C]raclopride PET study showed blunted DA release with a methylphenidate challenge in recently detoxified OUD patients compared to healthy controls (7). This hypodopaminergic response may be explained by dynorphin-mediated withdrawal. This is consistent with a rodent study that found chronic exposure and subsequent withdrawal from morphine led to prolonged (15 day) decreases in spontaneous dopaminergic neuron activity (216). This hypodopaminergic state may underlie dysphoria that drives compulsive drug-seeking (216).

Interestingly, post-mortem brain samples of heroin abusers showed lower levels of PDYN mRNA expression in the amygdalar nucleus of the periamygdaloid cortex compared to controls (217). Further, a post-mortem study reported elevated dynorphin levels in heroin abusers with reduced striatal PDYN mRNA expression, suggesting upregulation of PDYN mRNA translation despite reduced PDYN mRNA levels (126). These results corroborate findings of reduced PDYN mRNA expression and elevated expression of the brain stress marker, CRF, in the periamygdaloid cortex of heroin-dependent rats that were euthanized following 24 h of abstinence (217). Increased CRF may reflect the dynorphin-mediated withdrawal response in the heroin-dependent rats despite seemingly reduced *PDYN* expression (217).

Preclinical studies have found that KOP receptor agonists, including salvinorin A, cause KOP receptor internalization *in vitro* (218, 219). A [11C]GR103545 PET study in rodents found that a dose of 0.60 mg/kg of salvinorin A resulted in a prolonged decrease in [11C]GR103545 binding that persisted even after salvinorin A had cleared from the brain, consistent with KOP receptor internalization (220). This study provides insight into the neurochemical adaptations to KOP receptor agonist exposure, which may contribute to opioid tolerance (18).

### *OPRK1* Polymorphisms

A few *OPRK1* polymorphisms have been described in the context of SUDs, although the majority of them are silent and have no effect on gene expression (221). One example is rs1051660 (G36T), a synonymous SNP in exon 2 (153). These polymorphisms may affect KOP receptor signaling indirectly by altering mRNA stability or translation (222).

*PDYN* polymorphisms are associated with aberrant dynorphin expression and signaling (223) that may contribute to dysphoria and relapse during opioid withdrawal (155). Intronic variants may alter gene expression *via* splicing mechanisms or may be in linkage disequilibrium with neighboring variants that have more direct downstream effects (146, 224). Mutations within the 3' tail of mRNA transcripts could alter important sequences like the polyadenylate tail and may disrupt transcription termination (225), translation, and stability of mRNA (226–228). For example, rs910080, a polymorphism in the 3' untranslated region of *PDYN*, is in high linkage disequilibrium with two other 3' untranslated region SNPs, rs910079 and rs2235749; in a post-mortem analysis, this haplotype block was associated with levels of PDYN expression in the striatum (229). Other polymorphisms may alter gene expression directly. The 68-base pair variable number tandem repeat (VNTR) polymorphism, rs35286281, ranges from two to five repeats in the promoter region of *PDYN*, with each repeat containing one binding site for a transcription factor (230, 231). Thus, high dynorphin expression alleles (H alleles) contain three or more repeats and are associated with higher *PDYN* transcription and translation compared to low dynorphin expression alleles (L alleles) with one or two repeats (230).

## Genetic Association Studies: *OPRK1*, *PDYN*, and OUD

There has been little consensus regarding the role of *OPRK1* polymorphisms in OUD. The minor alleles of two intronic polymorphisms, rs997917 and rs6985606, were reported as risk factors for OUD in an Iranian population (154) but were not associated with OUD in a European American population (136). These conflicting findings are likely explained by ethnicity-dependent effects. Interestingly, the rs6473797 minor allele was found to be protective against OUD in a Caucasian population (130), but not in an Iranian population (154). However, rs6473797 did associate with withdrawal severity among OUD patients who underwent naloxone-precipitated withdrawal in an American population of mixed ethnicities (147). Additionally, Wang et al. (232) found that two *OPRK1* haplotype blocks associated with withdrawal symptoms such as joint aches, gooseflesh skin, and yawning in Taiwanese methadone-maintained OUD patients. Lastly, rs1051660 was initially linked to OUD (152), and this finding was replicated by Gerra et al. (153) in a Caucasian Italian population.

Given the critical role of dynorphin signaling in the negative emotion states of SUDs, several studies have examined *PDYN* polymorphisms in the context of OUD. One polymorphism, rs910080, has been associated with OUD across a wide range of ethnicities (139, 156–158). Additionally, there is evidence of sex effects on the association between another two *PDYN* polymorphisms and OUD. That is, both rs1997794 and rs1022563 were found to associate with OUD among European American females, but not males (158). In a prior study of Chinese females, Clarke et al. (159) found the rs1997794 minor allele associated with OUD. Further, these two polymorphisms were not associated with OUD in a study of Malaysian males (139). Together, these findings suggest sex- and ethnicity-specific effects of the *PDYN* genotype on susceptibility to OUD.

Two studies found that the H allele of the *PDYN* VNTR polymorphism was a risk factor for OUD in Chinese populations (155, 156). It was also associated with greater instances of withdrawal and subsequent relapse among heroin-dependent Chinese patients on methadone therapy (155). However, Hashemi et al. (157) did not find an association between the *PDYN* genotype and OUD in an Iranian population. While evidence exists that the H allele upregulates *PDYN* expression (230), further research is required to understand its functional consequences as it relates to OUD.

Despite preclinical and clinical evidence of KOP receptor signaling modulating anxiety and stress response (16, 205, 206, 210, 211, 233, 234), few studies have investigated the effects of *OPRK1* polymorphisms on personality or behavior. One study using the five-factor NEO found the minor allele at rs963549, in exon 3 of *OPRK1*, was associated with higher Neuroticism scores among participants with SUDs but not among healthy controls (235). While this SNP was found to not be a risk factor for SUDs in an Indian population (116), its effects may be ethnicity-dependent or potentially mediated by opioid use. Future studies on the functional effects of *OPRK1* polymorphisms and their associated changes in neurochemistry and behavior would clarify the link between KOP receptor signaling and OUD.

One study examining the effects of the *PDYN* VNTR polymorphism on behavior found that the L allele is associated with disinhibited behavior as assessed with the Zuckerman Sensation Seeking Scale (236). Given that higher scores on this scale correlate with a preference toward risky behavior, this finding suggests L allele carriers are at increased risk for SUDs, contradicting findings from genetic association studies described above (155, 156) but perhaps corroborating post-mortem findings of reduced *PDYN* expression in individuals with OUD (217).

## Molecular Imaging: KOP Receptor and OUD

At this point, no studies have used PET to examine *OPRK1* polymorphisms among patients with OUD. Only recently have radiotracers been developed to target KOP receptors, including the agonist tracers [$^{11}$C]GR103545 and [$^{11}$C]EKAP and the antagonist tracer [$^{11}$C]LY2795050. These radiotracers have been evaluated in primates (237–240) and humans (241–244).

In a [$^{11}$C]LY2795050 PET study, patients with AUD showed lower KOP receptor availability in the amygdala and pallidum compared to healthy controls (245). It is possible that the reduction in KOP receptor availability helps restore dopaminergic signaling and thus alleviates the aversive effects of drinking. However, reduced [$^{11}$C]LY2795050 specific binding to KOP receptors in AUD could also reflect increased competition for radiotracer binding from upregulation of dynorphin. Another [$^{11}$C]LY2795050 PET study found that healthy male subjects had greater KOP receptor availability in several brain regions including ACC, frontal cortex, insula, and ventral pallidum compared to females (246). According to the "simple occupation theory," the robustness of a drug response is directly proportional to the number of receptors occupied by the drug (247). This is consistent with the finding by Vijay et al. (246) that greater KOP receptor availability may mediate stronger responses to KOP receptor antagonists such as naltrexone treatment. Among patients with co-occurring cocaine and alcohol dependence, one study showed that naltrexone treatment reduced cocaine and alcohol use in men, but increased substance use in women (248). While sex differences in KOP receptor availability were not examined by Pettinati et al. (248), the authors suggest that receptor bioavailability and naltrexone treatment response may be sex-dependent. A potential non-neurochemical basis for the poorer treatment response in women compared to men is that women report higher rates of naltrexone-induced nausea, which results in lower medication compliance (249). However, it is important to note that other clinical studies found no sex differences of naltrexone treatment response in AUD (250, 251). Overall, these findings suggest that KOP receptor availability is associated with alcohol use and could potentially mediate the efficacy of KOP-targeted pharmacotherapies for AUD (245). Given the high comorbidity between AUD and OUD (252–254), these findings might have implications for opioid-antagonist treatment response in OUD.

## OPRD1

### *OPRD1* Background

*OPRD1* codes for DOP receptors, which are also involved in the negative affect and withdrawal stage of addiction, albeit with inverse effects than KOP receptors. Specifically, greater DOP receptor signaling leads to improvements in negative emotional states (255). DOP receptor agonists have demonstrated antidepressant and anxiolytic effects in rodent models (256, 257). DOP receptors are highly expressed in cortical and limbic areas such as the hippocampus and amygdala, as well as basal ganglia and hypothalamus (258–260). DOP receptors are located on presynaptic terminals of GABAergic interneurons and have region-specific effects on cAMP production (261). While striatal DOP receptor activation is inhibitory and results in increased extracellular dopamine (262), DOP receptors located in the olfactory bulb, medial prefrontal cortex, and primary cultures of hippocampal neurons stimulate cAMP production thereby inhibiting dopamine release (263–265).

Studies suggest DOP receptors modulate the rewarding effects of drugs of abuse. Le Merrer et al. (197) report DOP receptor knockout has no effect on morphine self-administration but does impair place conditioning in mice. In another rodent study, DOP receptor knockout resulted in reduced morphine reward and tolerance (266). Further, DOP receptor antagonists block sensitization to conditioned rewarding effects of opioids (267), whereas agonists enhance conditioned place preference to morphine (268). In a mouse model of OUD, DOP receptor knockout was associated with increased anhedonia and dysphoria during heroin abstinence compared to the wild-type genotype (269). Thus, *OPRD1* polymorphisms that alter DOP receptor signaling may influence opioid withdrawal-associated stress response and relapse.

### *OPRD1* Polymorphisms

Several polymorphisms of *OPRD1* have been studied in the context of SUDs. One, rs1042114 (G80T), results in an amino acid substitution from cysteine to phenylalanine in the N-terminus of the DOP receptor, and is proposed to disrupt DOP receptor maturation, leading to increased internalization of the receptor compared to wild type (270). The coding-region variant rs2234918 (T921C) is a synonymous polymorphism, that is, it does not cause a change in the coding amino acid, and has conflicting evidence for a role in OUD. Finally, rs569356, located in the promoter region, has been implicated in altered OPRD1 expression; Zhang et al. (271) found the G allele increased *OPRD1* transcription in transfected cell lines. Few other *OPRD1* polymorphisms have been described in terms of their functional effects; however, several have been assessed in genetic association studies.

### Genetic Association Studies: *OPRD1* and OUD

Two polymorphisms in the coding region of *OPRD1* have been associated with OUD. The rs1042114 polymorphism has been found to be a risk factor for OUD in Malaysian males (139) and in Caucasian populations (136, 140). However, Nelson et al. (137) did not replicate these findings in Australian OUD patients. Rs2234918, a synonymous *OPRD1* polymorphism, has also been studied in OUD with conflicting findings. The minor C allele of this polymorphism was initially reported as a risk factor for OUD in a German (142) and Chinese population (272). However, several studies have failed to replicate this association (130, 136, 140, 143) including a study that examined a German population but used a family-based association approach to control for population stratification (144). Thus, it is uncertain what role, if any, these *OPRD1* polymorphisms play in increasing vulnerability to OUD.

Several polymorphisms in intron 1 of *OPRD1* have been studied in OUD, although their functional effects remain largely unknown. Two studies found an association between rs2236861 and OUD among Caucasian patients (137, 150). Levran et al. (130) also found that the rs2236861 minor allele increases the risk of heroin dependence; however, the association did not survive multiple testing, perhaps due to a small sample size. Another intron 1 polymorphism, rs2236857, was associated with OUD in Iranian- and European-descent populations (130, 137, 146). However, Zhang et al. (136) were unable to replicate this association in a study of European Americans. Interestingly, among Chinese OUD patients, carriers of the rs2236857 minor allele were found to have higher subjective stress responses than non-carriers as assessed with the Life Event Questionnaire (272). This suggests that *OPRD1* polymorphisms may disrupt stress responses that increase addiction vulnerabilities. The minor allele of rs581111, located in intron 1, has also been reported as a risk factor for OUD among Australians (137) and African Americans but not European Americans (140). Additionally, the minor allele of rs581111 has been associated with poor response to buprenorphine treatment among Caucasian females, but not males, suggesting ethnicity- and sex-dependent influences on genetic associations (145). Lastly, the minor allele of an *OPRD1* intron 1 polymorphism, rs3766951, was reported as a risk factor for OUD in Caucasian populations (130, 137).

In addition, several studies have investigated the effects of *OPRD1* polymorphisms on treatment outcomes in OUD. For example, the major allele of rs678849 has been associated with higher relapse rates among African American OUD patients undergoing buprenorphine treatment, as indicated by positive opioid urine tests (148, 149). Interestingly, the major allele was initially associated with lower relapse rates among African American OUD patients on methadone treatment (148), but this association was not replicated (149). Jones et al. (147) reported an association between rs678849 and abstinence-induced opioid withdrawal severity; however, it did not withstand a multivariate analysis. While the mechanism of action is unknown, these findings suggest that rs678849 may affect OUD treatment outcomes by potentially mediating withdrawal symptoms.

Several other *OPRD1* polymorphisms have been studied in association with OUD with conflicting results as seen in **Table 1**.

*OPRD1* polymorphisms have also been associated with behaviors related to the negative affect and withdrawal stage of OUD. In one study of Pakistani OUD patients, the minor G allele of rs569356 was strongly associated with increased serum cortisol levels, a marker of stress response (273). Given the preclinical evidence that this minor allele may increase *OPRD1* transcription (271), the minor G allele may affect DOP receptor expression and stress responses that could contribute to OUD. While Zhang et al. (136) found a nominally significant association between rs569356 and OUD in a European American population, no significant association was found in Australian and Pakistani populations (137, 273).

### Molecular Imaging: DOP Receptor and OUD

No PET studies have examined neurochemical differences between carriers of *OPRD1* polymorphisms in OUD. The only DOP-selective radiotracer that has been developed for PET imaging in humans is N1'-([$^{11}$C]methyl)naltrindole ([$^{11}$C]MeNTI) (274).

PET studies investigating DOP receptor availability in healthy controls and AUD patients may provide insight into the functional effects of *OPRD1* polymorphisms in OUD. One [$^{11}$C]MeNTl PET study found that patients with AUD had slightly greater DOP receptor availability compared to healthy controls in the cingulate, amygdala, insula, ventral striatum, putamen, caudate nucleus, globus pallidus, and thalamus; however, group differences did not reach statistical significance (275). Within the AUD group, DOP receptor availability in the caudate showed a positive association with recent alcohol drinking (275). However, Weerts et al. (275) did not report associations between DOP receptor availability and other behavioral measures of alcohol dependence or withdrawal. Another PET study in abstinent AUD patients demonstrated that while naltrexone completely blocked MOP receptor radioligand binding, it only partially blocked [$^{11}$C]MeNTl binding and there was high interindividual variability in DOP receptor blockade (276). These findings could underlie interindividual differences in responses to naltrexone treatment in AUD that could translate to naltrexone treatment responses in OUD.

Additionally, one [$^{11}$C]MeNTl PET study found a negative correlation between mesolimbic DOP receptor availability and total cortisol output over a 4-h period following naloxone in healthy controls, but not in recently abstinent AUD patients (277). Given that endogenous DOP receptor signaling improves negative emotional states (278), the dissociation of DOP receptor availability from naloxone-induced cortisol response in AUD may suggest that chronic alcohol abuse disrupts DOP-mediated stress signaling during alcohol withdrawal. Whether this is the case for OUD remains to be determined. Notably however, Lutz et al. (269) reported that DOP receptor signaling ameliorates opioid withdrawal in rodents, so together, these findings may suggest a shared mechanism for negative emotional states in opioid and alcohol withdrawal.

## OPRL1

### *OPRL1* Background

The nociceptin opioid peptide (NOP) receptor is an inhibitory GPCR encoded by the Opioid Receptor-Like 1 gene (*OPRL1*) that has MOP, KOP, and DOP receptor structure homology and similar signaling cascades (279). However, the NOP receptor is pharmacologically distinct from classical opioid receptors. The NOP receptor is activated by nociceptin, and its effects are not blocked by the universal opioid antagonist naloxone (280, 281). NOP receptors are distributed throughout the amygdala, hippocampus, thalamus, and cortical processing areas (282) and have roles in both analgesia and hyperalgesia [reviewed in (283) and (284)]. NOP receptor signaling is also involved in processes including stress, anxiety, depression, cognition, and addiction (285–289).

Given the distribution of NOP receptors along the limbic region (290), it follows that NOP signaling is tied to stress signaling. For example, central injections of nociceptin in rats result in increased plasma stress hormone levels, reflecting activation of the HPA axis (291). However, there is also evidence that NOP receptors in extrahypothalamic brain regions exert anti-stress effects. For example, nociceptin injections in the central nucleus of the amygdala reduce anxiety behaviors in rodents exposed to restraint stress (292). Further, body restraint stress upregulates NOP receptor mRNA in the central nucleus of the amygdala and basolateral amygdala (292). In an electrophysiological study, nociceptin blocked CRF-induced GABAergic transmission in slices from the central nucleus of the amygdala; these effects were more pronounced in neurons from ethanol-dependent rodents (293). Additionally, nociceptin injections in the bed nucleus of the stria terminalis block CRF-induced anxiety behaviors in rodents (294, 295). Thus, the role of NOP receptors in stress is likely complex and may be relevant in OUD, particularly due to the high co-occurrence of anxiety and SUDs [reviewed in (296)].

NOP receptor signaling also seems to have an anti-reward effect. In microdialysis studies, nociceptin administration was found to decrease extracellular DA levels in the NAc of anesthetized mice (297) and to decrease morphine-induced DA release in the NAc of rats (298). Further, in several rodent studies, NOP receptor agonists reduced conditioned place preference to alcohol, amphetamines, cocaine, and morphine, suggesting NOP receptor signaling may reduce the rewarding effects of these substances (299–304). However, Walker et al. (305) found nociceptin administration failed to reduce heroin self-administration in rodents. There is also preliminary evidence that the NOP receptor antagonist, LY2940094, could be efficacious in treating AUD in rodents and humans, perhaps by blocking stress-induced relapse (306, 307). While an initial post-mortem analysis demonstrated individuals with AUD had lower *OPRL1* expression in the central amygdala compared to controls (308), no difference in *OPRL1* expression was detected in another post-mortem study in individuals with SUDs including AUD (309). Thus, the NOP receptor is likely implicated in substance abuse and poses a potential therapeutic target, but further research is required to clarify its roles in reward and stress-related behaviors.

### *OPRL1* Polymorphisms

The functional effects of several *OPRL1* polymorphisms have been studied. For example, two adjacent SNPs in intron 1, rs6512305 and rs6090043, are in high linkage disequilibrium and there is evidence that variants in rs6090043 may alter transcription factor binding sites, which could affect *OPRL1* gene expression (161). Further, the minor G allele at rs6090041, another intron 1 variant, and the minor C allele at rs6090043 provide additional transcription factor binding sites that could result in increased *OPRL1* transcription and NOP receptor availability (161). Given that NOP receptor signaling has been implicated in decreasing drug reward, there may be a role of *OPRL1* polymorphisms in susceptibility to SUDs.

### Genetic Association Studies: *OPRL1* and OUD

Xuei et al. (160) assessed correlations between SUDs and polymorphisms in *OPRL1* as well as in the prepronociceptin gene (*PNOC*), which encodes the NOP receptor precursor, in a European American population; rs6512305 and rs6090043 were nominally associated with opioid dependence; however, no SNPs proved significant (160). Briant et al. (161) found that minor alleles at rs6090043 and rs6090041 were risk factors for OUD among Caucasians but not African Americans. One haplotype (AT) of these variants was found to be a risk factor in both Caucasians and African Americans, while another haplotype (GC) was a risk factor in Caucasians only (161). While there is preliminary evidence that *OPRL1* may influence vulnerability to OUD, further analysis is required to determine the potential ethnicity-dependent effects.

### Molecular Imaging: NOP Receptor and OUD

NOP receptor antagonist PET radioligands have been developed; [$^{11}$C]NOP-1A has been tested in humans (290, 310, 311) and [$^{18}$F]MK-0911 has been tested in rhesus monkeys (312). To date, no molecular imaging of NOP has been done in participants with OUD; however, studies of other SUDs may provide insight. Using [$^{11}$C]NOP-1A, Narendran et al. (313) found no difference in NOP receptor availability between healthy controls and recently abstinent AUD subjects, nor did NOP receptor availability correlate with clinical measures of addiction severity. This conflicts with preclinical evidence that NOP receptor signaling is involved with AUD (289, 299, 300, 308). However, the subjects with AUD in this study were abstinent for 16 to 54 days before the PET scan, and there is preclinical evidence that prolonged abstinence may recover NOP receptor levels in rats (313, 314). In another PET study, recently abstinent CUD participants demonstrated a significant increase in [$^{11}$C]NOP-1A distribution volume notably in the midbrain, ventral striatum, and cerebellum compared to healthy controls (315). This increased NOP receptor availability may reflect a compensatory response to increased CRF transmission or decreased endogenous nociceptin associated with CUD (315). Further studies are required to evaluate NOP in OUD, for while studies in CUD have shown upregulation in brain, studies in AUD showed no differences (313), which suggests that there might be differences between SUDs. Also, research is needed to clarify changes during the different stages of the addiction cycle and to assess if there is recovery of NOP receptor availability with treatment.

# THE DOPAMINE SYSTEM

## DRD2

### *DRD2* Background

The gene *DRD2* codes for D2R, an inhibitory GPCR distributed throughout the brain. Expression of D2R is concentrated in the basal ganglia nuclei, including the caudate, putamen, NAc, substantia nigra, and VTA, as shown in **Figure 1** (316). As such, D2R signaling plays an important role in cognition, reward, motivation, and drug addiction, including OUD (317, 318). MOP receptors are expressed on DA neurons in the reward pathway; thus, with opioid use, MOP receptor binding leads to a release of DA, which then binds striatal D2Rs, leading to a decrease in intracellular cAMP production (69, 319). This D2R signaling inhibits the indirect ventral striatal pathway, which is connected to punishment (320).

Ankyrin Repeat and Kinase Domain Containing 1 (*ANKK1*) is a gene directly downstream of *DRD2* on chromosome 11 that expresses a serine/threonine kinase (321). The protein product of *ANKK1* upregulates the expression of the transcription factor NF-κB (322). Increased NF-κB expression results in increased *DRD2* transcription (323).

Several studies have shown that OUD is associated with a disruption of the mesolimbic dopaminergic pathway, which underlies the behavioral response to opioids (4). Koob and Volkow (4) suggest that D2Rs contribute to drug seeking behaviors, but not drug reward directly (324, 325). A conditioned place preference study of *DRD2*-null mice demonstrated that D2Rs are in part responsible for the reinforcing nature of morphine (326).

Lower D2R levels observed in SUDs may reflect a homeostatic downregulation of D2R after excessive drug use (29), and some evidence exists that D2R levels increase after pronounced abstinence (327). Alternatively, lower D2R availability may be an inherent risk factor for drug abuse, even before the initiation of drug taking (328, 329).

### *DRD2* Polymorphisms

A wide range of *DRD2*/*ANKK1* polymorphisms have been studied in the context of SUDs. One of the most well studied of these SNPs is *Taq*IA, located on exon 8 of *ANKK1*, adjacent to *DRD2* (321). Many studies have supported the role of *Taq*IA in addictive behaviors including various SUDs, obesity, and pathological gambling (330–333). Thus, the *Taq*IA1 variant, which alters ANKK1 substrate binding specificity, could lead to decreased D2R expression downstream (321). Indeed, [$^{11}$C]raclopride and [$^{11}$C]NMB PET studies have shown that minor alleles of *ANKK1* *Taq*IA and *Taq*IB, a linked *DRD2* SNP, are associated with low D2R availability in healthy controls (334–336). However,

*Taq*IA is in linkage disequilibrium with several functional *DRD2* polymorphisms (337); thus, it is unclear if reduced D2R expression is associated with *Taq*IA directly.

Lesser studied *DRD2* variants may also contribute to OUD *via* a diminution of D2R expression (338). SNPs in the 5' untranslated region of *DRD2*, including rs1799732, an insertion/deletion (*Ins/Del*) variant at position -141, have been shown to cause decreased promoter strength in an *in vitro* -141C *Del* luciferase construct (339). While one [11C]FLB-457 PET study found no association between rs1799732 and extrastriatal D2R in healthy volunteers (340), one [11C]raclopride PET study demonstrated higher striatal D2R availability in those with the combined minor variants of rs1799732, *Ins/Del* and *Del/Del*, compared to *Ins/Ins* (334). Until more studies are performed, the role of rs1799732 in D2R expression cannot be concluded.

Other *DRD2* polymorphisms produce splicing errors of the *DRD2* gene, resulting in altered D2R expression (341). For example, the minor allele of rs1076560, located in intron 6, is associated with a decreased ratio of short form D2 receptors (D2S) to long form receptors (D2L) (342). Preclinical studies have demonstrated that D2L knock-out mice have a loss of morphine preference in a conditioned place preference paradigm (343). Thus, this altered D2S/D2L ratio could help elucidate the mechanism of this SNP-OUD relationship. [123I]IBZM SPECT imaging revealed that in healthy volunteers, minor T allele carriers of this SNP showed lower levels of striatal D2R availability compared to G/G (344). However, another [123I]IBZM SPECT study in healthy volunteers did not replicate this finding (345). These findings may implicate *DRD2/ANKK1* polymorphisms in the lower D2R levels observed in individuals with OUD (6).

## Genetic Association Studies: *DRD2* and OUD

Several polymorphisms in *DRD2/ANKK1* have been suggested to predispose OUD, as outlined in **Table 2**. Indeed, a recent meta-analysis across 11 studies, with a total sample of 4,529 OUD patients and 4,168 healthy controls, found that the *Taq*IA1 allele is a risk factor for (OUD) (354). Further, several other minor alleles of *Taq*IA and *Taq*IB are more frequent among OUD patients compared to healthy controls (353, 355, 356, 360, 351).

There is less robust evidence for other *DRD2* polymorphisms in OUD. For example, despite preclinical evidence that rs1076560 may alter D2R expression, genetic association studies between rs1076560 and OUD have been inconsistent (44, 341, 348, 352, 354). In contrast, while the role of rs1799732 on D2R expression is uncertain, subjects with the minor variant have shown to be at higher risk for OUD in the Jordanian Arabic population (352).

The extent to which *DRD2* polymorphisms affect the response to MOUD in patients with OUD is inconsistent across studies. Lawford et al. (372) first reported that the *Taq*IA1 allele was associated with poorer treatment outcomes among Caucasian patients on methadone maintenance therapy. Since then, no group has replicated these findings in Caucasian populations (44, 134, 358, 361). Similarly, no association was found between *Taq*IB and methadone maintenance therapy response nor *Taq*IA and buprenorphine maintenance therapy response (44, 272). However, Crettol et al. (134) did report an association with rs6277 and patients' response to methadone maintenance therapy; patients with the major CC genotype were more likely to abuse illicit opioids on methadone therapy than those with CT or TT genotype. Interestingly, in two [11C]raclopride PET studies, the major C allele of rs6277 was associated with lower striatal D2R availability in healthy volunteers (373, 374), while another [11C]FLB457 PET study found the C allele predicted high extrastriatal D2R availability across the cortex and hypothalamus (340). However, several studies found no association between rs6277 and OUD (44, 134). Further, Doehring et al. (44) found no relationship between rs6277 and methadone maintenance therapy response. Instead, this group found that minor allele carriers of a different polymorphism, rs6275, required greater methadone doses than non-carriers and took longer to reach their maximum methadone dose (44). Thus, genetic studies suggest a role of *DRD2* polymorphisms in treatment response in OUD; however, they remain inconsistent and difficult to replicate.

Several studies have investigated the role of *DRD2* variants on behaviors associated with OUD. The tridimensional personality questionnaire scores personality on harm avoidance, novelty seeking, and reward dependence (375). These scores are used to calculate a borderline index using the equation: borderline index = harm avoidance + novelty seeking – reward dependence (376). Borderline index reflects borderline personality trait, characterized by a fear of abandonment, self-injurious behaviors, and emotional dysregulation (376, 377) (DSM-5). A recent study found that OUD patients had higher harm avoidance and novelty seeking scores and lower reward dependence scores, and thus a higher borderline index, than healthy volunteers (356). Further, Huang et al. (272) found that borderline index scores are inversely correlated with methadone dose, indicating the relevance of borderline index score in OUD treatment. These personality scores have not shown associations with *Taq*IA or *Taq*IB polymorphisms (272, 356). However, the -141C *Del* polymorphism (rs1799732) is associated with higher harm avoidance scores among OUD patients (356). In contrast, Gerra et al. (377) found that OUD patients had lower harm avoidance scores compared to CUD patients and healthy volunteers. However, this study reported that both CUD and OUD patients had higher novelty seeking scores and lower reward dependence scores than healthy volunteers (378). Therefore, this difference in harm avoidance could be rooted in genetic differences between the groups, as -141C *Del* is associated with higher harm avoidance scores in OUD, though Gerra et al. (378) did not report the genetic composition of their cohort (356).

## Molecular Imaging: D2R and OUD

[11C]raclopride and [123I]IBZM are widely used radiolabeled D2R antagonists differing *via* regioselectivity used to study D2R distribution, with additional affinity to D3Rs (D2-like inhibitory receptors) (379–381). [11C]NMB is another radiotracer used to study D2R availability with higher affinity for D2Rs over D3Rs than [11C]raclopride and [123I]IBZM (382, 383). Lastly, [11C]FLB-457 is a high-affinity radioligand that targets extrastriatal D2Rs and D3Rs (384).

In contrast to other SUDs, less is certain about D2R availability in OUD. In one [11C]raclopride PET study, OUD participants showed lower D2R availability compared to healthy controls (6). In this

**TABLE 2** | Polymorphisms associated with OUD in the dopamine system and imaging correlates.

| Gene | Polymorphism | Location | Findings | Author | Year | n | Ethnicity | Imaging Correlates |
|---|---|---|---|---|---|---|---|---|
| ***DRD1*** | **rs10078866** | Promoter | No significant association with OUD | Zhu et al. (346) | 2013 | 939 | Han Chinese | |
| | | | | Liu et al. (53) | 2013 | 739 | Han Chinese | |
| | **rs10078714** | Promoter | No significant association with OUD | Liu et al. (53) | 2013 | 739 | Han Chinese | |
| | **rs1799914** | Exon 1 | No significant association with OUD | Zhu et al. (346) | 2013 | 939 | Han Chinese | |
| | **rs265975** | 3' Near | Risk factor for OUD | *Jacobs et al. (347) | 2014 | 286 | Caucasian | |
| | **rs265973** | 3' Near | Risk factor for OUD | *Jacobs et al. (347) | 2014 | 286 | Caucasian | |
| | **rs686** | 3' UTR | Risk factor for OUD | Jacobs et al. (347) | 2013 | 187 | African American | |
| | | | No significant association with OUD | Zhu et al. (346) | 2013 | 939 | Han Chinese | |
| | | | | Liu et al. (53) | 2013 | 739 | Han Chinese | |
| | | | | Levran et al. (348) | 2015 | 801 | African American | |
| | | | | Levran et al. (349) | 2009 | 369 | African American | |
| | **rs267418** | 3' UTR | No significant association with OUD | Peng et al. (350) | 2013 | 739 | Han Chinese | |
| | **rs6882300** | 3' UTR | No significant association with OUD | Peng et al. (350) | 2013 | 739 | Han Chinese | |
| | **rs2168631** | 3' UTR | No significant association with OUD | Peng et al. (350) | 2013 | 739 | Han Chinese | |
| | **rs5326** | 5' UTR | Risk factor for OUD | *Levran et al. (349) | 2009 | 369 | African American | |
| | | | | Liu et al. (53) | 2013 | 739 | Han Chinese | |
| | | | No significant association with OUD | Zhu et al. (346) | 2013 | 939 | Han Chinese | |
| | | | | Peng et al. (350) | 2013 | 739 | Han Chinese | |
| | **rs4532** | 5' UTR | No significant association with OUD | Zhu et al. (346) | 2013 | 939 | Han Chinese | |
| | | | | Peng et al. (350) | 2013 | 739 | Han Chinese | |
| | | | | Liu et al. (53) | 2013 | 739 | Han Chinese | |
| | | | No significant association with methadone dose | Crettol et al. (134) | 2008 | 455 | Caucasian | |
| | **rs4867798** | 5' UTR | No significant association with OUD | Zhu et al. (346) | 2013 | 939 | Han Chinese | |
| | | | | Liu et al. (53) | 2013 | 739 | Han Chinese | |
| | **rs10063995** | 5' UTR | No significant association with OUD | Zhu et al. (346) | 2013 | 939 | Han Chinese | |
| | **rs265981** | 5' UTR | Protective against OUD | Liu et al. (53) | 2013 | 739 | Han Chinese | |
| ***DRD2*** | **rs6275** | Exon 7 | Risk factor for OUD | Wang et al. (351) | 2016 | 633 | Han Chinese | |
| | | | Higher methadone dose | Doehring et al. (44) | 2009 | 184 | Caucasian | |
| | | | No significant association with OUD | Al-eitan et al. (352) | 2012 | 425 | Jordanian Arabic | |
| | | | | Doehring et al. (44) | 2009 | 184 | Caucasian | |
| | **rs6277** | Exon 7 | Higher response rates to methadone treatment | Crettol et al. (134) | 2008 | 455 | Caucasian | |
| | | | No significant association with OUD | Doehring et al. (44) | 2009 | 184 | Caucasian | |
| | | | | Crettol et al. (134) | 2008 | 455 | Caucasian | |
| | **rs1801028** | Exon 7 | No significant association with OUD | Doehring et al. (44) | 2009 | 184 | Caucasian | |
| | **rs1125394** | Intron 1 | Risk factor for OUD | Wang et al. (351) | 2016 | 633 | Han Chinese | |
| | | | | Al-eitan et al. (352) | 2012 | 425 | Jordanian Arabic | |
| | **rs17115583** | Intron 1 | Protective against OUD | Wang et al. (351) | 2016 | 633 | Han Chinese | |
| | **rs1079597 (taqIB)** | Intron 1 | Risk factor for OUD | Tsou et al. (353) | 2017 | 950 | Han Chinese | -Low D2R availability in healthy controls (334, 336*) |
| | | | | *Zhang et al. (354) | 2018 | 593 | Han Chinese | |
| | | | | Xu et al. (355) | 2004 | 799 | Chinese | |
| | | | | Wang et al. (351) | 2016 | 633 | Han Chinese | |
| | | | | Vereczkei et al. (337) | 2013 | 858 | Central European | |
| | | | No significant association with methadone dose | Huang et al. (272) | 2016 | 138 | Taiwanese | |
| | **rs4648319** | Intron 1 | Risk factor for OUD | Tsou et al. (353) | 2017 | 950 | Han Chinese | |
| | **rs4648317** | Intron 1 | No significant association with OUD | Doehring et al. (44) | 2009 | 184 | Caucasian | |
| | **rs7350522** | Intron 1 | No significant association with OUD | Wang et al. (351) | 2016 | 633 | Han Chinese | |
| | **rs2075654** | Intron 2 | Risk factor for OUD | Al-eitan et al. (352) | 2012 | 425 | Jordanian Arabic | |
| | **rs2734836** | Intron 2 | Risk factor for OUD | Al-eitan et al. (352) | 2012 | 425 | Jordanian Arabic | |

*(Continued)*

study, all OUD patients actively used heroin and most, but not all, were also on methadone therapy (6). In another [$^{11}$C]raclopride PET study, recently detoxed OUD patients showed lower D2R availability than healthy controls (7). These patients also demonstrated lower levels of DA release in response to a methylphenidate challenge in comparison to healthy controls (7). In a [$^{123}$I]IBZM SPECT study, the OUD patients were abstinent without maintenance therapy anywhere from 1 to 24 weeks (318). Zijlstra et al. (318) observed a negative correlation in length of opioid use history with striatal D2R availability. In contrast, two [$^{11}$C]raclopride studies observed no differences in D2R availability between OUD patients receiving methadone therapy and healthy controls (19, 20). These findings suggest the potential therapeutic benefit of MOUD in restoring neurochemical imbalances resulting from substance abuse. These results demand further investigation into the relationship between OUD and D2R availability, particularly in the context of MOUD.

**TABLE 2 |** Continued

| Gene | Polymorphism | Location | Findings | Author | Year | n | Ethnicity | Imaging Correlates |
|---|---|---|---|---|---|---|---|---|
| | **rs1800498 (taqID)** | Intron 2 | Risk factor for OUD | Tsou et al. (353) | 2017 | 950 | Han Chinese | |
| | | | | *Xu et al. (355) | 2004 | 799 | Chinese | |
| | | | No significant association with OUD | Vereczkei et al. (337) | 2013 | 858 | Central European | |
| | | | | Doehring et al. (44) | 2009 | 184 | Caucasian | |
| | | | | Xu et al. (355) | 2004 | 663 | German | |
| | **rs2283265** | Intron 4 | Risk factor for OUD | Al-eitan et al. (352) | 2012 | 425 | Jordanian Arabic | |
| | | | | *Levran et al. (348) | 2015 | 801 | African American | |
| | | | No significant association with OUD | Zhang et al. (354) | 2018 | 593 | Han Chinese | |
| | **rs1076560** | Intron 6 | Risk factor for OUD | Al-eitan et al. (352) | 2012 | 425 | Jordanian Arabic | -Lower levels of striatal D2R availability in healthy controls (344) |
| | | | | Doehring et al. (44) | 2009 | 184 | Caucasian | |
| | | | | Clarke et al. (341) | 2014 | 2649 | African American and European American | |
| | | | | *Levran et al. (348) | 2015 | 801 | African American | -No association with striatal D2R availability in healthy controls (345) |
| | | | No significant association with OUD | Zhang et al. (354) | 2018 | 593 | Han Chinese | |
| | **rs2734842** | 3' Near | Risk factor for OUD | *Zhang et al. (354) | 2018 | 593 | Han Chinese | |
| | **rs2242591** | 3' Flanking Region | Risk factor for OUD | *Zhang et al. (354) | 2018 | 593 | Han Chinese | |
| | **rs6278** | 3' UTR | Risk factor for OUD | *Zhang et al. (354) | 2018 | 593 | Han Chinese | |
| | **rs6279** | 3' UTR | Risk factor for OUD | *Zhang et al. (354) | 2018 | 593 | Han Chinese | |
| | **rs1799732** | 5'- UTR | Risk factor for OUD (C deletion) | Al-eitan et al. (352) | 2012 | 425 | Jordanian Arabic | -Combined minor variants associated with higher striatal D2R availability in healthy controls (334) -No association with extrastriatal D2R in healthy controls (340) |
| | | | No significant association with OUD | Teh et al. (356) | 2012 | 93 | Han Chinese | |
| | | | | Zhang et al. (354) | 2018 | 593 | Han Chinese | |
| | | | | Doehring et al. (44) | 2009 | 184 | Caucasian | |
| | **rs12364283** | 5' UTR | No significant association with OUD | Doehring et al. (44) | 2009 | 184 | Caucasian | |
| | **rs1799978** | 5' UTR | No significant association with OUD | Doehring et al. (44) | 2009 | 184 | Caucasian | |
| | | | | Teh et al. (41) | 2012 | 93 | Han Chinese | |
| | | | Risk factor for OUD | *Hung et al. (357) | 2011 | 321 | Han Chinese | |
| | | | Higher methadone doses | Hung et al. (357) | 2011 | 321 | Han Chinese | |
| | | | No significant association with relapse rates on methadone treatment | Bawor et al. (358) | 2015 | 240 | Mixed | |
| | | | | Doehring et al. (44) | 2009 | 184 | Caucasian | |
| *ANKK1* | **rs4938013** | Exon 2 | Risk factor for OUD | Nelson et al. (359) | 2013 | 3485 | Caucasian | |
| | | | | *Zhang et al. (354) | 2018 | 593 | Han Chinese | |
| | **rs7118900** | Exon 5 | Risk factor for OUD | *Zhang et al. (354) | 2018 | 593 | Han Chinese | |
| | | | | *Levran et al. (348) | 2015 | 801 | African American | |
| | **rs1800497 (taqIA)** | Exon 8 | Risk factor for OUD | Teh et al. (356) | 2012 | 93 | Han Chinese | -Low D2R availability in healthy controls (334, 335, 336*) |
| | | | | Hou and Li (360) | 2009 | 1030 | Chinese/East Asian | |
| | | | | *Vereczkei et al. (337) | 2013 | 858 | Central European | |
| | | | | Tsou et al. (353) | 2017 | 950 | Han Chinese | |
| | | | | *Zhang et al. (354) | 2018 | 593 | Han Chinese | |
| | | | | *Doehring et al. (44) | 2009 | 184 | Caucasian | |
| | | | No significant association with OUD | Al-eitan et al. (352) | 2012 | 425 | Jordanian Arabic | |

*(Continued)*

**TABLE 2** | Continued

| Gene | Polymorphism | Location | Findings | Author | Year | n | Ethnicity | Imaging Correlates |
|---|---|---|---|---|---|---|---|---|
| | | | | Barratt et al. (361) | 2006 | 166 | Mixed | |
| | | | No significant association with methadone dose | Crettol et al. (134) | 2008 | 455 | Caucasian | |
| | | | No significant association with methadone or buprenorphine therapy success | Barratt et al. (361) | 2006 | 166 | Mixed | |
| | | | Improved withdrawal among methadone-maintained patients | Barratt et al. (361) | 2006 | 166 | Mixed | |
| | **rs877138** | 5'- Flanking Region | Risk factor for OUD | Nelson et al. (359) | 2013 | 3485 | Caucasian | |
| *DAT1* | **9-repeat VNTR** | 3' UTR | Risk factor for OUD | Galeeva et al. (362) | 2002 | 287 | Caucasian males | -Higher striatal DAT availability (363–365) -No association with striatal DAT availability (366, 367) |
| | | | No significant association with OUD | Hou and Li (360) | 2009 | 1030 | Han Chinese | |
| | | | | Yeh et al. (368) | 2010 | 1046 | Han Chinese | |
| | **10-repeat VNTR** | 3' UTR | Risk factor for OUD | Ornoy et al. (369) | 2016 | 158 | Israeli Jewish Females | -Higher striatal DAT availability (370, 371) -No association with striatal DAT availability (366, 367) |

*SNP associations refer to the minor allele.*
**Nominal significance.*

# DRD1

## *DRD1* Background

The D1R is the most abundant DA receptor in the brain (380). Coded by *DRD1*, this excitatory GPCR is widespread, but most densely expressed in the dorsal striatum, hippocampus, amygdala, and neocortex, as illustrated in **Figure 1** (385–388). D1Rs influence learning and memory *via* association with N-methyl-D-aspartate (NMDA)-mediated long-term potentiation as well as impact D2R-mediated events and regulate addiction-associated behaviors such as impulsivity (389–396). D1Rs are important mediators of several reward-related processes and there is evidence that D1Rs are required and sufficient for drug reward and conditioning (397, 398).

D1R function is relevant in OUD because DA release triggered by opioid-induced MOP receptor activation indirectly stimulates D1Rs and associated reward circuitry (69). While one post-mortem study showed lower D1R mRNA levels in the putamen and NAc shell in OUD subjects relative to controls (347), another postmortem analysis showed higher D1R mRNA and protein expression in VTA, NAc, and amygdala in the brains of opioid abusers compared to controls (399). This difference may be attributed to the difference in populations studied. Where Sadat-Shirazi et al. (399) studied patients who exclusively abused opioids, Jacobs et al. (347) included polysubstance users.

In addition, pharmacological manipulations of D1Rs in preclinical models of OUD demonstrate alterations in behaviors associated with dependence and withdrawal. For example, infusion of D1R agonist SKF 38393 into the NAc enhances, while antagonist SCH 23390 blunts, conditioned place preference in morphine-addicted rats (400). Additionally, infusions of SCH 23390 into the NAc core reduced cue-induced heroin-seeking in dependent rats (401). Furthermore, D1R agonist SKF 82958 relieved naloxone-precipitated withdrawal symptoms in morphine-dependent rats (402). These findings highlight the importance of D1Rs in OUD and correspond with other SUD models. For example, SCH 23390 infusion blocks reinstatement of cocaine-seeking in rats, while D1R agonist SKF 81297 reinstates cocaine-seeking (403, 404). In addition to pharmacological D1R blockade, D1R knock-out mice fail to self-administer cocaine (397). In models of AUD, NAc shell infusions of SCH 23390 blunt, while infusions of D1R agonist A-77636 enhance, ethanol self-administration in alcohol-preferring rats (405).

D1 and MOP receptors directly colocalize into hetero-oligomers in the rat cortex and striatum (including accumbens nucleus), regions of importance in reward and locomotor activity. Together, they promote locomotor sensitization in rats chronically treated with morphine, suggesting this association may be involved in the long-term neuronal changes associated with addiction (406, 407).

## *DRD1* Polymorphisms

While less attention has been given to variations in *DRD1* than *DRD2/ANKK1*, there are several functional polymorphisms that have been studied in the context of SUDs. One study demonstrated that rs5326A, located in the 5' untranslated region, correlated with decreased *DRD1* promoter strength in an *in vitro* luciferase model (408). Other *DRD1* polymorphisms may increase vulnerability to OUD by interacting with the glutamatergic system in the brain. Homer scaffold protein 1 (*HOMER1*) encodes HOMER1, a postsynaptic protein that facilitates glutamatergic transmission (409). Excitatory glutamatergic signaling has been shown to underlie the persistent compulsion to use drugs, suggesting SNPs disrupting this gene interaction may be relevant in OUD (410). In a post-mortem analysis of Caucasian samples, the *DRD1* polymorphism rs265973 associated with HOMER1 expression in the striatum (347). Interestingly, the minor T allele associated with higher levels of striatal HOMER1 mRNA among the OUD cohort, but associated with lower levels of striatal HOMER1 mRNA in the control cohort (347). Thus, it is possible *HOMER1*-associated genetic variants disrupt glutamatergic and dopaminergic signaling and contribute to OUD.

### Genetic Association Studies: *DRD1* and OUD

Preliminary findings suggest a role of *DRD1* SNPs in OUD, as outlined in **Table 2**. For example, Liu et al. (411) found that two SNPs located in the 5' untranslated region of *DRD1*, major allele rs265981G and minor allele rs5326A, associated with OUD in a Han Chinese population. Levran et al. (348, 349) also found a trend toward an association between rs5326A and OUD in an African American sample. However, other groups were unable to replicate these findings (346, 350). Jacobs et al. (347) found a nominally significant association between *DRD1* SNP rs265973 and OUD among Caucasians, but not African Americans. This provides further evidence of an association between *HOMER1* and OUD, perhaps with ethnicity-dependent effects.

Several studies demonstrate that *DRD1* variants associate with the duration of transition from the first use to dependence of opioids (346, 350). The duration of transition from the first use to dependence is of clinical significance; patients with a more rapid transition to dependence have poorer treatment outcomes and more severe SUDs (412, 413). Zhu et al. (346) found that the minor alleles of rs686 and rs4532 associated with a longer transition period. Peng et al. (350) were unable to replicate the rs4532 association, but found that homozygotes for the major alleles of rs5326 and rs6882300 had an accelerated transition to OUD. Interestingly, while these SNPS associated with the transition from first use to dependence, neither study found that they were associated with increased risk for OUD (346, 350).

*DRD1* variants have also been implicated in subjective ratings of pleasure in response to opioids, both upon first use and after dependence (346). Typically, the pleasurable feeling associated with opioids increases with duration of use: most patients report a negative response upon their first use and a euphoric response after dependence (133, 346). This suggests that chronic opioid use induces changes to reward-related circuitry. One potential mechanism is through D1R-mediated phosphorylation of NMDA, contributing to long-term potentiation (414). *DRD1* variants have been associated with this reward sensitization process in a Han Chinese population (346). This study revealed that *DRD1* SNPs that modulate the subjective response to opioids upon first use are distinct from those that do so after dependence. Specifically, the minor alleles of rs5326, rs10063995, and rs10078866 are associated with a non-pleasurable first use of opioids, but are not associated with the subjective response after dependence. Conversely, the minor variants of rs686 and rs4532 are associated with less pleasurable responses to opioids after dependence, but are not associated with the initial response (346). Findings from a rat study indicate that there is a reward-switching mechanism in opioid response within the basolateral amygdala in which D1R signaling is associated with reward upon first use and D2R signaling with reward after dependence (415). Thus, it is possible that rs686 and rs4532 associate with less pleasurable opioid responses after dependence by modulating D2R activity.

### Molecular Imaging: D1R and OUD

No molecular imaging studies have yet assessed D1R availability in OUD or in *DRD1* polymorphism carriers. Few studies have examined the relationship between other SUDs and D1R levels. [$^{11}$C]NNC 112 and [$^{11}$C]SCH 23390 are radiolabeled D1R antagonists that differentially distribute throughout the brain; however, both display high affinity in the striatum and extrastriatal regions (416–418). In one [$^{11}$C]NNC 112 study, D1R availability in CUD patients was not significantly different than in healthy controls (419). In contrast, studies utilizing [$^{11}$C]SCH 23390 PET reveal individuals with tobacco use disorder have lower D1R availability than healthy controls (420, 421). These limited findings highlight the need for increased investigation into D1R availability in addiction.

## DAT1

### *DAT1* Background

DAT are plasma membrane proteins essential for the clearance of DA from the synapse; they play a critical role in regulating DA neurotransmission, especially in the striatum (422–426). DAT harness the electrochemical gradient to transport two sodium ions with a DA molecule into the cell, thus regulating extracellular DA concentrations (423). DAT are coded by *DAT1*, a gene widely studied for its role in substance abuse (427).

### *DAT1* Polymorphisms

The most studied polymorphisms of *DAT1* are VNTRs in the 3' untranslated region, which may affect DAT expression (428–431). The most common variants are those with 9 or 10 repeats of the 40 base pair sequence (432) and multiple molecular imaging studies have investigated their functional effects. In several [$^{123}$I]β-CIT SPECT studies, 9-repeat VTNR carriers demonstrated higher striatal DAT availability than the 10-repeat homozygotes (363–365). In contrast, two [$^{123}$I]β-CIT SPECT studies found those homozygous for the 10-repeat allele had higher striatal DAT density compared to non-10-repeat carriers (370, 371). Finally, Martinez et al. (366) and Lynch et al. (367) found no effect of VNTR polymorphisms on striatal DAT expression in a [$^{123}$I]β-CIT SPECT and [$^{99m}$Tc]TRODAT-1 study, respectively. Lastly, Guindalini et al. (433) found that the rare 6-repeat VNTR genotype reduced DAT1 expression *in vitro*, particularly when cocaine was added to the culture. However, the effects of the 6-repeat VNTR polymorphism on *DAT1* availability has not been assessed *in vivo* with PET methodology. Thus, further research is required to determine these polymorphisms' functional effects on DAT expression and availability.

### Genetic Association Studies: *DAT1* and OUD

Genetic association studies of *DAT1* and OUD have yielded inconsistent results. While Galeeva et al. (362) found an association between 9-repeat VNTR allele and OUD in an ethnic Russian and Tartar male population, later studies in Han Chinese populations did not observe any association (360, 368). Ornoy et al. (369) examined the heritability of *DAT1* ADHD risk alleles in Sephardic and Ashkenazi Jewish heroin-dependent individuals and their children. They found that mothers with OUD were more likely to be carriers of the *DAT1* 10-repeat allele than mothers without OUD. This association was not seen in fathers and was not explained by prevalence of ADHD among mothers with the polymorphism. Further, the children of heroin-dependent parents were more likely to inherit the 10-repeat allele than children of healthy volunteers (369). However, it is unclear how these VNTR polymorphisms impact DAT availability and thus vulnerability to OUD, as molecular imaging studies have conflicting results (363–367, 370, 371).

Polymorphisms in *DAT1* have been associated with other SUDs, which may provide insight into their functional effects on DA signaling in addiction. *DAT1* VNTR has been associated with OUD (362) as well as AUD in Western European and Japanese populations (47, 434). A meta-analysis also found that the 9-repeat VNTR was associated with increased withdrawal severity in AUD (435). The 6-repeat VNTR genotype was found to be a risk factor for CUD, but this variant has not yet been studied in OUD (45). Thus, it seems that *DAT1* VNTR polymorphisms may affect DAT expression and contribute to SUDs.

Evidence suggests that the number of VNTR in patients with OUD influences their response to treatment. In each study, a "poor" treatment outcome indicates continued heroin use or treatment drop-out, whereas a "successful" outcome indicates cessation of illicit opioid use. In patients receiving buprenorphine therapy, carriers of the 10-repeat VNTR allele had poor outcomes more often than successful outcomes (436). Conversely, 6-, 7-, and 11-repeat VNTR allele carriers had successful outcomes in response to buprenorphine therapy more often than not (436). Gerra et al. (436) suggest that these variations in *DAT1* may modulate buprenorphine-associated DA transmission and thus affect treatment success. In a study of both oral and implanted naltrexone therapy, Krupitsky et al. (437) found that OUD patients with the 9-repeat VNTR allele had poor outcomes more often than successful ones on both forms of naltrexone. Thus, genotyping *DAT1* VNTR could be useful in OUD therapy selection.

While van Gestel et al. (438) reported an association between *DAT1* VNTR polymorphisms and novelty seeking, a personality trait associated with SUDs (439), other studies have failed to replicate this finding (440, 441).

### Molecular Imaging: DAT and OUD

Several molecular imaging studies have assessed DAT availability in SUDs utilizing DAT-sensitive tracers including [$^{99m}$Tc]TRODAT-1, [$^{123}$I]β-CIT, [11C]WIN 35,428, [11C]cocaine, and [$^{11}$C]CFT. There is evidence from molecular imaging studies that DAT availability is altered in SUDs. For example, CUD is associated with higher striatal DAT concentrations compared to healthy controls (54, 55), while methamphetamine-dependent individuals demonstrate lower striatal DAT availability compared to healthy controls (51, 57, 58). Alcohol and tobacco dependence have also been associated with lower striatal DAT levels (59, 60–62); however, other studies have observed no association between DAT levels and alcohol and tobacco dependency (22, 442). Although varied, these results overall suggest that DAT plays a role in SUDs.

PET and SPECT studies suggest that OUD is associated with decreased DAT availability. Chronic heroin users, detoxed abstainers, and methadone-maintained patients all present lower striatal DAT levels than healthy controls (48–53). A [$^{99m}$Tc]TRODAT-1 SPECT study comparing DAT concentrations between recently detoxed heroin-dependent patients and recently detoxed methamphetamine-dependent patients showed that both had lower striatal DAT availability than healthy controls and had no differences between them (51). In contrast, Cosgrove et al. (443) utilizing [$^{123}$I]β-CIT SPECT imaging, reported no differences in striatal DAT levels between heroin users and healthy controls, though they acknowledged the limitations of their small sample sizes (443).

DAT availability may also vary based on the use of MOUD. For example, one [$^{11}$C]CFT PET study reported methadone-maintained OUD patients showed lower DAT availability in the bilateral putamen than abstinent OUD patients, with both presenting lower striatal DAT availability compared to healthy controls (49). Further, while methadone-maintained patients showed lower DAT availability in caudate and putamen compared to controls, abstinent OUD patients showed lower DAT availability in the caudate only, suggesting that abstinence from opioids may partially recover DAT availability (49). However, a [$^{99m}$Tc]TRODAT-1 SPECT study found similar striatal DAT availability between methadone-maintained and abstinent OUD patients (50). This discrepancy may be due to methodological differences; in one study, patients were at least 6 months abstinent (49), while in the other, patients were abstinent for only 3 months or less (50). In a within-subjects [$^{99m}$Tc]TRODAT-1 SPECT study, Liu et al. (53) observed a 14–17% increase in DAT levels in the caudate and putamen of 64 heroin-dependent patients after 6 months of treatment with traditional Chinese Jitai tablets, an herbal remedy associated with withdrawal mitigation. No significant increase in DAT levels was observed in the placebo-treated group. However, even among the medication group, DAT availability was not restored to that of healthy control levels (53). Thus, further studies are required to determine the effects of MOUD compared to sustained abstinence on DAT availability.

## CONCLUSION

Preclinical and clinical studies have demonstrated the importance of the opioid and DA systems in SUDs, including OUD. Polymorphisms within these systems have functional consequences that may influence a number of modalities in addiction, including vulnerabilities, addiction severity, treatment response, and relapse rates. PET and SPECT methodology allow for the study of these receptor systems in both healthy and substance-dependent populations and provide insight into the neurobiology of OUD.

Within the opioid system, the MOP receptor has been most closely studied in the context of OUD. The minor allele of the *OPRM1* rs1799971 SNP has been widely linked to a reduction in

MOP receptor availability (100–105). The implications of this in OUD, however, remain elusive; findings from genetic association studies are varied and seem largely ethnicity-dependent (109). The KOP and NOP receptors have also been studied in relation to OUD; both play important roles in the dysphoric effects of drug abuse seen during withdrawal, including modulating activation of the HPA axis (16, 291, 294, 295, 444). A number of polymorphisms in *OPRK1* have been associated with OUD and opioid withdrawal severity (147, 155, 156, 232). Similarly, VNTR polymorphisms in *PDYN* have been correlated with opioid withdrawal, suggesting the importance of dynorphin-KOP receptor signaling system in the mediation of stress-induced withdrawal and compulsive drug-seeking (155). Lastly, genetic variants in both *PDYN* and *OPRL1* have been associated with personality traits and behaviors associated with SUDs, another indication of their roles in OUD (235, 236, 445). The DOP receptor has an inverse function to the KOP receptor, in that DOP receptor activation improves negative emotional states (255). While several *OPRD1* polymorphisms correlated with heroin dependence (130, 136, 138–141, 146, 150), it is likely that the effects are ethnicity-dependent, as several other studies found no significant associations between *OPRD1* polymorphisms and OUD (137, 140, 144).

The DA system has several well-studied polymorphisms that have been linked with OUD and other SUDs. For example, polymorphisms in *DRD2/ANKK1*, in particular the *Taq*IA and *Taq*IB SNPs, may result in lower D2R availability (321, 334, 335) and have been associated with addictive behaviors including OUD (330, 332, 354, 446, 447). Less studied *DRD2* polymorphisms may also affect D2R expression (341, 344) but results have been varied. Additionally, *DRD2* polymorphisms may associate with response to medications for OUD; however, there are conflicting reports and further research is required (44, 134, 272, 335, 358, 361, 372). Fewer conclusions can be drawn about *DRD1*; for example, several *DRD1* polymorphisms were initially associated with a rapid transition from first opioid use to opioid dependence, but the results could not be replicated (346, 350). Lastly, lower DAT availability has also been associated with OUD (48–53). Both the 9- and 10-repeat VNTR alleles have been associated with lower DAT availability (363–365, 370, 351); thus, more studies are required to pinpoint the effects of the different repeat VNTR polymorphisms in OUD.

While there is strong preliminary evidence of the role of genetic variants in the DA and opioid systems in OUD, more molecular imaging studies are required in individuals with OUD. In particular, studies utilizing PET tracers that target the less-studied opioid receptors, D1R, D3R, and DAT, would greatly contribute to our understanding of the complex interplay between these receptors in opioid addiction. For instance, as of yet, no imaging studies have examined DOP, KOP, NOP, D1, or D3 receptors in individuals with OUD. One of the most important molecular imaging research questions in OUD is how the different MOUD may alter the dopamine and opioid receptor systems and if these changes are associated with higher rates of successful abstinence. Current imaging studies largely group abstinent and medication-maintained OUD participants together and compare to healthy controls; however, analyses between OUD subgroups would shed light on any neurochemical benefits of MOUD. This would help inform treatment and ultimately improve outcomes for those suffering from OUD. Additionally, opioid receptor antagonist challenge studies would help assess the interaction between drugs like naloxone and semi-synthetic or synthetic opioids, improving safety and efficacy of overdose reversal and prevention. Finally, molecular imaging studies examining the effects of polymorphisms in the DA and opioid systems would help elucidate the genetic components of OUD. The literature relating to genetic association studies in OUD does suggest that certain polymorphisms are risk factors for OUD or may affect treatment outcomes. However, given that these associations are largely ethnicity-dependent, it is important to replicate these findings. Finally, there seem to be sex effects both on genetic association studies and PET/SPECT findings; therefore, future studies could investigate the sex differences in development and outcome of OUD. Further investigation into the underlying genetic factors of OUD and treatment response is critical to help curb the opioid crisis by means of addiction prevention, novel pharmacological targets, and precision treatment.

## AUTHOR CONTRIBUTIONS

PM, CW, NV, and G-JW contributed to the conception and design of the study. JB, DK, DF, and CK conducted a literature search and wrote the first draft. All authors contributed to manuscript revision, and read and approved the submitted version.

## ACKNOWLEDGMENTS

This work was accomplished with support from the National Institute on Alcohol Abuse and Alcoholism (Y1AA-3009). We also thank Dr. Marta Pecina for her counsel in constructing receptor distribution images using the Allen Brain Atlas.

## REFERENCES

1. Kolodny A, Courtwright DT, Hwang CS, Kreiner P, Eadie JL, Clark TW, et al. The prescription opioid and heroin crisis: a public health approach to an epidemic of addiction. *Annu Rev Public Health* (2015) 36:559–74. doi: 10.1146/annurev-publhealth-031914-122957
2. Volkow ND, Jones EB, Einstein EB, Wargo EM. Prevention and treatment of opioid misuse and addiction: a review. *JAMA Psychiatry* (2019) 76(2):208–16. doi: 10.1001/jamapsychiatry.2018.3126
3. Centers for Disease Control and Prevention. Annual surveillance report of drug-related risks and outcomes—United States. surveillance special report 2. centers for disease control and prevention, U.S. Department of Health and Human Services. (2018).
4. Koob GF, Volkow ND. Neurobiology of addiction: a neurocircuitry analysis. *Lancet Psychiatry* (2016) 3(8):760–73. doi: 10.1016/S2215-0366(16)00104-8
5. Volkow ND, Koob GF, McLellan AT. Neurobiologic advances from the brain disease model of addiction. *N Engl J Med* (2016) 374(4):363–71. doi: 10.1056/NEJMra1511480
6. Wang GJ, Volkow ND, Fowler JS, Logan J, Abumrad NN, Hitzemann RJ, et al. Dopamine D2 receptor availability in opiate-dependent subjects before and after naloxone-precipitated withdrawal. *Neuropsychopharmacology* (1997) 16(2):174–82. doi: 10.1016/S0893-133X(96)00184-4

7. Martinez D, Saccone PA, Liu F, Slifstein M, Orlowska D, Grassetti A, et al. Deficits in dopamine D(2) receptors and presynaptic dopamine in heroin dependence: commonalities and differences with other types of addiction. *Biol Psychiatry* (2012) 71(3):192–8. doi: 10.1016/j.biopsych.2011.08.024
8. Hou H, Wang C, Jia S, Hu S, Tian M. Brain dopaminergic system changes in drug addiction: a review of positron emission tomography findings. *Neurosci Bull* (2014) 30(5):765–76. doi: 10.1007/s12264-014-1469-5
9. Volkow ND, Wang GJ, Fowler JS, Tomasi D. Addiction circuitry in the human brain. *Annu Rev Pharmacol Toxicol* (2012b) 52:321–36. doi: 10.1146/annurev-pharmtox-010611-134625
10. Volkow ND, Wang GJ, Telang F, Fowler JS, Logan J, Wong C, et al. Sleep deprivation decreases binding of [11C]raclopride to dopamine D2/D3 receptors in the human brain. *J Neurosci* (2008) 28(34):8454–61. doi: 10.1523/JNEUROSCI.1443-08.2008
11. Volkow ND, Tomasi D, Wang GJ, Telang F, Fowler JS, Logan J, et al. Evidence that sleep deprivation downregulates dopamine D2R in ventral striatum in the human brain. *J Neurosci* (2012a) 32(19):6711–7. doi: 10.1523/JNEUROSCI.0045-12.2012
12. Wiers CE, Shumay E, Cabrera E, Shokri-Kojori E, Gladwin TE, Skarda E, et al. Reduced sleep duration mediates decreases in striatal D2/D3 receptor availability in cocaine abusers. *Transl Psychiatry* (2016) 6:e752. doi: 10.1038/tp.2016.14
13. Martinez D, Orlowska D, Narendran R, Slifstein M, Liu F, Kumar D, et al. Dopamine type 2/3 receptor availability in the striatum and social status in human volunteers. *Biol Psychiatry* (2010) 67(3):275–8. doi: 10.1016/j.biopsych.2009.07.037
14. Wiers CE, Shokri-Kojori E, Cabrera E, Cunningham S, Wong C, Tomasi D, et al. Socioeconomic status is associated with striatal dopamine D2/D3 receptors in healthy volunteers but not in cocaine abusers. *Neurosci Lett* (2016) 617:27–31. doi: 10.1016/j.neulet.2016.01.056
15. Berro LF, Frussa-Filho R, Tufik S, Andersen ML. Relationships between sleep and addiction: the role of drug-environment conditioning. *Med Hypotheses* (2014) 82(3):374–6. doi: 10.1016/j.mehy.2013.12.026
16. Land BB, Bruchas MR, Lemos JC, Xu M, Melief EJ, Chavkin C. The dysphoric component of stress is encoded by activation of the dynorphin kappa-opioid system. *J Neurosci* (2008) 28:407–14. doi: 10.1523/JNEUROSCI.4458-07.2008
17. Redila VA, Chavkin C. Stress-induced reinstatement of cocaine seeking is mediated by the kappa opioid system. *Psychopharmacology* (2008) 200:59–70. doi: 10.1007/s00213-008-1122-y
18. McLaughlin JP, Myers LC, Zarek PE, Caron MG, Lefkowitz RJ, Czyzyk TA, et al. Prolonged kappa opioid receptor phosphorylation mediated by G-protein receptor kinase underlies sustained analgesic tolerance. *Biol Chem* (2004) 279(3):1810–8. doi: 10.1074/jbc.M305796200
19. Daglish MRC, Williams TM, Wilson SJ, Taylor LG, Eap CB, Augsburger M, et al. Brain dopamine response in human opioid addiction. *Br J Psychiatry* (2008) 193(1):65–72. doi: 10.1192/bjp.bp.107.041228
20. Watson BJ, Taylor LG, Reid AG, Wilson SJ, Stokes PR, Brooks DJ, et al. Investigating expectation and reward in human opioid addiction with [11C] raclopride PET. *Addict Biol* (2014) 19:1032–40. doi: 10.1111/adb.12073
21. Rommelspacher H, Raeder C, Kaulen P, Bruning G. Adaptive changes of dopamine-D2 receptors in rat brain following ethanol withdrawal: a quantitative autoradiographic investigation. *Alcohol* (1992) 9:355–62. doi: 10.1016/0741-8329(92)90032-6
22. Volkow ND, Wang GJ, Fowler JS, Logan J, Hitzemann R, Ding YS, et al. Decreases in dopamine receptors but not in dopamine transporters in alcoholics. *Alcohol Clin Exp Res* (1996) 20(9):1594–8. doi: 10.1111/j.1530-0277.1996.tb05936.x
23. Syvälahti EK, Hietala J, Röyttä M, Grönroos J. Decrease in the number of rat brain dopamine and muscarinic receptors after chronic alcohol intake. *Pharmacol Toxicol* (1988) 62:4,210–2. doi: 10.1111/j.1600-0773.1988.tb01874.x
24. Martinez D, Gil R, Slifstein M, Hwang DR, Huang Y, Perez A, et al. Alcohol dependence is associated with blunted dopamine transmission in the ventral striatum. *Biol Psychiatry* (2005) 58(10):779–86. doi: 10.1016/j.biopsych.2005.04.044
25. Volkow ND, Wang GJ, Telang F, Fowler JS, Logan J, Jayne M, et al. Profound decreases in dopamine release in striatum in detoxified alcoholics: possible orbitofrontal involvement. *J Neurosci* (2007) 27:12700–6. doi: 10.1523/JNEUROSCI.3371-07.2007
26. Yoder KK, Albrecht DS, Dzemidzic M, Normandin MD, Federici LM, Graves T, et al. Differences in IV alcohol-induced dopamine release in the ventral striatum of social drinkers and nontreatment-seeking alcoholics. *Drug Alcohol Depend* (2016) 160:163–9. doi: 10.1016/j.drugalcdep.2016.01.001
27. Feltmann K, Borroto-Escuela DO, Rüegg J, Pinton L, de Oliveira Sergio T, Narváez M, et al. Effects of long-term alcohol drinking on the dopamine D2 receptor: gene expression and heteroreceptor complexes in the striatum in rats. *Alcohol Clin Exp Res* (2018) 42(2):338–51. doi: 10.1111/acer.13568
28. Hirth N, Meinhardt MW, Noori HR, Salgado H, Torres-Ramirez O, Uhrig S, et al. Convergent evidence from alcohol-dependent humans and rats for a hyperdopaminergic state in protracted abstinence. *Proc Natl Acad Sci U S A* (2016) 113(11):3024–9. doi: 10.1073/pnas.1506012113
29. Volkow ND, Wise RA, Baler R. The dopamine motive system: implications for drug and food addiction. *Nat Rev Neurosci* (2017) 18:12,741–752. doi: 10.1038/nrn.2017.130
30. Crist RC, Reiner BC, Berrettini WH. A review of opioid addiction genetics. *Curr Opin Psychol* (2019) 27:31–5. doi: 10.1016/j.copsyc.2018.07.014
31. Kreek MJ, Bart G, Lilly C, Laforge KS, Nielsen DA. Pharmacogenetics and human molecular genetics of opiate and cocaine addictions and their treatments. *Pharmacol Rev* (2005) 57:1–26. doi 10.1124/pr.57.1.1
32. Merikangas KR, Stolar M, Stevens DE, Goulet J, Preisig MA, Fenton B, et al. Familial transmission of substance use disorders. *Arch Gen Psychiatry* (1998) 55:973–9. doi: 10.1001/archpsyc.55.11.973
33. Drgon T, Zhang PW, Johnson C, Walther D, Hess J, Nino M, et al. Genome wide association for addiction: replicated results and comparisons of two analytic approaches. *PLoS One* (2010) 5(1):e8832. doi: 10 1371/journal.pone.0008832
34. Bierut LJ, Madden PA, Breslau N, Johnson EO, Hatsukami D, Pomerleau OF, et al. Novel genes identified in a high density genome wide association study for nicotine dependence Hum. *Mol Genet* (2006) 16(1):24–35. doi: 10.1093/hmg/ddl441
35. Rutter JL. Symbiotic relationship of pharmacogenetics and drugs of abuse. *Aaps J* (2006) 8(1):E174–84. doi: 10.1208/aapsj080121
36. Chamorro AJ, Marcos M, Mirón-Canelo JA, Pastor I, González-Sarmiento R, Laso FJ. Association of μ-opioid receptor (OPRM1) gene polymorphism with response to naltrexone in alcohol dependence: a systematic review and meta-analysis. *Addict Biol* (2012) 17(3):505–12. doi: 10.1111/j.1369-1600.2012.00442.x
37. Anton RF, Oroszi G, O'Malley S, Couper D, Swift R, Pettinati H, et al. An evaluation of mu-opioid receptor (OPRM1) as a predictor of naltrexone response in the treatment of alcohol dependence: results from the Combined Pharmacotherapies and Behavioral Interventions for Alcohol Dependence (COMBINE) study. *Arch Gen Psychiatry* (2008) 65:135–44. doi: 10.1001/archpsyc.65.2.135
38. Ray LA, Hutchison KE. Effects of naltrexone on alcohol sensitivity and genetic moderators of medication response: a double-blind placebo-controlled study. *Arch Gen Psychiatry* (2007) 64(9):1069–77. doi: 10.1001/archpsyc.64.9.1069
39. Oslin DW, Leong SH, Lynch KG, Berrettini W, O'Brien CP, Gordon AJ, et al. Naltrexone vs placebo for the treatment of alcohol dependence: a randomized clinical trial. *JAMA Psychiatry* (2015) 72(5):430–7. doi: 10.1001/jamapsychiatry.2014.3053
40. Zhang H, Luo X, Kranzler HR, Lappalainen J, Yang B-Z, Krupitsky E, et al. Association between two μ-opioid receptor gene (OPRM1) haplotype blocks and drug or alcohol dependence. *Hum Mol Genet* (2006) 15(6):807–19. doi: 10.1093/hmg/ddl024
41. Lerman C, Berrettini W, Pinto A, Patterson F, Crystal-Mansour S, Wileyto EP, et al. Changes in food reward following smoking cessation: a pharmacogenetic investigation. *Psychopharmacology* (2004) 174:571–7. doi: 10.1007/s00213-004-1823-9
42. Ray R, Jepson C, Wileyto EP, Dahl JP, Patterson F, Rukstalis M, et al. Genetic variation in mu-opioid-receptor-interacting proteins and smoking cessation in a nicotine replacement therapy trial. *Nicotine Tob Res* (2007) 9:1237–41. doi: 10.1080/14622200701648367
43. Le Foll B, Gallo A, Le Strat Y, Lu L, Gorwood P. Genetics of dopamine receptors and drug addiction: a comprehensive review. *Behav Pharmacol* (2009) 20(1):1–17. doi: 10.1097/FBP.0b013e3283242f05
44. Doehring A, Hentig NV, Graff J, Salamat S, Schmidt M, Geisslinger G, et al. Genetic variants altering dopamine D2 receptor expression or function modulate the risk of opiate addiction and the dosage requirements of

methadone substitution. *Pharmacogenet Genomics* (2009) 19(6):407–14. doi: 10.1097/FPC.0b013e328320a3fd
45. Stolf AR, Müller D, Schuch JB, Akutagava-Martins GC, Guimaraes LSP, Szobot CM, et al. Association between the intron 8 VNTR polymorphism of the DAT1 gene and crack cocaine addiction. *Neuropsychobiology* (2017) 75(3):141–4. doi: 10.1159/000485128
46. Muramatsu T, Higuchi S. Dopamine transporter gene polymorphism and alcoholism. *Biochem Biophys Res Commun* (1995) 211:28–32. doi: 10.1006/bbrc.1995.1773
47. Sander T, Harms H, Podschus J, Finckh U, Nickel B, Rolfs A, et al. Allelic association of a dopamine transporter gene polymorphism in alcohol dependence with withdrawal seizures or delirium. *Biol Psychiatry* (1997) 41(3):299–304. doi: 10.1016/S0006-3223(96)00044-3
48. Jia SW, Wang W, Liu Y, Wu ZM. Neuroimaging studies of brain corpus striatum changes among heroin-dependent patients treated with herbal medicine, U'finerTM capsule. *Addict Biol* (2005) 10(3):293–7. doi: 10.1080/13556210500222456
49. Shi J, Zhao LY, Copersino ML, Fang YX, Chen Y, Tian J, et al. PET imaging of dopamine transporter and drug craving during methadone maintenance treatment and after prolonged abstinence in heroin users. *Eur J Pharmacol* (2008) 579(1–3):160–6. doi: 10.1016/j.ejphar.2007.09.042
50. Yeh TL, Chen KC, Lin SH, Lee IH, Chen PS, Yao WJ, et al. Availability of dopamine and serotonin transporters in opioid-dependent users-a two-isotope SPECT study. *Psychopharmacology* (2012) 220:1:55–64. doi: 10.1007/s00213-011-2454-6
51. Yuan J, Liu XD, Han M, Lv R, Bin, Wang YK, et al. Comparison of striatal dopamine transporter levels in chronic heroin-dependent and methamphetamine-dependent subjects. *Addict Biol* (2017) 22(1):229–34. doi: 10.1111/adb.12271
52. Zaaijer ER, Van Dijk L, De Bruin K, Goudriaan AE, Lammers LA, Koeter MWJ, et al. Effect of extended-release naltrexone on striatal dopamine transporter availability, depression and anhedonia in heroin-dependent patients. *Psychopharmacology* (2015) 232(14):2597–607. doi: 10.1007/s00213-015-3891-4
53. Liu Y, Han M, Liu X, Deng Y, Li Y, Yuan J, et al. Dopamine transporter availability in heroin-dependent subjects and controls: longitudinal changes during abstinence and the effects of Jitai tablets treatment. *Psychopharmacology* (2013) 230(2):235–44. doi: 10.1007/s00213-013-3148-z
54. Crits-Christoph P, Newberg A, Wintering N, Ploessl K, Gibbons MBC, Ring-Kurtz S, et al. Dopamine transporter levels in cocaine dependent subjects. *Drug Alcohol Depend* (2008) 98(1–2):70–6. doi: 10.1016/j.drugalcdep.2008.04.014
55. Malison RT, Best SE, Van Dyck CH, McCance EF, Wallace EA, Lamelle M, et al. Elevated striatal dopamine transporters during acute cocaine abstinence as measured by [123I]β-CIT SPECT. *Am J Psychiatry* (1998) 155(6):832–4. doi: 10.1176/ajp.155.6.832
56. Volkow ND, Chang L, Wang GJ, Fowler JS, Ding YS, Sedler M, et al. Low level of brain dopamine D2 receptors in methamphetamine abusers: association with metabolism in the orbitofrontal cortex. *Am J Psychiatry* (2001) 158(12):2015–21. doi: 10.1176/appi.ajp.158.12.2015
57. Volkow ND, Wang GJ, Smith L, Fowler JS, Telang F, Logan J, et al. Recovery of dopamine transporters with methamphetamine detoxification is not linked to changes in dopamine release. *Neuroimage* (2015) 121:20–8. doi: 10.1016/j.neuroimage.2015.07.035
58. McCann UD, Wong DF, Yokoi F, Villemagne V, Dannals RF, Ricaurte GA. Reduced striatal dopamine transporter density in abstinent methamphetamine and methcathinone users: evidence from positron emission tomography studies with [11 C]WIN-35,428. *J Neurosci* (1998) 18(20):8417–22. doi: 10.1523/JNEUROSCI.18-20-08417.1998
59. Laine TPJ, Ahonen A, Räsänen P, Tiihonen J. Dopamine transporter availability and depressive symptoms during alcohol withdrawal. *Psychiatry Res Neuroimag* (1999) 90(3):153–7. doi: 10.1016/S0925-4927(99)00019-0
60. Krause KH, Dresel SH, Krause J, Kung HF, Tatsch K, Ackenheil M. Stimulant-like action of nicotine on striatal dopamine transporter in the brain of adults with attention deficit hyperactivity disorder. *Int J Neuropsychopharmacol* (2002) 5(2):111–3. doi: 10.1017/S1461145702002821
61. Yang YK, Yao WJ, Yeh TL, Lee IH, Chen PS, Lu RB, et al. Decreased dopamine transporter availability in male smokers - A dual isotope SPECT study. *Prog Neuropsychopharmacol Biol Psychiatry* (2008) 32(1):274–9. doi: 10.1016/j.pnpbp.2007.08.018
62. Leroy C, Karila L, Martinot JL, Lukasiewicz M, Duchesnay E, Comtat C, et al. Striatal and extrastriatal dopamine transporter in cannabis and tobacco addiction: a high-resolution PET study. *Addict Biol* (2012) 17(6):981–90. doi: 10.1111/j.1369-1600.2011.00356.x
63. Moningka H, Lichenstein S, Worhunsky PD, DeVito EE, Scheinost D, Yip SW. Can neuroimaging help combat the opioid epidemic? a systematic review of clinical and pharmacological challenge fMRI studies with recommendations for future research. *Neuropsychopharmacology* (2019) 44(2):259–73. doi: 10.1038/s41386-018-0232-4
64. Fareed A, Kim J, Ketchen B, Kwak WJ, Wang D, Shongo-Hiango H, et al. Effect of heroin use on changes of brain functions as measured by functional magnetic resonance imaging, a systematic review. *J Addict Dis* (2017) 36(2):105–16. doi: 10.1080/10550887.2017.1280898
65. Ieong HF, Yuan Z. Resting-state neuroimaging and neuropsychological findings in opioid use disorder during abstinence: a review. *Front Hum Neurosci* (2017) 11:169. doi: 10.3389/fnhum.2017.00169
66. Wollman SC, Alhassoon OM, Hall MG, Stern MJ, Connors EJ, Kimmel CL, et al. Gray matter abnormalities in opioid-dependent patients: a neuroimaging meta-analysis. *Am J Drug Alcohol Abuse* (2017) 43:5,505–517. doi: 10.1080/00952990.2016.1245312
67. Kieffer BL, Gavériaux-Ruff C. Exploring the opioid system by gene knockout. *Prog Neurobiol* (2002) 66(5):285–306. doi: 10.1016/S0301-0082(02)00008-4
68. Matthes HWD, Maldonado R, Simonin F, Valverde O, Slowe S, Kitchen I, et al. Loss of morphine-induced analgesia, reward effect and withdrawal symptoms in mice lacking the μ-opioid-receptor gene. *Nature* (1996) 383:819–23. doi: 10.1038/383819a0
69. Johnson SW, North RA. Opioids excite dopamine neurons by hyperpolarization of local interneurons. *J Neurosci* (1992) 12(2):483–8. doi: 10.1523/JNEUROSCI.12-02-00483.1992
70. Gysling K, Wang RY. Morphine-induced activation of A10 dopamine neurons in the rat. *Brain Res* (1983) 277:119–27. doi: 10.1016/0006-8993(83)90913-7
71. Jalabert M, Bourdy R, Courtin J, Veinante P, Manzoni OJ, Barrot M, et al. Neuronal circuits underlying acute morphine action on dopamine neurons. *Proc Natl Acad Sci U S A* (2011) 108(39):16446–50. doi: 10.1073/pnas.1105418108
72. Jhou TC, Xu SP, Lee MR, Gallen CL, Ikemoto S. Mapping of reinforcing and analgesic effects of the mu opioid agonist endomorphin-1 in the ventral midbrain of the rat. *Psychopharmacology* (2012) 224(2):303–12. doi: 10.1007/s00213-012-2753-6
73. Matsui A, Jarvie BC, Robinson BG, Hentges ST, Williams JT. Separate GABA afferents to dopamine neurons mediate acute action of opioids, development of tolerance, and expression of withdrawal. *Neuron* (2014) 82(6):1346–56. doi: 10.1016/j.neuron.2014.04.030
74. Hnasko TS, Sotak BN, Palmiter RD. Morphine reward in dopamine-deficient mice. *Nature* (2005) 438(7069):854–7. doi: 10.1038/nature04172
75. Nader K, van der Kooy D. Deprivation state switches the neurobiological substrates mediating opiate reward in the ventral tegmental area. *J Neurosci* (1997) 17(1):383–90. doi: 10.1523/JNEUROSCI.17-01-00383.1997
76. Bolger GT, Skolnick P, Rice KC, Weissman BA. Differential regulation of mu-opiate receptors in heroin- and morphine-dependent rats. *FEBS Lett* (1988) 234(1):22–6. doi: 10.1016/0014-5793(88)81294-8
77. Belcheva MM, Barg J, McHale RJ, Dawn S, Ho MT, Ignatova E, et al. Differential down- and up-regulation of rat brain opioid receptor types and subtypes by buprenorphine. *Mol Pharmacol* (1993) 44:173–9.
78. Tempel A, Espinoza K. Morphine-induced downregulation of mu-opioid receptors in neonatal rat brain. *Brain Res* (1992) 469:129–33. doi: 10.1016/0165-3806(88)90176-9
79. Yu Y, Zhang L, Yin X, Sun H, Uhl GR, Wang JB. Mu opioid receptor phosphorylation, desensitization, and ligand efficacy. *J Biol Chem* (1997) 272:28869–74. doi: 10.1074/jbc.272.46.28869
80. Keith DE, Anton B, Murray SR, Zaki PA, Chu PC, Lissin DV, et al. mu-Opioid receptor internalization: opiate drugs have differential effects on a conserved endocytic mechanism *in vitro* and in the mammalian brain. *Mol Pharmacol* (1998) 53:377–84. doi: 10.1124/mol.53.3.377
81. Von Zastrow M, Svingos A, Haberstock-Debic H, Evans C. Regulated endocytosis of opioid receptors: cellular mechanisms and proposed roles in physiological adaptation to opiate drugs. *Curr Opin Neurobiol* (2003) 13:348–53. doi: 10.1016/S0959-4388(03)00069-2

82. Blanchet C, Sollini M, Luscher C. Two distinct forms of desensitization of G-protein coupled inwardly rectifying potassium currents evoked by alkaloid and peptide mu-opioid receptor agonists. *Mol Cell Neurosci* (2003) 24:517–23. doi: 10.1016/S1044-7431(03)00173-8
83. Arden JR, Segredo V, Wang Z, Lameh J, Sadée W. Phosphorylation and agonist-specific intracellular trafficking of an epitope-tagged mu-opioid receptor expressed in HEK 293 cells. *J Neurochem* (1995) 65:1636–45. doi: 10.1046/j.1471-4159.1995.65041636.x
84. Keith DE, Murray SR, Zaki PA, Chu PC, Lissin DV, Kang L, et al. Morphine activates opioid receptors without causing their rapid internalization. *J Biol Chem* (1996) 277:19021–4. doi: 10.1074/jbc.271.32.19021
85. Whistler JL, Chuang HH, Chu P, Jan LY, von Zastrow M. Functional dissociation of mu opioid receptor signaling and endocytosis: implications for the biology of opiate tolerance and addiction. *Neuron* (1999) 23:737–46. doi: 10.1016/S0896-6273(01)80032-5
86. Martini L, Whistler JL. The role of mu opioid receptor desensitization and endocytosis in morphine tolerance and dependence. *Curr Opin Neurobiol* (2007) 17(5):556–64. doi: 10.1016/j.conb.2007.10.004
87. Zaki PA, Keith DE Jr, Brine GA, Carroll FI, Evans CJ. The role of G protein activation in agonist-dependent mu-opioid receptor internalization. *JPET* (2000) 292(3):1127–34.
88. Kieffer BL, Evans CJ. Opioid tolerance—in search of a holy grail. *Cell* (2002) 108:5:587–90. doi: 10.1016/S0092-8674(02)00666-9
89. Bailey CP, Couch D, Johnson E, Griffiths K, Kelly E, Henderson G. μ-Opioid receptor desensitization in mature rat neurons: lack of interaction between DAMGO and morphine. *J Neurosci* (2003) 33:10515–20. doi: 10.1523/JNEUROSCI.23-33-10515.2003
90. Rankovic Z, Brust TF, Bohn LM. Biased agonism: an emerging paradigm in GPCR drug discovery. *Bioorg Med Chem Lett* (2016) 26:241–50. doi: 10.1016/j.bmcl.2015.12.024
91. Urban JD, Clarke WP, von Zastrow M, Nichols DE, Kobilka B, Weinstein H, et al. Functional selectivity and classical concepts of quantitative pharmacology. *J Pharmacol Exp Ther* (2007) 320:1–13. doi: 10.1124/jpet.106.104463
92. Schmid CL, Kennedy NM, Ross NC, Lovell KM, Yue Z, Morgenweck J, Bias factor and therapeutic window correlate to predict safer opioid analgesics. *Cell* (2017) 171(5):1165–1175.e13. doi: 10.1016/j.cell.2017.10.035
93. Raehal KM, Walker JK, Bohn LM. Morphine side effects in beta-arrestin 2 knockout mice. *J Pharmacol Exp Ther* (2005) 314(3):1195–201. doi: 10.1124/jpet.105.087254
94. Bohn LM, Lefkowitz RJ, Gainetdinov RR, Peppel K, Caron MG, Lin FT. Enhanced morphine analgesia in mice lacking beta-arrestin 2. *Science* (1999) 286:2495–8. doi: 10.1126/science.286.5449.2495
95. Bu H, Liu X, Tian X, Yang H, Gao F. Enhancement of morphine analgesia and prevention of morphine tolerance by downregulation of β-arrestin 2 with antigene RNAs in mice. *Int J Neurosci* (2015) 125(1):56–65. doi: 10.3109/00207454.2014.896913
96. Beardsley PM, Zhang Y. Synthetic Opioids. *Handb Exp Pharmacol* (2018) 252:353–81. doi: 10.1007/164_2018_149
97. Crist RC, Berrettini WH. Pharmacogenetics of OPRM1. *Pharmacol Biochem Behav* (2014) 2014:25–33. doi: 10.1016/j.pbb.2013.10.018
98. Kasai S, Ikeda K. Pharmacogenomics of the human μ-opioid receptor. *Pharmacogenomics* (2011) 12:1305–20. doi: 10.2217/pgs.11.68
99. Yuferov V, Levran O, Proudnikov D, Nielsen DA, Kreek MJ. Search for genetic markers and functional variants involved in the development of opiate and cocaine addiction and treatment. *Ann NY Acad Sci* (2010) 1187:184–207. doi: 10.1111/j.1749-6632.2009.05275.x
100. Beyer A, Koch T, Schroder H, Schulz S, Höllt V. Effect of the A118G polymorphism on binding affinity, potency and agonist-mediated endocytosis, desensitization, and resensitization of the human mu-opioid receptor. *J Neurochem* (2004) 89:553–60. doi: 10.1111/j.1471-4159.2004.02340.x
101. Kroslak T, LaForge KS, Gianotti RJ, Ho A, Nielsen DA, Kreek MJ. The single nucleotide polymorphism A118G alters functional properties of the human mu opioid receptor. *J Neurochem* (2007) 103:1,77–87. doi: 10.1111/j.1471-4159.2007.04738.x
102. Robinson JE, Vardy E, DiBerto JF, Chefer VI, White KL, Fish EW, et al. Receptor reserve moderates mesolimbic responses to opioids in a humanized mouse model of the OPRM1 A118G polymorphism. *Neuropsychopharmacology* (2015) 40(11):2614–22. doi: 10.1038/npp.2015.109
103. Zhang Y, Wang D, Johnson AD, Papp AC, Sadée W. Allelic expression imbalance of human mu opioid receptor (OPRM1) caused by variant A118G. *J Biol Chem* (2005) 280(38):,32618–24. doi: 10.1074/jbc.M504942200
104. Weerts EM, McCaul ME, Kuwabara H, Yang X, Xu X, Dannals RF, et al. Influence of OPRM1 Asn40Asp variant (A118G) on [11C]carfentanil binding potential: preliminary findings in human subjects. *Int J Neuropsychopharmacol* (2013) 16(1):47–53. doi: 10.1017/S146114571200017X
105. Peciña M, Love T, Stohler CS, Goldman D, Zubieta JK. Effects of the Mu opioid receptor polymorphism (OPRM1 A118G) on pain regulation, placebo effects and associated personality trait measures. *Neuropsychopharmacology* (2015) 40(4):957–65. doi: 10.1038/npp.2014.272
106. Oertel BG, Doehring A, Roskam B, Kettner M, Hackmann N, Ferreiros N, et al. Genetic-epigenetic interaction modulates μ-opioid receptor regulation. *Human Mol Genet* (2012) 21(21):4751–60. doi: 10.1093/hmg/dds314
107. Bond C, LaForge KS, Tian M, Melia D, Zhang S, Borg L, et al. Single-nucleotide polymorphism in the human mu opioid receptor gene alters beta-endorphin binding and activity: possible implications for opiate addiction. *Proc Natl Acad Sci U S A* (1998) 95:9608–13. doi: 10.1073/pnas.95.16.9608
108. Befort K, Filliol D, Decaillot FM, Gavériaux-Ruff C, Hoehe MR, Kieffer BL. A single nucleotide polymorphic mutation in the human mu-opioid receptor severely impairs receptor signaling. *J Biol Chem* (2001) 276:3130–7. doi: 10.1074/jbc.M006352200
109. Haerian BS, Haerian MS. OPRM1 rs1799971 polymorphism and opioid dependence: evidence from a meta-analysis. *Pharmacogenomics* (2013) 14(7):813–24. doi: 10.2217/pgs.13.57
110. Woodcock EA, Lundahl LH, Burmeister M, Greenwald MK. Functional mu opioid receptor polymorphism (OPRM1 A118G) associated with heroin use outcomes in Caucasian males: a pilot study. *Am J Addict* (2015) 24(4):329–35. doi: 10.1111/ajad.12187
111. Szeto CYK, Tang NLS, Lee DTS, Stadlin A. Association between μ opioid receptor gene polymorphisms and Chinese heroin addicts. *Neuroreport* (2001) 12:1103–6. doi: 10.1097/00001756-200105080-00011
112. Gelernter J, Kranzler H, Cubells J. Genetics of two μ opioid receptor gene (OPRM1) exon 1 polymorphisms: population studies, and allele frequencies in alcohol- and drug-dependent subjects. *Mol Psychiatry* (1999) 4:476–83. doi: 10.1038/sj.mp.4000556
113. Clarke TK, Crist RC, Kampman KM, Dackis CA, Pettinati HM, O'Brien CP, et al. Low frequency genetic variants in the μ-opioid receptor (OPRM1) affect risk for addiction to heroin and cocaine. *Neurosci Lett* (2013) 10(542):71–5. doi: 10.1016/j.neulet.2013.02.018
114. Shi J, Hui L, Xu Y, Wang F, Huang W, Hu G. Sequence variations in the mu-opioid receptor gene (OPRM1) associated with human addiction to heroin. *Hum Mutat* (2002) 19:459–60. doi: 10.1002/humu.9026
115. Xu J, Lu Z, Xu M, Pan L, Deng Y, Xie X, et al. A heroin addiction severity-associated intronic single nucleotide polymorphism modulates alternative pre-mRNA splicing of the μ opioid receptor gene OPRM1 *via* hnRNPH interactions. *J Neurosci* (2014) 34(33):11048–66. doi: 10.1523/JNEUROSCI.3986-13.2014
116. Kumar D, Chakraborty J, Das S. Epistatic effects between variants of κ-opioid receptor gene and A118G of μ-opioid receptor gene increase susceptibility to addiction in Indian population. *Prog Neuropsychopharmacol Biol Psychiatry* (2012) 36:225–30. doi: 10.1016/j.pnpbp.2011.10.018
117. Nuechterlein EB, Ni L, Domino EF, Zubieta JK. Nicotine-specific and non-specific effects of cigarette smoking on endogenous opioid mechanisms. Prog Neuropsychopharmacol. *Biol Psychiatry* (2016) 69:69–77. doi: 10.1016/j.pnpbp.2016.04.006
118. Domino EF, Hirasawa-Fujita M, Ni L, Guthrie SK, Zubieta JK. Regional brain [(11)C]carfentanil binding following tobacco smoking. *Prog Neuropsychopharmacol Biol Psychiatry* (2015) 59:100–4. doi: 10.1016/j.pnpbp.2015.01.007
119. Ray R, Ruparel K, Newberg A, Wileyto EP, Loughead JW, Divgi C, et al. Human mu opioid receptor (OPRM1 A118G) polymorphism is associated with brain mu-opioid receptor binding potential in smokers. *Proc Natl Acad Sci U S A* (2011) 108(22):9268–73. doi: 10.1073/pnas.1018699108
120. Domino EF, Evans CL, Ni L, Guthrie SK, Koeppe RA, Zubieta JK. Tobacco smoking produces greater striatal dopamine release in G-allele carriers with mu opioid receptor A118G polymorphism. *Prog Neuropsychopharmacol Biol Psychiatry* (2012) 38(2):236–40. doi: 10.1016/j.pnpbp.2012.04.003

121. Kapur S, Sharad S, Singh RA, Gupta AK. A118G polymorphism in μ opioid receptor gene (oprm1): association with opiate addiction in subjects of Indian origin. *J Integr Neurosci* (2007) 6(4):511–22. doi: 10.1142/S0219635207001635
122. Deb I, Chakraborty J, Gangopadhyay PK, Choudhury SR, Das S. Single-nucleotide polymorphism (A118G) in exon 1 of OPRM1 gene causes alteration in downstream signaling by μ-opioid receptor and may contribute to the genetic risk for addiction. *J Neurochem* (2010) 112:486–96. doi: 10.1111/j.1471-4159.2009.06472.x
123. Tan E-C, Tan C-H, Karupathivan U, Yap EPH. μ opioid receptor gene polymorphisms and heroin dependence in Asian populations. *Neuroreport* (2003) 14:569–72. doi: 10.1097/00001756-200303240-00008
124. Nagaya D, Ramanathan S, Ravichandran M, Navaratnam V. A118G μ opioid receptor polymorphism among drug addicts in Malaysia. *J Integr Neurosci* (2012) 11:117–22. doi: 10.1142/S0219635212500082
125. Bart G, Heilig M, LaForge KS, Pollak L, Leal SM, Ott J, et al. Substantial attributable risk related to a functional μ-opioid receptor gene polymorphism in association with heroin addiction in central Sweden. *Mol Psychiatry* (2004) 9:547–9. doi: 10.1038/sj.mp.4001504
126. Drakenberg K, Nikoshkov A, Horváth MC, Fagergren P, Gharibyan A, Saarelainen K, et al. Mu opioid receptor A118G polymorphism in association with striatal opioid neuropeptide gene expression in heroin abusers. *Proc Natl Acad Sci U S A* (2006) 103(20):7883–8. doi: 10.1073/pnas.0600871103
127. Luo X, Kranzlet HR, Zhao H, Gelernter J. Haplotypes at the OPRM1 locus are associated with susceptibility to substance dependence in European-Americans. *Am J Med Genet* (2003) 120B:97–108. doi: 10.1002/ajmg.b.20034
128. Crowley JJ, Oslin DW, Patkar AA, Gottheil E, DeMaria PA Jr, O'Brien CP, et al. A genetic association study of the μ opioid receptor and severe opioid dependence. *Psychiatr Genet* (2003) 13:169–73. doi: 10.1097/00041444-200309000-00006
129. Franke P, Wang T, Nöthen MM, Knapp M, Neidt H, Albrecht S, et al. Nonreplication of association between μ-opioid-receptor gene (OPRM1) A118G polymorphism and substance dependence. *Am J Med Genet* (2001) 105(1):114–9. doi: 10.1002/1096-8628(20010108)105:1< 114::AID-AJMG1074>3.3.CO;2-C
130. Levran O, Londono D, O'Hara K, Nielsen DA, Peles E, Rotrosen J, et al. Genetic susceptibility to heroin addiction: a candidate gene association study. *Genes Brain Behav* (2008) 7:720–9. doi: 10.1111/j.1601-183X.2008.00410.x
131. Nikolov MA, Beltcheva O, Galabova A, Ljubenova A, Jankova E, Gergov G, et al. No evidence of association between 118A > G OPRM1 polymorphism and heroin dependence in a large Bulgarian case-control sample. *Drug Alcohol Depend* (2011) 117(1):62–5. doi: 10.1016/j.drugalcdep.2010.12.026
132. Li T, Liu X, Zhu ZH, Zhao J, Hu X, Sham PC, et al. Association analysis of polymorphisms in the μ opioid gene and heroin abuse in Chinese. *Addict Biol* (2000) 5:181–6. doi: 10.1080/13556210050003775
133. Zhang D, Shao C, Shao M, Yan P, Wang Y, Liu Y, et al. Effect of mu-opioid receptor gene polymorphisms on heroin-induced subjective responses in a Chinese population. *Biol Psychiatry* (2007) 61(11):1244–51. doi: 10.1016/j.biopsych.2006.07.012
134. Crettol S, Besson J, Croquette-Krokar M, Hämmig R, Gothuey I, Monnat M, et al. Association of dopamine and opioid receptor genetic polymorphisms with response to methadone maintenance treatment. *Prog Neuropsychopharmacol Biol Psychiatry* (2008) 32(7):1722–7. doi: 10.1016/j.pnpbp.2008.07.009
135. Levran O, Peles E, Randesi M, da Rosa JC, Adelson M, Kreek MJ. The μ-opioid receptor nonsynonymous variant 118A > G is associated with prolonged abstinence from heroin without agonist treatment. *Pharmacogenomics* (2017) 18(15):1387–91. doi: 10.2217/pgs-2017-0092
136. Zhang H, Kranzler HR, Yang BZ, Luo X, Gelernter J. The OPRD1 and OPRK1 loci in alcohol or drug dependence: OPRD1 variation modulates substance dependence risk. *Mol Psychiatry* (2008) 13:531–43. doi: 10.1038/sj.mp.4002035
137. Nelson EC, Lynskey MT, Heath AC, Wray N, Agrawal A, Shand FL, et al. Association of OPRD1 polymorphisms with heroin dependence in a large case-control series. *Addict Biol* (2014) 19(1):111–21. doi: 10.1111/j.1369-1600.2012.00445.x
138. Gao X, Wang Y, Lang M, Yuan L, Reece AS, Wang W. Contribution of genetic polymorphisms and haplotypes in DRD2, BDNF, and opioid receptors to heroin dependence and endophenotypes among the Han Chinese. *OMICS* (2017) 21(7):404–12. doi: 10.1089/omi.2017.0057
139. Nagaya D, Zahari Z, Saleem M, Yahaya BH, Tan SC, Yusoff NM. An analysis of genetic association in opioid dependence susceptibility. *J Clin Pharm Ther* (2018) 43(1):80–6. doi: 10.1111/jcpt.12585
140. Crist RC, Ambrose-Lanci LM, Vaswani M, Clarke TK, Zeng A, Yuan C, et al. Case-control association analysis of polymorphisms in the delta-opioid receptor, OPRD1, with cocaine and opioid addicted populations. *Drug Alcohol Depend* (2013) 127:122–8. doi: 10.1016/j.drugalcdep.2012.06.023
141. Huang CC, Kuo SC, Yeh TC, Yeh YW, Chen CY, Liang CS, et al. OPRD1 gene affects disease vulnerability and environmental stress in patients with heroin dependence in Han Chinese. *Prog Neuropsychopharmacol Biol Psychiatry* (2018) 89:109–16. doi: 10.1016/j.pnpbp.2018.08.028
142. Mayer P, Rochlitz H, Rauch E, Rommelspacher H, Hasse HE, Schmidt S, et al. Association between a delta opioid receptor gene polymorphism and heroin dependence in man. *Neuroreport* (1997) 8:2547–50. doi: 10.1097/00001756-199707280-00025
143. Xu K, Liu XH, Nagarajan S, Gu XY, Goldman D. Relationship of the delta-opioid receptor gene to heroin abuse in a large Chinese case/control sample. *Am J Med Genet* (2002) 110:45–50. doi: 10.1002/ajmg.10374
144. Franke P, Nöthen MM, Wang T, Neidt H, Knapp M, Lichtermann D, et al. Human delta-opioid receptor gene and susceptibility to heroin and alcohol dependence. *Am J Med Genet* (1999) 88:462–4. doi: 10.1002/(SICI)1096-8628(19991015)88:5<462::AID-AJMG4>3.0.CO;2-S
145. Clarke TK, Crist RC, Ang A, Ambrose-Lanci LM, Lohoff FW, Saxon AJ, et al. Genetic variation in OPRD1 and the response to treatment for opioid dependence with buprenorphine in European-American females. *Pharmacogenomics J* (2014a) 14(3):303–8. doi: 10.1038/tpj.2013.30
146. Sharafshah A, Fazel H, Albonaim A, Omarmeli V, Rezaei S, Mirzajani E, et al. Association of OPRD1 gene variants with opioid dependence in addicted male individuals undergoing methadone treatment in the north of Iran. *J Psychoactive Drugs* (2017) 49(3):242–51. doi: 10.1080/02791072.2017.1290303
147. Jones JD, Luba RR, Vogelman JL, Comer SD. Searching for evidence of genetic mediation of opioid withdrawal by opioid receptor gene polymorphisms. *Am J Addict* (2016) 25(1):41–8. doi: 10.1111/ajad.12316
148. Crist RC, Clarke TK, Ang A, Ambrose-Lanci LM, Lohoff FW, Saxon AJ, et al. An intronic variant in OPRD1 predicts treatment outcome for opioid dependence in African-Americans. *Neuropsychopharmacology* (2013) 38(10):2003–10. doi: 10.1038/npp.2013.99
149. Crist RC, Phillips KA, Furnari MA, Moran LM, Doyle GA, McNicholas LF, et al. Replication of the pharmacogenetic effect of rs678849 on buprenorphine efficacy in African-Americans with opioid use disorder. *Pharmacogenomics J* (2018) 19:260–68. doi: 10.1038/s41397-018-0065-x
150. Beer B, Erb R, Pavlic M, Ulmer H, Giacomuzzi S, Riemer Y, et al. Association of polymorphisms in pharmacogenetic candidate genes (OPRD1, GAL, ABCB1, OPRM1) with opioid dependence in European population: a case-control study. *PLoS One* (2013) 8(9):e75359. doi: 10.1371/journal.pone.0075359
151. Luo R, Li X, Qin S, Luo Z, Luo X, Hu P, et al. Impact of SNP–SNP interaction among ABCB1, ARRB2, DRD1 and OPRD1 on methadone dosage requirement in Han Chinese patients. *Pharmacogenomics* (2017) 18(18):1659–70. doi: 10.2217/pgs-2017-0072
152. Yuferov V, Fussella D, LaForgea KS, Nielsena DA, Gordonb D, Hoa A, et al. Redefinition of the human kappa opioid receptor gene (OPRK1) structure and association of haplotypes with opiate addiction. *Pharmacogenetics* (2004) 14(12):793–804. doi: 10.1097/00008571-200412000-00002
153. Gerra G, Leonardi C, Cortese E, D'Amore A, Lucchini A, Strepparola G, et al. Human kappa opioid receptor gene (OPRK1) polymorphism is associated with opiate addiction. *Am J Med Genet B Neuropsychiatr Genet* (2007) 144B(6):771–5. doi: 10.1002/ajmg.b.30510
154. Albonaim A, Fazel H, Sharafshah A, Omarmeli V, Rezaei S, Ajamian F, et al. Association of OPRK1 gene polymorphisms with opioid dependence in addicted men undergoing methadone treatment in an Iranian population. *J Addict Dis* (2017) 36(4):227–35. doi: 10.1080/10550887.2017.1361724
155. Yuanyuan J, Rui S, Hua T, Jingjing C, Cuola D, Yuhui S, et al. Genetic association analyses and meta-analysis of Dynorphin-Kappa Opioid system potential functional variants with heroin dependence. *Neurosci Lett* (2018) 685:75–82. doi: 10.1016/j.neulet.2018.08.023

156. Wei SG, Zhu YS, Lai JH, Xue HX, Chai ZQ, Li SB. Association between heroin dependence and prodynorphin gene polymorphisms. *Brain Res Bull* (2011) 85:238–42. doi: 10.1016/j.brainresbull.2011.02.010
157. Hashemi M, Shakiba M, Sanaei S, Shahkar G, Rezaei M, Mojahed A, et al. Evaluation of prodynorphin gene polymorphisms and their association with heroin addiction in a sample of the southeast Iranian population. *Mol Biol Res Commun* (2018) 7(1):1–6. doi: 10.22099/mbrc.2017.27182.1294
158. Clarke T-K, Ambrose-Lanci L, Ferraro TN, Berrettini WH, Kampman KM, Dackis CA, et al. Genetic association analyses of PDYN polymorphisms with heroin and cocaine addiction. *Genes Brain Behav* (2012) 2012(11):415–23. doi: 10.1111/j.1601-183X.2012.00785.x
159. Clarke TK, Krause K, Li T, Schumann G. An association of prodynorphin polymorphisms and opioid dependence in females in a Chinese population. *Addict Biol* (2009) 14:366–70. doi: 10.1111/j.1369-1600.2009.00151.x
160. Xuei X, Flury-Wetherill L, Almasy L, Bierut L, Tischfield J, Schuckit M, et al. Association analysis of genes encoding the nociceptin receptor (OPRL1) and its endogenous ligand (PNOC) with alcohol or illicit drug dependence. *Addict Biol* (2008) 13(1):80–7. doi: 10.1111/j.1369-1600.2007.00082.x
161. Briant JA, Nielsen DA, Proudnikov D, Londono D, Ho A, Ott J, et al. Evidence for association of two variants of the nociceptin/orphanin FQ receptor gene OPRL1 with vulnerability to develop opiate addiction in Caucasians. *Psychiatr Genet* (2010) 20(2):65–72. doi: 10.1097/YPG.0b013e32833511f6
162. Browne CA, Erickson RL, Blendy JA, Lucki I. Genetic variation in the behavioral effects of buprenorphine in female mice derived from a murine model of the OPRM1 A118G polymorphism. *Neuropharmacology* (2017) 117:401–7. doi: 10.1016/j.neuropharm.2017.02.005
163. Muriel J, Margarit C, Planelles B, Serralta MJ, Puga C, Inda MD, et al. OPRM1 influence on and effectiveness of an individualized treatment plan for prescription opioid use disorder patients. *Ann N Y Acad Sci* (2018) 1425:82–94. doi: 10.1111/nyas.13735
164. Wu WD, Wang Y, Fang YM, Zhou HY. Polymorphism of the micro-opioid receptor gene (OPRM1 118A > G) affects fentanyl-induced analgesia during anesthesia and recovery. *Mol Diagn Ther* (2009) 13:331–7. doi: 10.1007/BF03256337
165. Oueslati B, Moula O, Ghachem R. The impact of OPRM1's genetic polymorphisms on methadone maintenance treatment in opioid addicts: a systematic review. *Pharmacogenomics* (2018) 19(8):741–7. doi: 10.2217/pgs-2018-0017
166. Wand GS, Mangold D, El Deiry S, McCaul ME, Hoover D. Family history of alcoholism and hypothalamic opioidergic activity. *Arch Gen Psychiatry* (1998) 55:1114–9. doi: 10.1001/archpsyc.55.12.1114
167. Schluger JH, Ho A, Borg L, Porter M, Maniar S, Gunduz M, et al. Nalmefene causes greater hypothalamic–pituitary–adrenal axis activation than naloxone in normal volunteers: implications for the treatment of alcoholism. *Alcohol Clin Exp Res* (1998) 22:1430–6. doi: 10.1111/j.1530-0277.1998.tb03931.x
168. Chong RY, Oswald L, Yang X, Uhart M, Lin PI, Wand GS. The mu-opioid receptor polymorphism A118G predicts cortisol responses to naloxone and stress. *Neuropsychopharmacology* (2006) 31:204–11. doi: 10.1038/sj.npp.1300856
169. Hernandez-Avila CA, Wand G, Luo X, Gelernter J, Kranzler HR. Association between the cortisol response to opioid blockade and the Asn40Asp polymorphism at the mu-opioid receptor locus (OPRM1). *Am J Med Genet* (2003) 118:60–5. doi: 10.1002/ajmg.b.10054
170. Wand GS, McCaul M, Yang X, Reynolds J, Gotjen D, Lee S, et al. The mu-opioid receptor gene polymorphism (A118G) alters HPA axis activation induced by opioid receptor blockade. *Neuropsychopharmacology* (2002) 26:106–14. doi: 10.1016/S0893-133X(01)00294-9
171. Belcher AM, Volkow ND, Moeller GF, Ferre S. Personality traits and vulnerability or resilience to substance use disorders. *Trends Cogn Sci* (2014) 18(4):211–7. doi: 10.1016/j.tics.2014.01.010
172. McCrae RR, Costa PT, Jr. Updating Norman's "Adequate Taxonomy": intelligence and personality dimensions in natural language and in questionnaires. *J Pers Soc Psychol* (1985) 49(3):710–21. doi: 10.1037//0022-3514.49.3.710
173. Martin ED, Sher KJ. Family history of alcoholism, alcohol-use disorders and the 5-factor model of personality. *J Stud Alcohol* (1994) 55:81–90. doi: 10.15288/jsa.1994.55.81
174. Ball SA, Tennen H, Poling JC, Kranzler HR, Rounsaville BJ. Personality, temperament, and character dimensions and the DSM-IV personality disorders in substance abusers. *J Abnorm Psychol* (1997) 106:545–53. doi: 10.1037/0021-843X.106.4.545
175. Terracciano A, Costa PT. Smoking and the five-factor model of personality. *Addiction* (2004) 99:472–81. doi: 10.1111/j.1360-0443.2004.00687.x
176. Raketic D, Barisic JV, Svetozarevic SM, Gazibara T, Tepavcevic DK, Milovanovic SD. Five-factor model personality profiles: the differences between alcohol and opiate addiction among females. *Psychiatr Danub* (2017) 29(1):74–80. doi: 10.24869/psyd.2017.74
177. Carter JA, Herbst JH, Stoller KB, King VL, Kidorf MS, Costa PT Jr, et al. Short-term stability of NEO-PI-R personality trait scores in opioid-dependent outpatients. *Psychol Addict Behav* (2001) 15(3):255–60. doi: 10.1037//0893-164X.15.3.255
178. Kornør H, Nordvik H. Five-factor model personality traits in opioid dependence. *BMC Psychiatry* (2007) 6(7):37. doi: 10.1186/1471-244X-7-37
179. McCrae RR, John OP. An introduction to the five-factor model and its applications. *J Pers Disord* (1992) 60(2):175–215. doi: 10.1111/j.1467-6494.1992.tb00970.x
180. Hernandez-Avila CA, Covault J, Gelernter J, Kranzler, HR. Association study of personality factors and the Asn40Asp polymorphism at the mu-opioid receptor gene (OPRM1). *Psychiatr Genet* (2004) 14(2):89–92. doi: 10.1097/01.ypg.0000107931.32051.c7
181. Love TM, Stohler CS, Zubieta JK. Positron emission tomography measures of endogenous opioid neurotransmission and impulsiveness traits in humans. *Arch Gen Psychiatry* (2009) 66(10):1124–34. doi: 10.1001/archgenpsychiatry.2009.134
182. Smith GT, Fischer S, Cyders MA, Annus AM, Spillane NS, McCarthy DM. On the validity and utility of discriminating among impulsivity-like traits. *Assessment* (2007) 14(2):155–70. doi: 10.1177/1073191106295527
183. Fischer S, Anderson KG, Smith GT. Coping with distress by eating or drinking: role of trait urgency and expectancies. *Psychol Addict Behav* (2004) 18(3):269–74. doi: 10.1037/0893-164X.18.3.269
184. Frost JJ, Mayberg HS, Sadzot B, Dannals RF, Lever JR, Ravert HT, et al. Comparison of [11C]diprenorphine and [11C]carfentanil binding to opiate receptors in humans by positron emission tomography. *J Cereb Blood Flow Metab* (2001) 10(4):484–92. doi: 10.1038/jcbfm.1990.90
185. Kling MA, Carson RE, Borg L, Zametkin A, Matochik JA, Schluger J, et al. Opioid receptor imaging with positron emission tomography and [(18)F]cyclofoxy in long-term, methadone-treated former heroin addicts. *J Pharmacol Exp Ther* (2000) 295(3):1070–6.
186. Rothman RB, McLean S. An examination of the opiate receptor subtypes labeled by [3H]cycloFOXY: an opiate antagonist suitable for positron emission tomography. *Biol Psychiatry* (1988) 23(5):435–58. doi: 10.1016/0006-3223(88)90016-9
187. Hiller JM, Fan LQ. Laminar distribution of the multiple opioid receptors in the human cerebral cortex. *Neurochem Res* (1996) 21(11):1333–45. doi: 10.1007/BF02532374
188. Cohen RM, Andreason PJ, Doudet DJ, Carson RE, Sunderland T. Opiate receptor avidity and cerebral blood flow in Alzheimer's disease. *J Neurol Sci* (1997) 148(2):171–80. doi: 10.1016/S0022-510X(96)05315-4
189. Lewis JW, Husbands SM. The orvinols and related opioids—high affinity ligands with diverse efficacy profiles. *Curr Pharm Des* (2004) 10:717–32. doi: 10.2174/1381612043453027
190. Negus SS, Bidlack JM, Mello NK, Furness MS, Rice KC, Brandt MR. Delta opioid antagonist effects of buprenorphine in rhesus monkeys. *Behav Pharmacol* (2002) 13:557–70. doi: 10.1097/00008877-200211000-00005
191. Richards ML, Sadee W. *In vivo* opiate receptor binding of oripavines to mu, delta and kappa sites in rat brain as determined by an ex vivo labeling method. *Eur J Pharmacol* (1985) 114:343–53. doi: 10.1016/0014-2999(85)90379-6
192. Greenwald M, Johanson CE, Bueller J, Chang Y, Moody DE, Kilbourn M, et al. Buprenorphine duration of action: mu-opioid receptor availability and pharmacokinetic and behavioral indices. *Biol Psychiatry* (2007) 61(1):101–10. doi: 10.1016/j.biopsych.2006.04.043
193. Kuhlman JJ Jr, Lalani S, Magluilo J Jr, Levine B, Darwin WD. Human pharmacokinetics of intravenous, sublingual, and buccal buprenorphine. *J Clin Pharmacol* (1997) 37:31–7. doi: 10.1093/jat/20.6.369
194. Greenwald MK, Johanson CE, Moody DE, Woods JH, Kilbourn MR, Koeppe RA, et al. Effects of buprenorphine maintenance dose on mu-opioid receptor availability, plasma concentrations, and antagonist blockade in

heroin-dependent volunteers. *Neuropsychopharmacology* (2003) 28(11):2000–9. doi: 10.1038/sj.npp.1300251
195. Zubieta J, Greenwald MK, Lombardi U, Woods JH, Kilbourn MR, Jewett DM, et al. Buprenorphine-induced changes in μ-opioid receptor availability in male heroin-dependent volunteers: a preliminary study. *Neuropsychopharmacology* (2000) 23(3):326–34. doi: 10.1016/S0893-133X(00)00110-X
196. Al-Hasani R, Bruchas MR. Molecular mechanisms of opioid receptor-dependent signaling and behavior. *Anesthesiology* (2011) 115(6):1363–81. doi: 10.1097/ALN.0b013e318238bba6
197. Le Merrer J, Becker JA, Befort K, Kieffer BL. Reward processing by the opioid system in the brain. *Physiol Rev* (2009) 89(4):1379–412. doi: 10.1152/physrev.00005.2009
198. Minami M, Satoh M. Molecular biology of the opioid receptors: structures, functions and distributions. *Neurosci Res* (1995) 23(2):121–45. doi: 10.1016/0168-0102(95)00933-K
199. Simonin F, Gavériaux-Ruff C, Befort K, Matthes H, Lannes B, Micheletti G, et al. kappa-Opioid receptor in humans: cDNA and genomic cloning, chromosomal assignment, functional expression, pharmacology, and expression pattern in the central nervous system. *Proc Natl Acad Sci U S A* (1995) 92(15):7006–10. doi: 10.1073/pnas.92.15.7006
200. Meng F, Xie GX, Thompson RC, Mansour A, Goldstein A, Watson SJ, et al. Cloning and pharmacological characterization of a rat kappa opioid receptor. *Proc Natl Acad Sci U S A* (1993) 90(21):9954–8. doi: 10.1073/pnas.90.21.9954
201. Mansour A, Fox CA, Akil H, Watson SJ. Opioid-receptor mRNA expression in the rat CNS: anatomical and functional implications. *Trends Neurosci* (1995) 18(1):22–9. doi: 10.1016/0166-2236(95)93946-U
202. Attali B, Saya D, Vogel Z. Kappa-opiate agonists inhibit adenylate cyclase and produce heterologous desensitization in rat spinal cord. *J Neurochem* (1989) 52(2):360–9. doi: 10.1111/j.1471-4159.1989.tb09130.x
203. Lawrence DM, Bidlack JM. The kappa opioid receptor expressed on the mouse R1.1 thymoma cell line is coupled to adenylyl cyclase through a pertussis toxin-sensitive guanine nucleotide-binding regulatory protein. *J Pharmacol Exp Ther* (1993) 266(3):1678–83.
204. Tallent M, Dichter MA, Bell GI, Reisine T. The cloned kappa opioid receptor couples to an N-type calcium current in undifferentiated PC-12 cells. *Neuroscience* (1994) 63(4):1033–40. doi: 10.1016/0306-4522(94)90570-3
205. Pfeiffer A, Brantl V, Herz A, Emrich HM. Psychotomimesis mediated by kappa opiate receptors. *Science* (1986) 233:774–6. doi: 10.1126/science.3016896
206. Gonzalez D, Riba J, Bouso JC, Gomez-Jarabo G, Barbanoj MJ. Pattern of use and subjective effects of *Salvia divinorum* among recreational users. *Drug Alcohol Depend* (2006) 85:157–62. doi: 10.1016/j.drugalcdep.2006.04.001
207. Knoll AT, Meloni EG, Thomas JB, Carroll FI, Carlezon WA, Jr. Anxiolytic-like effects of kappa-opioid receptor antagonists in models of unlearned and learned fear in rats. *J Pharmacol Exp Ther* (2007) 323:838–45. doi: 10.1124/jpet.107.127415
208. Valdez GR, Harshberger E. κ opioid regulation of anxiety-like behavior during acute ethanol withdrawal. *Pharmacol Biochem Behav* (2012) 102:1,44–7. doi: 10.1016/j.pbb.2012.03.019
209. Wang YJ, Hang A, Lu YC, Long Y, Zan GY, Li XP, et al. κ Opioid receptor activation in different brain regions differentially modulates anxiety-related behaviors in mice. *Neuropharmacology* (2016) 110(Pt A):92–101. doi: 10.1016/j.neuropharm.2016.04.022
210. Schlosburg JE, Whitfield TW Jr, Park PE, Crawford EF, George O, Vendruscolo LF, et al. Long-term antagonism of κ opioid receptors prevents escalation of and increased motivation for heroin intake. *J Neurosci* (2013) 33(49):19384–92. doi: 10.1523/JNEUROSCI.1979-13.2013
211. Sedki F, Eigenmann K, Gelinas J, Schouela N, Courchesne S, Shalev U. A role for kappa-, but not mu-opioid, receptor activation in acute food deprivation-induced reinstatement of heroin seeking in rats. *Addict Biol* (2015) 20(3):423–32. doi: 10.1111/adb.12133
212. Shirayama Y, Ishida H, Iwata M, Hazama G, Kawahara R, Duman RS. Stress increases dynorphin immunoreactivity in limbic brain regions and dynorphin antagonism produces antidepressant-like effects. *J Neurochem* (2004) 90:1258–68. doi: 10.1111/j.1471-4159.2004.02589.x
213. Schwarzer C. 30 years of dynorphins—new insights on their functions in neuropsychiatric diseases. *Pharmacol Therap* (2009) 123:353–70. doi: 10.1016/j.pharmthera.2009.05.006
214. Massaly N, Morón JA, Al-Hasani R. A trigger for opioid misuse: chronic pain and stress dysregulate the mesolimbic pathway and kappa opioid system. *Front Neurosci* (2016) 10:480. doi: 10.3389/fnins.2016.00480
215. Koob GF. Addiction is a reward deficit and stress surfeit disorder. *Front Psychiatry* (2013) 4:72. doi: 10.3389/fpsyt.2013.00072
216. Diana M, Pistis M, Muntoni A, Gessa G. Profound decrease of mesolimbic dopaminergic neuronal activity in morphine withdrawn rats. *J Pharmacol Exp Ther* (1995) 272(2):781–5.
217. Anderson SA, Michaelides M, Zarnegar P, Ren Y, Fagergren P, Thanos PK, et al. Impaired periamygdaloid-cortex prodynorphin is characteristic of opiate addiction and depression. *J Clin Invest* (2013) 123(12):5334–41. doi: 10.1172/JCI70395
218. Liu-Chen LY. Agonist-induced regulation and trafficking of kappa opioid receptors. *Life Sci* (2004) 75(5):511–36. doi: 10.1016/j.lfs.2003.10.041
219. Wang Y, Tang K, Inan S, Siebert D, Holzgrabe U, Lee DY, et al. Comparison of pharmacological activities of three distinct kappa ligands (Salvinorin A, TRK-820 and 3FLB) on kappa opioid receptors *in vitro* and their antipruritic and antinociceptive activities *in vivo*. *J Pharmacol Exp Ther* (2005) 312(1):220–30. doi: 10.1124/jpet.104.073668
220. Placzek MS, Van de Bittner GC, Wey HY, Lukas SE, Hooker JM. Immediate and persistent effects of salvinorin A on the kappa opioid receptor in rodents, monitored *in vivo* with PET. *Neuropsychopharmacology* (2015) 40(13):2865–72. doi: 10.1038/npp.2015.159
221. Mayer P, Hollt V. Pharmacogenetics of opioid receptors and addiction. *Pharmacogenet Genomics* (2006) 16(1):1–7. doi: 10.1097/01.fpc.0000182781.87932.0d
222. Wei LN, Hu X, Bi J, Loh H. Post-transcriptional regulation of mouse kappa-opioid receptor expression. *Mol Pharmacol* (2000) 57(2):401–8.
223. Votinov M, Pripfl J, Windischberger C, Kalcher K, Zimprich A, Zimprich F, et al. A genetic polymorphism of the endogenous opioid dynorphin modulates monetary reward anticipation in the corticostriatal loop. *PLoS One* (2014) 9(2):e89954. doi: 10.1371/journal.pone.0089954
224. Lomelin D, Jorgenson E, Risch N. Human genetic variation recognizes functional elements in noncoding sequence. *Genome Res* (2018) 20(3):311–9. doi: 10.1101/gr.094151.109
225. Colgan D, Manley J. Mechanism and regulation of mRNA polyadenylation. *Genes Dev* (1997) 11:2755–66. doi: 10.1101/gad.11.21.2755
226. Ford LP, Bagga PS, Wilusz J. The poly(A) tail inhibits the assembly of a 3′-to-5′ exonuclease in an *in vitro* RNA stability system. *Mol Cell Biol* (1997) 17:398–406. doi: 10.1128/MCB.17.1.398
227. Preiss T, Hentze MW. Dual function of the messenger RNA cap structure in poly(A)-tail-promoted translation in yeast. *Nature* (1998) 392:516–20. doi: 10.1038/33192
228. Sachs A, Sarnow P, Hentze M. Starting at the beginning, middle, and end: translation initiation in eukaryotes. *Cell* (1997) 89:831–8. doi: 10.1016/S0092-8674(00)80268-8
229. Yuferov V, Ji F, Nielsen DA, Levran O, Ho A, Morgello S, et al. A functional haplotype implicated in vulnerability to develop cocaine dependence is associated with reduced PDYN expression in human brain. *Neuropsychopharmacology* (2008) 34:1185. doi: 10.1038/npp.2008.187
230. Zimprich A, Kraus J, Wöltje M, Mayer P, Rauch E, Höllt V. An allelic variation in the human prodynorphin gene promoter alters stimulus-induced expression. *J Neurochem* (2000) 74:472–7. doi: 10.1046/j.1471-4159.2000.740472.x
231. Saify K, Saadat I, Saadat M. Association between VNTR polymorphism in promoter region of prodynorphin (PDYN) gene and heroin dependence. *Psychiatry Res* (2014) 219(3):690–2. doi: 10.1016/j.psychres.2014.06.048
232. Wang SC, Tsou HH, Chung RH, Chang YS, Fang CP, Chen CH, et al. The association of genetic polymorphisms in the κ-opioid receptor 1 gene with body weight, alcohol use, and withdrawal symptoms in patients with methadone maintenance. *J Clin Psychopharmacol* (2014) 34:205–11. doi: 10.1097/JCP.0000000000000082
233. Bruchas MR, Land BB, Lemos JC, Chavkin C. CRF1-R activation of the dynorphin/kappa opioid system in the mouse basolateral amygdala mediates anxiety-like behavior. *PLoS One* (2009) 4:e8528. doi: 10.1371/journal.pone.0008528
234. Kastenberger I, Lutsch C, Herzog H, Schwarzer C. Influence of sex and genetic background on anxiety-related and stress-induced behaviour of prodynorphin-deficient mice. *PLoS One* (2012) 7:3,e34251. doi: 10.1371/journal.pone.0034251

235. Luo X, Zuo L, Kranzler H, Zhang H, Wang S, Gelernter J. Multiple OPR genes influence personality traits in substance dependent and healthy subjects in two American populations. *Am J Med Genet B Neuropsychiatr Genet* (2008) 147B(7):1028–39. doi: 10.1002/ajmg.b.30701

236. Flory JD, Pytte CL, Hurd Y, Ferrell RE, Manuck SB. Alcohol dependence, disinhibited behavior and variation in the prodynorphin gene. *Biol Psychol* (2011) 88(1):51–6. doi: 10.1016/j.biopsycho.2011.06.007

237. Talbot PS, Narendran R, Butelman ER, Huang Y, Ngo K, Slifstein M, et al. 11C-GR103545, a radiotracer for imaging kappa-opioid receptors *in vivo* with PET: synthesis and evaluation in baboons. *J Nucl Med* (2005) 46(3):484–94.

238. Tomasi G, Nabulsi N, Zheng MQ, Weinzimmer D, Ropchan J, Blumberg L, et al. Determination of *in vivo* Bmax and Kd for 11C-GR103545, an agonist PET tracer for κ-opioid receptors: a study in nonhuman primates. *J Nucl Med* (2013) 54(4):600–8. doi: 10.2967/jnumed.112.112672

239. Kim SJ, Zheng MQ, Nabulsi N, Labaree D, Ropchan J, Najafzadeh S, et al. Determination of the *in vivo* selectivity of a new κ-opioid receptor antagonist PET tracer 11C-LY2795050 in the rhesus monkey. *J Nucl Med* (2013) 54(9):1668–74. doi: 10.2967/jnumed.112.118877

240. Li S, Zheng MQ, Naganawa M, Kim S, Gao H, Kapinos M, et al. Development and *in vivo* evaluation of a novel kappa opioid receptor agonist as PET radiotracer with superior imaging characteristics. *J Nucl Med* (2019) 60(7):1023–30. doi: 10.2967/jnumed.118.220517

241. Naganawa M, Jacobsen LK, Zheng MQ, Lin SF, Banerjee A, Byon W, et al. Evaluation of the agonist PET radioligand [$^{11}$C]GR103545 to image kappa opioid receptor in humans: kinetic model selection, test-retest reproducibility and receptor occupancy by the antagonist PF-04455242. *Neuroimage* (2014a) 99:69–79. doi: 10.1016/j.neuroimage.2014.05.033

242. Naganawa M, Zheng MQ, Nabulsi N, Tomasi G, Henry S, Lin SF, et al. Kinetic modeling of (11)C-LY2795050, a novel antagonist radiotracer for PET imaging of the kappa opioid receptor in humans. *J Cereb Blood Flow Metab* (2014b) 34(11):1818–25. doi: 10.1038/jcbfm.2014.150

243. Naganawa M, Zheng MQ, Henry S, Nabulsi N, Lin SF, Ropchan J, et al. Test-retest reproducibility of binding parameters in humans with 11C-LY2795050, an antagonist PET radiotracer for the κ opioid receptor. *J Nucl Med* (2015) 56(2):243–8. doi: 10.2967/jnumed.114.147975

244. Matuskey D, Dias M, Naganawa M, Pittman B, Henry S, Li S, et al. Social status and demographic effects of the kappa opioid receptor: a PET imaging study with a novel agonist radiotracer in healthy volunteers. *Neuropsychopharmacology* (2019) 44:1714–19. doi: 10.1038/s41386-019-0379-7

245. Vijay A, Cavallo D, Goldberg A, de Laat B, Nabulsi N, Huang Y, et al. PET imaging reveals lower kappa opioid receptor availability in alcoholics but no effect of age. *Neuropsychopharmacology* (2018) 43(13):2539–47. doi: 10.1038/s41386-018-0199-1

246. Vijay A, Wang S, Worhunsky P, Zheng MQ, Nabulsi N, Ropchan J, et al. PET imaging reveals sex differences in kappa opioid receptor availability in humans, *in vivo. Am J Nucl Med Mol Imaging* (2016) 6:4,205–14.

247. Clark AJ. The mode of action of drugs on cells. *Nature* (1933) 132:695. doi: 10.1038/132695d0

248. Pettinati HM, Kampman KM, Lynch KG, Suh JJ, Dackis CA, Oslin DW, et al. Gender differences with high-dose naltrexone in patients with co-occurring cocaine and alcohol dependence. *J Subst Abuse Treat* (2007) 34(4):378–90. doi: 10.1016/j.jsat.2007.05.011

249. O'Malley SS, Krishnan-Sarin S, Farren C, O'Connor PG. Naltrexone-induced nausea in patients treated for alcohol dependence: clinical predictors and evidence for opioid-mediated effects. *J Clin Psychopharmacol* (2000) 20:69–76. doi: 10.1097/00004714-200002000-00012

250. Baros A, Latham P, Anton R. Naltrexone and cognitive behavioral therapy for the treatment of alcohol dependence: do sex differences exist? *Alcohol Clin Exp Res* (2008) 32:771–6. doi: 10.1111/j.1530-0277.2008.00633.x

251. Greenfield SF, Pettinati HM, O'Malley S, Randall PK, Randall CL. Gender differences in alcohol treatment: an analysis of outcome from the COMBINE study. *Alcohol Clin Exp Res* (2010) 34(10):1803–12. doi: 10.1111/j.1530-0277.2010.01267.x

252. Saxon AJ. The unmet challenges of co-occurring alcohol and opioid use. *Alcohol Clin Exp Res* (2018) 42:1406–7. doi: 10.1111/acer.13797

253. Hughes A, Williams MR, Lipari RN, Bose J, Copello EAP, Kroutil LA. Prescription drug use and misuse in the United States: Results from the 2015 National Survey on Drug Use and Health. *NSDUH Data Rev* (2016). Retrieved from http://www.samhsa.gov/data/.

254. Kerridge B. Nonmedical prescription opioid use and DSM-5 nonmedical prescription opioid use disorder in the United States. *Drug Alcohol Depen* (2016) 156:47–56. doi: 10.1016/j.drugalcdep.2015.08.026

255. Pradhan AA, Befort K, Nozaki C, Gavériaux-Ruff C, Kieffer BL. The delta opioid receptor: an evolving target for the treatment of brain disorders. *Trends Pharmacol Sci* (2011) 32(10):581–90. doi: 10.1016/j.tips.2011.06.008

256. Saitoh A, Kimura Y, Suzuki T, Kawai K, Nagase H, Kamei J. Potential anxiolytic and antidepressant-like activities of SNC80, a selective delta-opioid agonist, in behavioral models in rodents. *J Pharmacol Sci* (2004) 95:374–80. doi: 10.1254/jphs.FPJ04014X

257. Jutkiewicz EM, Rice KC, Traynor JR, Woods JH. Separation of the convulsions and antidepressant-like effects produced by the delta-opioid agonist SNC80 in rats. *Psychopharmacology (Berl)* (2005) 182:588–96. doi: 10.1007/s00213-005-0138-9

258. Simonin F, Befort K, Gavériaux-Ruff C, Matthes H, Nappey V, Lannes B, et al. The human delta-opioid receptor: genomic organization, cDNA cloning, functional expression, and distribution in human brain. *Mol Pharmacol* (1994) 46:6,1015–21.

259. Peckys D, Landwehrmeyer GB. Expression of mu, kappa, and delta opioid receptor messenger RNA in the human CNS: a 33P *in situ* hybridization study. *Neuroscience* (1999) 88(4):1093–135. doi: 10.1016/S0306-4522(98)00251-6

260. Peng J, Sarkar S, Chang SL. Opioid receptor expression in human brain and peripheral tissues using absolute quantitative real-time RT-PCR. *Drug Alcohol Depend* (2012) 124(3):223–8. doi: 10.1016/j.drugalcdep.2012.01.013

261. Rezaï X, Faget L, Bednarek E, Schwab Y, Kieffer BL, Massotte D. Mouse δ opioid receptors are located on presynaptic afferents to hippocampal pyramidal cells. *Cell Mol Neurobiol* (2012) 32:509–16. doi: 10.1007/s10571-011-9791-1

262. Hirose N, Murakawa K, Takada K, Oi Y, Suzuki T, Nagase H, et al. Interactions among mu- and delta-opioid receptors, especially putative delta1- and delta2-opioid receptors, promote dopamine release in the nucleus accumbens. *Neuroscience* (2005) 135(1):213–25. doi: 10.1016/j.neuroscience.2005.03.065

263. Onali P, Olianas MC. G protein activation and cyclic AMP modulation by naloxone benzoylhydrazone in distinct layers of rat olfactory bulb. *Br J Pharmacol* (2004) 143:638–48. doi: 10.1038/sj.bjp.0705951

264. Olianas MC, Dedoni S, Olianas A, Onali P. δ-Opioid receptors stimulate the metabolic sensor AMP-activated protein kinase through coincident signaling with G(q/11)-coupled receptors. *Mol Pharmacol* (2012) 81:154–65. doi: 10.1124/mol.111.075267

265. Yao L, Fan P, Jiang Z, Mailliard WS, Gordon AS, Diamond I. Addicting drugs utilize a synergistic molecular mechanism in common requiring adenosine and Gi-beta gamma dimers. *Proc Natl Acad Sci U S A* (2003) 100:14379–84. doi: 10.1073/pnas.2336093100

266. Chefer VI, Shippenberg TS. Augmentation of morphine-induced sensitization but reduction in morphine tolerance and reward in delta-opioid receptor knockout mice. *Neuropsychopharmacology* (2009) 34(4):887–98. doi: 10.1038/npp.2008.128

267. Shippenberg TS, Chefer VI, Thompson AC. Delta-opioid receptor antagonists prevent sensitization to the conditioned rewarding effects of morphine. *Biol Psychiatry* (2009) 65:2,169–74. doi: 10.1016/j.biopsych.2008.09.009

268. Suzuki T, Tsuji M, Mori T, Misawa M, Endoh T, Nagase H. Effect of the highly selective and nonpeptide delta opioid receptor agonist TAN-67 on the morphine-induced place preference in mice. *J Pharmacol Exp Ther* (1996) 279:1,177–85.

269. Lutz PE, Ayranci G, Chu-Sin-Chung P, Matifas A, Koebel P, Filliol D, et al. Distinct mu, delta, and kappa opioid receptor mechanisms underlie low sociability and depressive-like behaviors during heroin abstinence. *Neuropsychopharmacology* (2014) 39(11):2694–705. doi: 10.1038/npp.2014.126

270. Leskela TT, Markkanen PM, Alahuhta IA, Tuusa JT, Petaja-Repo UE. Phe27Cys polymorphism alters the maturation and subcellular localization of the human delta opioid receptor. *Traffic* (2009) 10(1):116–29. doi: 10.1111/j.1600-0854.2008.00846.x

271. Zhang H, Gelernter J, Gruen JR, Kranzler HR, Herman AI, Simen AA. Functional impact of a single-nucleotide polymorphism in the OPRD1 promoter region. *J Hum Genet* (2010) 55:278. doi: 10.1038/jhg.2010.22\
272. Huang MW, Chiang TA, Lo PY, Huang CS. Relationship among methadone dose, polymorphisms of dopamine D2 receptor and tri-dimensional personality questionnaire in heroin-addicted patients. *Behav Brain Funct* (2016) 12(1):24. doi: 10.1186/s12993-016-0109-9
273. Rashid F, Zafar MM, Ahmed I, Jabeen S, Ahmad MS, Minhas NM, et al. Association of OPRD1 rs569356 SNP with stress response in opioid addicts. Presented at 20th European Congress of Endocrinology, Barcelona, Spain. Endocrine Abstracts (2018). 56 P669. doi: 10.1530/endoabs.56.P669
274. Madar I, Lever JR, Kinter CM, Scheffel U, Ravert HT, Musachio JL, et al. Imaging of δ opioid receptors in human brain by N1′- ([11C] methyl)naltrindole and PET. *Synapse* (1996) 24:19–28. doi: 10.1002/(SICI)1098-2396(199609)24:1<19::AID-SYN3>3.0.CO;2-J
275. Weerts EM, Wand GS, Kuwabara H, Munro CA, Dannals RF, Hilton J, et al. Positron emission tomography imaging of mu- and delta-opioid receptor binding in alcohol-dependent and healthy control subjects. *Alcohol Clin Exp Res* (2011) 35:2162–73. doi: 10.1111/j.1530-0277.2011.01565.x
276. Weerts EM, Kim YK, Wand GS, Dannals RF, Lee JS, Frost JJ, et al. Differences in δ- and μ-opioid receptor blockade measured by positron emission tomography in naltrexone-treated recently abstinent alcohol-dependent subjects. *Neuropsychopharmacology* (2007) 33:653. doi: 10.1038/sj.npp.1301440
277. Wand GS, Weerts EM, Kuwabara H, Wong DF, Xu X, McCaul ME. The relationship between naloxone-induced cortisol and delta opioid receptor availability in mesolimbic structures is disrupted in alcohol-dependent subjects. *Addict Biol* (2013) 18:181–92. doi: 10.1111/j.1369-1600.2011.00430.x
278. Nieto MM, Guen SLE, Kieffer BL, Roques BP, Noble F. Physiological control of emotion-related behaviors by endogenous enkephalins involves essentially the delta opioid receptors. *Neuroscience* (2005) 135:305–13. doi: 10.1016/j.neuroscience.2005.06.025
279. Mollereau C, Parmentier M, Mailleux P, Butour JL, Moisand C, Chalon P, et al. ORL1, a novel member of the opioid receptor family. Cloning, functional expression and localization. *FEBS Lett* (1994) 341(1):33–8. doi: 10.1016/0014-5793(94)80235-1
280. Meunier JC, Mollereau C, Toll L, Suandeau C, Moisand C, Alvinerie P, et al. Isolation and structure of the endogenous agonist of opioid receptor-like ORL1 receptor. *Nature* (1995) 377:532–5. doi: 10.1038/377532a0
281. Reinscheid RK, Nothacker HP, Bourson A, Ardati A, Henningsen RA, Bunzow JR, et al. Orphanin FQ: a neuropeptide that activates an opioidlike G protein-coupled receptor. *Science* (1995) 270(5237):792–4. doi: 10.1126/science.270.5237.792
282. Mollereau C, Mouledous L. Tissue distribution of the opioid receptor-like (ORL1) receptor. *Peptides* (2000) 21:907–17. doi: 10.1016/S0196-9781(00)00227-8
283. Mika J, Obara I, Przewlocka B. The role of nociceptin and dynorphin in chronic pain: implications of neuro-glial interaction. *Neuropeptides* (2011) 45(4):247–61. doi: 10.1016/j.npep.2011.03.002
284. Chiou LC, Liao YY, Fan PC, Kuo PH, Wang CH, Riemer C, et al. Nociceptin/orphanin FQ peptide receptors: pharmacology and clinical implications. *Curr Drug Targets* (2007) 8(1):117–35. doi: 10.2174/138945007779315605
285. Jenck F, Wichmann J, Dautzenberg, FM, Moreau JL, Ouagazzal AM, Martin JR, et al. A synthetic agonist at the orphanin FQ/nociceptin receptor ORL1: anxiolytic profile in the rat. *Proc Natl Acad Sci U S A* (2000) 97(9):4938–43. doi: 10.1073/pnas.090514397
286. Gavioli EC, Vaughan CW, Marzola G, Guerrini R, Mitchell VA, Zucchini S, et al. Antidepressant-like effects of the nociceptin/orphanin FQ receptor antagonist UFP-101: new evidence from rats and mice. Naunyn Schmiedebergs. *Arch Pharmacol* (2004) 369:547–53. doi: 10.1007/s00210-004-0939-0
287. Martin-Fardon R, Zorrilla EP, Ciccocioppo R, Weiss F. Role of innate and drug-induced dysregulation of brain stress and arousal systems in addiction: focus on corticotropin-releasing factor, nociceptin/orphanin FQ, and orexin/hypocretin. *Brain Res* (2010) 1314:145–61. doi: 10.1016/j.brainres.2009.12.027
288. Nabeshima T, Noda Y, Mamiya T. The role of nociceptin in cognition. *Brain Res* (1999) 848(1–2):167–73. doi: 10.1016/S0006-8993(99)01906-X
289. Sakoori K, Murphy NP. Endogenous nociceptin (orphanin FQ) suppresses basal hedonic state and acute reward responses to methamphetamine and ethanol, but facilitates chronic responses. *Neuropsychopharmacology* (2008) 33:877–91. doi: 10.1038/sj.npp.1301459
290. Lohith TG, Zoghbi SS, Morse CL, Araneta MF, Barth VN, Goebl NA, et al. Brain and whole-body imaging of nociceptin/orphanin FQ peptide receptor in humans using the PET ligand 11C-NOP-1A. *J Nucl Med* (2012) 53(3):385–92. doi: 10.2967/jnumed.111.097162
291. Devine DP, Watson SJ, Akil H. Nociceptin/orphanin FQ regulates neuroendocrine function of the limbic–hypothalamic–pituitary–adrenal axis. *Neuroscience* (2001) 102(3):541–53. doi: 10.1016/S0306-4522(00)00517-0
292. Ciccocioppo R, de Guglielmo G, Hansson AC, Ubaldi M, Kallupi M, Cruz MT, et al. Restraint stress alters nociceptin/orphanin FQ and CRF systems in the rat central amygdala: significance for anxiety-like behaviors. *J Neurosci* (2014) 34(2):363–72. doi: 10.1523/JNEUROSCI.2400-13.2014
293. Cruz MT, Herman MA, Kallupi M, Roberto M. Nociceptin/orphanin FQ blockade of corticotropin-releasing factor-induced gamma-aminobutyric acid release in central amygdala is enhanced after chronic ethanol exposure. *Biol Psychiatry* (2012) 71(8):666–76. doi: 10.1016/j.biopsych.2011.10.032
294. Ciccocioppo R, Fedeli A, Economidou D, Policani F, Weiss F, Massi M. The bed nucleus is a neuroanatomical substrate for the anorectic effect of corticotropin-releasing factor and for its reversal by nociceptin/orphanin FQ. *J Neurosci* (2003) 23(28):9445–51. doi: 10.1523/JNEUROSCI.23-28-09445.2003
295. Rodi D, Zucchini S, Simonato M, Cifani C, Massi M, Polidori C. Functional antagonism between nociceptin/orphanin FQ (N/OFQ) and corticotropin-releasing factor (CRF) in the rat brain: evidence for involvement of the bed nucleus of the stria terminalis. *Psychopharmacology (Berl)* (2008) 196(4):523–31. doi: 10.1007/s00213-007-0985-7
296. Vorspan F, Mehtelli W, Dupuy G, Bloch V, Lépine JP. Anxiety and substance use disorders: co-occurrence and clinical issues. *Curr Psychiatry Rep* (2015) 17(2):4. doi: 10.1007/s11920-014-0544-y
297. Murphy NP, Ly HT, Maidment NT. Intracerebroventricular orphanin FQ/nociceptin suppresses dopamine release in the nucleus accumbens of anaesthetized rats. *Neuroscience* (1996) 75:1–4. doi: 10.1016/0306-4522(96)00322-3
298. Di Giannuario A, Pieretti S, Catalani A, Loizzo A. Orphanin FQ reduces morphine-induced dopamine release in the nucleus accumbens: a microdialysis study in rats. *Neurosci Lett* (1999) 272(3):183–6. doi: 10.1016/S0304-3940(99)00579-0
299. Ciccocioppo R, Panocka I, Polidori C, Regoli D, Massi M. Effect of nociceptin on alcohol intake in alcohol-preferring rats. *Psychopharmacology (Berl)* (1999) 141:220–4. doi: 10.1007/s002130050828
300. Kuzmin A, Sandin J, Terenius L, Ogren SO. Acquisition, expression, and reinstatement of ethanol-induced conditioned place preference in mice: effects of opioid receptor-like 1 receptor agonists and naloxone. *J Pharmacol Exp Ther* (2003) 304:310–8. doi: 10.1124/jpet.102.041350
301. Kotlinska J, Rafalski P, Biala G, Dylag T, Rolka K, Silberring J. Nociceptin inhibits acquisition of amphetamine-induced place preference and sensitization to stereotypy in rats. *Eur J Pharmacol* (2003) 474:233–9. doi: 10.1016/S0014-2999(03)02081-8
302. Kotlinska J, Wichmann J, Legowska A, Rolka K, Silberring J. Orphanin FQ/nociceptin but not Ro 65-6570 inhibits the expression of cocaine-induced conditioned place preference. *Behav Pharmacol* (2002) 13:229–35. doi: 10.1097/00008877-200205000-00006
303. Sakoori K, Murphy NP. Central administration of nociceptin/orphanin FQ blocks the acquisition of conditioned place preference to morphine and cocaine, but not conditioned place aversion to naloxone in mice. *Psychopharmacology (Berl)* (2004) 172:129–36. doi: 10.1007/s00213-003-1643-3
304. Ciccocioppo R, Angeletti S, Sanna PP, Weiss F, Massi M. Effect of nociceptin/orphanin FQ on the rewarding properties of morphine. *Eur J Pharmacol* (2000) 404:153–9. doi: 10.1016/S0014-2999(00)00590-2
305. Walker JR, Spina M, Terenius L, Koob GF. Nociceptin fails to affect heroin self-administration in the rat. *Neuroreport* (1998) 9:2243–7. doi: 10.1097/00001756-199807130-00017
306. Rorick-Kehn LM, Ciccocioppo R, Wong CJ, Witkin JM, Martinez-Grau MA, Stopponi S, et al. A novel, orally bioavailable nociceptin receptor antagonist, LY2940094, reduces ethanol self-administration and ethanol seeking in animal models. *Alcohol Clin Exp Res* (2016) 40(5):945–54. doi: 10.1111/acer.13052

307. Post A, Smart TS, Jackson K, Mann J, Mohs R, Rorick-Kehn L, et al. Proof-of-concept study to assess the nociceptin receptor antagonist LY2940094 as a new treatment for alcohol dependence. *Alcohol Clin Exp Res* (2016) 40(9):1935–44. doi: 10.1111/acer.13147
308. Kuzmin A, Bazov I, Sheedy D, Garrick T, Harper C, Bakalkin G. Expression of pronociceptin and its receptor is downregulated in the brain of human alcoholics. *Brain Res* (2009) 1305(Suppl):S80–5. doi: 10.1016/j.brainres.2009.05.067
309. Lutz PE, Zhou Y, Labbe A, Mechawar N, Turecki G. Decreased expression of nociceptin/orphanin FQ in the dorsal anterior cingulate cortex of suicides. *Eur Neuropsychopharmacol* (2015) 25:11,2008–14. doi: 10.1016/j.euroneuro.2015.08.015
310. Pike VW, Rash KS, Chen Z, Pedregal C, Statnick MA, Kimura Y, et al. Synthesis and evaluation of radioligands for imaging brain nociceptin/orphanin FQ peptide (NOP) receptors with positron emission tomography. *J Med Chem* (2011) 54(8):2687–700. doi: 10.1021/jm101487v
311. Lohith TG, Zoghbi SS, Morse CL, Araneta MD, Barth VN, Goebl NA, et al. Retest imaging of [11C]NOP-1A binding to nociceptin/orphanin FQ peptide (NOP) receptors in the brain of healthy humans. *Neuroimage* (2014) 87:89–95. doi: 10.1016/j.neuroimage.2013.10.068
312. Hostetler ED, Sanabria-Bohórquez S, Eng W, Joshi AD, Patel S, Gibson RE, et al. Evaluation of [$^{18}$F]MK-0911, a positron emission tomography (PET) tracer for opioid receptor-like 1 (ORL1), in rhesus monkey and human. *Neuroimage* (2013) 68:1–10. doi: 10.1016/j.neuroimage.2012.11.053
313. Narendran R, Ciccocioppo R, Lopresti B, Paris J, Himes ML, Mason NS. Nociceptin receptors in alcohol use disorders: a positron emission tomography study using [11C]NOP-1A. *Biol Psychiatry* (2018) 84(10):708–14. doi: 10.1016/j.biopsych.2017.05.019
314. Lindholm S, Ploj K, Franck J, Nylander I. Nociceptin/orphanin FQ tissue concentration in the rat brain. Effects of repeated ethanol administration at various post-treatment intervals. *Prog Neuropsychopharmacol Biol Psychiatry* (2002) 26(2):303–6. doi: 10.1016/S0278-5846(01)00270-6
315. Narendran R, Tollefson S, Himes ML, Paris J, Lopresti B, Ciccocioppo R, et al. Nociceptin receptors upregulated in cocaine use disorder: a positron emission tomography imaging study using [11C]NOP-1A. *Am J Psychiatry* (2019) 176(6):468–76. doi: 10.1176/appi.ajp.2019.18081007
316. Gerfen CR, Engber TM, Mahan LC, Susel Z, Chase TN, Monsma FJ Jr, et al. D1 and D2 dopamine receptor-regulated gene expression of striatonigral and striatopallidal neurons. *Science* (1990) 250(4986):1429–32. doi: 10.1126/science.2147780
317. Trifilieff P, Feng B, Urizar E, Winiger V, Ward RD, Taylor KM, et al. Increasing dopamine D2 receptor expression in the adult nucleus accumbens enhances motivation. *Mol Psychiatry* (2013) 18(9):1025–33. doi: 10.1038/mp.2013.57
318. Zijlstra F, Booij J, van den Brink W, Franken IHA. Striatal dopamine D2 receptor binding and dopamine release during cue-elicited craving in recently abstinent opiate-dependent males. *Eur Neuropsychopharmacol* (2008) 18(4):262–70. doi: 10.1016/j.euroneuro.2007.11.002
319. Usiello A, Baik JH, Rougé-Pont F, Picetti R, Dierich A, LeMeur M, et al. Distinct functions of the two isoforms of dopamine D2 receptors. *Nature* (2000) 408:6809,199–203. doi: 10.1038/35041572
320. Volkow ND, Morales M. The brain on drugs: from reward to addiction. *Cell* (2015) 162(4):712–25. doi: 10.1016/j.cell.2015.07.046
321. Neville MJ, Johnstone EC, Walton RT. Identification and characterization of ANKK1: a novel kinase gene closely linked to DRD2 on chromosome band 11q23.1. *Hum Mutat* (2004) 23(6):540–5. doi: 10.1002/humu.20039
322. Meylan E, Tschopp J. The RIP kinases: crucial integrators of cellular stress. *Trends Biochem Sci* (2005) 30(3):151–9. doi: 10.1016/j.tibs.2005.01.003
323. Bontempi S, Fiorentini C, Busi C, Guerra N, Spano P, Missale C. Identification and characterization of two nuclear factor-kappaB sites in the regulatory region of the dopamine D2 receptor. *Endocrinology* (2007) 148(5):2563–70. doi: 10.1210/en.2006-1618
324. Norman AB, Tabet MR, Norman MK, Fey BK, Tsibulsky VL, Millard RW. The affinity of D2-like dopamine receptor antagonists determines the time to maximal effect on cocaine self-administration. *J Pharmacol Exp Ther* (2011) 338(2):724–8. doi: 10.1124/jpet.111.183244
325. Caine SB, Negus SS, Mello NK, Patel S, Bristow L, Kulagowski J, et al. Role of dopamine D2-like receptors in cocaine self-administration: studies with D2 receptor mutant mice and novel D2 receptor antagonists. *J Neurosci* (2002) 22(7):2977–88. doi: 10.1523/JNEUROSCI.22-07-02977.2002
326. Maldonado R, Saiardi A, Valverde O, Samad TA, Roques BP, Borrelli E. Absence of opiate rewarding effects in mice lacking dopamine D2 receptors. *Nature* (1997) 388:6642,586–9. doi: 10.1038/41567
327. Rominger A, Cumming P, Xiong G, Koller G, Boning G, Wulff M, et al. [18F]fallypride PET measurement of striatal and extrastriatal dopamine D 2/3 receptor availability in recently abstinent alcoholics. *Addict Biol* (2012) 17(2):490–503. doi: 10.1111/j.1369-1600.2011.00355.x
328. Volkow ND, Wang GJ, Fowler JS, Thanos PP, Logan J, Gatley SJ, et al. Brain DA D2 receptors predict reinforcing effects of stimulants in humans: replication study. *Synapse* (2002) 46:2,79–82. doi: 10.1002/syn.10137
329. Volkow ND, Wang GJ, Fowler JS, Logan J, Gatley SJ, Gifford A, et al. Prediction of reinforcing responses to psychostimulants in humans by brain dopamine D2 receptor levels. *Am J Psychiatry* (1999) 156(9):1440–3. doi: 10.1176/ajp.156.9.1440
330. Blum K, Noble EP, Sheridan PJ, Montgomery A, Ritchie T, Jagadeeswaran P, et al. Allelic association of human dopamine D2 receptor gene in alcoholism. *JAMA* (1990) 263(15):2055–60. doi: 10.1001/jama.263.15.2055
331. Noble EP, Blum K, Khalsa ME, Ritchie T, Montgomery A, Wood RC, et al. Allelic association of the D2 dopamine receptor gene with cocaine dependence. *Drug Alcohol Depend* (1993) 33(3):271–85. Erratum in: Drug Alcohol Depend. 34:1,83-4. doi: 10.1016/0376-8716(93)90113-5
332. Comings DE, Rosenthal RJ, Lesieur HR, Rugle LJ, Muhleman D, Chiu C, et al. A study of the dopamine D2 receptor gene in pathological gambling. *Pharmacogenetics* (1996) 6(3):223–34. doi: 10.1097/00008571-199606000-00004
333. Blum K, Braverman ER, Wood RC, Gill J, Li C, Chen TJ, et al. Increased prevalence of the Taq I A1 allele of the dopamine receptor gene (DRD2) in obesity with comorbid substance use disorder: a preliminary report. *Pharmacogenetics* (1996a) 6(4):297–305. doi: 10.1097/00008571-199608000-00003
334. Jönsson EG, Nöthen MM, Grünhage F, Farde L, Nakashima Y, Propping P, et al. Polymorphisms in the dopamine D2 receptor gene and their relationships to striatal dopamine receptor density of healthy volunteers. *Mol Psychiatry* (1999) 4(3):290–6. doi: 10.1038/sj.mp.4000532
335. Eisenstein SA, Bogdan R, Love-Gregory L, Corral-Frías NS, Koller JM, Black KJ, et al. Prediction of striatal D2 receptor binding by DRD2/ANKK1 TaqIA allele status. *Synapse* (2016) 70(10):418–31. doi: 10.1002/syn.21916
336. Wiers CE, Towb PC, Hodgkinson CA, Shen PH, Freeman C, Miller G, et al. Association of genetic ancestry with striatal dopamine D2/D3 receptor availability. *Mol Psychiatry* (2018) 23:8,1711–1716. doi: 10.1038/mp.2017.208
337. Vereczkei A, Demetrovics Z, Szekely A, Sarkozy P, Antal P, Szilagyi A, et al. Multivariate analysis of dopaminergic gene variants as risk factors of heroin dependence. *PLoS One* (2013) 8(6):e66592. doi: 10.1371/journal.pone.0066592
338. Ritchie T, Noble EP. Association of seven polymorphisms of the D2 dopamine receptor gene with brain receptor-binding characteristics. *Neurochem Res* (2003) 28(1):73–82. doi: 10.1023/A:1021648128758
339. Arinami T, Gao M, Hamaguchi H, Toru M. A functional polymorphism in the promoter region of the dopamine D2 receptor gene is associated with schizophrenia. *Human Mol Genet* (1997) 6(4):577–82. doi: 10.1093/hmg/6.4.577
340. Hirvonen MM, Lumme V, Hirvonen J, Pesonen U, Någren K, Vahlberg T, et al. C957T polymorphism of the human dopamine D2 receptor gene predicts extrastriatal dopamine receptor availability *in vivo*. *Prog Neuropsychopharmacol Biol Psychiatry* (2009) 33(4):630–6. doi: 10.1016/j.pnpbp.2009.02.021
341. Clarke TK, Weiss AR, Ferarro TN, Kampman KM, Dackis CA, Pettinati HM, et al. The dopamine receptor D2 (DRD2) SNP rs1076560 is associated with opioid addiction. *Ann Hum Genet* (2014b) 78(1):33–9. doi: 10.1111/ahg.12046
342. Moyer RA, Wang D, Papp AC, Smith RM, Duque L, Mash DC, et al. Intronic polymorphisms affecting alternative splicing of human dopamine D2 receptor are associated with cocaine abuse. *Neuropsychopharmacology* (2011) 36(4):753–62. doi: 10.1038/npp.2010.208
343. Smith JW, Fetsko LA, Xu R, Wang Y. Dopamine D2L receptor knockout mice display deficits in positive and negative reinforcing properties of morphine and in avoidance learning. *Neuroscience* (2002) 4:755–65:113. doi: 10.1016/S0306-4522(02)00257-9

344. Bertolino A, Taurisano P, Pisciotta NM, Blasi G, Fazio L, Romano R, et al. Genetically determined measures of striatal D2 signaling predict prefrontal activity during working memory performance. *PLoS ONE* (2010) 5:2. doi: 10.1371/journal.pone.0009348
345. Taurisano P, Romano R, Mancini M, Giorgio A, DiAntonucci LA, Fazio L, et al. Prefronto-striatal physiology is associated with schizotypy and is modulated by a functional variant of DRD2. *Front Behav Neurosci* (2014) 8:235. doi: 10.3389/fnbeh.2014.00235
346. Zhu F, Yan CX, Wen YC, Wang J, Bi J, Zhao YL, et al. Dopamine D1 receptor gene variation modulates opioid dependence risk by affecting transition to addiction. *PLoS One* (2013) 8(8):e70805. doi: 10.1371/journal.pone.0070805
347. Jacobs MM, Ökvist A, Horvath M, Keller E, Bannon MJ, Morgello S, et al. Dopamine receptor D1 and postsynaptic density gene variants associate with opiate abuse and striatal expression levels. *Mol Psychiatry* (2013) 18(11):1205–10. doi: 10.1038/mp.2012.140
348. Levran O, Randesi M, da Rosa JC, Ott J, Rotrosen J, Adelson M, et al. Overlapping dopaminergic pathway genetic susceptibility to heroin and cocaine addictions in African Americans. *Ann Hum Genet* (2015) 79(3):188–98. doi: 10.1111/ahg.12104
349. Levran O, Londono D, O'Hara K, Randesi M, Rotrosen J, Casadonte P, et al. Heroin addiction in African Americans: a hypothesis-driven association study. *Genes Brain Behav* (2009) 5:531–40. doi: 10.1111/j.1601-183X.2009.00501.x
350. Peng S, Du J, Jiang H, Fu Y, Chen H, Sun H, et al. The dopamine receptor D1 gene is associated with the length of interval between first heroin use and onset of dependence in Chinese Han heroin addicts. *J Neural Transm (Vienna)* (2013) 120(11):1591–8. doi: 10.1007/s00702-013-1029-6
351. Wang N, Zhang JB, Zhao J, Cai XT, Zhu YS, Li SB. Association between dopamine D2 receptor gene polymorphisms and the risk of heroin dependence. *Genet Mol Res* (2016) 15:4. doi: 10.4238/gmr15048772
352. Al-Eitan LN, Jaradat SA, Hulse GK, Tay GK. Custom genotyping for substance addiction susceptibility genes in Jordanians of Arab descent. *BMC Res Notes* (2012) 5:497. doi: 10.1186/1756-0500-5-497
353. Tsou CC, Chou HW, Ho PS, Kuo SC, Chen CY, Huang CC, et al. DRD2 and ANKK1 genes associate with late-onset heroin dependence in men. *World J Biol Psychiatry* (2017) 25:1–11. doi: 10.1080/15622975.2017.1372630
354. Zhang J, Yan P, Li Y, Cai X, Yang Z, Miao X, et al. A 35.8 kilobases haplotype spanning ANKK1 and DRD2 is associated with heroin dependence in Han Chinese males. *Brain Res* (2018) 1688:54–64. doi: 10.1016/j.brainres.2018.03.017
355. Xu K, Lichtermann D, Lipsky RH, Franke P, Liu X, Hu Y, et al. Association of specific haplotypes of D2 dopamine receptor gene with vulnerability to heroin dependence in 2 distinct populations. *Arch Gen Psychiatry* (2004) 61(6):597–606. doi: 10.1001/archpsyc.61.6.597
356. Teh LK, Izuddin AF MHFH, Zakaria ZA, Salleh MZ. Tridimensional personalities and polymorphism of dopamine D2 receptor among heroin addicts. *Biol Res Nurs* (2012) 14(2):188–96. doi: 10.1177/1099800411405030
357. Hung CC, Chiou MH, Huang BH, Hsieh YW, Hsieh TJ, Huang CL, et al. Impact of genetic polymorphisms in ABCB1, CYP2B6, OPRM1, ANKK1 and DRD2 genes on methadone therapy in Han Chinese patients. *Pharmacogenomics* (2011) 12(11):1525–33. doi: 10.2217/pgs.11.96
358. Bawor M, Dennis BB, Tan C, Pare G, Varenbut M, Daiter J, et al. Contribution of BDNF and DRD2 genetic polymorphisms to continued opioid use in patients receiving methadone treatment for opioid use disorder: an observational study. *Addict Sci Clin Pract* (2015) 10:19. doi: 10.1186/s13722-015-0040-7
359. Nelson EC, Lynskey MT, Heath AC, Wray N, Agrawal A, Shand FL, et al. ANKK1, TTC12, and NCAM1 polymorphisms and heroin dependence: importance of considering drug exposure. *JAMA Psychiatry* (2013) 70(3):325–33. doi: 10.1001/jamapsychiatry.2013.282
360. Hou QF, Li SB. Potential association of DRD2 and DAT1 genetic variation with heroin dependence. *Neurosci Lett* (2009) 464(2):127–30. doi: 10.1016/j.neulet.2009.08.004
361. Barratt DT, Coller JK, Somogyi AA. Association between the DRD2 A1 allele and response to methadone and buprenorphine maintenance treatments. *Am J Med Genet B Neuropsychiatr Genet* (2006) 141B(4):323–31. doi: 10.1002/ajmg.b.30319
362. Galeeva AR, Gareeva AE, Iur'ev EB, Khusnutdinova EK. VNTR polymorphisms of the serotonin transporter and dopamine transporter genes in male opiate addicts. *Mol Biol (Mosk)* (2002) 36(4):593–8. doi: 10.1023/A:1019883806620
363. Jacobsen LK, Staley JK, Zoghbi SS, Seibyl JP, Kosten TR, Innis RB, et al. Prediction of dopamine transporter binding availability by genotype: a preliminary report. *Am J Psychiatry* (2000) 157(10):1700–3. doi: 10.1176/appi.ajp.157.10.1700
364. Van Dyck CH, Malison RT, Jacobsen LK, Seibyl JP, Staley JK, Laruelle M, et al. Increased dopamine transporter availability associated with the 9-repeat allele of the SLC6A3 gene. *J Nucl Med* (2005) 46:5,745–51.
365. Van de Giessen EM, de Win MML, Tanck MWT, van den Brink W, Baas F, Booij J. Striatal dopamine transporter availability associated with polymorphisms in the dopamine transporter gene SLC6A3. *J Nucl Med* (2008) 50(1):45–52. doi: 10.2967/jnumed.108.053652
366. Martinez D, Gelernter J, Abi-Dargham A, van Dyck CH, Kegeles L, Innis RB, et al. The variable number of tandem repeats polymorphism of the dopamine transporter gene is not associated with significant change in dopamine transporter phenotype in humans. *Neuropsychopharmacology* (2001) 24(5):553–60. doi: 10.1016/S0893-133X(00)00216-5
367. Lynch DR, Mozley PD, Sokol S, Maas NM, Balcer LJ, Siderowf AD. Lack of effect of polymorphisms in dopamine metabolism related genes on imaging of TRODAT-1 in striatum of asymptomatic volunteers and patients with Parkinson's disease. *Mov Disord* (2003) 18(7):804–12. doi: 10.1002/mds.10430
368. Yeh YW, Lu RB, Tao PL, Shih MC, Lin WW, Huang SY. Neither single-marker nor haplotype analyses support an association between the dopamine transporter gene and heroin dependence in Han Chinese. *Genes Brain Behav* (2010) 9:6,638–47. doi: 10.1111/j.1601-183X.2010.00597.x
369. Ornoy A, Finkel-Pekarsky V, Peles E, Adelson M, Schreiber S, Ebstein PR. ADHD risk alleles associated with opiate addiction: study of addicted parents and their children. *Pediatr Res* (2016) 80(2):228–36. doi: 10.1038/pr.2016.78
370. Heinz A, Goldman D, Jones DW, Palmour R, Hommer D, Gorey JG, et al. Genotype influences *in vivo* dopamine transporter availability in human striatum. *Neuropsychopharmacology* (2000) 22:133–9. doi: 10.1016/S0893-133X(99)00099-8
371. Cheon KA, Ryu YH, Kim JW, Cho DY. The homozygosity for 10-repeat allele at dopamine transporter gene and dopamine transporter density in Korean children with attention deficit hyperactivity disorder: relating to treatment response to methylphenidate. *Eur Neuropsychopharmacol* (2005) 15:95–101. doi: 10.1016/j.euroneuro.2004.06.004
372. Lawford BR, Young RM, Noble EP, Sargent J, Rowell J, Shadforth S, et al. The D(2) dopamine receptor A(1) allele and opioid dependence: association with heroin use and response to methadone treatment. *Am J Med Genet* (2000) 96(5):592–8. doi: 10.1002/1096-8628(20001009)96:5<592::AID-AJMG3>3.0.CO;2-Y
373. Hirvonen M, Laakso A, Någren K, Rinne JO, Pohjalainen T, Hietala J. C957T polymorphism of the dopamine D2 receptor (DRD2) gene affects striatal DRD2 availability *in vivo*. *Mol Psychiatry* (2004) 9(12):1060–1. doi: 10.1038/sj.mp.4001561
374. Smith CT, Dang LC, Buckholtz JW, Tetreault AM, Cowan RL, Kessler RM, et al. The impact of common dopamine D2 receptor gene polymorphisms on D2/3 receptor availability: C957T as a key determinant in putamen and ventral striatum. *Transl Psychiatry* (2017) 7:e1091. doi: 10.1038/tp.2017.45
375. Cloninger CR. A systematic method for clinical description and classification of personality variants. A proposal. *Arch Gen Psychiatry* (1987) 44(6):573–88. doi: 10.1001/archpsyc.1987.01800180093014
376. Huang WL, Lin YH, Kuo TB, Chang LR, Chen YZ, Yang CC. Methadone-mediated autonomic functioning of male patients with heroin dependence: the influence of borderline personality pattern. *PLoS One* (2012) 7(5):e37464. doi: 10.1371/journal.pone.0037464
377. American Psychiatric Association. Substance use disorders. In: *Diagnostic and statistical manual of mental disorders.*, 5th ed. American Psychiatric Publishing (2013). doi: 10.1176/appi.books.9780890425596
378. Gerra G, Bertacca S, Zaimovic A, Pirani M, Branchi B, Ferri M. Relationship of personality traits and drug of choice by cocaine addicts and heroin addicts. *Subst Use Misuse* (2008) 43(3-4):317–30. doi: 10.1080/10826080701202726
379. Hall H, Köhler C, Gawell L, Farde L, Sedvall G. Raclopride, a new selective ligand for the dopamine-D2receptors. *Prog Neuropsychopharmacol Biol Psychiatry* (1988) 12(5):559–68. doi: 10.1016/0278-5846(88)90001-2
380. Kung HF, Alavi A, Chang W, Kung MP, Keyes JW Jr, Velchik MG, et al. *In vivo* SPECT imaging of CNS D-2 dopamine receptors: initial studies with iodine-123-IBZM in humans. *J Nucl Med* (1990) 31(5):573–9.

381. Videbk C, Toska K, Scheideler MA, Paulson OB, Knudsen GM. SPECT tracer [123I]IBZM has similar affinity to dopamine D2 and D3 receptors. *Synapse* (2000) 38(3):338–42. doi: 10.1002/1098-2396(20001201)38:3<338::AID-SYN13>3.0.CO;2-N

382. Suehiro M, Dannals RF, Scheffel U, Stathis M, Wilson AA, Ravert HT, et al. *In vivo* labeling of the dopamine D2 receptor with N-11C-methyl-benperidol. *J Nucl Med* (1990) 31:12,2015–21.

383. Moerlein SM, Perlmutter JS, Markham J, Welch MJ. *In vivo* kinetics of [18F](N-methyl)benperidol: a novel PET tracer for assessment of dopaminergic D2-like receptor binding. *J Cereb Blood Flow Metab* (1997) 17(8):833–45. doi: 10.1097/00004647-199708000-00002

384. Halldin C, Farde L, Högberg T, Mohell N, Hall H, Suhara T, et al. Carbon-11-FLB 457: a radioligand for extrastriatal D2 dopamine receptors. *J Nucl Med* (1995) 36(7):1275–81.

385. Hall H, Sedvall G, Magnusson O, Kopp J, Halldin C, Farde L. Distribution of D1- and D2-dopamine receptors, and dopamine and its metabolites in the human brain. *Neuropsychopharmacology* (1994) 11(4):245–56. doi: 10.1038/sj.npp.1380111

386. Kebabian JW, Calne DB. Multiple receptors for dopamine. *Nature* (1979) 277:5692,93–6. doi: 10.1038/277093a0

387. Stoof JC, Kebabian JW. Opposing roles for D-1 and D-2 dopamine receptors in efflux of cyclic AMP from rat neostriatum. *Nature* (1981) 294(5839):366–8. doi: 10.1038/294366a0

388. Palacios JM, Camps M, Cortés R, Probst A. Mapping dopamine receptors in the human brain. *J Neural Transm Suppl* (1988) 27:227–35. doi: 10.1007/978-3-7091-8954-2_20

389. Beninger RJ, Miller R. Dopamine D1-like receptors and reward-related incentive learning. *Neurosci Biobehav Rev* (1998) 22(2):335–45. doi: 10.1016/S0149-7634(97)00019-5

390. Andrzejewski ME, Spencer RC, Kelley AE. Instrumental learning, but not performance, requires dopamine D1-receptor activation in the amygdala. *Neuroscience* (2005) 135(2):335–45. doi: 10.1016/j.neuroscience.2005.06.038

391. Tran AH, Tamura R, Uwano T, Kobayashi T, Katsuki M, Ono T. Dopamine D1 receptors involved in locomotor activity and accumbens neural responses to prediction of reward associated with place. *Proc Natl Acad Sci* (2005) 102(6):2117–22. doi: 10.1073/pnas.0409726102

392. van Gaalen MM, van Koten R, Schoffelmeer AN, Vanderschuren LJ. Critical involvement of dopaminergic neurotransmission in impulsive decision making. *Biol Psychiatry* (2006) 60(1):66–73. doi: 10.1016/j.biopsych.2005.06.005

393. Gurden H, Takita M, Jay TM. Essential role of D1 but not D2 receptors in the NMDA receptor-dependent long-term potentiation at hippocampal-prefrontal cortex synapses *in vivo*. *J Neurosci* (2000) 20(22):106RC–. doi: 10.1523/JNEUROSCI.20-22-j0003.2000

394. Jung E-Y, Shim I. Differential DAergic control of D1 and D2 receptor agonist over locomotor activity and GABA level in the striatum. *Exp Neurobiol* (2011) 20(3):153. doi: 10.5607/en.2011.20.3.153

395. Molloy AG, Waddington JL. Behavioural responses to the selective D1-dopamine receptor agonist R-SK&F 38393 and the selective D2-agonist RU 24213 in young compared with aged rats. *Br J Pharmacol* (1988) 95(2):335–42. doi: 10.1111/j.1476-5381.1988.tb11651.x

396. Eagle DM, Wong JCK, Allan ME, Mar AC, Theobald DE, Robbins TW. Contrasting roles for dopamine D1 and D2 receptor subtypes in the dorsomedial striatum but not the nucleus accumbens core during behavioral inhibition in the stop-signal task in rats. *J Neurosci* (2011) 31(20):7349–56. doi: 10.1523/JNEUROSCI.6182-10.2011

397. Caine SB, Thomsen M, Gabriel KI, Berkowitz JS, Gold LH, Koob GF, et al. Lack of self-administration of cocaine in dopamine D1 receptor knock-out mice. *J Neurosci* (2007) 27:13140–50. doi: 10.1523/JNEUROSCI.2284-07.2007

398. Zweifel LS, Parker JG, Lobb CJ, Rainwater A, Wall VZ, Fadok JP, et al. Disruption of NMDAR-dependent burst firing by dopamine neurons provides selective assessment of phasic dopamine-dependent behavior. *Proc Natl Acad Sci U S A* (2009) 106:7281–8. doi: 10.1073/pnas.0813415106

399. Sadat-Shirazi MS, Zarrindast MR, Daneshparvar H, Ziaie A, Fekri M, Abbasnezhad E, et al. Alteration of dopamine receptors subtypes in the brain of opioid abusers: a postmortem study in Iran. *Neurosci Lett* (2018) 687:169–76. doi: 10.1016/j.neulet.2018.09.043

400. Zarrindast MR, Azami BN, Rostami P, Rezayof A. Repeated administration of dopaminergic agents in the nucleus accumbens and morphine-induced place preference. *Behav Brain Res* (2006) 169(2):248–55. doi: 10.1016/j.bbr.2006.01.011

401. Bossert JM, Poles GC, Wihbey KA, Koya E, Shaham Y. Differential effects of blockade of dopamine D1-family receptors in nucleus accumbens core or shell on reinstatement of heroin seeking induced by contextual and discrete cues. *J Neurosci* (2007) 27(46):12655–63. doi: 10.1523/JNEUROSCI.3926-07.2007

402. Chartoff EH, Mague SD, Barhight MF, Smith AM, Carlezon WA. Behavioral and molecular effects of dopamine D1 receptor stimulation during naloxone-precipitated morphine withdrawal. *J Neurosci* (2006) 26(24):6450–7. doi: 10.1523/JNEUROSCI.0491-06.2006

403. Anderson SM, Bari AA, Pierce RC. Administration of the D1-like dopamine receptor antagonist SCH-23390 into the medial nucleus accumbens shell attenuates cocaine priming-induced reinstatement of drug-seeking behavior in rats. *Psychopharmacology (Berl)* (2003) 168(1-2):132–8. doi: 10.1007/s00213-002-1298-5

404. Bachtell RK, Whisler K, Karanian D, Self DW. Effects of intra-nucleus accumbens shell administration of dopamine agonists and antagonists on cocaine-taking and cocaine-seeking behaviors in the rat. *Psychopharmacology (Berl)* (2005) 183(1):41–53. doi: 10.1007/s00213-005-0133-1

405. Hauser SR, Deehan GA Jr, Dhaher R, Knight CP, Wilden JA, McBride WJ, et al. D1 receptors in the nucleus accumbens-shell, but not the core, are involved in mediating ethanol-seeking behavior of alcohol-preferring (P) rats. *Neuroscience* (2015) 295:243–51. doi: 10.1016/j.neuroscience.2015.03.030

406. Tao YM, Yu C, Wang WS, Hou YY, Xu XJ, Chi ZQ, et al. Heteromers of μ opioid and dopamine D1 receptors modulate opioid-induced locomotor sensitization in a dopamine-independent manner. *Br J Pharmacol* (2017) 174(17):2842–61. doi: 10.1111/bph.13908

407. Juhasz JR, Hasbi A, Rashid AJ, So CH, George SR, O'Dowd BF. Mu-opioid receptor heterooligomer formation with the dopamine D1 receptor as directly visualized in living cells. *Eur J Pharmacol* (2008) 581(3):235–43. doi: 10.1016/j.ejphar.2007.11.060

408. Tsang J, Fullard JF, Giakoumaki SG, Katsel P, Katsel P, Karagiorga VE, et al. The relationship between dopamine receptor D1 and cognitive performance. *NPJ Schizophr* (2015) 1:14002. doi: 10.1038/npjschz.2014.2

409. Thomas U. Modulation of synaptic signalling complexes by Homer proteins. *J Neurochem* (2002) 81(3):407–13. doi: 10.1046/j.1471-4159.2002.00869.x

410. Kalivas PW, Volkow ND. The neural basis of addiction: a pathology of motivation and choice. *Am J Psychiatry* (2005) 162(8):1403–13. doi: 10.1176/appi.ajp.162.8.1403

411. Liu JH, Zhong HJ, Dang J, Peng L, Zhu YS. Single-nucleotide polymorphisms in dopamine receptor D1 are associated with heroin dependence but not impulsive behavior. *Genet Mol Res* (2015) 14:2,4041–50. doi: 10.4238/2015.April.27.19

412. Behrendt S, Wittchen HU, Höfler M, Lieb R, Beesdo K. Transitions from first substance use to substance use disorders in adolescence: is early onset associated with a rapid escalation? *Drug Alcohol Depend* (2009) 99(1-3):68–78. doi: 10.1016/j.drugalcdep.2008.06.014

413. Sartor CE, Lynskey MT, Bucholz KK, Madden PA, Martin NG, Heath AC. Timing of first alcohol use and alcohol dependence: evidence of common genetic influences. *Addiction* (2009) 104(9s):1512–8. doi: 10.1111/j.1360-0443.2009.02648.x

414. Dudman JT, Eaton ME, Rajadhyaksha A, Macías W, Taher M, Barczak A, et al. Dopamine D1 receptors mediate CREB phosphorylation *via* phosphorylation of the NMDA receptor at Ser897-NR1. *J Neurochem* (2003) 87(4):922–34. doi: 10.1046/j.1471-4159.2003.02067.x

415. Lintas A, Chi N, Lauzon NM, Bishop SF, Gholizadeh S, Sun N, et al. Identification of a dopamine receptor-mediated opiate reward memory switch in the basolateral amygdala-nucleus accumbens circuit. *J Neurosci* (2011) 31(31):11172–83. doi: 10.1523/JNEUROSCI.1781-11.2011

416. Andersen PH, Grønvald FC, Hohlweg R, Hansen LB, Guddal E, Braestrup C, et al. NNC-112, NNC-687 and NNC-756, new selective and highly potent dopamine D1 receptor antagonists. *Eur J Pharmacol* (1992) 219(1):45–52. doi: 10.1016/0014-2999(92)90578-R

417. Abi-Dargham A, Martinez D, Mawlawi O, Simpson N, Hwang DR, Slifstein M, et al. Measurement of striatal and extrastriatal dopamine D1 receptor binding potential with [11C]NNC 112 in humans: validation and

reproducibility. *J Cereb Blood Flow Metab* (2000) 20(2):225–43. doi: 10.1097/00004647-200002000-00003

418. Sedvall G, Farde L, Barnett A, Hall H, Halldin C. 11C-SCH 39166, a selective ligand for visualization of dopamine-D1 receptor binding in the monkey brain using PET. *Psychopharmacology (Berl)* (1991) 103(2):150–3. doi: 10.1007/BF02244195
419. Martinez D, Slifstein M, Narendran R, Foltin RW, Broft A, Hwang DR, et al. Dopamine D1 receptors in cocaine dependence measured with PET and the choice to self-administer cocaine. *Neuropsychopharmacology* (2009) 34(7):1774–82. doi: 10.1038/npp.2008.235
420. Yasuno F, Ota M, Ando K, Ando T, Maeda J, Ichimiya T, et al. Role of ventral striatal dopamine D1 receptor in cigarette craving. *Biol Psychiatry* (2007) 61(11):1252–9. doi: 10.1016/j.biopsych.2006.06.028
421. Dagher A, Bleicher C, Aston JA, Gunn RN, Clarke PB, Cumming P. Reduced dopamine D1 receptor binding in the ventral striatum of cigarette smokers. *Synapse* (2001) 42(1):48–53. doi: 10.1002/syn.1098
422. Dubol M, Trichard C, Leroy C, Sandu AL, Rahim M, Granger B, et al. Dopamine transporter and reward anticipation in a dimensional perspective: a multimodal brain imaging study. *Neuropsychopharmacology* (2018) 43(4):820–7. doi: 10.1038/npp.2017.183
423. Mulvihill KG. Presynaptic regulation of dopamine release: role of the DAT and VMAT2 transporters. *Neurochem Int* (2019) 122:94–105. doi: 10.1016/j.neuint.2018.11.004
424. Sotnikova TD, Beaulieu JM, Gainetdinov RR, Caron MG. Molecular biology, pharmacology and functional role of the plasma membrane dopamine transporter. *CNS Neurol Disord Drug Targets* (2006) 5(1):45–56. doi: 10.2174/187152706784111579
425. Schmitz Y, Benoit-Marand M, Gonon F, Sulzer D. Presynaptic regulation of dopaminergic neurotransmission. *J Neurochem* (2003) 87(2):273–89. doi: 10.1046/j.1471-4159.2003.02050.x
426. Sesack SR, Hawrylak VA, Guido MA, Levey AI. Cellular and subcellular localization of the dopamine transporter in rat cortex. *Adv Pharmacol* (1998) 42:171–4. doi: 10.1016/S1054-3589(08)60720-6
427. Sweitzer MM, Donny EC, Hariri AR. Imaging genetics and the neurobiological basis of individual differences in vulnerability to addiction. *Drug Alcohol Depend* (2012) 123(1):S59–71. doi: 10.1016/j.drugalcdep.2012.01.017
428. VanNess SH, Owens MJ, Kilts CD. The variable number of tandem repeats element in DAT1 regulates *in vitro* dopamine transporter density. BMC. *Genetics* (2005) 6:1–11. doi: 10.1186/1471-2156-6-55
429. Fuke S, Suo S, Takahashi N, Koike H, Sasagawa N, Ishiura S. The VNTR polymorphism of the human dopamine transporter (DAT1) gene affects gene expression. *Pharmacogenomics J* (2001) 1(2):152–6. doi: 10.1038/sj.tpj.6500026
430. Bannon MJ, Michelhaugh SK, Wang J, Sacchetti P. The human dopamine transporter gene: gene organization, transcriptional regulation, and potential involvement in neuropsychiatric disorders. Eur. *Neuropsychopharmacol* (2001) 11:449–55. doi: 10.1016/S0924-977X(01)00122-5
431. Nakamura Y, Koyama K, Matsushima M. VNTR (variable number of tandem repeat) sequences as transcriptional, translational, or functional regulators. *J Hum Genet* (1998) 43:149–52. doi: 10.1007/s100380050059
432. Mitchell RJ, Howlett S, Earl L, White NG, McComb J, Schanfield MS, Distribution of the 3′ VNTR polymorphism in the human dopamine transporter gene in world populations. *Hum Biol* (2000) 72:295–304.
433. Guindalini C, Howard M, Haddley K, Laranjeira R, Collier D, Ammar N, et al. A dopamine transporter gene functional variant associated with cocaine abuse in a Brazilian sample. *Proc Natl Acad Sci U S A* (2006) 103(12):4552–7. doi: 10.1073/pnas.0504789103
434. Ueno S, Nakamura M, Mikami M, Kondoh K, Ishiguro H, Arinami T, et al. Identification of a novel polymorphism of the human dopamine transporter (DAT1) gene and the significant association with alcoholism. *Mol Psychiatry* (1999) 4(6):552–7. doi: 10.1038/sj.mp.4000562
435. Du Y, Nie Y, Li Y, Wan YJ. The association between the SLC6A3 VNTR 9-repeat allele and alcoholism-a meta-analysis. *Alcohol Clin Exp Res* (2011) 35(9):1625–34. doi: 10.1111/j.1530-0277.2011.01509.x
436. Gerra G, Somaini L, Leonardi C, Cortese E, Maremmani I, Manfredini M, et al. Association between gene variants and response to buprenorphine maintenance treatment. *Psychiatry Res* (2014) 215(1):202–7. doi: 10.1016/j.psychres.2013.11.001
437. Krupitsky EM, Kibitov AO, Blokhina EA, Verbitskaya EV, Brodyansky VM, Alekseeva NP, et al. Stabilization of remission in patients with opioid dependence with naltrexone implant: a pharmacogenetic approach. *Zh Nevrol Psikhiatr Im S S Korsakova* (2015) 115(4 Pt 2):14–23. doi: 10.17116/jnevro20151154214-23
438. van Gestel S, Forsegren T, Claes S, Del-Favero J, van Duijn GM, Sluijs S, et al. Epistatic effect of genes from the dopamine and serotonin systems on the temperament traits of novelty seeking and harm avoidance. *Mol Psychiatry* (2002) 7:448–50. doi: 10.1038/sj.mp.4001005
439. Bardo MT, Donohew R, Harrington NG. Psychobiology of novelty seeking and drug seeking behavior. *Behav Brain Res* (1996) 77:23–43. doi: 10.1016/0166-4328(95)00203-0
440. Chmielowiec J, Chmielowiec K, Suchanecka A, Trybek G, Mroczek B, Małecka I, et al. Associations between the dopamine D4 receptor and DAT1 dopamine transporter genes polymorphisms and personality traits in addicted patients. *Int J Environ Res Public Health* (2018) 15(10):2076. doi: 10.3390/ijerph15102076
441. Kim SJ, Kim YS, Kim CH, Lee HS. Lack of association between polymorphism of the dopamine receptor D4 and dopamine transporter genes and personality in a Korean population. *Yonsei Med J* (2006) 47:787–92. doi: 10.3349/ymj.2006.47.6.787
442. Staley JK, Krishnan-Sarin S, Zoghbi S, Tamagnan G, Fujita M, Seibyl JP, et al. Sex differences in [123I]β-CIT SPECT measures of dopamine and serotonin transporter availability in healthy smokers and nonsmokers. *Synapse* (2001) 41(4):275–84. doi: 10.1002/syn.1084
443. Cosgrove KP, Tellez-Jacques K, Pittman B, Petrakis I, Baldwin RM, Tamagnan G, et al. Dopamine and serotonin transporter availability in chronic heroin users: A [123I]β-CIT SPECT imaging study. *Psychiatry Res Neuroimag* (2010) 184(3):192–5. doi: 10.1016/j.pscychresns.2010.08.001
444. Knoll AT, Carlezon WA, Jr. Dynorphin, stress, and depression. *Brain Res* (2010) 1314:56–73. doi: 10.1016/j.brainres.2009.09.074
445. Andero R, Brothers SP, Jovanovic T, Chen YT, Salah-Uddin H, Cameron M, et al. Amygdala-dependent fear is regulated by Oprl1 in mice and humans with PTSD. *Sci Transl Med* (2013) 5(188):188ra73. doi: 10.1126/scitranslmed.3005656
446. Uhl G, Blum K, Noble E, Smith S. Substance abuse vulnerability and D2 receptor genes. *Trends Neurosci* (1993) 16(3):83–8. doi: 10.1016/0166-2236(93)90128-9
447. Blum K, Sheridan PJ, Wood RC, Braverman ER, Chen TJ, Cull JG, et al. The D2 dopamine receptor gene as a determinant of reward deficiency syndrome. *J R Soc Med* (1996b) 89(7):396–400. doi: 10.1177/014107689608900711

13

# Improvement of Emotional Empathy and Cluster B Personality Disorder Symptoms Associated with Decreased Cocaine use Severity

*Matthias Vonmoos[1*‡], Christoph Eisenegger[2†‡], Oliver G. Bosch[1,3], Katrin H. Preller[1], Lea M. Hulka[1], Markus Baumgartner[4], Erich Seifritz[3,5] and Boris B. Quednow[1,5*‡]*

*[1] Experimental and Clinical Pharmacopsychology, Department of Psychiatry, Psychotherapy and Psychosomatics, Psychiatric Hospital of the University of Zurich, Zurich, Switzerland, [2] Neuropsychopharmacology and Biopsychology Unit, Department of Basic Psychological Research and Research Methods, Faculty of Psychology, University of Vienna, Vienna, Austria, [3] Department of Psychiatry, Psychotherapy and Psychosomatics, Psychiatric Hospital of the University of Zurich, Zurich, Switzerland, [4] Center of Forensic Hairanalytics, Institute of Forensic Medicine, University of Zurich, Zurich, Switzerland, [5] Neuroscience Center Zurich, University and ETH Zurich, Zurich, Switzerland*

***Correspondence:***
*Boris B. Quednow*
*quednow@bli.uzh.ch*
*Matthias Vonmoos*
*matthias.vonmoos@bli.uzh.ch*

*†Christoph Eisenegger passed away on February 27th, 2017.*
*‡These authors have contributed equally to this work.*

**Aims:** Chronic cocaine users display impaired social cognitive abilities, reduced prosocial behavior, and pronounced cluster B personality disorder (PD) symptoms all contributing to their social dysfunctions in daily life. These social dysfunctions have been proposed as a major factor for maintenance and relapse of stimulant use disorders in general. However, little is known about the reversibility of social cognitive deficits and socially problematic personality facets when stimulant use is reduced or ceased. Therefore, we examined the relation between changing intensity of cocaine use and the development of sociocognitive functioning and cluster B PD symptomatology over the course of 1 year.

**Methods:** Social cognition, social decision-making, and cluster B PD symptoms were assessed in 38 cocaine users (19 with increased and 19 with decreased use) and 48 stimulant-naive healthy controls at baseline and at 1-year follow-up. Cocaine use severity was objectively determined by quantitative 6-month hair analyses. The categorization of the two cocaine user groups was based on a combination of absolute (± 0.5 ng/mg) and relative (± 10%) changes in the cocaine hair concentration between baseline and the 1-year follow-up. Social cognition was assessed using the Multifaceted Empathy Test (MET) and the Movie for the Assessment of Social Cognition (MASC). A combined Distribution/Dictator Game was applied for assessing social decision-making. Cluster B PD symptoms were measured by a Structured Clinical Interview for DSM-IV Axis II Disorders (SCID-II) PD questionnaire according to *Diagnostic and Statistical Manual of Mental Disorders*, 4th edition (DSM-IV).

**Results:** Increased cocaine use was linked to worsened empathy, while decreased cocaine use went along with improved emotional empathy. Moreover, whereas decreased cocaine use was associated with reduced severity of self-reported cluster B PD symptoms, these symptoms remained largely stable in *increasers*. In contrast to a significant reduction of prosocial behavior at baseline in the combined cocaine user group, specifically *decreasers* were not statistically distinguishable from controls at the follow-up.

**Conclusions:** Sociocognitive deficits and cluster B PD symptoms of chronic cocaine users are adaptable over time as they covary with the increase or decrease in cocaine use. Hence, abstinence orientation and training of social cognition and interaction might improve social functioning, and should therefore be important therapeutic elements in cocaine addiction treatment.

**Keywords: cocaine, stimulants, social cognition, empathy, Theory-of-Mind, social decision-making, cognition, personality disorder**

## INTRODUCTION

Neurocognitive deficits such as impaired attention, memory, and executive functions related to chronic cocaine use are well documented (1–3) and a risk factor for poor treatment outcomes (4, 5). While some studies investigated the linkage between these neurocognitive deficits and cocaine abstinence (6), only one study yet investigated the longitudinal relationship between cognitive impairments and changing cocaine use (7). In sum, these studies indicate that basal cognitive deficits in cocaine users seem to be largely drug-induced, remain stable during the first weeks of abstinence but likely improve after some months (8).

While nonsocial cognitive functions have been studied well during the last two decades, the systematic assessment of sociocognitive functioning in cocaine users has only recently emerged. Per definition, the concept of social cognition comprises not only abilities enabling the dynamic interaction with our social environments and include emotional and mental perspective-taking functions such as emotion recognition, emotional empathy (EE), and *Theory-of-Mind*, but also interactive abilities such as social decision-making (SDM), moral behavior, and social network behavior (9, 10). As daily-life social functioning strongly depends on intact social cognition and as the deteriorative impact of sociocognitive impairments on development, progress, and prognosis on other psychiatric disorders such as schizophrenia is well known (11), a close relationship between sociocognitive functioning and the origin and course of stimulant use disorders has been proposed (12–15). Accordingly, we previously demonstrated smaller social networks (16), reduced EE (16), altered SDM (17), stronger detachment from social norms (14), and impaired emotion recognition from voices (18) in recreational and dependent cocaine user groups. Moreover, dependent cocaine users made more errors than controls in a video-based *Theory-of-Mind* task, with recreational cocaine users performing intermediate between the two groups (16). Finally, cocaine users show also blunted neuronal responses to implicit and explicit forms of social reward (19, 20). Notably, all these studies were implemented with a cross-sectional design, but no study has investigated the longitudinal development of sociocognitive functioning so far. Thus, it is unclear if sociocognitive impairments are predisposed or drug-induced and if they are reversible upon prolonged abstinence or reduction of drug use.

As social cognition is the sum of those processes that allow individuals to interact in interpersonal contexts (21), disturbed sociocognitive functioning leads to aberrant social behavior and, in excessive forms, to deviant personality characteristics and impaired interpersonal functioning (22, 23). Notably, cocaine-addicted individuals show an increased risk for concurrent cluster B personality disorders (PDs), mainly of the antisocial and borderline types (24, 25). A cluster B PD comorbidity is largely influential for cocaine addiction severity and treatment outcomes including pronounced executive function deficits (26), more intense cocaine intake, lower rates of treatment applications, and decreased probability of cocaine addiction remission (27, 28). Additionally, it was demonstrated that impulsivity and gambling decision-making, which are both closely related to cluster B PD pathologies (22, 29), covary with changes in the intensity of cocaine use over 1 year (30). Nonetheless, the longitudinal relation between cocaine use intensity and cluster B PD symptomatology has also not been investigated to date.

In sum, only little is known about the temporal dynamics between cocaine use intensity and sociocognitive functioning. Hence, in order to investigate whether the described sociocognitive impairments and comorbid cluster B PD symptomatology in chronic cocaine users are modulated by the increase or decrease in cocaine abuse, we performed a longitudinal study with an interval of 1 year. Thereby, we compared 48 psychostimulant-naive controls with 19 cocaine users with decreased use (*decreasers*) and 19 cocaine users with increased use (*increasers*) after a 1-year interval. To objectively assess the severity and change in cocaine use and to control for co-use of other drugs, we performed quantitative hair and urine toxicology analyses at baseline and follow-up. Considering our previous results from the present sample that changes in basal cognitive functions and impulsivity clearly covary with cocaine use intensity over time (7, 30), we hypothesized that escalating cocaine use is also associated with aggravation of sociocognitive impairments and more cluster B PD symptoms within 1 year. *Vice versa*, we also expected that reduced cocaine use is linked to a reduction of sociocognitive deficits and cluster B PD symptomatology. To test these hypotheses, we expect significant time × group interactions specifically between *decreasers* and *increasers*. Given that at baseline cocaine users displayed significant alterations in EE, social network size, prosocial behavior in money distribution games, *Theory-of-Mind*, and cluster B PD symptoms (14, 16, 17), the longitudinal analysis was focused solely on these parameters.

# METHODS

## Participants

From a baseline sample of 234 participants (96 healthy stimulant-naive controls, 138 cocaine users) (3, 16, 17), 48 healthy stimulant-naive controls and 38 chronic cocaine users were included in the present longitudinal study. This subsample has been published twice previously but with different outcome measures (7, 30). From the baseline sample, 102 participants could not be measured at the follow-up because of unavailability (i.e., not responding to the invitation, loss of interest, lack of time, death), 27 participants had to be excluded from the final analyses as hair analyses revealed drug use not allowed by our exclusion criteria (e.g., polysubstance use, change in drug preferences), and 19 cocaine users did not meet our cocaine use criteria [see also the cocaine user group assignment below; for further recruitment and selection details, please see Ref. (7)].

At baseline, general exclusion criteria were clinically significant somatic diseases, neurological disorders, head injuries, family history of schizophrenia/obsessive-compulsive disorder/bipolar disorder, or any medication affecting the central nervous system. Additional exclusion criteria for controls were *Diagnostic and Statistical Manual of Mental Disorders*, 4th edition (DSM-IV) axis I psychiatric disorders (excluding nicotine dependence) and regular illegal drug use (>15 lifetime occasions, except for recreational cannabis use). Additional exclusion criteria for cocaine users were a history of heroin use, polysubstance use, or DSM-IV axis I psychiatric disorders (except for cocaine, nicotine, cannabis, and alcohol abuse/dependence, attention deficit hyperactivity disorder, and a previous episode of an affective disorder). At baseline, inclusion criteria for cocaine users were cocaine use of >0.5 g per month, cocaine as primary drug, and an abstinence duration of <6 months. Participants were asked to abstain from illegal substances for at least 72 h and from alcohol for 24 h before the test sessions. Compliance with these instructions was controlled by urine screenings (semiquantitative enzyme multiplied immunoassay method). The study was approved by the Cantonal Ethics Committee of Zurich. All participants provided written informed-consent statements and were compensated for their participation.

## Cocaine User Group Assignment

The categorization of the two cocaine user groups was based on changes of cocaine concentration in hair samples as determined by liquid chromatography–tandem mass spectrometry [for technical details, see Ref. (3)]. If possible, 6-cm hair samples were drawn covering the previous drug use of approximately 6 months. Cocaine users were categorized based on a combination of absolute (±0.5 ng/mg) and relative (>10% increase/decrease) changes in the hair concentration of $\text{cocaine}_{\text{total}}$ between baseline and the 1-year follow-up (7, 30, 31). According to these criteria, cocaine users were divided into three equally sized groups: 19 cocaine *increasers* [mean ± SD: +30.4 ± 61.9 ng/mg (+297%), range: +0.5 to +268.5 ng/mg (+20% to +5,374%)], 19 cocaine *decreasers* [−10.6 ± 26.7 ng/mg (−72%), −116.9 to −0.6 ng/mg (−100% to −12%)]), and 19 users with a relatively low and stable cocaine use pattern who did not meet both criteria [−0.1 ± 0.5 ng/mg (−2%), −1.9 to +0.5 ng/mg (−100% to +720%)], and, thus, were not further analyzed in this study [for further details, see Ref. (7)].

## Procedure

At baseline, self-reported drug use was assessed with a structured and standardized Interview for Psychotropic Drug Consumption (32), attention deficit hyperactivity disorder (ADHD) symptoms were assessed with the ADHD Self-Rating Scale (ADHD-SR) (33), and the Structured Clinical Interview for DSM-IV axis I disorders (SCID-I) (34) was carried out by trained psychologists.

The test battery was assessed at baseline and follow-up and included the Multifaceted Empathy Test (MET) (35) assessing EE, the Movie for the Assessment of Social Cognition (MASC) (36) for the measurement of *Theory-of-Mind*, a Distribution/Dictator Game (37, 38) for the determination of prosocial behavior, the Social Network Questionnaire (SNQ) (39) measuring the social network size, and the SCID-II questionnaire (40) in order to ascertain cluster B PD symptoms. More detailed test descriptions published already in our previous work (16, 17) are given in **Methods S1.**

## Statistical Analysis

Effect sizes and power analyses were calculated with G*Power 3.1 (41). As our previous analyses showed an effect size of ${}_{p}\eta^2 = 0.12$ (Cohen's f = 0.37) and a power of 99% for the significant interaction in the domain of working memory between *decreasers* and *increasers* (two groups, $p < .05$, two measurements) for the present sample (7), we assumed a more conservative effect size of ${}_{p}\eta^2 = 0.06$ (f = 0.25) and calculated a still acceptable power of 86% for the detection of significant interactions in sociocognitive functions in the present sample.

In order to reduce data quantity [see also Ref. (17)], we computed an SDM composite score that was derived by averaging z-transformed payoffs for the other player in the Distribution and Dictator Game (payoffs B) according to the means and standard deviations of the control group. Because of a strong correlation of the explicit and implicit EE scores from the MET in the total sample ($r = 0.86$, $p < .001$), we further integrated both parameters by adding them up into a single MET EE score. The SCID-II Cluster B symptom score was calculated by summing up the dimensional values from histrionic, narcissistic, borderline, and antisocial PD.

Group differences in demographic data and drug use patterns were analyzed by means of Pearson's chi-squared tests, analyses of variance (ANOVA), or independent Student's t-tests. For the longitudinal analysis and in order to investigate group differences over all groups, we performed a multiple linear regression (forced entry) with the test score change values ($\Delta = t2 - t1$) as dependent variables and four preselected independent variables: age, sex, ADHS-SR score, and dummy-coded (zero/one) group contrasts. The two demographic variables were included because previous findings suggest a linkage between advancing age and fairness in stimulant users (17) and due to known gender effects in social cognition/functioning (42, 43). Moreover, because ADHD has previously been linked to cognitive and sociocognitive performance in cocaine users (3, 16, 44), this variable was further included as a predictor into the regression model. To compare the groups, cocaine *increasers* acted as the reference group. To further analyze test score changes within the single groups (value t2 vs. value t1), we applied dependent Student's t-tests ($t_{dep}$). To compare the effect of changing cocaine use, we applied independent Student's t-tests ($t_{ind}$) between controls and a combined cocaine user sample (CCU = *increasers* + *decreasers*) at baseline as well as between controls, cocaine *increasers*, and cocaine *decreasers* at the follow-up. Notably, at baseline, cocaine *increasers* and *decreasers* showed comparable baseline values in all reported test parameters (MET, MASC, SDM, SNQ, SCID-II Cluster B) differing only with very small effect sizes ($t_{ind}(32–35) = 0.05–0.34$, p = .99–.74, d = 0.00–0.11). In the test parameter analysis, frequency data were analyzed by the Fisher–Freeman–Halton Exact Test (FET) (45). To test for test–retest effects, we applied the Pearson product-moment correlation analyses. The confirmatory statistical comparisons were carried out on a significance level of $p < .05$ (two-tailed).

## RESULTS

*Demographic characteristics and drug use:* As shown before (7, 30), the three experimental groups did not significantly differ regarding age, sex distribution, verbal IQ, years of education, length of study interval (**Table 1**), and socioeconomic status (**Table S1**). Still, cocaine-using groups showed significantly higher BDI and ADHD-SR sum scores than controls at baseline (7, 30). Whereas at baseline both cocaine user groups showed comparable cocaine use severity, the $cocaine_{total}$ hair concentrations for *increasers* (~3-fold increase) and *decreasers* (reduction by the factor 3.5) were significantly different at follow-up. Moreover, hair data revealed a clear preference for cocaine use compared to other illegal drugs. Finally, in both user groups, 8 of 19 participants sought psychiatric or psychological treatment during the study interval. The other cocaine users did not report any related treatment between baseline and follow-up.

*Emotional empathy*: The introduced predictors explained a significant amount of variance of the EE change scores in the multiple regression analysis [$F(5,80) = 2.68$, $p < .05$, $R^2 = .14$; **Table 2**]. The strongest predictors were sex ($\beta = -0.25$, $p < .05$) and the group contrast cocaine *increasers* vs. *decreasers* ($\beta = -0.25$, $p < .05$; **Figure 1**). *Post hoc* analyses showed that controls and the combined cocaine user (CCU) group showed a nonsignificant difference in EE with a small to moderate effect size at baseline [$t_{ind}(84) = 1.78$, p = .08, d = 0.39]. Whereas in the 1-year interval, *increasers* slightly reduced their already hampered EE [$t_{dep}(18) = 1.19$, p = .25 d = 0.27], and cocaine *decreasers* moderately improved their ability to respond empathically [$t_{dep}(18) = 1.80$, p = .09, d = 0.41]. Notably, controls remained largely stable in EE [$t_{dep}(47) = 0.98$, p = .33, d = 0.14]. Accordingly, at follow-up, controls differed significantly from the *increaser* group [$t_{ind}(25) = 2.14$, $p < .05$, d = 0.64], whereas the difference between controls and *decreasers* was strongly reduced [$t_{ind}(65) = 0.40$, p = .69, d = 0.11]. Finally, at follow-up, *increasers* and *decreasers* displayed a nonsignificant group difference of moderate effect size [$t_{ind}(36) = 1.69$, p = .10, d = 0.56].

*Theory-of-Mind*: The applied multiple regression model could not predict the MASC total error change scores (**Table 2**). At the phenomenological level, both cocaine user groups displayed small test–retest improvements [*increasers*: $t_{dep}(18) = 1.12$, p = .28, d = 0.26; *decreasers*: $t_{dep}(17) = 0.60$, p = .56, d = 0.14], while the control group showed pronounced improvements [$t_{dep}(47) = 4.68$, $p < .001$, d = 0.68; **Figure 2**).

*Social interaction*: The multiple regression model was also not able to predict the SDM composite change score (**Table 2**). From the phenomenological perspective, controls and *increasers* acted less prosocial (giving less money to the opponent), while *decreasers* remained stable but, with that, came closer to the controls (**Figure 3**). Exploratory *post hoc* analyses confirmed that controls and CCU significantly differed at baseline [$t_{ind}(65) = 2.51$, $p < .05$, d = 0.56]. At follow-up, controls and *increasers* still display a moderate group difference [$t_{ind}(65) = 1.92$, p = .06, d = 0.50], whereas the group difference between controls and *decreasers* was reduced to a small effect size [$t_{ind}(64) = 0.98$, p = .33, d = 0.26]. In addition, we analyzed behavioral changes between baseline and follow-up (more prosocial decisions, more self-serving decisions, similar decision) only in cocaine users and found that about two-thirds of the *increasers* (58% = 11/19) but only one-third of the *decreasers* (33% = 6/18) showed more self-serving decisions at follow-up (p = .40; FET; **Figure S1**).

*Social network size:* Regarding the SNQ total network size, the multiple regression model could again not substantially predict the change scores (**Table 2**, **Figure 4**). Interestingly, during the 1-year interval, all three groups reported a substantial and moderate social network reduction of about 2.5 contacts [controls: $t_{dep}(47) = 3.75$, $p < .001$, d = 0.54; *increasers*: $t_{dep}(17) = 1.94$, p = .70, d = 0.46; *decreasers*: $t_{dep}(17) = 3.09$, $p < .01$, d = 0.73].

*Cluster B PD*: The regression model significantly explained the variance in cluster B PD symptom change [$F(5,77) = 3.25$, $p < .01$, $R^2 = .17$; **Table 2**]. This change score was best predicted by the ADHS-SR score ($\beta = -0.32$, $p < .01$) and the group contrasts cocaine *increasers* vs. *decreasers* ($\beta = 0.34$, $p < .01$) and cocaine *increasers* vs. controls ($\beta = 0.31$, $p < .01$). Importantly, the CCU group showed at baseline significantly more cluster B PD symptoms than the controls [$t_{ind}(81) = 4.40$, $p < .001$, d = 0.96; **Figure 5**]. Whereas controls [$t_{dep}(47) = 4.91$, $p < .001$, d = 0.71] and *decreasers* [$t_{dep}(17) = 3.55$, $p < .01$, d = 0.84] had significantly lower symptom scores after the 1-year interval period, the amount of symptoms for the *increaser* group remained largely stable [$t_{dep}(16) = 0.52$, p = .61, d = 0.13]. Accordingly, at follow-up, controls differed strongly from the *increasers* [$t_{ind}(19) = 4.70$, $p < .001$, d = 1.58] and from the *decreasers* [$t_{ind}(22) = 3.11$, $p < .01$, d = 0.96]. Interestingly, already after 1 year of different cocaine use, *increasers* and *decreasers* displayed a moderate to strong group difference in cluster B PD symptoms at follow-up [$t_{ind}(33) = 1.85$, p = .07, d = 0.63]. Of note, approximately three quarters of the *decreasers* (13/18) displayed lower cluster B PD scores, while more than half of the cocaine *increasers* (9/17) showed even more symptoms at follow-up ($p < .05$; FET; **Figure S2**).

Remarkably, the interaction effect on cluster B PD symptoms was mainly driven by changes in the narcissistic and borderline subscores and less by the histrionic and surprisingly also not by the antisocial subscore (see **Figure S3a–d**). Both the narcissistic

**TABLE 1** | Demographic data and pattern of cocaine use.

| | Baseline (t1) | | | | | | 1-year follow-up (t2)[m] | | | | | |
|---|---|---|---|---|---|---|---|---|---|---|---|---|
| | Controls (n = 48) | Cocaine Increaser (n = 19) | Cocaine Decreaser (n = 19) | $F/\chi^2/T$ | df, $df_{err}$ | p | Controls (n = 48) | Cocaine Increaser (n = 19) | Cocaine Decreaser (n = 19) | $F/\chi^2/T$ | df, $df_{err}$ | p |
| Age, years | 30.3 (8.9) | 31.5 (9.4) | 31.4 (8.3) | .20[a] | 2,83 | .82 | | | | | | |
| Sex (f/m) | 16/32 | 3/16 | 5/14 | 2.11[b] | 2 | .35 | | | | | | |
| Verbal IQ (MWT-B)[d] | 107.6 (10.0) | 102.9 (9.7) | 103.8 (7.1) | 2.20[a] | 2,83 | .12 | | | | | | |
| Education, years | 10.8 (1.8) | 10.4 (1.8) | 10.0 (1.5) | 1.30[a] | 2,83 | .28 | | | | | | |
| ADHD-SR score (0-22) | 7.7 (5.2) | 13.5 (9.4)** | 14.1 (6.8)** | 8.83[a] | 2,83 | **<.001** | | | | | | |
| ADHD DSM IV (y/n)[e] | 0/48 | 4/15 | 3/16 | 7.02[b] | 2 | **.03** | | | | | | |
| Weeks between t1 and t2 | 58.2 (10.1) | 59.3 (12.1) | 61.9 (14.5) | .69[a] | 2,83 | .50 | | | | | | |
| BDI score (0–63) | 3.5 (3.3) | 7.3 (8.0)* | 8.7 (6.5)** | 7.53[a] | 2,83 | **<.001** | | | | | | |
| BDI depression (y/n)[g] | 0/48 | 1/18 | 1/18 | 2.59[b] | 2 | .27 | | | | | | |
| **Cocaine** | | | | | | | | | | | | |
| Times per week[h] | – | 1.6 (1.8) | 1.0 (1.3) | 1.17[c] | 36 | .25 | – | 1.1 (0.8) | 0.3 (0.3) | 3.85[c] | 36 | **<.001** |
| Grams per week[h] | – | 2.0 (2.5) | 1.7 (2.3) | .41[c] | 36 | .68 | – | 1.6 (2.5) | 0.4 (0.4) | 2.18[c] | 36 | **.04** |
| Years of use | – | 7.0 (5.5) | 8.2 (5.4) | .68[c] | 36 | .50 | – | 8.9 (5.4) | 9.7 (5.2) | .45[c] | 36 | .65 |
| Age of cocaine onset | – | 24.5 (8.1) | 23.1 (5.2) | .61[c] | 36 | .54 | | | | | | |
| Max. dose (g/day)[k] | – | 4.7 (4.4) | 5.9 (6.4) | .71[c] | 36 | .48 | – | 3.7 (2.5) | 3.1 (2.8) | .63[c] | 36 | .53 |
| Cumulative dose (g)[k] | – | 1182 (1635) | 3698 (8585) | 1.25[c] | 36 | .22 | – | 91 (119) | 49 (89) | 1.25[c] | 36 | .22 |
| Last consumption (days) | – | 18.5 (25.1) | 16.8 (14.6) | .29[c] | 36 | .77 | – | 7.0 (6.3) | 81.4 (145.1) | 2.23[c] | 36 | **.03** |
| Cocaine craving (0–70)[i] | – | 19.8 (9.5) | 17.7 (7.2) | .79[c] | 36 | .44 | – | 20.5 (10.8) | 15.8 (6.2) | 1.66[c] | 36 | .11 |
| Hair analysis (ng/mg)[l] | | | | | | | | | | | | |
| $Cocaine_{total}$ | – | 10.3 (29.2) | 14.9 (32.2) | .46[c] | 36 | .65 | – | 40.7 (76.1) | 4.2 (8.2) | 2.08[c] | 36 | **.05** |
| Cocaine | – | 8.2 (23.3) | 11.4 (23.9) | .42[c] | 36 | .68 | – | 31.7 (56.5) | 3.1 (5.9) | 2.19[c] | 36 | **.03** |
| Benzoylecgonine | – | 1.9 (5.5) | 3.1 (7.6) | .58[c] | 36 | .56 | – | 8.3 (19.6) | 1.0 (2.2) | 1.62[c] | 36 | .11 |
| Cocaethylene | – | 1.0 (2.8) | 0.9 (2.8) | .11[c] | 36 | .91 | – | 1.2 (2.1) | 0.3 (1.0) | 1.56[c] | 36 | .13 |
| $Norcocaine_t$ | – | 0.2 (0.5) | 0.4 (0.8) | .83[c] | 36 | .41 | – | 0.6 (1.4) | 0.1 (0.1) | 1.71[c] | 36 | .10 |
| Urine toxicology (n/p)[k] | 48/0 | 14/5 | 16/3 | .63[b] | 1 | .43 | 48/0 | 7/12 | 18/1 | 14.15[b] | 1 | **<.001** |
| **Alcohol**[n] | | | | | | | | | | | | |
| Grams per week[h] | 119.9 (136.8) | 169.4 (129.2) | 155.3 (146.4) | 1.07[a] | 2,83 | .35 | 104.3 (88.6) | 259.7 (244.5)*** | 127.4 (141.4)° | 7.71[a] | 2,83 | **<.001** |
| Years of use | 13.3 (8.8) | 13.7 (7.6) | 12.0 (7.3) | .23[a] | 2,83 | .79 | 14.0 (8.7) | 14.8 (7.5) | 12.6 (7.9) | .34[a] | 2,83 | .71 |
| **Nicotine**[n] | | | | | | | | | | | | |
| Smoking (y/n)[f] | 37/11 | 14/5 | 14/5 | .13[b] | 2 | .94 | 40/8 | 15/4 | 13/6 | 1.83[b] | 2 | .40 |
| Cigarettes per day[h] | 8.7 (8.7) | 12.8 (11.2) | 9.5 (8.2) | 1.38[a] | 2,83 | .26 | 8.2 (8.7) | 13.4 (12.0) | 8.2 (7.8) | 2.31[a] | 2,83 | .11 |
| Years of use | 9.3 (8.3) | 10.4 (8.9) | 12.7 (10.3) | .95[a] | 2,83 | .39 | 10.5 (8.8) | 12.5 (8.6) | 12.6 (9.9) | .56[a] | 2,83 | .57 |
| **Cannabis**[n] | | | | | | | | | | | | |
| Grams per week[h] | 0.6 (1.6) | 3.3 (8.9) | 1.2 (2.3) | 2.38[a] | 2,83 | .10 | 0.5 (1.6) | 2.1 (4.6) | 1.1 (2.7) | 2.28[a] | 2,83 | .11 |
| Years of use | 4.5 (4.9) | 9.5 (8.5)* | 10.1 (9.7)* | 5.92[a] | 2,83 | **.004** | 4.6 (5.9) | 10.5 (9.8)* | 8.6 (9.7) | 4.64[a] | 2,83 | **.01** |
| Cumulative dose (grams) | 980 (3985) | 3199 (5899) | 2606 (6359) | 1.61[a] | 2,83 | .21 | 53.4 (180) | 217.8 (526.5) | 84.7 (189.6) | 2.15[a] | 2,83 | .12 |
| Last consumption (days)[j] | 30.3 (1.6);n = 22 | 10.0 (0.4);n = 14 | 25.4 (1.1);n = 12 | 2.19[a] | 2,45 | .12 | 36.5 (1.5);n = 22 | 9.7 (0.4);n = 13 | 50.8 (2.1);n = 10 | 1.20[a] | 2,42 | .31 |
| Urine toxicology (n/p)[k] | 42/6 | 15/4 | 14/5 | 2.03[b] | 2 | .36 | 42/6 | 7/12 | 15/4 | 18.61[b] | 2 | **<.001** |
| **Amphetamine**[n] | | | | | | | | | | | | |
| Grams per week[h] | 0.0 (0.1) | 0.1 (0.1)** | 0.0 (0.1) | 5.18[a] | 2,83 | **.008** | 0.0 (0.0) | 0.1 (0.2)** | 0.0 (0.1) | 5.89[a] | 2,83 | **.004** |
| Years of use | 0.0 (0.0) | 3.3 (4.0)*** | 1.3 (3.1)° | 13.73[a] | 2,83 | **<.001** | 0.1 (0.5) | 3.2 (4.9)** | 2.7 (5.5)* | 7.46[a] | 2,83 | **.001** |
| Cumulative dose (grams) | 0.0 (0.1) | 56.0 (177.6)* | 16.2 (35.9) | 2.99[a] | 2,83 | .06 | 0.0 (0.1) | 4.4 (8.9)** | 1.4 (3.5) | 6.47[a] | 2,83 | **.002** |
| Last consumption (days)[j] | 121.6 (5.1);n = 1 | 73.6 (3.1);n = 10 | 90.9 (3.8);n = 3 | .29[a] | 2,11 | .75 | 17.5 (0.7);n = 1 | 35.7 (1.5);n = 8 | 99.8 (4.2);n = 4 | 1.48[a] | 2,10 | .27 |
| Hair analysis (ng/mg) | 0.0 (0.0) | 0.1 (0.2)* | 0.0 (0.0) | 4.35[a] | 2,83 | **.02** | 0.0 (0.0) | 0.1 (0.2) | 0.1 (0.2) | 2.89[a] | 2,83 | .06 |

*(Continued)*

**TABLE 1** | Continued

| | Baseline (t1) | | | | | | 1-year follow-up (t2)[m] | | | | | |
|---|---|---|---|---|---|---|---|---|---|---|---|---|
| | Controls (n = 48) | Cocaine Increaser (n = 19) | Cocaine Decreaser (n = 19) | $F/\chi^2/T$ | df, $df_{err}$ | p | Controls (n = 48) | Cocaine Increaser (n = 19) | Cocaine Decreaser (n = 19) | $F/\chi^2/T$ | df, $df_{err}$ | p |
| **MDMA**[n] | | | | | | | | | | | | |
| Tablets per week[h] | 0.0 (0.0) | 0.0 (0.1)*** | 0.0 (0.0)° | 7.42[a] | 2,83 | **.001** | 0.0 (0.0) | 0.4 (0.9)** | 0.0 (0.0)° | 5.54[a] | 2,83 | **.006** |
| Years of use | 0.3 (1.0) | 3.5 (4.5)*** | 2.4 (4.6)* | 8.42[a] | 2,83 | **<.001** | 0.2 (1.4) | 3.8 (5.5)** | 3.2 (5.6)* | 7.78[a] | 2,83 | **<.001** |
| Cumulative dose (tablets) | 1.3 (4.0) | 108.8 (249.7)** | 18.7 (46.2) | 5.71[a] | 2,83 | **.005** | 0.2 (0.8) | 17.0 (49.3)* | 2.8 (5.2) | 3.67[a] | 2,83 | **.03** |
| Last consumption (days)[j] | 5.0 (0.2);n = 1 | 89.9 (3.7);n = 7 | 40.2 (1.7);n = 4 | 1.63[a] | 2,9 | .25 | 91.2 (3.8);n = 3 | 41.6 (1.7);n = 6 | 47.8 (2.0);n = 5 | 1.11[a] | 2,11 | .36 |
| Hair analysis (ng/mg) | 0.0 (0.0) | 0.3 (0.7) | 0.4 (1.5) | 2.23[a] | 2,83 | .11 | 0.0 (0.0) | 0.5 (0.8)*** | 0.1 (0.3) | 7.87[a] | 2,83 | **<.001** |
| **GHB**[n] | | | | | | | | | | | | |
| Cumulative dose (pipettes) | 0.0 (0.0) | 0.5 (0.7) | 0.5 (1.7) | 3.36[a] | 2,83 | **.04** | 0.0 (0.0) | 0.0 (0.0) | 0.0 (0.0) | – | – | – |
| **Hallucinogens**[n] | | | | | | | | | | | | |
| Cumulative dose (times) | 0.9 (2.2) | 27.9 (72.8)* | 9.9 (22.9) | 3.92[a] | 2,83 | **.02** | 0.0 (0.0) | 1.1 (1.6)*** | 0.6 (1.5) | 8.57[a] | 2,83 | **<.001** |
| **Methlyphenidate**[n] | | | | | | | | | | | | |
| Cumulative dose (tablets) | 0.0 (0.0) | 20.2 (60.4)* | 0.5 (2.3) | 3.76[a] | 2,83 | **.03** | 0.0 (0.1) | 67.7 (239.5) | 0.3 (0.6) | 2.72[a] | 2,83 | .07 |
| Hair analysis (ng/mg) | 0.0 (0.0) | 0.0 (0.1) | 0.0 (0.0) | 1.80[a] | 2,83 | .17 | 0.0 (0.0) | 0.1 (0.2)* | 0.0 (0.0) | 3.62[a] | 2,83 | **.03** |

*Means and standard deviations. Significant p values are shown in bold.*

[a]*ANOVA (all groups, with significant Sidak post hoc test vs. control group: *p < .05; **p < .01; ***p < .001; vs. cocaine increaser: °p < .05).*

[b] *$\chi^2$-test (all groups/cocaine users only) for frequency data.*

[c]*Independent t-test (cocaine users only).*

[d]*Verbal IQ was assessed by the Mehrfachwahl Wortschatz Intelligenztest (46).*

[e]*ADHD-SR, ADHD self-rating scale (cutoff DSM-IV criteria) (33).*

[f]*Smoking habits were assessed by the Fagerstroem Test of Nicotine Dependence (47).*

[g]*BDI, Beck Depression Inventory (cutoff ≥ 18) (48).*

[h]*Average use during the last 6 months.*

[i]*Craving for cocaine was assessed by the Brief-CCQ (49).*

[j]*Last consumption is averaged only for persons who used the drug in the last 6 months.*

[k]*Urine toxicology (neg/pos) are based on the cutoff value for cocaine = 150 ng/ml and for tetrahydrocannabinol 50 ng/ml (50). The $\chi^2$-test for cocaine includes only cocaine users; the $\chi^2$-test for cannabis includes controls and cocaine users.*

[l]*Hair samples were voluntary and data are missing for three controls.*

[m]*Parameters at follow-up refer to the 1-year period between t1 and t2.*

[n]*At baseline, average use during the last 6 months. Use frequency, duration of use, and cumulative doses are averaged within the total group.*

**TABLE 2** | Multiple regression analyses.

| | Emotional empathy Δ MET Emotional empathy | | | Theory-of-Mind Δ MASC total errors | | | Social interaction Δ SDM composite score | | | Social network Δ SNQ network size | | | Personality disorder Δ SCID-II Cluster B | | |
|---|---|---|---|---|---|---|---|---|---|---|---|---|---|---|---|
| | B | SE | β | B | SE | β | B | SE | β | B | SE | β | B | SE | β |
| Constant | 1.55 | 1.14 | | −1.85 | 2.02 | | −0.26 | 0.45 | | −0.73 | 2.72 | | −1.01 | 2.80 | |
| Age | 0.04 | 0.03 | 0.14 | 0.06 | 0.05 | 0.14 | −0.01 | 0.01 | −0.08 | −0.04 | 0.06 | −0.08 | 0.02 | 0.06 | 0.04 |
| Sex | −1.16 | 0.50 | −0.25* | −0.99 | 0.86 | −0.12 | 0.09 | 0.20 | 0.05 | −0.56 | 1.20 | −0.05 | −0.71 | 1.23 | −0.06 |
| ADHD-SR score | −0.05 | 0.03 | −0.16 | −0.07 | 0.06 | −0.14 | 0.00 | 0.01 | −0.01 | 0.04 | 0.08 | 0.05 | −0.24 | 0.08 | −0.32** |
| Controls vs. cocaine increaser | −0.26 | 0.59 | −0.05 | 1.71 | 1.03 | 0.20 | 0.03 | 0.24 | 0.01 | 0.35 | 1.43 | 0.03 | 4.00 | 1.49 | 0.31** |
| Cocaine decreaser vs. cocaine increaser | −1.30 | 0.66 | −0.25* | −0.51 | 1.17 | −0.06 | −0.31 | 0.27 | −0.16 | 0.54 | 1.63 | 0.05 | 4.43 | 1.69 | 0.34** |
| $R^2$ | | 0.14 | | | 0.10 | | | 0.03 | | | 0.01 | | | 0.17 | |
| F | | 2.68* | | | 1.67 | | | 0.57 | | | 0.22 | | | 3.25** | |

*Multiple linear regression with the independent variables age, sex, ADHD-SR score, and dummy coded (zero, one) group variables. To compare the groups, cocaine increaser acted as the reference group. Dependent variables are change values (Δ = value at t2 – value at t1).*

*B, unstandardized regression coefficient; SE, unstandardized standard error; β, standardized beta.*

*(*)p < .10; *p < .05; **p < .01; ***p < .001.*

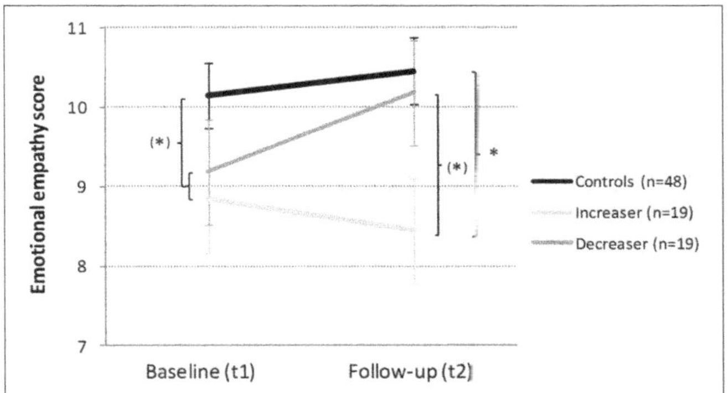


**FIGURE 1** | Development of emotional empathy in cocaine *increasers*, *decreasers*, and stimulant-naive controls within 1 year. Mean emotional empathy sum scores and standard errors. At baseline, controls vs combined cocaine user (CCU) (= Ø of increaser and decreaser). Independent Student's t-tests are shown if p < .10. (*)p < .10; *p < .05.

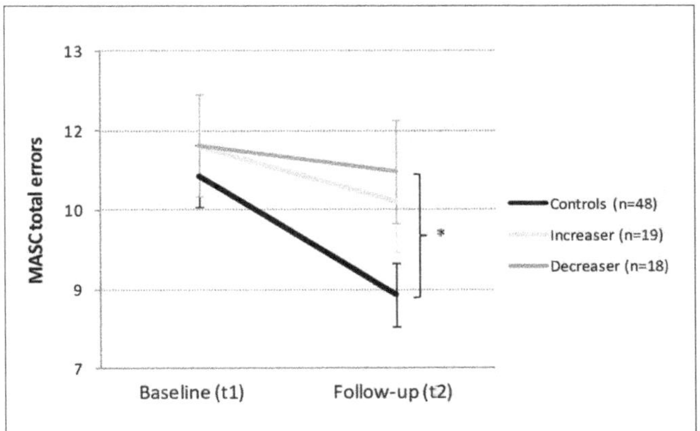


**FIGURE 2** | Development of the *Theory-of-Mind* in cocaine *increasers*, *decreasers*, and stimulant-naive controls within 1 year. Mean Movie for the Assessment of Social Cognition (MASC) total errors and standard errors. At baseline, controls vs CCU (= Ø of increaser and decreaser). Independent Student's t-tests are shown if p < .10. *p < .05.

and the borderline subscores revealed significant regression models (**Table S2**), but only the borderline subscore was significantly predicted by the group contrast cocaine *increasers* vs. *decreasers* (β = 0.40, p < .01). Compared to baseline, less symptoms occurred in controls [$t_{dep}(47) = 4.99$, p < .001, d = 0.72] and *decreasers* [$t_{dep}(17) = 3.16$, p < .01, d = 0.75] at follow-up, while symptoms remained stable in *increasers* [$t_{dep}(16) = 0.18$, p = .86, d = 0.04], resulting in a strong group effect between *increasers* and *decreasers* [$t_{ind}(33) = 2.57$, p < .05, d = 0.87] at follow-up.

*Change in alcohol use*: As not only cocaine but also alcohol intake was increased in *increasers* (see **Table 1**), the change in alcohol consumption was considered in additional multiple regression models. However, alcohol change was not significant in any of the main regression models (p-values ranged from .222 to .659) shown in **Table 2**, while the interaction effects and also the explained variances remained stable, indicating that changes in alcohol consumption have not impacted our main results.

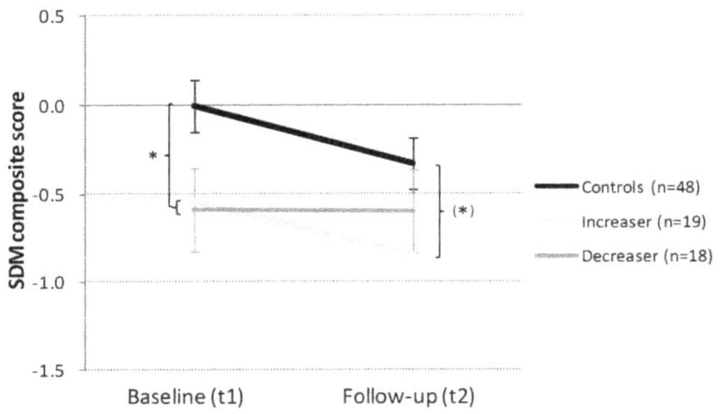


**FIGURE 3 |** Development of social interaction in cocaine *increasers*, *decreasers*, and stimulant-naive controls within 1 year. Mean social decision-making (SDM) composite z-scores and standard errors. At baseline, controls vs CCU (= Ø of increaser and decreaser). Independent Student's t-tests are shown if p < .10. (*)p < .10; *p < .05.

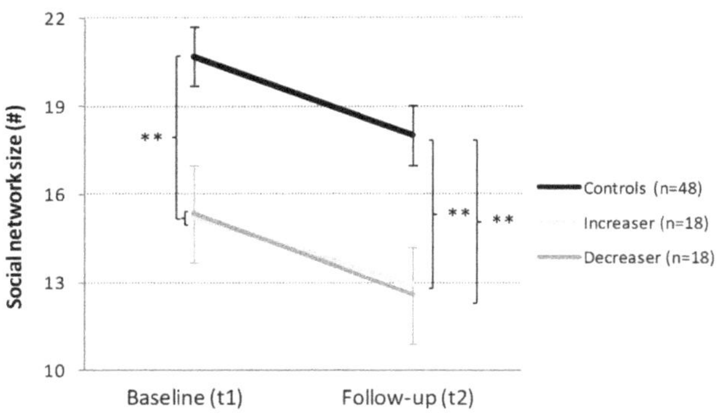


**FIGURE 4 |** Development of social network size in cocaine *increasers*, *decreasers*, and stimulant-naive controls within 1 year. Mean total network size and standard errors. At baseline, controls vs CCU (= Ø of increaser and decreaser). Independent Student's t-tests are shown if p < .10. **p < .01.

*Test–retest reliability*: In the total sample, all dependent variables displayed acceptable to good test–retest reliabilities (**Table 3**). Interestingly, in the SDM paradigm, controls and CCU differed significantly in their test–retest reliability (z = −3.25; p < .001): While in controls the SDM score showed hardly acceptable reliability (r = 0.48; p < .001), it was good in the cocaine users (r = 0.85; p < .001).

## DISCUSSION

The present longitudinal study investigated the change of social cognition, social interaction, and socially relevant cluster B PD symptoms in healthy controls and relatively pure and non-help-seeking chronic cocaine users who clearly increased or decreased their cocaine consumption during a 1-year study interval. The most striking findings were that i) improved EE correlated with

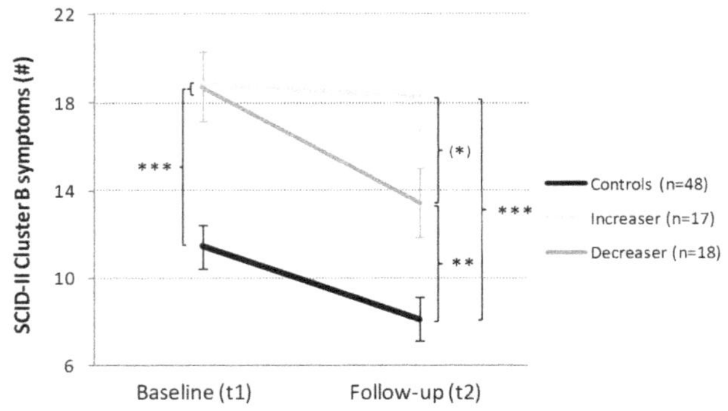


**FIGURE 5 |** Development of Structured Clinical Interview for DSM-IV Axis II Disorders (SCID-II) Cluster B in cocaine *increasers*, *decreasers*, and stimulant-naive controls within 1 year. Mean SCID-II Cluster B symptoms and standard errors. At baseline, controls vs CCU (= Ø of increaser and decreaser). Independent Student's t-tests are shown if p < .10. (*)p < .10; **p < .01; ***p < .001.

**TABLE 3 |** One-year test–retest reliability between baseline and 1-year follow-up in controls and cocaine users.

| | Controls (n = 48) | Combined cocaine users (n = 38) | Total sample (n = 86) |
|---|---|---|---|
| MET Emotional empathy score | 0.66*** | 0.79*** | 0.74*** |
| MASC total errors | 0.67*** | 0.60*** | 0.63*** |
| SDM composite score | 0.48*** | 0.85*** | 0.70*** |
| SNQ network size | 0.75*** | 0.81*** | 0.80*** |
| SCID-II Cluster B symptoms | 0.68*** | 0.74*** | 0.77*** |

*Pearson's product-moment correlation. Significance level: ***p < .001.*

decreased cocaine consumption, whereas increased cocaine use severity was linked to less EE; and ii) cluster B PD symptom burden was lowered in *decreasers,* whereas *increasers* showed stable severity in these symptoms. Additionally, during the study interval, we found an approximation between controls and *decreasers* regarding their prosocial behavior, while the large gap between *increasers* and controls remained. Moreover, neither the *Theory-of-Mind* Task (MASC) nor the social network size showed interactions with changing cocaine use, indicating that mental perspective-taking (sometimes also interpreted as *cognitive empathy*) and the number of social contacts in the last months were not affected by changing drug use during the study interval.

Importantly, the present analysis of smaller (longitudinal) subgroups from our larger cross-sectional ZuCo²St sample published previously (14, 16, 17) still showed significantly reduced prosocial behavior, a smaller social network, and strongly elevated cluster B personality symptoms in the total group of cocaine users at baseline, indicating that these indicators of social functioning were robustly altered in this population. The EE score of the MET showed only a statistical trend between cocaine users and controls at baseline, but the present effect size (d = 0.39) was in the range of the previously reported effect sizes of the larger cross-sectional sample of recreational and dependent cocaine users (d = 0.39–0.64), suggesting rather a deficiency of power than a lack of reliability. This assumption is further supported by the fact that the MET EE score showed good test–retest reliability scores. Moreover, the MASC did not show any baseline group differences in the present subsample of cocaine users underscoring our previous conclusion that mainly very severe cocaine users with a putative ADHD comorbidity show disturbances in this task (16, 44).

While sociocognitive functions represent basic abilities in perspective-taking and interaction, more conventional psychopathology is aiming at the identification and quantification of symptoms in psychiatric disorders (51). As such, the research on the relationship between PDs and cocaine use is of special interest, as the differentiation between predispositions vs. drug-induced effects merges with the question if these pathologies are reversible or not. In our longitudinal investigation, we found that *decreasers* of cocaine consumption also significantly improved in cluster B PD symptoms during 1 year, whereas the increasers showed a stable PD symptom burden. This is insofar interesting as in both user groups 8 of 19 participants sought psychiatric treatment in the interval, but only *decreasers* improved in some social functions and socially relevant PD symptoms.

In general, PDs are defined as typical constellations of impaired subjective and behavioral traits that result in suffering of the affected individual and/or society (52). These personality traits are regarded as relatively stable across time and consistent across situations (diagnostically mandatory) (53–56). Moreover, cluster B PDs show a higher stability over 12 to 18 years than the other clusters (57). However, studies also found considerable variability of PD symptoms across individuals over time (58, 59), questioning the trait-like character of the disorder. An early study showed changes in PD symptoms related to treatment in substance-dependent patients (60). Interestingly, clusters A and C profited most, while cluster B changes were only observed in patients with borderline PD. In patients with cocaine addiction, cluster B PDs are the most frequent and these patients have the most severe courses of illness including worst treatment outcomes (24, 26–28, 61, 62). Therefore, cluster B PD symptoms are likely personality features that increase the risk for cocaine use and the development of an addiction. However, as seen in the present study, cluster B PD symptom load is nevertheless variable and reduction of consumption leads to a substantial improvement in these symptoms. Consequently, a reduction of cluster B PD symptom burden again increases likelihood of successful treatment, offering the patient an opportunity to leave the vicious circle of addiction.

The suggested consumption-dependent variability of social behavior as well as cluster B symptoms are well in line with our previous analyses from this sample that not only basal cognitive functions such as working memory but also self-reported impulsivity improve with a strong reduction of cocaine use, while they are worsened with increased cocaine consumption (7, 30). The present data and the previous analyses from this sample are also in accordance with our recent results from an independent longitudinal investigation showing that decreased cortical thickness (CT) of several regions within the prefrontal cortex of cocaine users can improve after a strong reduction of cocaine use, while sustained use went along with a further decrease in prefrontal CT during the study interval (63). Importantly, the cortical changes were correlated with cognitive changes, i.e., improved CT as associated with enhanced sustained attention (63). Thus, the overall pattern of change shown by longitudinal data supports our assumption that sociocognitive impairments of cocaine users are at least in part drug-induced and that neuroplastic changes in brain regions and neurotransmitter systems involved in social cognition, social interaction, and social reward processing contribute to a further decrease in social contact and social support leading to an increase in social isolation, aggression, and depressive symptoms. This ends in a further reduction of social reward resources, ongoing social withdrawal, and the establishment of cocaine as the main source of reward resulting in the maintenance of stimulant use and recurrent relapses (15).

While EE is more a perceptive social cognition ability, social decision-making (here assessed with a combined Distribution/Dictator Game) is a form of socially interactive behavior. In our previous cross-sectional analysis sample, cocaine users cared more about efficiency than about fairness compared to healthy controls at baseline (17). This was previously interpreted as predisposition of stimulant use (15), as such fairness preferences and severity of cocaine use were not correlated (17). Intriguingly, utilitarian and opportunistic attitudes assessed with the Machiavellianism Questionnaire (MACH-IV) were also increased in cocaine users compared to controls and were shown to be stable and independent of changing cocaine use (14). However, our data indicated a shift toward improved prosocial behavior in cocaine *decreasers* indicating space for enhancement potential by treatment. Conclusively, SDM deficits in cocaine users likely have both a trait and a state component, and it might be worse to specifically target the state component in therapy in order to improve the treatment outcome.

## Limitations

When interpreting the present results, some limitations of our study have to be considered: i) The total sample size is moderate for a longitudinal analysis. Moreover, the test–retest reliabilities of the applied social cognition tasks and questionnaire have a broad range (in controls: r = 0.48–0.75; in cocaine users: r = 0.60–0.85; in the total sample: r = 0.63–0.80). As a consequence of both, the shown interaction effects are not very strong (in terms of p-values). However, to our knowledge, these are the only existing longitudinal samples of chronic cocaine users with objectively verified increasing and decreasing cocaine use (by hair testing). Moreover, the included individuals were preferably pure cocaine users with little axis-I psychiatric comorbidities. We therefore think that the carefully selected and homogeneous sample has nonetheless sufficient explanatory power. ii) In the context of our hypotheses, we attribute the changes in behavior to the changes in cocaine consumption. However, we cannot rule out if other changes in the lives of our cocaine users (e.g., positive or negative changes in their social environment) not assessed by our test battery may have impacted both drug use and social functioning. Future studies should therefore assess more information on the social life of cocaine users beyond simple parameters such as social network size (e.g., social media use).

## Conclusions

The aim of this longitudinal study was to investigate whether cocaine use is associated with permanent or reversible alterations of social cognition and interaction as well as cluster B PD symptoms. We found that specific social dysfunctions and PD symptoms are variable over time as they seem to depend on variations in cocaine use. Thus, strong reduction of cocaine use within only 1 year seems to positively affect social dysfunctions that are assumed to be crucial factor in the maintenance of stimulant addiction (15, 64). From our perspective, the shown positive effects of reduced cocaine use clearly favor abstinence-orientated treatment approaches of cocaine addiction. Furthermore, having the strong impact of social cognitive abilities as well as prosocial behavior and attitudes on the patient–therapist relationships in mind (15), future developments in the psychotherapy of cocaine addictions should consider trainings specifically of social skills and cognitions in order to improve treatment outcome.

## AUTHOR CONTRIBUTIONS

BQ and MV had full access to all the data in the study and take responsibility for the integrity of the data and the accuracy of the data analysis. CE and BQ contributed to the study concept and design. CE, MV, OB, KP, LH, MB, and BQ contributed to the acquisition, analysis, or interpretation of data. OB, CE, MV, and BQ contributed to the drafting of the manuscript. All authors contributed to the critical revision of the manuscript for important intellectual content. MV and BQ conducted the statistical analysis. ES and BQ obtained funding. KP, LH, MV, and ES contributed to the administrative, technical, or material support. ES and BQ were in charge of supervision.

## ACKNOWLEDGMENTS

This article is in tribute to our esteemed friend and colleague Prof. Christoph Eisenegger, who passed away so suddenly and unexpectedly during the time we worked on this article. We are grateful to Alex Gamma for the critical discussion of the present data. Moreover, we thank Daniela Jenni and Kathrin Küpeli for their excellent support.

## REFERENCES

1. Jovanovski D, Erb S, Zakzanis KK. Neurocognitive deficits in cocaine users: a quantitative review of the evidence. *J Clin Exp Neuropsychol* (2005) 27(2):189–204. doi: 10.1080/13803390490515694
2. Spronk DB, van Wel JH, Ramaekers JG, Verkes RJ. Characterizing the cognitive effects of cocaine: a comprehensive review. *Neurosci Biobehav Rev* (2013) 37(8):1838–59. doi: 10.1016/j.neubiorev.2013.07.003
3. Vonmoos M, Hulka LM, Preller KH, Jenni D, Baumgartner MR, Stohler R, et al. Cognitive dysfunctions in recreational and dependent cocaine users: role of attention-deficit hyperactivity disorder, craving and early age at onset. *Br J Psychiatry* (2013) 203(1):35–43. doi: 10.1192/bjp.bp.112.118091
4. Aharonovich E, Nunes E, Hasin D. Cognitive impairment, retention and abstinence among cocaine abusers in cognitive-behavioral treatment. *Drug Alcohol Depend* (2003) 71(2):207–11. doi: 10.1016/S0376-8716(03)00092-9
5. Aharonovich E, Hasin DS, Brooks AC, Liu X, Bisaga A, Nunes EV. Cognitive deficits predict low treatment retention in cocaine dependent patients. *Drug Alcohol Depend* (2006) 81(3):313–22. doi: 10.1016/j.drugalcdep.2005.08.003
6. Potvin S, Stavro K, Rizkallah E, Pelletier J. Cocaine and cognition: a systematic quantitative review. *J Addict Med* (2014) 8(5):368–76. doi: 10.1097/ADM.0000000000000066
7. Vonmoos M, Hulka LM, Preller KH, Minder F, Baumgartner MR, Quednow BB. Cognitive impairment in cocaine users is drug-induced but partially reversible: evidence from a longitudinal study. *Neuropsychopharmacology* (2014) 39(9):2200–10. doi: 10.1038/npp.2014.71
8. Vonmoos M, Quednow BB. Cognitive dysfunctions in chronic cocaine users. In: Preedy VR. *The neuroscience of cocaine*. San Diego: Academic Press (2017). p. 395–405. doi: 10.1016/B978-0-12-803750-8.00040-3
9. Rilling JK, Sanfey AG. The neuroscience of social decision-making. *Annu Rev Psychol* (2011) 62:23–48. doi: 10.1146/annurev.psych.121208.131647
10. Lieberman MD. Social cognitive neuroscience: a review of core processes. *Annu Rev Psychol* (2007) 58:259–89. doi: 10.1146/annurev.psych.58.110405.085654
11. Couture SM, Penn DL, Roberts DL. The functional significance of social cognition in schizophrenia: a review. *Schizophr Bull* (2006) 32 Suppl 1:S44–63. doi: 10.1093/schbul/sbl029
12. Homer BD, Solomon TM, Moeller RW, Mascia A, DeRaleau L, Halkitis PN. Methamphetamine abuse and impairment of social functioning: a review of the underlying neurophysiological causes and behavioral implications. *Psychol Bull* (2008) 134(2):301–10. doi: 10.1037/0033-2909.134.2.301
13. Volkow ND, Baler RD, Goldstein RZ. Addiction: pulling at the neural threads of social behaviors. *Neuron* (2011) 69(4):599–602. doi: 10.1016/j.neuron.2011.01.027
14. Quednow BB, Hulka LM, Preller KH, Baumgartner MR, Eisenegger C, Vonmoos M. Stable self-serving personality traits in recreational and dependent cocaine users. *PLoS One* (2017) 12(3):e0172853. doi: 10.1371/journal.pone.0172853
15. Quednow BB. Social cognition and interaction in stimulant use disorders. *Curr Opin Behav Sci* (2017) 13:55–62. doi: 10.1016/j.cobeha.2016.10.001
16. Preller KH, Hulka LM, Vonmoos M, Jenni D, Baumgartner MR, Seifritz E, et al. Impaired emotional empathy and related social network deficits in cocaine users. *Addict Biol* (2014) 19(3):452–66. doi: 10.1111/adb.12070
17. Hulka LM, Eisenegger C, Preller KH, Vonmoos M, Jenni D, Bendrick K, et al. Altered social and non-social decision-making in recreational and dependent cocaine users. *Psychol Med* (2014) 44(5):1015–28. doi: 10.1017/S0033291713001839
18. Hulka LM, Preller KH, Vonmoos M, Broicher SD, Quednow BB. Cocaine users manifest impaired prosodic and cross-modal emotion processing. *Front Psychiatry* (2013) 4:98. doi: 10.3389/fpsyt.2013.00098
19. Preller KH, Herdener M, Schilbach L, Stampfli P, Hulka LM, Vonmoos M, et al. Functional changes of the reward system underlie blunted response to social gaze in cocaine users. *Proc Natl Acad Sci U S A* (2014) 111(7):2842–7. doi: 10.1073/pnas.1317090111
20. Tobler PN, Preller KH, Campbell-Meiklejohn DK, Kirschner M, Kraehenmann R, Stampfli P, et al. Shared neural basis of social and non-social reward deficits in chronic cocaine users. *Soc Cogn Affect Neurosci* (2016) 11(6):1017–25. doi: 10.1093/scan/nsw030
21. Frith CD, Frith U. Social cognition in humans. *Curr Biol* (2007) 17(16):R724–32. doi: 10.1016/j.cub.2007.05.068

22. Roepke S, Vater A, Preißler S, Heekeren HR, Dziobek I. Social cognition in borderline personality disorder. *Front Neurosci* (2012) 6:195. doi: 10.3389/fnins.2012.00195
23. Ruiz-Tagle A, Costanzo E, De Achával D, Guinjoan S. Social cognition in a clinical sample of personality disorder patients. *Front Psychiatry* (2015) 6:75. doi: 10.3389/fpsyt.2015.00075
24. Chen KW, Banducci AN, Guller L, Macatee RJ, Lavelle A, Daughters SB, et al. An examination of psychiatric comorbidities as a function of gender and substance type within an inpatient substance use treatment program. *Drug Alcohol Depend* (2011) 118(2–3):92–9. doi: 10.1016/j.drugalcdep.2011.03.003
25. Fernandez-Montalvo J, Lorea I. Comorbilidad de la adicción a la cocaína con los trastornos de la personalidad. *An Sist Sanit Navar* (2007) 30(2):225–31. doi: 10.4321/S1137-66272007000300007
26. Albein-Urios N, Martinez-Gonzalez JM, Lozano-Rojas O, Verdejo-Garcia A. Executive functions in cocaine-dependent patients with Cluster B and Cluster C personality disorders. *Neuropsychology* (2014) 28(1):84–90. doi: 10.1037/neu0000007
27. Ford JD, Gelernter J, DeVoe JS, Zhang W, Weiss RD, Brady K, et al. Association of psychiatric and substance use disorder comorbidity with cocaine dependence severity and treatment utilization in cocaine-dependent individuals. *Drug Alcohol Depend* (2009) 99(1–3):193–203. doi: 10.1016/j.drugalcdep.2008.07.004
28. Lopez-Quintero C, Hasin DS, de Los Cobos JP, Pines A, Wang S, Grant BF, et al. Probability and predictors of remission from life-time nicotine, alcohol, cannabis or cocaine dependence: results from the National Epidemiologic Survey on Alcohol and Related Conditions. *Addiction* (2011) 106(3):657–69. doi: 10.1111/j.1360-0443.2010.03194.x
29. Bagby RM, Vachon DD, Bulmash E, Quilty LC. Personality disorders and pathological gambling: a review and re-examination of prevalence rates. *J Pers Disord* (2008) 22(2):191–207. doi: 10.1521/pedi.2008.22.2.191
30. Hulka LM, Vonmoos M, Preller KH, Baumgartner MR, Seifritz E, Gamma A, et al. Changes in cocaine consumption are associated with fluctuations in self-reported impulsivity and gambling decision-making. *Psychol Med* (2015) 45(14):3097–110. doi: 10.1017/S0033291715001063
31. Hoelzle C, Scheufler F, Uhl M, Sachs H, Thieme D. Application of discriminant analysis to differentiate between incorporation of cocaine and its congeners into hair and contamination. *Forensic Sci Int* (2008) 176(1):13–8. doi: 10.1016/j.forsciint.2007.07.020
32. Quednow BB, Kuhn KU, Hoenig K, Maier W, Wagner M. Prepulse inhibition and habituation of acoustic startle response in male MDMA ('ecstasy') users, cannabis users, and healthy controls. *Neuropsychopharmacology* (2004) 29(5):982–90. doi: 10.1038/sj.npp.1300396
33. Roesler M, Retz W, Retz-Junginger P, Thome J, Supprian T, Nissen T, et al. Instrumente zur Diagnostik der Aufmerksamkeitsdefizit-/Hyperaktivitätsstörung (ADHS) im Erwachsenenalter. *Nervenarzt* (2004) 75:888–95. doi: 10.1007/s00115-003-1622-2
34. American Psychiatric Association (APA). *Diagnostic and statistical manual of mental disorders: DSM-IV*. In: Washington D, editor. *American Psychiatric Association (APA).*, 4th ed. Washington, DC: American Psychiatric Association (APA) (1994).
35. Dziobek I, Rogers K, Fleck S, Bahnemann M, Heekeren HR, Wolf OT, et al. Dissociation of cognitive and emotional empathy in adults with Asperger syndrome using the Multifaceted Empathy Test (MET). *J Autism Dev Disord* (2008) 38(3):464–73. doi: 10.1007/s10803-007-0486-x
36. Dziobek I, Fleck S, Kalbe E, Rogers K, Hassenstab J, Brand M, et al. Introducing MASC: a movie for the assessment of social cognition. *J Autism Dev Disord* (2006) 36(5):623–36. doi: 10.1007/s10803-006-0107-0
37. Charness G, Rabin M. Understanding social preferences with simple tests. *Q J Econ* (2002) 117(3):817–69. doi: 10.1162/003355302760193904
38. Engelmann D, Strobel M. Inequality aversion, efficiency, and maximin preferences in simple distribution experiments. *Am Econ Rev* (2004) 94(4):857–69. doi: 10.1257/0002828042002741
39. Linden M, Lischka A-M, Popien C, Golombek J. Der multidimensionale Sozialkontakt Kreis (MuSK)—ein Interviewverfahren zur Erfassung des sozialen Netzes in der klinischen Praxis. [The multidimensional social contact circle—an interview for the assessment of the social network in Clinicle Practical]. *Z Med Psychol* (2007) 16(3):135–43.
40. Fydrich T, Renneberg B, Schmitz B, Wittchen H-U. SKID-II Strukturiertes Klinisches Interview für DSM-IV, Achse II: Persönlichkeitsstörungen. In: *[SCID-II Structured Clinical Interview for DSM-IV, Axis II: Personality Disorders]*. Goettingen: Hogrefe (1997).
41. Faul F, Erdfelder E, Lang AG, Buchner A. G*Power 3: a flexible statistical power analysis program for the social, behavioral, and biomedical sciences. *Behav Res Methods* (2007) 39(2):175–91. doi: 10 3758/BF03193146
42. Christov-Moore L, Simpson EA, Coude G, Grigaityte K, Iacoboni M, Ferrari PF. Empathy: gender effects in brain and behavior. *Neurosci Biobehav Rev* (2014) 46 Pt 4:604–27. doi: 10.1016/j.neubiorev.2014.09.001
43. Kret ME, De Gelder B. A review on sex differences in processing emotional signals. *Neuropsychologia* (2012) 50(7):1211–21. doi: 10.1016/j.neuropsychologia.2011.12.022
44. Wunderli MD, Vonmoos M, Niedecker SM, Hulka LM, Preller KH, Baumgartner MR, et al. Cognitive and emotional impairments in adults with attention-deficit/hyperactivity disorder and cocaine use. *Drug Alcohol Depend* (2016) 163:92–9. doi: 10.1016/j.drugalcdep.2016.03.026
45. Freeman GH, Halton JH. Note on an exact treatment of contingency, goodness of fit and other problems of significance. *Biometrika* (1951) 38(1/2):141–9. doi: 10.2307/2332323
46. Lehrl S. *Mehrfachwahl-Wortschatz-Intelligenztest. MWT-B*. 4th ed. Balingen: Spitta (1999).
47. Heatherton TF, Kozlowski LT, Frecker RC, Fagerstrom KO. The Fagerstrom Test for Nicotine Dependence: a revision of the Fagerstrom Tolerance Questionnaire. *Br J Addict* (1991) 86(9):1119–27. doi: 10.1111/j.1360-0443.1991.tb01879.x
48. Hautzinger M, Bailer M, Worall H, Keller F. Beck-Depressions-Inventar (BDI). Bearbeitung der deutschen Ausgabe. Testhandbuch. In: *Beck Depression Inventory. Test manual.*, 2nd ed. Bern, Göttingen, Toronto, Seattle: Huber (1994).
49. Sussner BD, Smelson DA, Rodrigues S, Kline A, Losonczy M, Ziedonis D. The validity and reliability of a brief measure of cocaine craving. *Drug Alcohol Depend* (2006) 83(3):233–7. doi: 10.1016/j.drugalcdep.2005.11.022
50. Substance Abuse and Mental Health Services Administration. Mandatory guidelines for federal workplace drug testing programs. *Fed Regist* (2008) 73(228):71858–907.
51. Jaspers K. *Allgemeine Psychopathologie*. 9th ed. Berlin, Heidelberg, New York: Springer-Verlag (1973).
52. American Psychiatric Association (APA). *Diagnostic and statistical manual of mental disorders*. 5th ed. Washington, DC: American Psychiatric Association (APA) (2013) doi: 10.1176/appi.books.9780890425596
53. Lenzenweger MF. Stability and change in personality disorder features: the longitudinal study of personality disorders. *Arch Gen Psychiatry* (1999) 56(11):1009–15. doi: 10.1001/archpsyc.56.11 1009
54. Hopwood CJ, Morey LC, Donnellan MB, Samuel DB, Grilo CM, McGlashan TH, et al. Ten-year rank-order stability of personality traits and disorders in a clinical sample. *J Pers* (2013) 81(3):335–44. doi: 10.1111/j.1467-6494.2012.00801.x
55. Shea MT, Stout R, Gunderson J, Morey LC, Grilo CM, McGlashan T, et al. Short-term diagnostic stability of schizotypal, borderline, avoidant, and obsessive-compulsive personality disorders. *Am J Psychiatry* (2002) 159(12):2036–41. doi: 10.1176/appi.ajp.159.12.2036
56. Grilo CM, Sanislow CA, Gunderson JG, Pagano ME, Yen S, Zanarini MC, et al. Two-year stability and change of schizotypal, borderline, avoidant, and obsessive-compulsive personality disorders. *J Consult Clin Psychol* (2004) 72(5):767–75. doi: 10.1037/0022-006X.72.5.767
57. Nestadt G, Di C, Samuels JF, Bienvenu OJ, Reti IM, Costa P, et al. The stability of DSM personality disorders over twelve to eighteen years. *J Psychiatr Res* (2010) 44(1):1–7. doi: 10.1016/j.jpsychires.2009.06.009
58. Durbin CE, Klein DN. Ten-year stability of personality disorders among outpatients with mood disorders. *J Abnorm Psychol* (2006) 115(1):75–84. doi: 10.1037/0021-843X.115.1.75
59. Lenzenweger MF, Johnson MD, Willett JB. Individual growth curve analysis illuminates stability and change in personality disorder features: the longitudinal study of personality disorders. *Arch Gen Psychiatry* (2004) 61(10):1015–24. doi: 10.1001/archpsyc.61.10.1015
60. de Groot MH, Franken IH, van der Meer CW, Hendriks VM. Stability and change in dimensional ratings of personality disorders in drug abuse patients during treatment. *J Subst Abuse Treat* (2003) 24(2):115–20. doi: 10.1016/S0740-5472(02)00351-3
61. Harro J. Neuropsychiatric adverse effects of amphetamine and methamphetamine. *Int Rev Neurobiol* (2015) 120:179–204. doi: 10.1016/bs.irn.2015.02.004

# 14

# Prehabilitation in Alcohol Dependence as a Treatment Model for Sustainable Outcomes: A Narrative Review of Literature on the Risks Associated with Detoxification, from Animal Models to Human Translational Research

*Christos Kouimtsidis[1]*, Theodora Duka[2], Emily Palmer[1] and Anne Lingford-Hughes[1]*

*[1] Centre for Psychiatry, Imperial College London, London, United Kingdom, [2] Sussex Addiction Research and Intervention Centre (SARIC), School of Psychology, University of Sussex, Brighton, United Kingdom*

***Correspondence:***
*Christos Kouimtsidis*
*christos.kouimtsidis1@nhs.net*

In this review paper, we discuss how the overarching concept of prehabilitation is applicable to alcohol dependence. Central to prehabilitation are the concepts of expected harm, risks, and proactive planning to eliminate the harm or cope with the risks. We review the evidence from animal models, psychological experimental studies, as well as pharmacological studies, on the potential risks and harms associated with medically assisted alcohol detoxification and the current treatment paradigm for alcohol dependence. Animal models provide an approximation mostly of the physical aspect of alcohol withdrawal and detoxification process and make predictions about the development of the phenomena in humans. Despite their limitations, these models provide good evidence that withdrawal from chronic ethanol use induces cognitive impairment, which is worsened by repeated bouts of withdrawal and that these impairments are dependent on the duration of alcohol withdrawal. Initial clinical observations with alcohol-dependent patients confirmed increased incidence of seizures. In recent years, accumulating evidence suggests that patients who have had repeated episodes of withdrawal also show changes in their affect, increased craving, as well as significant deterioration of cognitive abilities, when compared to patients with fewer withdrawals. Alcohol dependence is associated with tolerance and withdrawal, with neuroadaptations in γ-Aminobutyric Acid-A Receptor (GABA-A) and glutamatergic *N*-methyl-D-aspartate (NMDA) receptors playing key roles. It is suggested that dysregulation of the NMDA receptor system underpins alcohol-related memory impairments. Finally, we discuss the Structured Preparation for Alcohol Detoxification (SPADe) as an example of how prehabilitation has been applied in clinical practice. We discuss the importance of partial control over drinking as an interim step toward abstinence and early introduction of lifestyle changes for both the patient and the immediate environment prior to detoxification and while the patient is still drinking.

**Keywords: alcohol dependence, prehabilitation, withdrawal, detoxification, animal models, human research**

## INTRODUCTION

The concept of pre-habilitation has been introduced in the field of orthopedics and describes a set of exercises and training routines for certain groups of patients with the aim to maximize physical strength and reduce the risk of expected harm or frequent injuries, therefore taking a proactive rather than a reactive approach. The concept is applied in surgery with the aim of preparing patients for a surgical intervention. It is a strategy for proactive management of risk factors associated with the surgical intervention. The approach is therefore described as a shift away from an impairment-driven reactive model and as an opportunity for introducing proactive sustainable and appropriate lifestyle changes (1).

Central to the successful implementation of pre-habilitation are the concepts of expected harm or risk and proactive planning. Both concepts are considered to be crucial determinants of the interaction between humans and the environment in general, associated with human evolution and the progress from hunting to agriculture, structured communities, and human civilization. Planning is crucial in all aspects of everyday life. The ability to predict or anticipate certain harm or assess certain risks is associated with the human ability of learning from experience, modify behavioral responses, and develop long-term and sustainable response strategies. To that effect, planning in advance of anticipation of risks can be considered as an essential strategy associated with individual survival and progress. Planning should not been viewed as a barrier for improvisation and innovation; on the contrary, it provides a stable environment for progress and positive change to take place.

The term "alcohol dependence" was first introduced in 1976 (2) and was used in both International Classification of Diseases (ICD-10) classification systems (3) and the *Diagnostic and Statistical Manual of Mental Disorders, Fourth Edition* (*DSM-IV*) (4). In *DSM-5*, dependence is now conceptualized on a continuum with abuse, such that a single disorder is now called alcohol use disorder (AUD) with mild, moderate, and severe sub-classifications (5). Alcohol withdrawal syndrome is a collection of symptoms that occur after an alcohol-dependent individual stops consumption (6). Withdrawal from alcohol has been associated with cognitive impairments in recovering alcohol-dependent patients and furthermore the risk of relapse after withdrawal is associated with cognitive deficit (7, 8).

In this paper, we introduce the concept of pre-habilitation and its role in the clinical management of alcohol dependence. The approach has many aspects that overlap with other clinical management interventions, such as harm reduction and opioid substitution treatment. The overall aim is to reduce medical and other associated risks in a safe environment and to empower the individual to achieve the psychosocial changes required for recovery and social reintegration. Here, we focus on alcohol detoxification and withdrawal, given that it poses substantial risks to cognitive function. We review the evidence from animal studies, human psychological experimental studies, and imaging studies. We have conducted a narrative review of preclinical and clinical evidence regarding alcohol withdrawal or detoxification using online resources, e.g., PubMed and Google Scholar, and that were published in English prior to September 2018. For the preclinical evidence, we have focused the review on studies using cognitive behavioral paradigms rather than those on physical withdrawal symptoms, e.g., seizures. For the clinical review, we have focused on neuroimaging studies of relevant neurobiological processes. We also discuss the limitations of current pharmacological interventions. Finally, we discuss, in some detail, an example of a clinical implementation of the model. In this paper, we have chosen to use the older and longer established term "patient" rather than client or service user. This choice does not refer to a scientific or philosophical position.

## CURRENTLY RECOMMENDED TREATMENT PARADIGM TO MANAGE ALCOHOL DETOXIFICATION

Current clinical guidelines suggest that medically assisted withdrawal or detoxification is generally required for the treatment of moderate to severe alcohol dependence. This should be planned and the importance of providing structured aftercare is emphasized (9). Medically assisted detoxification is required to minimize the risks of withdrawal-related symptoms and complications.

The guidelines suggest that the patient prepares for detoxification by attending sessions at a specialist service to enhance and maintain motivation to change and develop a plan for structured aftercare (9). As described, the latter is considered important to ensure effective treatment. What is delivered however may vary widely with sessions not necessarily providing structured preparation to address issues such as stabilizing the amount of drinking, enhancing partial control over drinking, promoting early lifestyle changes, or empowering changes within the immediate family or social environment.

Detoxification may be medically assisted as an outpatient in the community or as an inpatient in a general hospital or a specialist unit. The choice between these two detoxification settings depends on health risk factors and the availability of social support to mitigate these risk factors during the detoxification process, and it is usually made by the health professionals (9). Medically assisted detoxification is discussed in more detail in Section 6 below.

Structured aftercare (also referred to as rehabilitation) is considered by clinical guidelines as the most important component of the current treatment paradigm, with strong evidence for its effectiveness (9). It is recommended that the structured aftercare that follows detoxification be delivered within a Cognitive Behavioral Therapy approach, either on an individual basis or *via* membership of a Relapse Prevention Group, alongside family interventions. It is highly recommended that patients engage with peer-support or mutual aid groups, such as Alcoholics Anonymous or SMART Recovery. Pharmacological interventions such as acamprosate, naltrexone, or disulfiram are also recommended. The existing evidence does not favor outpatient over inpatient detoxification, or residential aftercare treatment over community treatment, or longer versus shorter duration residential aftercare treatment programs (9). However, access to residential aftercare programs is recommended for homeless individuals, and efforts should be made to address accommodation issues prior to discharge (9).

Two of the long-term challenges for professionals (both academics and clinicians) involved in the treatment of alcohol dependence are the definition of successful outcome as well as the high relapse rate. For example, statistics from Public Health England for the period 2017–2018 suggest that 61% of clients complete treatment successfully (i.e., are free from dependence, which could mean abstinence but not necessarily), the same proportion as the previous year (10). This number provides an indication of how successful treatment is but is dependent on the definition of successful treatment, the severity of presenting problem, and the time when completion and exit are reported. Other indicators such as maintenance of abstinence for 6 months and 12 months for alcohol-dependent patients could enhance our understanding of the effectiveness of the current treatment paradigm. Our local data suggest that only 60% of patients who have completed planned detoxification have been engaged in aftercare interventions, which are considered to be essential for long-term recovery (11). This ratio has improved to 82% when a pre-habilitation approach has been implemented, such as participation in the Abstinence Preparation Group (see Section 7 below) (12). There may be several explanations for this improvement, including benefits of participating in a group or more specific theory-based factors such as regaining of partial control over drinking and early lifestyle changes (12).

In summary, current treatment guidelines advocate avoidance of unplanned and urgent detoxifications as they do not lead to sustainable outcomes with regard to drinking behaviors (9). They put emphasis on the provision of psychological treatment following detoxification and promotion of participation in peer-support interventions (9). Given the challenges in improving treatment outcomes, we consider that the main shortfalls of these guidelines are that (1) the only therapeutic input prior to detoxification is restricted to motivation enhancement and preparation of an aftercare plan without any theory-based structured intervention to manage the risks expected once alcohol is withdrawn, and (2) a large proportion of patients completing detoxification do not engage with any evidence-based aftercare to reduce the risk for relapse. Given that the majority of psychological interventions may not have an immediate effect, and the high risk of relapse during the first 3 months post-detoxification, we need to consider an alternative approach such as pre-habilitation to reduce the risk of relapse. Furthermore, the fact that these interventions are taking place during a period of mood dysregulation, which is the result of the detoxification itself, might compromise their effect.

## LEARNING AND HABIT DEVELOPMENT IN HUMANS

Humans have the ability to test out a new behavior as a solution to a challenge and—depending on the results (e.g., reward)—to either consolidate or abandon this behavior. Consolidated rewarding behaviors then become repeated in similar (or different) situations and, over time, become automatized. This leads to the fast replication of such behaviors—a bypassing of the conscious and careful consideration of pros and cons—since the analysis of their efficacy has already been done, in the past, and proven successful (13). The ability to automatize successful behaviors allows humans to continue with further learning and the accumulation of new skills and expertise. This ability to bypass the conscious decision-making control mechanism confers the advantage of fast and successful responses to dangerous environmental stimuli, but it has a major disadvantage: humans are not able to monitor the appropriateness of the behavior or assess the possible need for behavioral modification (13).

Whenever an automatized behavior requires modification, the learning process must be slowed down, in order to allow for the decision-making process to again become conscious. This does not refer to a meta-cognitive process, but rather to the creation of time and space between the high-risk situation and the behavioral response. In other words, implicit cognitions must again become explicit if the individual is to regain conscious control in order to modify the extant behavior. It is easier to undertake this reversal process (14) in a safe, practice-friendly environment, where those factors necessitating the fast reproduction of a behavioral response may be kept under control. Factors such as stress, threat, or uncomfortable physical symptoms typically provoke instinctive responses of a habitual nature. Humans tend to think more clearly and laterally when they can explore alternative solutions without facing immediate threat or being subject to stress.

### The Expected Risk in Alcohol Dependence

In the case of drinking (as well as other substance misuse), this leads to the state whereby habitual drinking dominates all other behaviors and becomes repeated despite the person's awareness of its loss of effectiveness and the accumulation of evidence of the associated harm. This leads the person into the paradox of wanting (implicit activation of need) although not liking (conscious desire and choice) drinking (15). From a psychological perspective, all explicit cognitions—such as positive and negative expectancies of the effect of drinking—which were conscious and under the control of the individual, are rendered implicit, and bypass the conscious decision-making pathway fuelling the continuation of drinking (13). This phenomenon is described as "loss of control", an underlying theme common to 9 out of the 11 criteria of Alcohol Use Disorder in *DSM-5* (5), three out of six criteria for alcohol dependence in ICD 10 (3), and one of three in ICD 11.

In the sections below, we discuss the risks associated with alcohol withdrawal and medication-assisted detoxification interventions. We review the evidence from animal models, pharmacological studies, and psychological experimental studies to explore risks such as cognitive impairment, stress sensitivity, the limitations of medication-based protective roles, as well as limitations of the existing treatment paradigm of planned detoxification and rehabilitation.

## ANIMAL MODELS OF ALCOHOL WITHDRAWAL AND DETOXIFICATION ON COGNITIVE IMPACT

Animal models have been used to try and understand the phenomenon of alcohol withdrawal and specifically to determine if repeated withdrawals particularly have an impact on cognitive function. Animal models have several advantages in alcohol research. They may be used to study determinants of alcohol-related behavior where there are ethical issues with carrying out such research in humans due to risks in giving volunteers or patients addictive harmful substances (16).

Further, animal models are used because animals have similar genetic, biochemical, and physiological compositions to humans. Therefore, research using animals can inform the understanding of the human condition and help lead to the development of new therapeutics. Some of the current medications approved for the treatment of alcohol use disorders (e.g., naltrexone and acamprosate) were developed using animal models (16). However, animal models do not represent the entire complex disorder; instead, they allow the study of component features of the condition and help provide evidence for the determinants of such behaviors (17).

There are currently several different methods used to model ethanol (alcohol) dependence in rodents such as forced consumption in drinking water, ethanol containing liquid diet, ethanol vapor inhalation, and repeated intraperitoneal or intragastric administration (18). In addition to route of administration, the length of ethanol exposure varies between models of alcohol use, e.g., from a 4-day chronic intermittent exposure (19) or a 6-month chronic model (20). The variation in both administration and duration of chronic ethanol administration complicates the interpretation of results. All of these models aim to mimic the neuroadaptations in the brain, which lead to tolerance and physical dependence of alcohol. A key issue with these models is the forced exposure to ethanol, which doesn't accurately represent the compulsive element of the human experience of alcohol dependency despite efforts to assess operant re-enforcing and conditioned responses (16). Induction of alcohol dependency in animals is considered to be successful if withdrawal symptoms are present upon cessation of exposure (18). However, this is representative only of a physical dependency and lacks the complexity of all the environmental and psychosocial influences that contribute to the complex human experience of alcohol addiction.

Animal models of alcohol consumption have also been developed to reflect voluntary alcohol consumption such as the two-bottle choice test, using gradually increasing concentrations of ethanol or adding sweeteners (17). Although preference tests are often influenced mainly by taste, some animals show a preference for the pharmacological effects of alcohol, and this has allowed genetic manipulation to produce high or low alcohol preference breeds. Rodents will voluntarily consume up to 40% ethanol (16). For the study of alcohol withdrawal, these voluntary consumption paradigms are often not sufficient because consumption levels are not high enough to induce withdrawal symptoms. Another limitation of these procedures is the difficultly to determine an animal's motivation to seek alcohol. Motivation to consume alcohol can be best demonstrated by an operant task model (such as lever pressing to receive alcohol in which the number of presses required increases) or a conditioned place preference task [for a detailed description, see (21)].

### The Impact of Withdrawal on Cognition

Physical withdrawal symptoms are similar in humans and animals and include tremors, agitation, rigidity, spontaneous seizures, audio sensitivity, handling-induced seizure sensitivity, and weight loss (22). However, alcohol withdrawal induces much more than just physical symptoms with low mood and anxiety evident. This negative affective state is thought to contribute to the risk of relapse in alcohol dependence and is therefore a critical area of study (these effects in humans are discussed in detail in Section 5 below). Withdrawal is thought to induce these effects *via* neuroadaptations from chronic ethanol's exposure on brain areas that control fear and memory. For this review, we focused on the studies assessing the impact on withdrawal from chronic alcohol exposure on cognitive function in rodents, which are summarized in **Table 1**. This table shows evidence that cognitive deficits are seen in animal models of withdrawal, that this deficit can worsen with repeated withdrawal, and finally that this cognitive impact varies with the length of the withdrawal period.

### The Presence of Cognitive Impact

The experiments in **Table 1** used behavioral paradigms following a variety of chronic alcohol models to assess cognitive function including the elevated plus maze, the T maze, social interaction, and conditioned fear response learning. These have been used to demonstrate withdrawal-induced impairments in learning (19, 31), cognitive flexibility (26), memory (20, 24, 25, 31, 36), sociability (38), as well as increasing anxiety (23, 27) and sleep disruption (35). In addition to the previously described limitations associated with animal models of chronic alcohol consumption and withdrawal, these studies are also subject to the limitations of the behavioral paradigms used. For example, several studies that illustrate the effect of ethanol withdrawal on inducing anxiety in rodents use paradigms such as the elevated plus maze, the light–dark box, and the open field (18). Measures used in these paradigms such as line crossings or % of time spent in the center, can be influenced by impaired locomotion of the animal, as well as anxiety, and therefore these results may lack construct validity. However, taken together, given the multiple cognitive defects assessed, it can be concluded that alcohol withdrawal may induce some cognitive impairment.

### The Effect of Multiple Withdrawals

Several of the studies described in **Table 1** indicate the worsening of withdrawal symptoms given multiple withdrawal episodes, which is consistent with the clinical picture. The best documented example of this phenomenon in rodents is the frequency of seizures following several detoxifications: known as the kindling

**TABLE 1** | The effects of withdrawal on cognition; a summary of research using animal models.

| Reference | Animal | Species | Gender | Age/weight | Chronic alcohol model | Daily alcohol intake | Withdrawal period | Cognitive testing/measure | Cognitive deficit present |
|---|---|---|---|---|---|---|---|---|---|
| (23) | Rat | Lister hooded | Male | 250–300 g | Ethanol-containing diet for 24 days 2 × 3-day withdrawal episodes | 13–14 g/kg | 2 weeks<br>2 weeks<br>2 weeks + 1 month | Negative patterning task<br>Contextual fear conditioning via a foot shock<br>Spatial learning in the Barnes maze | YES<br>NO<br>NO |
| (24) | Rat | Sprague–Dawley | Male | 160–180 g | In drinking water as sole source of fluid (20%) 8, 18, and 28 weeks | 12.2 to 9.7g/kg | 4 weeks | Eight arms radial maze (memory):<br>Spatial<br>Nonspatial | <br>YES<br>YES |
| (25) | Rat | Sprague–Dawley | Male | 200–250 g | 25% ethanol solution as the only source of fluid for 9 months (increasing concentrations from 10%) | 53–26 mg% | 2 weeks | Memory performance shuttle box:<br>Active avoidance<br>Passive avoidance | <br>NO<br>YES |
| (26) | Mouse | C57BL/6 | Male | At least 70 days old | Chronic intermittent ethanol exposure ethanol vapor (16 h/day for 4 days with 8-h periods of withdrawal) 3 consecutive cycles, with 3 days of withdrawal IP primer 1.6 g/kg | 175–225 mg/dl) | Up to 1 week | Behavioral attentional set-shifting task and reversal learning | YES |
| (27) | Rat | Wistar | Male | 250–280 g | 2 g/kg ethanol *via* gavage twice a day for 28 days | BAC up to 120 mg/dl | 5 days | Open field (exploratory behavior) | YES (lower frequency of rearing) |
| (28) | Rat | Hooded Lister | Male | 200–240 g | Nutritionally complete liquid diet 7% ethanol Single withdrawal, 24 consecutive days | 17.5 g/kg BAC 100 mg/dl | 12 days | Seizures (PTZ kindling)<br>Conditioned emotional response | YES<br>NO |
| | | | | | Nutritionally complete liquid diet 7% ethanol<br>Repeated withdrawal, 30 days, with two periods of 3 days, 11, and 21, in which they received control diet | | 12 days | Seizures (PTZ kindling)<br>Conditioned emotional response | YES (faster than either control or SWD rats)<br>NO ↓ |
| (19) | Rat | Sprague–Dawley | Male | 275–325 g | Catheters in the stomach 5 g/kg 25% in diluted nutritionally complete diet<br>Additional ethanol was administered every 8 h for 4 consecutive days | 7.6 g/kg | 4.5 days | Morris water maze (learning) | YES |
| (29) | Rat | Hooded Lister | Male | 200–240 g | Nutritionally complete liquid diet 7% ethanol<br>Single withdrawal, 24 consecutive days | 12.5 ± 0.8 g/kg | 2 weeks | Conditioned emotional response (fear conditioning low and high intensity):<br>Suppression<br>Extinction<br>Reversal | <br>NO<br>NO<br>NO |
| | | | | | Nutritionally complete liquid diet 7% ethanol<br>Repeated withdrawal, 30 days, with two periods of 3 days, 11, and 21, in which they received control diet | 12.9 ± 1.0 g/kg | 2 weeks | Conditioned emotional response (fear low–high intensity):<br>Suppression<br>Extinction<br>Reversal | <br>NO<br>YES<br>YES |
| (30) | Rat | Hooded Lister | Male | 200–240 g | Nutritionally complete liquid diet 7% ethanol<br>Single withdrawal, 24 consecutive days | 15.0 ± 0.4 g/kg | 2 weeks | Pavlovian-to-instrumental transfer | YES |

*(Continued)*

**TABLE 1** | Continued

| Reference | Animal | Species | Gender | Age/weight | Chronic alcohol model | Daily alcohol intake | Withdrawal period | Cognitive testing/measure | Cognitive deficit present |
|---|---|---|---|---|---|---|---|---|---|
| | | | | | Nutritionally complete liquid diet 7% ethanol<br>Repeated withdrawal, 30 days, with two periods of 3 days, 11, and 21, in which they received control diet | 15.3 ± 0.6 g/kg | | | YES |
| (31) | Mice | CD-1 | Male | 8 weeks | Only source of liquid increasing concentrations up to 20% ethanol<br>4 weeks | 0.20 ± 0.01 g/dl | 3 or 12 weeks after | T-Maze Foot shock Avoidance<br>Greek Cross Brightness Discrimination<br>Step-Down Passive Avoidance<br>Shuttle box Active Avoidance | NO<br>NO<br>NO<br>NO |
| | | | | | Only source of liquid increasing concentrations up to 20% ethanol<br>8 weeks | | | T-Maze Foot shock Avoidance<br>Greek Cross Brightness Discrimination<br>Step-Down Passive Avoidance<br>Shuttle box Active Avoidance | YES<br>YES<br>YES<br>YES |
| (32) | Mouse | C57BL/6J | Male | | Vapor exposure 16 h with 8-h break | 2.5–3.0 g/kg | 32 h | Odor cue conditioning influence on voluntary ethanol consumption 15% presented in a free choice situation with water 5 days | YES |
| (33) | Rat | Wistar | Male | 240–270 g | Nutritionally complete liquid diet as the sole source of nutrients.<br>All rats received the CON liquid diet for an initial 3 days then (6% v/v) for 14 days | 8.4–10.4 g/kg BEC 80.3 ± 7.5–132 ± 5.9 mg/dl | 8 h, 48 h and 72 h | Elevated plus maze. (anxiogenic-like effect)<br>Contextual fear conditioning (foot shock freezing) | YES (8 h only)<br>YES |
| (34) | Rats | Lister hooded | Male | 130–160 g<br>350–400 g | Nutritionally complete liquid diet 7% ethanol<br>Single withdrawal, 24 consecutive days | 18 g/kg Experiments 2 and 3 12.5 g/kg | 8 h | Elevated plus maze (anxiety)<br>Plasma corticosterone | YES<br>YES ↑ |
| | | | | | Nutritionally complete liquid diet 7% ethanol<br>Repeated withdrawal, 30 days, with two periods of 3 days, 11, and 21, in which they received control diet | | | Elevated plus maze (anxiety)<br>Plasma corticosterone | YES but no more than SWD<br>NO |
| (35) | Mouse | C57BL6/J | Male | 90–100 days<br>24–28 g | 4 bouts of 16-h exposure to EtOH vapor separated by 8-h periods of withdrawal | 64.76 ± 31.97 mg/dl | 4 days continuous | Electrophysiological recording from surgically implanted electrode:<br>Sleep time<br>Sleep architecture | <br>YES ↓<br>YES |
| (36) | Rat | Wistar | Male | 250–300 g | Self-administration continuous (24 h/day for 7 days/week) or intermittent (24 h/day for 3 days/week) access to alcohol (20%) using a two bottle choice procedure 5 months | <80 mg% | 24 h to 68 days | Working memory performance in a Y-maze and the delayed nonmatching-to-sample task (DNMS)<br>Elevated plus maze | YES (24–72 h) but not (16–68 days)<br>NO |
| (37) | Mouse | Swiss | Male | 8 weeks | 1–8 weeks of intermittent access to 20% 3 days/week 24–48 h between EtOH access days, two-bottle choice | 11.10–284.3 mg/dl | 6–8 h | Aggressive and nonaggressive behaviors with a conspecific | YES (aggression and decreased social contact) |
| (20) | Mouse | C57/BL6 | Male | 4 months at start | Source of liquid, concentrated solutions of ethanol 4% the 1st week, 8% the 2nd week, and 12% for 6 months | 15.34 ± 4.3 g/kg | Progressively withdrawn 1 week (1 W) | Working memory task. Spontaneous alternation was tested in a T-maze<br>Elevated plus maze | YES<br>YES |

*(Continued)*

TABLE 1 | Continued

| Reference | Animal | Species | Gender | Age/weight | Chronic alcohol model | Daily alcohol intake | Withdrawal period | Cognitive testing/measure | Cognitive deficit present |
|---|---|---|---|---|---|---|---|---|---|
| | | | | | | | 6 weeks (6 W) | Working memory task. Spontaneous alternation was tested in a T-maze | YES |
| | | | | | | | | Elevated plus maze | NO |
| (38) | Mouse | C57BL/6J | Male | At least 10 weeks old | Chronic intermittent vapor inhalation. 16 h separated by 8-h periods of withdrawal ip primer dose | 211.2 ± 25.0 | 3 to 10 days | Social Approach | NO |
| | | | | | | 208.8 ± 14.3 | | Novelty-Suppressed Feeding | YES ↑. |
| | | | | | | 211.2 ± 25.0 | | Digging | YES ↑ |
| | | | | | | 208.8 ± 14.3 | | Bottle Brush Tests | YES ↑ |
| | | DBA/2J | Male | At least 10 weeks old | Chronic intermittent vapor inhalation. 16 h separated by 8-h periods of withdrawal ip primer dose | 253.3 ± 16.0 | 3 to 10 days | Social Approach | YES |
| | | | | | | 173.3 ± 14.7 | | Novelty-Suppressed Feeding | NO |
| | | | | | | 169.5 ± 19.9 | | Digging | YES ↑ |
| | | | | | | 179.5 ± 22.3 | | Bottle Brush Tests | YES ↑ |

effect (39, 40). The kindling effect is defined by Pinel et al. as "the progressive intensification of elicited motor seizures that occurs during a series of convulsive stimulations"; this leads to increased susceptibility to convulsive seizures during alcohol withdrawal due to previous seizure-inducing withdrawals (39). The impact of multiple withdrawals also has a worsening effect on some of the associated cognitive impairments. This was demonstrated using rats fed an ethanol-containing diet (13–14 g/kg/day) for 24 days with two 3-day withdrawals compared with controls and with rats undergoing continuous ethanol treatment (23). These rats performed worse at negative patterning tasks but not spatial learning, which indicates that repeated withdrawals may affect some areas of cognition such as plasticity but not others. This differential effect of repeated withdrawals on only some cognitive defects is consistent with evidence that repeated withdrawals in rats compromised the acquisition of a conditioned fear response without impacting the recall of a previously learned fear association (29). These findings led to a hypothesis that multiple withdrawals induce aberrant neuronal plasticity, which gives rise to interesting predictions. Based on the idea that repeated withdrawal from alcohol results in repeated overactivity within glutamatergic systems (see below), it is possible that hyperactivation of glutamatergic systems would induce synaptic plasticity, leading to synaptic strength. If repeated withdrawals increase synaptic strengths, then stimulation of input pathways will have an enhanced effects on outputs, leading to certain excitability. However, if synapses are already strengthened, then the capacity for further plasticity will be reduced, leading to impaired learning of new associations (41, 42). However, further research is required to determine the underlying mechanism(s) behind multiple withdrawals reinforcing some but not all cognitive defects.

## The Duration of the Withdrawal Effect on Cognition

A key consideration is the duration of withdrawal from alcohol treatment. Some studies have looked at immediate effects of withdrawal after 8–24 h (23, 36, 37), while others assess cognitive defects present after a much longer period (several weeks) (25, 31). One key question is whether any cognitive impairment is long-lasting and/or persistent even following a significant period of abstinence. One study found that withdrawal caused significant working memory impairment during acute withdrawal (24–72 h) but not extended abstinence (16–68 days) (36). This contrasts with another study in mice in which short-term memory was not affected by withdrawal but learning and long-term memory were still impaired when tested 12 weeks after cessation of ethanol consumption (31). This suggests that withdrawal, while having a severe acute effect on cognition, may also cause long-lasting impairments. Therefore, the type of cognitive impairment present may also differ depending on the duration of abstinence.

### Proposed Mechanisms of Withdrawal-Induced Cognitive Dysfunction

There is much discussion about the mechanism by which withdrawal from chronic ethanol induces cognitive impairments.

Animal models have been used to link alcohol consumption with neurodegeneration and changing brain structure by neurotoxicity, reducing neurogenesis, and reducing the size of existing neurons. This has been related to dysfunctional behavior, which is suggestive of cognitive impairments (19). There have been several studies investigating the processes underlying these neurotoxicities. One such experiment in both rats and mice of both genders found increased levels of corticosterone in the brain tissue and plasma of both acutely (plasma) and prolonged (brain) withdrawn animals (43). Raised levels of corticosterone are known to cause neuronal damage, and it was therefore proposed as a potential mechanism underlying withdrawal-induced cognitive dysfunction. These raised corticosterone levels are thought to increase neuronal damage by potentiating excitatory transmission, inducing neuronal atrophy. Additionally, increased expression of NMDA receptors was found on the synaptic neurones of the medial prefrontal cortex, using a mouse model of chronic intermittent ethanol (26). This was also linked to a behavioral deficit in cognitive flexibility a week after the cessation of ethanol consumption. These findings suggest that the neuro-adaptive changes as a result of chronic alcohol consumption may contribute to withdrawal-induced dysfunction.

Other studies have focused on which brain areas are damaged during alcohol withdrawal, which may further inform how cognitive defects occur. For example, rat performance on a cognitive task was impaired by lesions of the basolateral amygdala (conditioned reinforcement and reinforcer devaluation) and central nucleus of the amygdala (Pavlovian-to-instrumental transfer) to identify which area is affected during single or repeated withdrawals. The result indicated that the central but not basolateral nucleus was affected during withdrawal. Similarity studies of mouse brains found that dendritic spine density was reduced in the lateral orbitofrontal cortex of mice following chronic intermittent exposure to ethanol (43). A comprehensive review of all relevant research is beyond the scope of this article; however, these examples provide evidence that the induction cognitive dysfunction following withdrawal is a complex process involving several brain regions. It is a vital area of research if we are to protect the brain, or at least limit the damage, in alcohol dependence.

### Conclusion From Animal Models

Ultimately, there are several different animal models of chronic alcohol consumption that are used to study the impact of withdrawal on cognition. While these models fail to replicate all the complexities of psychosocial and compulsive factors that occur in the human experience of withdrawal, these animal models provide good evidence that withdrawal from chronic ethanol induces cognitive impairment, that this impairment is worsened by repeated bouts of withdrawal, and that these impairments are dependent on the duration of alcohol withdrawal and abstinence. These animal models have led to the identification of neuroadaptations and increased levels of corticosterone as potential modifiers of cognitive deficits caused by withdrawal and which brain regions are vulnerable to or involved in these impairments. Understanding the risks of withdrawal and the underlying neurobiology is vital if we are to develop more effective therapies for reducing the damaging consequences of alcohol withdrawal.

## CONSEQUENCES OF REPEATED DETOXIFICATION OF PATIENTS DEPENDENT ON ALCOHOL

There is strong evidence that repeated detoxifications are associated with several cognitive and emotional impairments. Initial observations confirmed increased incidence of seizures (44–46). During recent years, accumulating evidence suggests that individuals who have experienced repeated episodes of withdrawal show changes to their affect, increased craving, as well as significant deterioration of cognitive abilities, when they are compared to patients with fewer withdrawals (47–49).

Several investigators had suggested that repeated episodes of detoxification increase the risk of withdrawal seizures. Further support to their suggestion came with the discovery of the differential response of alcohol-dependent patients to anxiety evoked by the noradrenergic alpha2 agonist, yohimbine, between those with two or more detoxifications compared to those with only one (50). These initial observations were followed by a plethora of experimental evidence showing that repeated experience of repeated detoxifications results not only in increased incidence of seizures and anxiety but also in increased craving and impaired inhibitory control of several behaviors in tasks (50, and in more detail below, e.g., 51, 52). Such tasks are challenging for high-order executive functions within problem solving or emotional evaluation contexts like reward seeking under conditions of incentive conflict, cognitive flexibility in an intra-extra dimensional shift, and reversal task and recognition of emotions in others.

Correspondingly, brain imaging shows that inaccurate performance on the cognitive tasks in alcohol dependence in humans who had experienced multiple detoxifications is associated with loss of gray matter in prefrontal regions; the loss of gray matter is positively correlated with the number of detoxifications. Evidence also suggests that the ability to recognize emotions in others (e.g., fearful faces) is associated with reduced connectivity between insula and prefrontal areas, but increased connectivity between insula and subcortical regions (colliculus) and between amygdala and other subcortical regions [e.g., bed nucleus of stria terminalis (BNST)].

Understanding the mechanisms that underlie the associations between repeated detoxifications and cognitive and emotional impairments as well as brain structure and functions alterations is mainly based on animal models [see previous section and (23)]. Additionally though, binge drinking (a tendency to drink excessively in one session leading to intoxication followed by abstinence) in young human adults has also been used as a model to explore possible predisposition to and early consequences of alcohol drinking in the form of repeated cycles (53–58).

Here, we will summarize the empirical evidence of the cognitive and behavioral deficits and their brain substrates associated with repeated detoxifications and how such deficits may increase vulnerability to relapse.

## Cognitive Control Processes Involved in Relapse

Increased urges to drink alcohol when induced by alcohol-associated stimuli and reduced ability to control the amount are recognized as the two basic processes of alcohol dependence. Inhibitory control is necessary for self-regulation. This is linked to executive function. Individuals who have low executive capacity or have damage to brain substrates subserving executive function display reduced ability for self-regulation and a greater susceptibility to behavior driven by stimulus and relapse (59, 60). Stimuli irrelevant to the present task or in contrast to the individual's current goals can diminish self-regulatory behavior in a stimulus-driven fashion and lead to relapse (61, 62). Other evidence, however, suggests that a stimulus-driven effect may be dependent on search goals driven by the individual's desire to consume alcohol (63). Several cognitive processes are considered to support self-regulation such as working memory and the ability to shift attention from previously relevant (but now irrelevant) stimuli (e.g., alcohol cues) to currently relevant factors (e.g., awareness of drinking consequences).

With the escalation of dependence, alcohol-associated stimuli become more salient and attract attention faster, thus diminishing the ability to inhibit the urge to drink. Such alcohol-associated attentional bias predicts relapse rates and treatment outcomes (64). Neuroimaging studies have provided strong evidence for the increased involvement of stimulus-driven networks (subcortical structures) and reduced involvement of brain substrates associated with cognitive control (65–67). Thus, as dependence progresses, relapse after several efforts to achieve and maintain abstinence becomes increasingly likely as distinct places, people, and paraphernalia associated with the reward offered by alcohol trigger an intense motivation within the addicted person to consume alcohol. As mentioned above, attentional processes (i.e., the ability to shift attention from previously relevant (but now irrelevant) stimuli to currently relevant factors may be crucial for self-regulation. Although impairments of cognitive control are associated with increased incidence of relapse in alcohol dependence, few studies have directly examined the possible impact of repeated detoxifications on cognitive control.

Alcohol-dependent individuals show impaired cognitive flexibility as measured in an intra–extra dimensional shift and reversal task (IED). This is associated with reduced volume of gray matter in a cluster within the inferior frontal gyrus (BA47) and the neighboring anterior insula. This is an area that shows reduced gray matter volume in alcohol-dependent patients and especially in those with a history of multiple detoxifications (52). The inferior frontal gyrus (IFG) is an area involved in inhibitory control. Observed decreased gray matter volume in this area suggests that decreased inhibitory control due to IFG damage may be linked with repeated relapses (68). Therefore, inhibitory control seems to modulate the translation of desire to drink into alcohol consumption and weakening of inhibitory control may lead to addiction (68). To that effect, strengthening inhibitory control may be an important cognitive strategy to prevent relapse (69).

## Social Competence as a Cause of Relapse: Brain Mechanisms

The cognitive deficits caused by reduced function of prefrontal brain areas (41, 42) in alcohol dependence, arising from repeated detoxifications, may not only contribute to inflexible behavior and perseveration of drinking but also to the impairments in social cognition, which is crucial for adaptive social interaction (70, 71).

Earlier studies have demonstrated that alcohol-dependent patients generally have reduced ability to recognize emotions expressed by facial expression in others (72–74). Our research has shown that such impairments may increase with greater numbers of detoxifications (75). Emotional recognition deficits are associated with less successful recovery (76, 77). A recent study that examined prospectively objective treatment outcomes found that alcohol-dependent patients who were poor in recognizing emotions in others were also more prone to relapse (78).

Neuroimaging findings have revealed brain changes associated with emotion recognition deficits most commonly in prefrontal cortex, amygdala, and insula brain areas (51, 52). The amygdala is the brain structure involved in processing of emotion (79) including the recognition of fearful facial expressions (80); the insula is associated not only with emotional processing but also with emotion regulation. Imaging the brain of alcohol-dependent patients during fear recognition in emotional facial expression of fear (74) revealed reduced connectivity between insula and prefrontal emotional regulatory regions (81–84). In particular, a reduced connectivity of insula with the anterior cingulate cortex (ACC), orbitofrontal cortex (OFC), and ventrolateral prefrontal cortex (VLPFC) was seen in alcohol-dependent patients with two or more detoxifications compared with either controls or patients with a single or no prior detoxification (51). Increased connectivity, also in patients with two or more detoxifications, was found between insula and a colliculus neuronal cluster, a region representing an important subcortical area for arousal mechanisms (85), as well as between amygdala and bed nucleus of stria terminalis (BNST). BNST has been identified as the key component area of stress-induced relapse in animal models of addiction (86). From these findings, it can be argued that increased connectivity in amygdala-related networks could lead to an increased emotional reactivity (84), whereas decreases in the network integrity of insula-related networks could lead to inappropriate analysis of the emotional input (87).

Importantly, the strength of connectivity between insula and areas involved in control of behavior and regulation of emotion (inferior frontal cortex, frontal pole) was negatively correlated with the number of detoxifications and with the ability to control drinking as evaluated by a self-rating questionnaire (ICQ; 51), suggesting a relationship between repeated detoxifications and the subjective perception of the ability to abstain. These findings further support that focusing treatment in reducing the impact of repeated experiences of detoxifications represents a reasonable approach.

## Incentive Conflict and Cognitive Control as a Cause of Relapse: Brain Mechanisms

From the above, it becomes clear that controlling drug taking depends on the ability of higher-level monitoring functions to interrupt the incentive process that is induced by the rewarding properties of the drug, but could also depend on the strengthening of the incentive process as addiction progresses (88).

Drug taking is considered as an impulsive choice for an immediate positive outcome based on previous hedonic experience or relief from pain or stress but on the possible expense of long-term health and social benefits. Alcohol dependence may impair processes that contribute to choice impulsivity (89), so that later consequences of drinking are not taken into account. For the alcohol-dependent patient trying for abstinence, the conflict between the desire to drink and the aim to abstain in order to avoid adverse consequences may be particularly strong, leading to erroneous choice at the time and a lapse.

We have studied aspects of the interaction between incentive learning and behavioral control using the incentive conflict task (ICT) (90). This is a version of negative patterning tasks used in cognitive psychology (91). When performing the ICT, subjects first learn that two independent discrete cues signal reward (money gains), and in this way, they acquire incentive properties. In a second phase, while the individual cues continue to signal reward, when presented together in a compound, they signal punishment (money losses). Participants have to learn to respond appropriately so that they respond to gain money when the stimuli are individually presented, but withhold responding to avoid money losses when the stimuli are presented in compound. The incentive conflict task is thus a task that puts demands on decision-making under conditions requiring conflict resolution. We have proposed that the task creates a conflict between abstaining and responding for reward, which is similar to that experienced by the patient before lapse. Therefore, the impaired ability of patients who have experienced multiple detoxifications to perform the task might reflect the consequences of the detoxification process itself on behavioral control.

As the number of previously experienced detoxifications increases, patients become increasingly impaired in withholding their responses in the condition of no reward, suggesting that the process of detoxification may engender brain changes that affect decision-making to avoid reward losses and lead to loss of control (90). This is consistent with deficits observed in a rodent version of the same task, in rats chronically exposed to alcohol (23). Importantly, in this well-controlled animal study, it was the number of withdrawal events ("detoxifications") that determined the extent of the deficit.

Neuroimaging of the ICT task with human control participants shows activation of several areas but most importantly those of the supplementary motor area, striatum (including putamen), gyrus rectus, ventromedial prefrontal cortex (vmPFC), and superior frontal gyrus areas, which are implicated in cognitive and emotional processing of reward (91–93) and regulatory control over a behavioral response (94, 95). Smaller gray matter volume in alcohol-dependent patients in the areas where dysregulated brain responses are seen during ICT have been reported, such as vmPFC and superior frontal gyrus, even more so in patients who had experienced more detoxifications. This is consistent with suggestions that these smaller volumes are "brain damage" associated with the detoxification experience. Further, the smaller volumes likely are associated with impairments in motivational decision-making, which involves the vmPFC (96, 97), and behavioral control, which involves the superior frontal gyrus (94, 95). Activation changes of vmPFC is shared with the gambling task (97), which resembles incentive conflict in requiring decision-making. Alcohol-dependent patients with several detoxifications also show impairments in this task (98). These findings are further supported by a study (99) that found that resolution of emotional conflict was associated with activation of an area that included the vmPFC.

Blunted response of the vmPFC in alcohol-dependent humans to the presentation of stress cues, a condition that the ICT also possibly generates, has been found to predict the incidence of relapse (100). Higher incidence of relapse with the possibility of trying to detoxify again leads to experience of multiple detoxifications found in our studies to be associated with smaller gray matter volume in vmPFC. Aberrant responsiveness to vmPFC to stress (101) is proposed to be associated with autonomic neural system dysfunction probably induced by the decreased ability of vmPFC to regulate emotional responses to stress or conflict situations. Prefrontal gyrus activation on the other hand may be more associated with the attentional and executive processes involved in inhibitory control that govern responding to ICT (94, 95, 102). Recent work on brain network efficiency of patients with alcohol dependence has identified, among other areas, the superior frontal gyrus area to show reduced nodal efficiency, supporting reduced ability of this area to carry out its functional activity (103).

The damage induced by alcohol—and detoxification—is not restricted to the areas identified in the ICT experiments. For example, the inferior frontal gyrus has been implicated in previous research during cognitive set switching (104) and also when resolving decision conflict during an instrumental learning task (105). Again, decreased inhibitory control due to IFG damage may support the occurrence of repeated relapses.

# BRAIN IMAGING OF ALCOHOL DETOXIFICATION IN HUMANS

Alcohol dependence is associated with tolerance and withdrawal with neuroadaptations in GABA-A and glutamatergic *N*-methyl-D-aspartate (NMDA) receptors playing key roles (106). Dysregulation of the NMDA receptor system is thought to underpin alcohol-related memory impairments (107).

## Imaging Glutamate in Humans

In humans, magnetic resonance spectroscopy (MRS) can be used to measure glutamate levels in the brain, albeit often with other metabolites and neurotransmitter and metabolic pools that cannot be robustly distinguished (108). A number of studies have reported greater glutamate levels in alcohol-dependent individuals during early withdrawal from alcohol.

One study reported greater MRS glutamate + glutamine (Glx) levels in the anterior cingulate cortex (ACC) at the start (day 1) of alcohol detoxification in alcohol-dependent individuals compared with controls, which normalized over the next 14 days (109). Benzodiazepines were used for treatment. Glx levels were not related to severity of alcohol withdrawal. Complementary preclinical translational studies showed that glutamate levels in the medial prefrontal cortex (mPFC) of ethanol-dependent rats were increased at 12 h of withdrawal compared with controls and during intoxication; the glutamate levels had declined by 60 h. A further study from the same group provided more evidence that a hyperglutamatergic state is associated with brain neurotoxicity. In both humans and rats, hippocampal glutamatergic function was found to be inversely related to volume, although notably, no differences were found with controls in either species (110). This may have been due to different methodology and lack of power to detect a group difference due to smaller hippocampal volume.

However, other studies have reported that human glutamate levels were lower in the ACC, dorsolateral prefrontal cortex (DLPFC), or parieto-occipital cortex (POC) 9 days after stopping drinking compared with "light drinkers" and normalized (i.e., increased) during the following month in ACC only (109). The authors suggested that their first time point may have missed the early elevation in glutamate reported by others and that, altogether, studies suggest that glutamate levels change during alcohol withdrawal and early abstinence. Although glutamate levels at the earlier time point were inversely associated with cognitive task performance, improved cognitive function was not related to any changes in glutamate or indeed other MRS markers [creatine, *N*-acetylaspartate (NAA), choline, and GABA]. Similarly, lower glutamine levels have been found in alcohol-dependent individuals who are still drinking, though breathalyzed negative at the time of the scan, compared with light drinkers (111). An inverse relationship between glutamate, but not glutamine, levels and number of heavy drinking days has been reported in ACC of alcohol-dependent participants but not light drinkers (18).

Higher levels of glutamate + glutamine in the nucleus accumbens and anterior cingulate have also been shown to be positively related to craving in recently detoxified alcohol-dependent individuals (112, 113). However higher levels have not always been reported in the anterior cingulate (112), which may suggest a differential rate of glutamatergic normalization in brain regions. No moderating effect of medication, e.g., diazepam or clomethiazole, was seen on glutamate levels and no relationship was seen with withdrawal symptoms (112). No cognitive measures were described in this study.

Although studies did not necessarily find any relationship of glutamate levels with clinical variables, this is likely due to the clinical heterogeneity of alcoholism in the small number of participants in these imaging studies. Due to the lack of appropriate longitudinal studies, it is not clear whether any differences in MRS-derived markers reflect the neurotoxicity or neuroadaptations from alcohol directly or predate alcohol consumption and increase the risk of an alcohol use disorder.

## Modulating Glutamatergic Function

In human alcohol-dependent individuals undergoing alcohol detoxification, those who received acamprosate compared with placebo resulted in a reduction in a glutamate:creatinine ratio between 4 and 25 days in the anterior cingulate (114). Diazepam was allowed if required during detoxification. It appears that any effect of acamprosate took a while to develop as it did not have an effect on alcohol withdrawal symptoms or on glutamate:creatinine ratio in the first few days of detox. Another study reported that glutamate levels were reduced after 4 weeks of acamprosate treatment compared with slight increases in those patients who did not receive acamprosate (113). The evidence from these studies is consistent with acamprosate having an "anti-glutamatergic" effect and that this likely underpins its clinical efficacy including reduction in craving. As no cognitive measures were obtained in the participants in either study, it is unclear if acamprosate did result in any cognitive benefits.

## Other MRS Markers

Other MRS markers of neuronal integrity and function have also been studied in alcohol use disorder. For example, evidence is not consistent with lower, higher, or no differences seen in the metabolite *N*-acetylaspartate (NAA), which is seen as a marker of neuronal integrity and function. This likely reflects the heterogeneity of the disorder and methodologies used. Nevertheless, there is evidence that NAA is lower as a result of heavy alcohol consumption, that it increases on stopping drinking, suggesting recovery, and that low thalamic NAA levels have been shown to be associated with poorer treatment outcomes at 3 months (115, 116).

## Imaging Inflammatory Response in Alcoholism

The inflammatory burden of alcohol consumption and dependence in regard to cognition is not well characterized in humans though it is likely to be an important target for treatment (115). Such inflammation may also contribute to alcoholism, increasing the risk of Alzheimer's disease (117). Positron emission tomography (PET) imaging studies assessing microglial activity with translocator protein (TSPO) tracers have shown lower, rather than higher, availability in abstinent alcoholics (106, 118, 119). Indeed one study showed that TSPO binding was positively correlated with verbal memory performance (118). Therefore, these studies suggest that lower glial density or an altered activation state with lower TSPO expression may contribute to cognitive impairment in alcoholism.

## Treatment of Alcohol Withdrawal/ Detoxification

As described, alcohol withdrawal and its complications develop as alcohol levels decrease and recurrent withdrawals result in increase in severity of symptoms due to kindling (120, 121). Such complications are also more likely in those alcohol-dependent patients who are hypoglycemic, hypokalemic, hypomagnesemic, or with infection or trauma (e.g., subdural hematoma) (120).

Treatment of alcohol withdrawal generally attenuates the risk of such consequences, but too frequently, alcohol dependence is missed due to lack of appropriate questioning or disclosure, so appropriate treatment is not started. Clearly, since delirium tremens and seizures reflect brain toxicity, there may also be an effect on cognition; thus, their prevention is paramount to protect brain function and optimize recovery. The reader is directed to clinical guidelines concerning more information regarding treatment of alcohol detoxification and prevention of complications (9, 122, 123).

Medically assisted alcohol withdrawal is generally treated with a reducing regimen of a benzodiazepine (e.g., chlordiazepoxide, diazepam, and lorazepam) (120, 122, 123). An alternative regimen is "symptom-triggered", where the benzodiazepine is given once symptoms meet a threshold for treatment. This requires regular monitoring of alcohol withdrawal symptoms with a validated scale [e.g., Clinical Institute Withdrawal Assessment for Alcohol (CIWA-Ar)] by appropriately trained staff and so is not suitable in all circumstances, e.g., a busy admissions unit or nonverbal patients. Other anticonvulsants may be used (e.g., carbamazepine and sodium valproate); however, a Cochrane review did not find evidence in favor of their use to treat alcohol withdrawal (124). It should be remembered that benzodiazepines are also effective anticonvulsants and therefore risk of alcohol-related seizures can be managed with sufficient doses rather than adding in another anticonvulsant (123).

Another important clinical intervention to reduce risk of brain toxicity is consideration of thiamine deficiency as this vitamin is a key co-factor in metabolism. Thiamine deficiency may present with "paresthesia" (pins and needles) in hands and feet with numbness and with Wernicke's encephalopathy (WE), which is a medical emergency. Clinicians are advised to be suspicious as the classic triad of confusion, ataxia, and ophthalmoplegia, suggesting the diagnosis of WE, are rarely seen together, whereas the first two symptoms are very commonly seen in alcoholism (123, 125). Clinically, thiamine deficiency and WE are generally only considered with alcohol detoxification when greater metabolic load increases the risk; however, it may occur at any time and in other addictions with poor diet and absorption. For those with WE or at risk of it, parenteral thiamine is required since absorption from oral thiamine is insufficient to replenish stores (122, 123, 125). Thus, giving thiamine appropriately is a critical intervention to protect brain function and prevent irreversible alcohol brain-related brain disorder.

As described, current clinical treatment with benzodiazepines may not be optimal in attenuating the hyperglutamatergic state of alcohol withdrawal. As described, MRS studies have shown that acamprosate reduces glutamate in the brain. Clinically, acamprosate appears to be well tolerated during alcohol detoxification, when added to benzodiazepines, though there is no impact on alcohol withdrawal symptoms as measured with the CIWA-Ar (114, 126). However, acamprosate during alcohol detoxification has been noted to improve sleep and reduce arousal levels (alpha slow-wave index) when assessed with magnetoencephalography (127). Therefore, it is unclear if acamprosate-related reduction in glutamatergic activity does improve cognitive outcomes either in the short term or in the longer term.

## EXAMPLES OF IMPLEMENTATION OF PRE-HABILITATION IN ALCOHOL DEPENDENCE

As described, the concept of pre-habilitation can be applied to the treatment of alcohol dependence, such as our model: "Structured Preparation for Alcohol Detoxification" (SPADe). Although SPADe has been applied on an individual basis, primarily it has been applied as an open, rolling group program, and described initially as Preparation for Alcohol Detox (PAD) and more recently as Abstinence Preparation Group (APG). The intervention may be regarded as a modified Cognitive Behavioral Therapy approach (128, 129), which is offered prior to detoxification and while the person is still drinking. The basic components of this treatment approach include (i) partial control over drinking, (ii) introduction of lifestyle changes for the individual, (iii) and the immediate family and social environment. Existing evaluations of SPADe treatment pathways suggest that about 72% of individuals with alcohol dependence presenting for treatment can engage and complete the pre-habilitation intervention (APG) (12).

### Partial Controlled Drinking

When presented as an alternative to lifelong abstinence as the sole treatment outcome (130), the concept of controlled drinking generates intense conflict within the field of addiction medicine. However, within clinical guidelines (9) controlled drinking within "healthy" limits may be considered as an appropriate treatment objective for harmful drinkers. For dependent drinkers, abstinence remains the preferred treatment objective (9).

The main aim of pre-habilitation is to pre-empt clinical withdrawal symptoms and the associated urges to drink. Within the SPADe treatment approach for alcohol dependence, controlled drinking is referred to as "partial" for two reasons: (i) it is an intermediate treatment stage rather than the final treatment aim, which is abstinence; and (ii) the amount and pattern of drinking are not within healthy limits. Therefore, within SPADe, the primary aim of the "partial controlled drinking" stage is to stabilize both the amount of alcohol consumed and the pattern of drinking. Alcohol is considered as "if it were a medication" with frequent and regular dosing to prevent the onset rather than to treat the appearance of withdrawal symptoms. This proactive elimination of symptoms is considered fundamental from a biological perspective, since it protects against acute brain dysregulation, which, in turn, might sensitize the brain, leading to an exaggeration of the negative impact associated with the disturbance of the brain homeostatic system. From a psychological perspective, it empowers the individual by restoring some control over decision-making and reducing the impulsivity associated with the experience and avoidance of cravings and withdrawal symptoms. Furthermore, partial controlled drinking provides a relatively stable environment for the individual—and their social group–to begin implementing lifestyle changes that lead to an increased sense of self-efficacy. This is considered the final mediating factor in social learning theory and cognitive behavioral treatment models (131).

The aim is to avoid substantial and dramatic reductions to the amount of alcohol consumed, which not only will prove unsustainable but might also lead to the precipitation of withdrawal symptoms, which could be life threatening. Thus, small sustainable changes are implemented, and once stability is achieved, a further gradual reduction of alcohol intake can be safely undertaken. In our experience, about half of the patients following this approach will be able to come off alcohol without the use of detoxification medication (12). This model of detoxification is called "guided self-detox", and alcohol is regarded as if it was a medication that is gradually discontinued.

### Early Introduction of Lifestyle Changes

The stabilization of drinking provides for a short period a relatively stable and safe environment for the patient, the immediate family, and the patient's social network to develop and test out lifestyle changes. Such early and gradual changes implemented within the individual's lifestyle are necessary to provide (i) a routine in everyday life that will protect against early relapse, (ii) a response to the void that alcohol detoxification would otherwise leave in its wake, (iii) a distraction strategy against the onset of craving, (iv) an enhancement of personal responsibility, (v) a de-mystification of alcohol and a challenge to the omnipotence of cravings or withdrawal symptoms, and, finally, (vi) protection against the acute sense of stress experienced in the early days of abstinence.

The involvement of family members and the immediate social support system in treatment helps in reframing the environment, modifying unrealistic expectations, and supports the gradual adaptation to the new family dynamics (following the removal of alcohol). It will help in managing the anxiety and difficult feelings/emotions associated with broken trust and promotes a partnership approach. Fundamentally, recovery is easier to achieve and more sustainable within a respectful, stress-free, and supportive environment. It is far easier for the patient to maintain abstinence (in particular during the first few weeks) within a family environment that is also abstinent, thus removing proximal cues/triggers (smell or sight of alcohol) as well more distant cues, such as elevated levels of stress or negative emotional states.

## CONCLUSION

In this review, we have described how alcohol detoxification is a neurobiologically challenging time for the brain and is associated with cognitive impairments that contribute to the high risk of relapse. Despite their limitations, animal models have demonstrated that alcohol withdrawals induce impairments in learning, cognitive flexibility, memory, sociability, increased levels of anxiety, and disrupting sleep. The evidence is mixed on the duration of these effects, suggesting that, potentially, in addition to the acute effects, there might be long-lasting impairments. Furthermore, repeated withdrawals may affect some areas of cognition such as plasticity but not all. Evidence supports roles for elevated levels of corticosterone or increased expression of NMDA receptors in neuro-adaptations underpinning alcohol withdrawal.

How does this evidence translate into human patients? There is evidence that with repeated detoxifications, withdrawal seizures, levels of anxiety, and experience of cravings increase, whereas inhibitory control of certain behaviors such as reward seeking, cognitive flexibility, and recognition of emotions in others is reduced. Furthermore, attentional bias towards alcohol-associated stimuli is increased and predicts relapse rates and poorer treatment outcomes.

The evidence from neuroimaging studies is unable to clarify whether any differences observed reflect the neurotoxicity or neuro-adaptations from alcohol directly or predate alcohol consumption and increase the risk of an alcohol use disorder. Nevertheless, it seems that current clinical treatment with benzodiazepines may not be optimal in attenuating the hyperglutamatergic state of alcohol withdrawal.

How could the above evidence guide our clinical practice? The evidence reviewed in this paper suggests that the process of detoxification from alcohol in humans seems to have a negative impact on cognitive functioning and create or worsen mood dysregulation. These effects are temporal, although the exact duration is not specific as multiple factors might have an effect beyond and above the severity of the baseline alcohol intake (chronicity, amount, and pattern). Nevertheless, given that this impact is anticipated, it is prudent to be prepared and proactive into managing the associated risks. To that effect, stabilization of the amount and pattern of drinking, empowerment of the individual patient and the immediate environment to prepare and implement lifestyle changes in advance of stopping alcohol, and furthermore the avoidance, if possible, of detoxification by a gradual withdrawal might prevent or provide protection against or increase the ability of the patient and the immediate environment to cope with them.

There is some evidence that people who had more than two detoxifications do worse than those who had less than two detoxifications. Although some of the cognitive impairment observed might be pre-existing (i.e., as part of increasing vulnerability to addiction), this evidence indicates that there might be an accumulating effect with worsening of outcomes and reduction of the possibility of achieving sustainable outcomes. If this evidence is correct and the hypotheses that repeated detoxifications have a long-term negative impact, then it is crucial to avoid repetition of detoxifications and approach each detox as if it would be the last one. A proactive approach within the spirit of pre-habilitation to maximize the chances of lifelong abstinence following detoxification is even more relevant.

Further, evidence presented suggests that the medication used at the moment does not protect from or necessarily reverse the negative cognitive impact and therefore is not optimal to reduce the risk of relapse and possible long-term accumulative negative effects of detoxifications. Until such medication is developed, active participation with aftercare interventions to maintain abstinence or at least keep drinking at low risk level is crucial and every effort should be made for patients to continue their treatment beyond the end of detoxification. A pre-habilitation approach that exposes and familiarizes patients to psychosocial interventions will enhance their ability to participate in aftercare interventions.

There are several clinical questions for which we require evidence. How many detoxifications should we offer within a specific period of time? How soon after a relapse should we offer another detoxification? Is there a washout period following a detoxification or are these effects permanent? Does this mean that, following two failed detoxifications, there is no further negative impact and therefore detoxification should be offered at any given opportunity? Given the above clinical uncertainties and the potential risks indicated by the reviewed evidence and until further evidence provides answers, a new treatment paradigm based on the principles of pre-habilitation in addition to rehabilitation seems to have major advantages in providing aspects of the rehabilitation treatment before detoxification. SPADe provides such a model, in which a structured Cognitive Behavior Therapy-based intervention, which aims to stabilize drinking, introduce early lifestyle changes, and involve immediate social system into proactive changes to support the early stages of abstinence, is consistent with pre-habilitation and is supported by preliminary evidence that might be effective (11, 12). It is important though to remind ourselves that one of the primary objectives of a pre-habilitation treatment paradigm is the empowerment of the person with the drinking problem and for the immediate social environment to take responsibility for the problem and be active agents of the solution. Structured interventions prior to detoxification should be offered within the spirit of pre-habilitation and not as a screening process to manage the ever-reducing budgets for inpatient detoxification as suggested in the most recent report of PHE (10). If implemented to screen patients, then such a use of pre-detoxification groups could create barriers into accessing treatment and compromise rather than enhance long-term treatment outcomes (10).

## AUTHOR CONTRIBUTIONS

CK: overall coordination of the manuscript with final editing and writing up of sections Introduction, Currently Recommended Treatment Paradigm to Manage Alcohol Detoxification, Learning and Habit Development in Humans, Examples of Implementation of Prehabilitation in Alcohol Dependence, and Conclusion. TD: written section Consequences of Repeated Detoxification of Patients Dependent on Alcohol; EP: written section Animal Models of Alcohol Withdrawal and Detoxification on Cognitive Impact; and AL-H: written section Brain Imaging of Alcohol Detoxification in Humans.

## REFERENCES


1. Wynter-Blyth V, Moorthy K. Prehabilitation: preparing patients for surgery. *BMJ* (2017) 358. doi: 10.1136/bmj.j3702
2. Edwards G, Gross MM. Alcohol dependence: provisional description of a clinical syndrome. *Br Med J* (1976) 1:1058–61. doi: 10.1136/bmj.1.6017.1058
3. *International statistical classification of diseases and related health problems. 10th revision*, Fifth edition, Geneva: World Health Organization (2016). II.ICD-10. ISBN: 978 92 4 154916 5
4. American Psychiatric Association (APA). *DSM-IV. Diagnostic and statistical manual of mental disorders. 4th ed.* Washington, DC: APA (1994).
5. Publication No NIH. 13–7999. (2016). https://pubs.niaaa.nih.gov/publications/dsmfactsheet/dsmfact.pdf.
6. De Witte P, Pinto E, Ansseau M, Verbanck P. Alcohol and withdrawal: from animal research to clinical issues. *Neurosci Biobehav Rev* (2003) 27:189–97. doi: 10.1016/S0149-7634(03)00030-7
7. Leber WR, Jenkins RL, Parsons OA. Recovery of visual-spatial learning and memory in chronic alcoholics. *J Clin Psychol* (1981) 37:192–7. doi: 10.1002/1097-4679(198101)37:1<192::AID-JCLP2270370140>3.0.CO;2-M
8. Noël X, Sferrazza R, Van Der Linden M, Paternot J, Verhas M, Hanak C, et al. Contribution of frontal cerebral blood flow measured by (99m)Tc-Bicisate spect and executive function deficits to predicting treatment outcome in alcohol-dependent patients. *Alcohol Alcohol* (2002) 37:347–54. doi: 10.1093/alcalc/37.4.347
9. *Alcohol use disorders: diagnosis, assessment and management of harmful drinking and alcohol dependence.* London: NICE (2011).
10. Public Health England. (Accessed accessed 11/01/2019). https://www.gov.uk/government/publications/substance-misuse-treatment-for-adults-statistics-2017-to-2018/alcohol-and-drug-treatment-for-adults-statistics-summary-2017-to-2018.
11. Kouimtsidis C, Ford L. A staged programme approach for alcohol dependence: cognitive behaviour therapy groups for detoxification preparation and aftercare; preliminary findings. Short report. *Drugs: Educ Prev Policy* (2011) 18(3):237–9. doi: 10.3109/09687637.2010.498392
12. Kouimtsidis C, Sharma E, Smith A, Charge KJ. Structured intervention to prepare dependent drinkers to achieve abstinence; results from a cohort evaluation for six months post detoxification. *J Substance Use* (2015) 21(3):331–4. doi: 10.3109/14659891.2015.1029020
13. Tiffany ST, Conklin CA. A cognitive processing model of alcohol craving and compulsive alcohol use. *Addiction* (2000) 95(8 Supplement 2):145–53. doi: 10.1046/j.1360-0443.95.8s2.3.x
14. Kouimtsidis C, Reynolds M, Drummond C, Davis P, Tarrier N. *Cognitive behavioural therapy in the treatment of addiction: a treatment planner for clinicians.* London: John Wiley and Sons Ltd (2007).
15. Robinson TE, Berridge KC. The psychology and neurobiology of addiction: an incentive-sensitization view. *Addiction* (2000) 95(Supplement 2):S91–S117. doi: 10.1046/j.1360-0443.95.8s2.19.x
16. Spanagel R. Alcohol addiction research: from animal models to clinics. *Best Pract Res Clin Gastroenterol* (2003) 17:507–18. doi: 10.1016/S1521-6918(03)00031-3
17. Tabakoff B, Hoffman PL. Animal models in alcohol research. *Alcohol Res Health: The journal of the National Institute on Alcohol Abuse and Alcoholism* (2000) 24:77–84.
18. Kliethermes CL. Anxiety-like behaviors following chronic ethanol exposure. *Neurosci Biobehav Rev* (2005) 28:837–50. doi: 10.1016/j.neubiorev.2004.11.001
19. Obernier JA, White AM, Swartzwelder HS, Crews FT. Cognitive deficits and CNS damage after a 4-day binge ethanol exposure in rats. *Pharmacol Biochem Behav* (2002) 72:521–32. doi: 10.1016/S0091-3057(02)00715-3
20. Dominguez G, Belzung C, Pierard C, David V, Henkous N, Decorte L, et al. Alcohol withdrawal induces long-lasting spatial working memory impairments: relationship with changes in corticosterone response in the prefrontal cortex. *Addict Biol* (2017) 22:898–910. doi: 10.1111/adb.12371
21. Blegen MB, Silva DE, Bock R, Morisot N, Ron D, Alvarez VA. Alcohol operant self-administration: investigating how alcohol-seeking behaviours predict drinking in mice using two operant approaches. *Alcohol* (2017) 67:23–36. doi: 10.1016/j.alcohol.2017.08.008
22. Pohorecky LA. Interaction of ethanol and stress: research with experimental animals–an update. *Alcohol Alcohol* (1990) 25:263–76. doi: 10.1093/oxfordjournals.alcalc.a045000
23. Borlikova GG, Elbers NA, Stephens DN. Repeated withdrawal from ethanol spares contextual fear conditioning and spatial learning but impairs negative patterning and induces over-responding: evidence for effect on frontal cortical but not hippocampal function? *Eur J Neurosci* (2006a) 24:205–16. doi: 10.1111/j.1460-9568.2006.04901.x
24. Arendt T, Allen Y, Marchbanks RM, Schugens MM, Sinden J, Lantos PL, et al. Cholinergic system and memory in the rat: effects of chronic ethanol, embryonic basal forebrain brain transplants and excitotoxic lesions of cholinergic basal forebrain projection system. *Neuroscience* (1989) 33:435–62. doi: 10.1016/0306-4522(89)90397-7
25. Melis F, Stancampiano R, Imperato A, Carta G, Fadda F. Chronic ethanol consumption in rats: correlation between memory performance and hippocampal acetylcholine release *in vivo*. *Neuroscience* (1996) 74:155–9. doi: 10.1016/0306-4522(96)00109-1
26. Kroener S, Mulholland PJ, New NN, Gass JT, Becker HC, Chandler LJ. Chronic alcohol exposure alters behavioral and synaptic plasticity of the rodent prefrontal cortex. *PLoS One* (2012) 7:e37541. doi: 10.1371/journal.pone.0037541

27. Hansen AW, Almeida FB, Bandiera S, Pulcinelli RR, Fragoso ALR, Schneider R Jr, et al. Taurine restores the exploratory behavior following alcohol withdrawal and decreases BDNF mRNA expression in the frontal cortex of chronic alcohol-treated rats. *Pharmacol Biochem Behav* (2017) 161:6–12. doi: 10.1016/j.pbb.2017.09.001
28. Stephens DN, Brown G, Duka T, Ripley T. Impaired fear conditioning but enhanced seizure sensitivity in rats given repeated experience of withdrawal from alcohol. *Eur J Neurosci* (2001) 14(12):2023–31. ISSN 0953-816X
29. Ripley TL, O'Shea M, Stephens DN. Repeated withdrawal from ethanol impairs acquisition but not expression of conditioned fear. *Eur J Neurosci* (2003) 18:441–48. doi: 10.1046/j.1460-9568.2003.02759.x
30. Ripley TL, Borlikova G, Lyons S, Stephens DN. Selective deficits in appetitive conditioning as a consequence of ethanol withdrawal. *Eur J Neurosci* (2004) 19(2):415–25.
31. Farr SA, Scherrer JF, Banks WA, Flood JF, Morley JE. Chronic ethanol consumption impairs learning and memory after cessation of ethanol. *Alcohol Clin Exp Res* (2005) 29:971–82. doi: 10.1097/01.ALC.0000171038.03371.56
32. Becker HC, Lopez MF. Increased ethanol drinking after repeated chronic ethanol exposure and withdrawal experience in C57BL/6 mice. *Alcohol Clin Exp Res* (2004) 28(12):1829–38.
33. Bertotto ME, Bustos SG, Molina VA, Martijena ID. Influence of ethanol withdrawal on fear memory: effect of D-cycloserine. *Neuroscience* (2006) 142(4):979–90. Epub 2006 Aug 23.
34. Borlikova GG, Le Merrer J, Stephens DN. Previous experience of ethanol withdrawal increases withdrawal-induced c-fos expression in limbic areas, but not withdrawal-induced anxiety and prevents withdrawal-induced elevations in plasma corticosterone. *Psychopharmacology (Berl)* (2006b) 185:188–200. doi: 10.1007/s00213-005-0301-3
35. Veatch LM. Disruptions in sleep time and sleep architecture in a mouse model of repeated ethanol withdrawal. *Alcohol Clin Exp Rese* (2006) 30:1214–22. doi: 10.1111/j.1530-0277.2006.00134.x
36. George O, Sanders C, Freiling J, Grigoryan E, Vu S, Allen CD, et al. Recruitment of medial prefrontal cortex neurons during alcohol withdrawal predicts cognitive impairment and excessive alcohol drinking. *Proc Natl Acad Sci U S A* (2012) 109:18156–61. doi: 10.1073/pnas.1116523109
37. Hwa LS, Nathanson AJ, Shimamoto A, Tayeh JK, Wilens AR, Holly EN, et al. Aggression and increased glutamate in the mPFC during withdrawal from intermittent alcohol in outbred mice. *Psychopharmacology* (2015) 232:2889–902. doi: 10.1007/s00213-015-3925-y
38. Sidhu H, Kreifeldt M, Contet C. Affective disturbances during withdrawal from chronic intermittent ethanol inhalation in C57BL/6J and DBA/2J male mice. *Alcohol Clin Exp Rese* (2018) 42:1281–90. doi: 10.1111/acer.13760
39. Pinel JPJ. Alcohol withdrawal seizures: implications of kindling. *Pharmacol Biochem Behav* (1980) 13:225–31. doi: 10.1016/S0091-3057(80)80034-7
40. Parsons OA, Stevens L. Previous alcohol intake and residual cognitive deficits in detoxified alcoholics and animals. *Alcohol Alcohol* (1986) 21:137–57.
41. Stephens DN, Duka T. Review. Cognitive and emotional consequences of binge drinking: role of amygdala and prefrontal cortex. *Philos Trans R Soc Lond B Biol Sci* (2008) 363:3169–79. doi: 10.1098/rstb.2008.0097
42. Stephens DN, Ripley TL, Borlikova G, Schubert M, Albrecht D, Hogarth L, et al. Repeated ethanol exposure and withdrawal impairs human fear conditioning and depresses long-term potentiation in rat amygdala and hippocampus. *Biol Psychiatry* (2005) 58:392–400. doi: 10.1016/j.biopsych.2005.04.025
43. Little HJ, Croft AP, O'Callaghan MJ, Brooks SP, Wang G, Shaw SG. Selective increases in regional brain glucocorticoid: a novel effect of chronic alcohol. *Neuroscience* (2008) 156:1017–27. doi: 10.1016/j.neuroscience.2008.08.029
44. McGuier NS, Padula AE, Lopez MF, Woodward JJ, Mulholland PJ. Withdrawal from chronic intermittent alcohol exposure increases dendritic spine density in the lateral orbitofrontal cortex of mice. *Alcohol* (2015) 49:21–7. doi: 10.1016/j.alcohol.2014.07.017
45. Baker TB, Cannon DS. Potentiation of ethanol withdrawal by prior dependence. *Psychopharmacology (Berl)* (1979) 60:105–10. doi: 10.1007/BF00432279
46. Brown ME, Anton RF, Malcolm R, Ballenger JC. Alcohol detoxification and withdrawal seizures: clinical support for a kindling hypothesis. *Biol Psychiatry* (1988) 23:507–14. doi: 10.1016/0006-3223(88)90023-6
47. Lechtenberg R, Worner TM. Relative kindling effect of detoxification and non-detoxification admissions in alcoholics. *Alcohol Alcohol* (1991) 26:221–5. doi: 10.1093/oxfordjournals.alcalc.a045104
48. Duka T, Townshend JM, Collier K, Stephens DN. Kindling of withdrawal: a study of craving and anxiety after multiple detoxifications in alcoholic inpatients. *Alcohol Clin Exp Res* (2002) 26:785–95. doi: 10.1111/j.1530-0277.2002.tb02606.x
49. Duka T, Townshend JM, Collier K, Stephens DN. Impairment in cognitive functions after multiple detoxifications in alcoholic inpatients. *Alcohol Clin Exp Res* (2003) 27:1563–72. doi: 10.1097/01.ALC.0000090142.11260.D7
50. Duka T, Gentry J, Malcolm R, Ripley TL, Borlikova G, Stephens DN, et al. Consequences of multiple withdrawals from alcohol. *Alcohol Clin Exp Res* (2004) 28:233–46. doi: 10.1097/01.ALC.0000113780.41701.81
51. O'Daly OG, Trick L, Scaife J, Marshall J, Ball D, Phillips ML, et al. Withdrawal-associated increases and decreases in functional neural connectivity associated with altered emotional regulation in alcoholism. *Neuropsychopharmacology* (2012) 37:2267–76. doi: 10.1038/npp.2012.77
52. Trick L, Kempton MJ, Steven CR, Williams SCR, Duka T. Impaired fear recognition and flexible behavior is associated with brain structural changes in alcoholic patients. *Addict Biol* (2014) 19:1041–54. doi: 10.1111/adb.12175
53. Krystal JH, Webb E, Grillon C, Cooney N, Casal L, Morgan CA, et al. Evidence of acoustic startle hyperreflexia in recently detoxified early onset male alcoholics: modulation by yohimbine and m-chlorophenylpiperazine (mCPP). *Psychopharmacology (Berl)* (1997) 131:207–15. doi: 10.1007/s002130050285
54. De Bellis MD, Narasimhan A, Thatcher DL, Keshavan MS, Soloff P, Clark DB. Prefrontal cortex, thalamus, and cerebellar volumes in adolescents and young adults with adolescent-onset alcohol use disorders and comorbid mental disorders. *Alcohol Clin Exp Res* (2005) 29:1590–600. doi: 10.1097/01.alc.0000179368.87886.76
55. Medina KL, Schweinsburg AD, Cohen-Zion M, Nagel BJ, Tapert SF. Effects of alcohol and combined marijuana and alcohol use during adolescence on hippocampal volume and asymmetry. *Neurotoxicol Teratol* (2007) 29:141–52. doi: 10.1016/j.ntt.2006.10.010
56. Nagel BJ, Schweinsburg AD, Phan V, Tapert SF. Reduced hippocampal volume among adolescents with alcohol use disorders without psychiatric comorbidity. *Psychiatry Res* (2005) 139:181–90. doi: 10.1016/j.pscychresns.2005.05.008
57. Sanchez-Roige S, Baro V, Trick L, Pena-Oliver Y, Stephens DN, Duka T. Exaggerated waiting impulsivity associated with human binge drinking, and high alcohol consumption in mice. *Neuropsychopharmacology: Official Publication of the American College of Neuropsychopharmacology* (2014) 39:2919–27. doi: 10.1038/npp.2014.151
58. Squeglia LM, Schweinsburg AD, Pulido C, Tapert SF. Adolescent binge drinking linked to abnormal spatial working memory brain activation: differential gender effects. *Alcohol Clin Exp Res* (2011) 35:1831–41. doi: 10.1111/j.1530-0277.2011.01527.x
59. Dretsch MN, Tipples J. Working memory involved in predicting future outcomes based on past experiences. *Brain Cogn* (2008) 66:83–90. doi: 10.1016/j.bandc.2007.05.006
60. Hofmann W, Gschwendner T, Friese M, Wiers RW, Schmitt M. Working memory capacity and self-regulatory behavior: toward an individual differences perspective on behavior determination by automatic versus controlled processes. *J Pers Soc Psychol* (2008) 95:962–77. doi: 10.1037/a0012705
61. Derryberry D, Rothbart MK. Reactive and effortful processes in the organization of temperament. *Dev Psychopathol* (1997) 9:633–52. doi: 10.1017/S0954579497001375
62. Mann T, Ward A. Attention, self-control, and health behaviors. *Curr Dir Psychol Sci* (2007) 16:280–3. doi: 10.1111/j.1467-8721.2007.00520.x
63. Brown CRH, Duka T, Forster S. Attentional capture by alcohol-related stimuli may be activated involuntarily by top-down search goals. *Psychopharmacology* (2018) 235:2087–99. doi: 10.1007/s00213-018-4906-8
64. Cox WM, Hogan LM, Kristian MR, Race JH. Alcohol attentional bias as a predictor of alcohol abusers' treatment outcome. *Drug Alcohol Depend* (2002) 68:237–43. doi: 10.1016/S0376-8716(02)00219-3
65. Hester R, Garavan H. Neural mechanisms underlying drug-related cue

distraction in active cocaine users. *Pharmacol Biochem Behav* (2009) 93:270–7. doi: 10.1016/j.pbb.2008.12.009

66. Luijten M, Veltman DJ, van den Brink W, Hester R, Field M, Smits M, et al. Neurobiological substrate of smoking-related attentional bias. *Neuroimage* (2011) 54:2374–81. doi: 10.1016/j.neuroimage.2010.09.064
67. Nikolaou K, Field M, Critchley H, Duka T. Acute alcohol effects on attentional bias are mediated by subcortical areas associated with arousal and salience attribution. *Neuropsychopharmacology* (2013) 38:1365–73. doi: 10.1038/npp.2013.34
68. Volkow ND, Fowler JS, Wang GJ. The addicted human brain: insights from imaging studies. *J Clin Invest* (2003) 111:1444–51. doi: 10.1172/JCI18533
69. Brewer JA, Worhunsky PD, Carroll KM, Rounsaville BJ, Potenza MN. Pretreatment brain activation during Stroop task is associated with outcomes in cocaine-dependent patients. *Biol Psychiatry* (2008) 64(11):998–1004. doi: 10.1016/j.biopsych.2008.05.024
70. Freeman CR, Wiers CE, Sloan ME, Zehra A, Ramirez V, Wang GJ, et al. Emotion recognition biases in alcohol use disorder. *Alcohol Clin Exp Rese* (2018) 42:1541–7. doi: 10.1111/acer.13802
71. Thoma P, Friedmann C, Suchan B. Empathy and social problem solving in alcohol dependence, mood disorders and selected personality disorders. *Neurosci Biobehav Rev* (2013) 37:448–70. doi: 10.1016/j.neubiorev.2013.01.024
72. Kornreich C, Blairy S, Philippot P, Hess U, Noel X, Streel E, et al. Deficits in recognition of emotional facial expression are still present in alcoholics after mid- to long-term abstinence. *J Stud Alcohol* (2001) 62:533–42. doi: 10.15288/jsa.2001.62.533
73. Kornreich C, Philippot P, Foisy ML, Blairy S, Raynaud E, Dan B, et al. Impaired emotional facial expression recognition is associated with interpersonal problems in alcoholism. *Alcohol Alcohol* (2002) 37:394–400. doi: 10.1093/alcalc/37.4.394
74. Maurage P, Campanella S, Philippot P, Charest I, Martin S, de Timary P. Impaired emotional facial expression decoding in alcoholism is also present for emotional prosody and body postures. *Alcohol Alcohol* (2009) 44:476–85. doi: 10.1093/alcalc/agp037
75. Townshend JM, Duka T. Mixed emotions: alcoholics' impairments in the recognition of specific emotional facial expressions. *Neuropsychologia* (2003) 41:773–82. doi: 10.1016/S0028-3932(02)00284-1
76. Charlet K, Schlagenhauf F, Richter A, Naundorf K, Dornhof L, Weinfurtner CE, et al. Neural activation during processing of aversive faces predicts treatment outcome in alcoholism. *Addict Biol* (2014) 19:439–51. doi: 10.1111/adb.12045
77. Maurage P, Campanella S. Experimental and clinical usefulness of crossmodal paradigms in psychiatry: an illustration from emotional processing in alcohol-dependence. *Front Hum Neurosci* (2013) 7:Article 394. doi: 10.3389/fnhum.2013.00394
78. Rupp C, Derntl B, Osthaus F, Kemmler G, Fleischhacker W. Impact of social cognition on alcohol dependence treatment outcome: poorer facial emotion recognition predicts relapse/dropout. *Alcohol Clin Exp Res* (2017) 41 (12):2197–206. doi: 10.1111/acer.13522
79. LeDoux JE. Emotion circuits in the brain. *Annu Rev Neurosci* (2000) 23:155–84. doi: 10.1146/annurev.neuro.23.1.155
80. Derntl B, Habel U, Windischberger C, Robinson S, Kryspin-Exner I, Gur RC, et al. General and specific responsiveness of the amygdala during explicit emotion recognition in females and males. *BMC Neurosci* (2009) 10:91. doi: 10.1186/1471-2202-10-91
81. Mesulam MM, Mufson EJ. Insula of the old world monkey. I. Architectonics in the insulo-orbito-temporal component of the paralimbic brain. *J Comp Neurol* (1982a) 212:1–22. doi: 10.1002/cne.902120102
82. Mesulam MM, Mufson EJ. Insula of the old world monkey. III: efferent cortical output and comments on function. *J Comp Neurol* (1982b) 212:38–52. doi: 10.1002/cne.902120104
83. Ongur D, Ferry AT, Price JL. Architectonic subdivision of the human orbital and medial prefrontal cortex. *J Comp Neurol* (2003) 460:425–49. doi: 10.1002/cne.10609
84. Liddell BJ, Brown KJ, Kemp AH, Barton MJ, Das P, Peduto A, et al. A direct brainstem–amygdala–cortical 'alarm' system for subliminal signals of fear. *Neuroimage* (2005) 24:235–43. doi: 10.1016/j.neuroimage.2004.08.016
85. Baas JM, Milstein J, Donlevy M, Grillon C. Brainstem correlates of defensive states in humans. *Biol Psychiatry* (2006) 59:588–93. doi: 10.1016/j.biopsych.2005.09.009
86. Aston-Jones G, Harris GC. Brain substrates for increased drug seeking during protracted withdrawal. *Neuropharmacology* (2004) 47(Suppl 1):167–79. doi: 10.1016/j.neuropharm.2004.06.020
87. Bechara A, Van Der Linden M. Decision-making and impulse control after frontal lobe injuries. *Curr Opin Neurol* (2005) 18:734–739.78. doi: 10.1097/01.wco.0000194141.56429.3c
88. Robinson TE, Berridge KC. The neural basis of drug craving: an incentive-sensitization theory of addiction. *Brain Res Rev* (1993) 18:247–91. doi: 10.1016/0165-0173(93)90013-P
89. Moselhy HF, Georgiou G, Kahn A. Frontal lobe changes in alcoholism: a review of the literature. *Alcohol Alcohol* (2001) 36:357–68. doi: 10.1093/alcalc/36.5.357
90. Duka T, Trick L, Nikolaou K, Gray MA, Kempton MJ, Williams H, et al. Unique brain areas associated with abstinence control are damaged in multiply detoxified alcoholics. *Biol Psychiatry* (2011) 70:545–52. doi: 10.1016/j.biopsych.2011.04.006
91. Bischoff-Grethe A, Hazeltine E, Bergren L, Ivry RB, Grafton ST. The influence of feedback valence in associative learning. *Neuroimage* (2009) 44:243–51. doi: 10.1016/j.neuroimage.2008.08.038
92. Elliott R, Agnew Z, Deakin JF. Medial orbitofrontal cortex codes relative rather than absolute value of financial rewards in humans. *Eur J Neurosci* (2008) 27:2213–8. doi: 10.1111/j.1460-9568.2008.06202.x
93. O'Doherty JP, Deichmann R, Critchley HD, Dolan RJ. Neural responses during anticipation of a primary taste reward. *Neuron* (2002) 33:815–26. doi: 10.1016/S0896-6273(02)00603-7
94. Floden D, Stuss DT. Inhibitory control is slowed in patients with right superior medial frontal damage. *J Cogn Neurosci* (2006) 18:1843–9. doi: 10.1162/jocn.2006.18.11.1843
95. Picton TW, Stuss DT, Alexander MP, Shallice T, Binns MA, Gillingham S. Effects of focal frontal lesions on response inhibition. *Cereb Cortex* (2007) 17:826–38. doi: 10.1093/cercor/bhk031
96. Bechara A. Neurobiology of decision-making: risk and reward. *Semin Clin Neuropsychiatry* (2001) 6:205–16. doi: 10.1053/scnp.2001.22927
97. Bechara A, Tranel D, Damasio H. Characterization of the decision-making deficit of patients with ventromedial prefrontal cortex lesions. *Brain* (2000) 123 (Pt 11):2189–202. doi: 10.1093/brain/123.11.2189
98. Loeber S, Duka T, Welzel H, Nakovics H, Heinz A, Flor H, et al. Impairment of cognitive abilities and decision making after chronic use of alcohol: the impact of multiple detoxifications. *Alcohol Alcohol* (2009) 44:372–81. doi: 10.1093/alcalc/agp030
99. Etkin A, Egner T, Peraza DM, Kandel ER, Hirsch J. Resolving emotional conflict: a role for the rostral anterior cingulate cortex in modulating activity in the amygdala. *Neuron* (2006) 51:871–82. doi: 10.1016/j.neuron.2006.07.029
100. Seo D, Lacadie CM, Tuit K, Hong KI, Constable RT, Sinha R. Disrupted ventromedial prefrontal function, alcohol craving, and subsequent relapse risk. *JAMA psychiatry* (2013) 70:727–39. doi: 10.1001/jamapsychiatry.2013.762
101. Blaine SK, Seo D, Sinha R. Peripheral and prefrontal stress system markers and risk of relapse in alcoholism. *Addict Biol* (2017) 22:468–78. doi: 10.1111/adb.12320
102. Goldberg II, Harel M, Malach R. When the brain loses its self: prefrontal inactivation during sensorimotor processing. *Neuron* (2006) 50:329–39. doi: 10.1016/j.neuron.2006.03.015
103. Wang Y, Zhao Y, Nie H, Liu C, Chen J. Disrupted brain network efficiency and decreased functional connectivity in multi-sensory modality regions in male patients with alcohol use disorder. *Front Hum Neurosci* (2018) 12:513. doi: 10.3389/fnhum.2018.00513
104. Kim C, Johnson NF, Cilles SE, Gold BT. Common and distinct mechanisms of cognitive flexibility in prefrontal cortex. *J Neurosci* (2011) 31:4771–9. doi: 10.1523/JNEUROSCI.5923-10.2011
105. Mitchell DG, Luo Q, Avny SB, Kasprzycki T, Gupta K, Chen G, et al. Adapting to dynamic stimulus-response values: differential contributions of inferior frontal, dorsomedial, and dorsolateral regions of prefrontal cortex to decision making. *J Neurosci* (2009) 29:10827–34. doi: 10.1523/JNEUROSCI.0963-09.2009
106. Most D, Ferguson L, Harris RA. Molecular basis of alcoholism. *Handb Clin Neurol* (2014) 125:89–111. doi: 10.1016/B978-0-444-62619-6.00006-9
107. Zorumski CF, Mennerick S, Izumi Y. Acute and chronic effects of ethanol on learning-related synaptic plasticity. *Alcohol* (2014) 48(1):1–17. doi: 10.1016/j.alcohol.2013.09.045

108. Myers JF, Nutt DJ, Lingford-Hughes AR. γ-Aminobutyric acid as a metabolite: interpreting magnetic resonance spectroscopy experiments. *J Psychopharmacol* (2016) 30(5):422–7. doi: 10.1177/0269881116639298
109. Mon A, Durazzo TC, Meyerhoff DJ. Glutamate, GABA, and other cortical metabolite concentrations during early abstinence from alcohol and their associations with neurocognitive changes. *Drug Alcohol Depend* (2012) 125(1–2):27–36. doi: 10.1016/j.drugalcdep.2012.03.012
110. Frischknecht U, Hermann D, Tunc-Skarka N, Wang GY, Sack M, van Eijk J, et al. Negative association between MR-spectroscopic glutamate markers and gray matter volume after alcohol withdrawal in the hippocampus: a translational study in humans and rats. *Alcohol Clin Exp Res* (2017) 41(2):323–33. doi: 10.1111/acer.13308
111. Prisciandaro JJ, Schacht JP, Prescot AP, Renshaw PF, Brown TR, Anton RF. Brain glutamate, GABA, and glutamine levels and associations with recent drinking in treatment-naïve individuals with Alcohol Use Disorder versus light drinkers. *Alcohol Clin Exp Res* (2018) 43(2):221–6. doi: 10.1111/acer.13931
112. Bauer J, Pedersen A, Scherbaum N, Bening J, Patschke J, Kugel H, et al. Craving in alcohol-dependent patients after detoxification is related to glutamatergic dysfunction in the nucleus accumbens and the anterior cingulate cortex. *Neuropsychopharmacology* (2013) 38(8):1401. doi: 10.1038/npp.2013.45
113. Frye MA, Hinton DJ, Karpyak VM, Biernacka JM, Gunderson LJ, Geske J, et al. Elevated glutamate levels in the left dorsolateral prefrontal cortex are associated with higher cravings for alcohol. *Alcohol Clin Exp Res* (2016) 40(8):1609–16. doi: 10.1111/acer.13131
114. Umhau JC, Momenan R, Schwandt ML, Singley E, Lifshitz M, Doty L, et al. Effect of acamprosate on magnetic resonance spectroscopy measures of central glutamate in detoxified alcohol-dependent individuals: a randomized controlled experimental medicine study. *Arch Gen Psychiatry* (2010) 67(10):1069–77. doi: 10.1001/archgenpsychiatry.2010.125
115. Zahr NM, Carr RA, Rohlfing T, Mayer D, Sullivan EV, Colrain IM, et al. Brain metabolite levels in recently sober individuals with alcohol use disorder: relation to drinking variables and relapse. *Psychiatry Res: Neuroimaging* (2016) 250:42–49. doi: 10.1016/j.pscychresns.2016.01.015
116. Zahr NM, Kaufman KL, Harper CG. Clinical and pathological features of alcohol-related brain damage. *Nat Rev Neurol* (2011) 7(5):284. doi: 10.1038/nrneurol.2011.42
117. Venkataraman A, Kalk N, Sewell G, Ritchie CW, Lingford-Hughes A. Alcohol and Alzheimer's disease—Does alcohol dependence contribute to beta-amyloid deposition, neuroinflammation and neurodegeneration in Alzheimer's disease? *Alcohol Alcohol* (2017) 52(2):151–8. doi: 10.1093/alcalc/agw092
118. Kalk N, Guo Q, Owen D, Cherian R, Erritzoe D, Gilmour A, et al. Decreased hippocampal translocator protein (18 kDa) expression in alcohol dependence: a [11C] PBR28 PET study. *Transl Psychiatry* (2017) 7(1):e996. doi: 10.1038/tp.2016.264
119. Hillmer A, Sandiego C, Hannestad J, Angarita G, Kumar A, McGovern E, et al. In vivo imaging of translocator protein, a marker of activated microglia, in alcohol dependence. *Mol Psychiatry* (2017) 22(12):1759. doi: 10.1038/mp.2017.10
120. Jesse S, Bråthen G, Ferrara M, Keindl M, Ben-Menachem E, Tanasescu R, et al. Alcohol withdrawal syndrome: mechanisms, manifestations, and management. *Acta Neurol Scand* (2017) 135(1):4–16. doi: 10.1111/ane.12671
121. Goodson CM, Clark BJ, Douglas IS. Predictors of severe alcohol withdrawal syndrome: a systematic review and meta-analysis. *Alcohol Clin Exp Res* (2014) 38(10):2664–77. doi: 10.1111/acer.12529
122. NICE. *Alcohol use disorders: diagnosis and clinical management of alcohol-related physical complications NICE clinical guideline 100 NICE.* London: National Institute for Health and Clinical Excellence (2010).
123. Lingford-Hughes AR, Welch S, Peters L, Nutt D. BAP updated guidelines: evidence-based guidelines for the pharmacological management of substance abuse, harmful use, addiction and comorbidity: recommendations from BAP. *J Psychopharmacol* (2012) 26(7):899–952. doi: 10.1177/0269881112444324
124. Minozzi S, Amato L, Vecchi S, Davoli M. Anticonvulsants for alcohol withdrawal. *Cochrane Database Syst Rev* (2010) 17(3)CD0050064. doi: 10.1002/14651858.CD005064.pub3
125. Caine D, Halliday G, Kril J, Harper C. Operational criteria for the classification of chronic alcoholics: identification of Wernicke's encephalopathy. *J Neurol Neurosurg Psychiatry* (1997) 62(1):51–60. doi: 10.1136/jnnp.62.1.51
126. Gual A, Lehert P. Acamprosate during and after acute alcohol withdrawal: a double-blind placebo-controlled study in Spain. *Alcohol Alcohol* (2001) 36(5):413–8. doi: 10.1093/alcalc/36.5.413
127. Boeijinga P, Parot P, Soufflet L, Landron F, Danel T, Gendre I, et al. Pharmacodynamic effects of acamprosate on markers of cerebral function in alcohol-dependent subjects administered as pretreatment and during alcohol abstinence. *Neuropsychobiology* (2004) 50(1):71–7. doi: 10.1159/000077944
128. Croxford A, Notley C, Maskrey V, Holland R, Kouimtsidis C. An exploratory qualitative study seeking participant views evaluating group Cognitive Behavioural Therapy group preparation for alcohol detoxification. *J Substance Use* (2015) 20(1):61–8. doi: 10.3109/14659891.2014.894590
129. Kouimtsidis C, Charge KJ, Moch JP, Stahl D. Abstinence Preparation Group Intervention for dependent alcohol users. How does it work? Results of a process study. *J Substance Use* (2017) 22 (2):149–55. doi: 10.3109/14659891.2016.1153164
130. Davies DL. Normal drinking in recovered alcohol addicts. *Q J Stud Alcohol* (1962) 23:94–104.
131. Kouimtsidis C, Stahl D, West R, Drummond C. Path analysis of cognitive behavioural models in substance misuse. What is the relationship between concepts involved? *J Substance Use* (2013) 19(6):399–404. doi: 10.3109/14659891.2013.837974

15

# A Novel Cognition-Guided Neurofeedback BCI Dataset on Nicotine Addiction

*Junjie Bu[1,2*†], Chang Liu[1†], Huixing Gou[1], Hefan Gan[1], Yan Cheng[3], Mengyuan Liu[3], Rui Ni[4], Zhen Liang[2], Guanbao Cui[5], Ginger Qinghong Zeng[1] and Xiaochu Zhang[1,3,5,6,7*]*

*[1] Department of Radiology, The First Affiliated Hospital of USTC, Hefei National Laboratory for Physical Sciences at the Microscale and School of Life Science, Division of Life Science and Medicine, University of Science and Technology of China, Hefei, China, [2] Department of Intelligent Medical Engineering, School of Biomedical Engineering, Anhui Medical University, Hefei, China, [3] Department of Psychology, School of Humanities and Social Science, University of Science and Technology of China, Hefei, China, [4] Department of Life Sciences, Imperial College London, London, United Kingdom, [5] Institute of Advanced Technology, University of Science and Technology of China, Hefei, China, [6] Hefei Medical Research Center on Alcohol Addiction, Anhui Mental Health Center, Hefei, China, [7] Academy of Psychology and Behavior, Tianjin Normal University, Tianjin, China*

***Correspondence:***
*Junjie Bu*
*bujunjie@ahmu.edu.cn*
*Xiaochu Zhang*
*zxcustc@ustc.edu.cn*

*†These authors have contributed equally to this work*

Compared with the traditional neurofeedback paradigm, the cognition-guided neurofeedback brain–computer interface (BCI) is a novel paradigm with significant effect on nicotine addiction. However, the cognition-guided neurofeedback BCI dataset is extremely lacking at present. This paper provides a BCI dataset based on a novel cognition-guided neurofeedback on nicotine addiction. Twenty-eight participants are recruited and involved in two visits of neurofeedback training. This cognition-guided neurofeedback includes two phases: an offline classifier construction and a real-time neurofeedback training. The original electroencephalogram (EEG) raw data of two phases are provided and evaluated in this paper. The event-related potential (ERP) amplitude and channel waveform suggest that our BCI dataset is of good quality and consistency. During neurofeedback training, the participants' smoking cue reactivity patterns have a significant reduction. The mean accuracy of the multivariate pattern analysis (MVPA) classifier can reach approximately 70%. This novel cognition-guided neurofeedback BCI dataset can be used to develop comparisons with other neurofeedback systems and provide a reference for the development of other BCI algorithms and neurofeedback paradigms on addiction.

**Keywords: brain-computer interface, cognition-guided neurofeedback, nicotine addiction, electro encephalogram, public dataset**

## INTRODUCTION

The brain–computer interface (BCI) is a hardware and software system integrated as the interface between the brain and the computer (Janapati et al., 2020). Considering time sensitivity and device portability, BCI system generally uses electroencephalogram (EEG), electrocorticogram (ECoG), functional magnetic resonance imaging (fMRI), functional near-infrared spectroscopy (fNIRS), magnetoencephalography (MEG), and positron emission tomography (PET) as imaging methods. Among them, EEG is the most widely used BCIs (Kwon et al., 2020). ECoG can collect purer signal than EEG, but it is invasive (Korostenskaja et al., 2014). Although fMRI and fNIRS have high spatial resolution, their temporal resolution is low (Cui et al., 2011). Besides, MEG and PET require large and expensive equipment and are not suitable for large-scale applications (Stam, 2010).

Nowadays, BCI system includes ERP, steady-state visually evoked potential (SSVEP), motor imagery (MI), and emotional BCI. In recent years, BCI-related fields have developed. Neurofeedback, as the predecessor of BCI, is applied to improve normal cognitive abilities, such as the enhancement of attention and working memory (Hsueh et al., 2016). It is also more and more used in the field of psychiatry studies, such as depression (Trambaiolli et al., 2021), anxiety (Gadea et al., 2020), addiction (Posson, 2019), etc.

Previous addiction-related neurofeedback datasets were usually based on fixed EEG or fMRI signals. Traditional EEG-based neurofeedback usually focuses on arousal/anxiety symptom in drug addiction by regulating α, α/θ, and sensorimotor rhythm (SMR)/β signals (Sokhadze et al., 2008). Real-time fMRI neurofeedback usually focuses on the activation of anterior cingulate cortex (ACC) or functional connectivity of bilateral ACC, medial prefrontal cortex (mPFC), orbitofrontal cortex (OFC), etc. (Martz et al., 2020). These datasets mentioned above have the following problems:

- No cognition task is performed to disclose the relationship between signals and behaviors/cognition components.
- Individual differences are not considered as all the subjects use a single and fixed signal to regulate the addiction behaviors.
- The efficacy of the traditional neurofeedback urges to be further improved in the treatment of addiction, as it is only rated as "probably efficacious."

Therefore, it is of vital importance to propose a novel neurofeedback paradigm.

We attempt to resolve the shortcomings of traditional neurofeedback by proposing the EEG cognition-guided neurofeedback based on a cue reactivity model. According to this model, when smokers are presented with visual, taste, or tactile cues related to smoking, they will have significant cue reactivity (physiological and physical reaction). Similar reactivity is found in healthy control subjects to non-drug evocative stimuli (Garavan et al., 2000). Cue reactivity leads to impulsive behavior in drug-seeking behavior as well as relapse (Chiamulera, 2005). The cue reactivity task is usually used to induce cue reactivity of participants. In our study, we used a smoking cue reactivity task to induce specific cue reactivity. Cue reactivity has multiple EEG features including both time- (e.g., P300, slow positive wave) and frequency-domain (e.g., alpha oscillation) features. Compared with the single signal, combing with multiple features (both time and frequency domain) using multivariate pattern analysis can better enhance sensitivity of detecting a particular brain activity pattern (Littel et al., 2012; Campanella et al., 2014). Our cognition-guided neurofeedback regulated the multiple signals induced by the specific cue reactivity. Therefore, the cognition-guided neurofeedback process included a specific addiction-related cognitive model (cue reactivity model). Based on this model, we performed the cognitive task (cue reactivity task) to obtain the specific addiction-related brain activities represented by multiple EEG features. In addition, this paradigm achieved a good intervention effect for smokers: the number of cigarettes consumed per day decreased 30.6, 38.2, and 27.4% compared with the baseline (pre-neurofeedback) at 1 week, 1 month, and 4 months follow-up (Bu et al., 2019). Our BCI dataset is based on a novel neurofeedback paradigm, which is closed loop, individualized, and MVPA based. Previous researchers have proposed a framework for cognitive neurofeedback in food cravings (Sokunbi, 2014; Ihssen et al., 2017) and cocaine addiction (Kirschner et al., 2018), but most of these studies are based on fMRI.

According to the cue reactivity model, smoking behavior enhances the conditional value of smoking cues, which is specifically reflected at two levels (**Supplementary Figure 1**):

- Bottom–up automatic processing to activate attentional functions.
- Top–down modulation of sensory inputting and motor controlling from cortical area.

According to conditioned reflex learning theory (Rees and Heather, 1995; Versace et al., 2017), the craving for cigarettes induced by smoking cues may partly relate to the conditioned reflex established by learning to associate smoking-related cues with smoking behavior (Karelitz, 2020). The reinforcement of smoking behavior also enhances the conditioned value of smoking cues, which automatically activates the attention function from the bottom to up. Besides, previous fMRI study has reported the regulation of cue-induced cravings from the top to down (Li et al., 2013).

Different from other neutral neurofeedback (for example, the height of the column is used for neurofeedback visual signals) (Zotev et al., 2014), we used an adaptive closed-loop method to develop our cognition-guided neurofeedback in the process of self-regulation training (Bu et al., 2019). The essence of this method is that when the participants' task performance decreased, the program would arouse the participants' attention and alertness by increasing the difficulty of the current task (deBettencourt et al., 2015). We established a mapping relationship between the probabilistic score and the 11 pictures (the probabilistic score was positively correlated with the desiring rating of the picture). Participants' brain activity state toward smoking cues was reflected as smoking-related pictures with different craving levels. At the same time, the picture would affect the brain activity pattern in the next trial, which was mapped to the corresponding smoking-related picture. In other words, we amplified the consequence of neurofeedback training: rewarding successful downregulation by reducing difficulty and punishing unsuccessful downregulation by increasing difficulty to activate participants' self-monitoring ability. By this way, an adaptable closed-loop effect was formed, which is one of the characteristics of our cognition-guided neurofeedback.

Neurofeedback intervention methods may produce different effects in different participants. Different visits of the same participant will also lead to different EEG signals (Gruzelier, 2014). Considering the individual differences of neurofeedback intervention and changeable craving of a specific participant, our neurofeedback paradigm built an individual model for each visit of each participant, which eliminated individual differences to a great extent. Each subject had exclusive classifier, and the regulated EEG signals (time and frequency domain) were obtained from his/her own cue reactivity task. The model used by the subject was reconstructed in the current cycle. Traditional neurofeedback regulated fixed signal, which may be not suitable in some subjects. Individual classification is one of the characteristics of our cognition-guided neurofeedback.

Traditional dependent neurofeedback usually includes single signal. There are also researches about neurofeedback based on network features, such as the algorithm based on common spatial pattern (CSP) and local characteristic-scale decomposition (LCD) developed by Ai et al. (2019). Addiction is a complex pattern of brain activity, rather than just being related to a certain electrical brain signal, such as P300 (Littel et al., 2012) and α power (Cui et al., 2013). The development of a classifier with more features or variables is particularly important. MVPA classifier is used to extract features of different dimensions from cue reactivity task (Zafar et al., 2017). This algorithm based on machine learning can detect the brain reactivity patterns in response to smoking and neutral stimulus more sensitively (Sitaram et al., 2017).

Our novel paradigm has a good performance and shows significant short- and long-term effects (Bu et al., 2019), but so far, there is a lack of novel neurofeedback-related datasets. Sharing these datasets online can facilitate comparison with other neurofeedback datasets, promote parameter optimization process, and help optimize the BCI algorithm. Single data may be limited. More datasets shared online can also be applied to big data models to get better results. In addition, BCI datasets are also instructive for BCI hardware development. In the field of psychiatry, more datasets on clinical nicotine addiction are needed to promote the study of addiction mechanisms, especially smoking cue reactivity mechanisms.

In this paper, we provide a novel dataset based on a cognition-guided, closed-loop, and individualized neurofeedback, which is based on MVPA classifier. The dataset includes EEG data of two phases: the cue reactivity task and the real-time neurofeedback training. In addition, we evaluated the quality of EEG data in our dataset by ERP and topographic map analysis. A linear correlation is used to indicate the trend of probabilistic score in neurofeedback training. Prediction accuracies of each participant are used to evaluate the classification power. The publication of novel cognition-guided neurofeedback dataset is of vital importance to the development of this field.

## MATERIALS AND METHODS

### Participants

In this study, 28 participants (male; mean age, 23.7 years) were recruited through online advertisements and posters by the criteria listed below. The score of Fagerstrom Test for Nicotine Dependence (FTND) of the 28 subjects were 4.6 ± 1.9 (mean ± SD, **Table 1**). Since there are only a few female smokers (2.7%) in China, we recruited only male participants for this experiment. This study was approved by the Human Ethics Committee of the University of Science and Technology of China (USTC). According our records, no participant reported uncomfortable feelings after neurofeedback training (Bu et al., 2019).

Selection criteria were as follows:

- Smoking 10 cigarettes or more per day for at least 2 years
- Right-handedness
- 18–40 years old
- Normal or corrected-to-normal vision
- Normal mental and physical health condition assessed by the Mini-International Neuropsychiatric Interview (MINI).

Exclusion criteria were as follows:

- Chronic neurological, psychiatric, or medical disease
- Taking any drugs in the past 3 months
- Unable to perform EEG for any reasons.

### Experimental Design

We developed a novel cognition-guided neurofeedback paradigm on nicotine addiction. Participants were involved in two continuous visits over 2 days. In each visit, participants experienced a two-phase procedure shown in **Figure 1C**: offline classifier construction and real-time EEG neurofeedback training.

Before the formal experiment, we prepared 330 pictures (210 × 180 pixels), including 150 smoking-related pictures (e.g., holding a cigarette in hand), 150 paired neutral pictures (e.g., holding a pencil in hand), and 30 pictures of animals (e.g., cat). The selection of these pictures mainly referred to the previous work on addiction of our laboratory (Zhang, 2011). To eliminate the possible impact of visual information, these smoking pictures and neutral pictures were matched as much as possible in terms of visual information such as background color, brightness, and object orientation. We recruited 20 participants to evaluate the craving degree of these pictures. The picture evaluation procedure is shown in **Figure 2A**. Eleven pictures were selected for real-time EEG neurofeedback training from 150 smoking-related pictures. They were listed in ascending order of the craving score given by the participants (**Figure 2B**).

**TABLE 1** | Demographic information of 28 participants.

| Characteristic | Value |
|---|---|
| Age (years) | 23.7 (3.8) |
| Education (years) | 14.8 (2.5) |
| Cigarettes (day) | 14.1 (4.5) |
| Cigarette use (years) | 7.1 (3.9) |
| FTND score | 4.6 (1.9) |

*Values were mean and values in parentheses were 1 standard deviation (SD).*

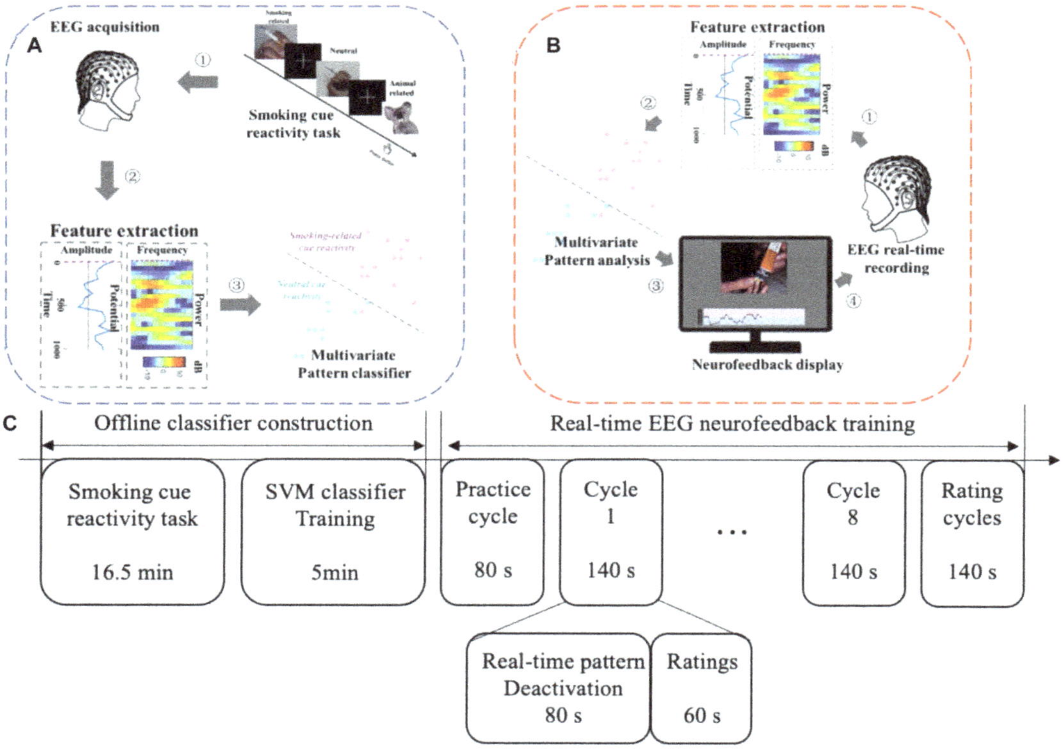


**FIGURE 1 |** Two phases for one neurofeedback visit: offline model construction and real-time neurofeedback training. **(A)** Offline classifier construction phase. **(B)** Real-time EEG neurofeedback training phase. **(C)** Experimental protocol in one visit. NF, neurofeedback.

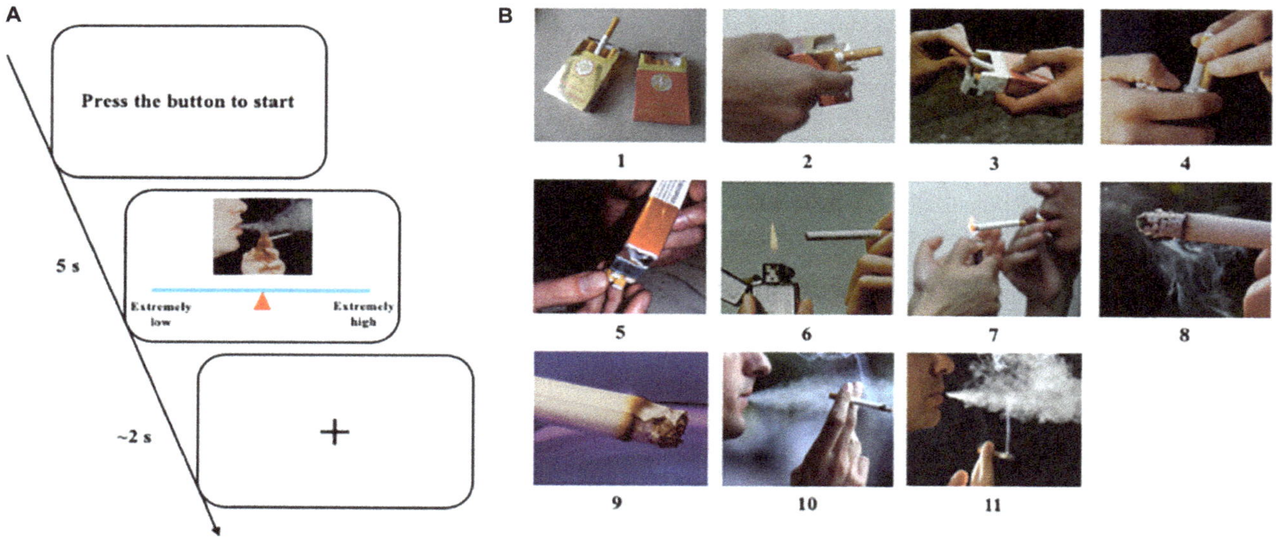


**FIGURE 2 |** Evaluation of nicotine related cues. **(A)** Picture evaluation protocol and procedure. Participants pressed the button to start a new trial. They had 5 s to move the mouse to change the position of the triangle on the line to give an appropriate score according to their craving to this picture. Then, they had about 2 s to rest and wait for the next trial. **(B)** Eleven selected pictures listed in ascending order of craving score.

### Offline Classifier Construction

Offline classifier construction consisted of two parts: the smoking cue reactivity task and the support vector machines (SVMs) classifier training (**Figure 1A**). EEG data collected from cue reactivity task were used to train the classifier.

The smoking cue reactivity task was block design. Three smoking and neutral blocks each were assessed in a pseudo-randomized order (neutral, smoking, smoking, neutral, smoking, and neutral). There were 55 trials in each block, and participants were requested to focus on the pictures as much as possible. Among them, 50 trials were smoking or neutral cues. Another five randomly distributed trials were animal cues, which were used to improve the concentration of participants on the task. They were asked to press the space button of the keyboard quickly and accurately when seeing animal cues (the main objects are animals, such as cats and dogs) and press the space button of the keyboard quickly and accurately. At the same time, EEG data were collected during each block. In the block interval, participants had 90 s of rest. The smoking cue reactivity program was written by Psychophysics Toolbox[1] for MATLAB (version 2016a, MathWorks Inc., Natick, MA, United States).

EEG data were processed offline in order to remove noise using EEGLAB (more details and parameters will be mentioned in *Data processing*). Permutation test was performed to extract features in time and frequency domain from the processed data ($\alpha$ = 0.05). Specifically, we compared EEG data collected from smoking and neutral blocks to obtain significantly different features in time (amplitude) and frequency (power) domain. These statistically significant features were transferred to cluster features via cluster-based statistic (maximum cluster-level mass) and imported into the classifier in the form of a column vector to train a personalized SVM classifier to recognize brain activity patterns in response to smoking stimuli. This step was calculated using the MATLAB function fitcsvm (Bu et al., 2019). Sixty channels (64 standard channels except for CB1, CB2, HEOG, and VEOG) were used to construct the model. In order to evaluate the classification effectiveness of the classifier, we used 20% of the trials to calculate the prediction accuracy in each cross-validation cycle. This step repeated five times for each participant.

### Real-Time EEG Neurofeedback Training

The neurofeedback training phase comprised eight same cycles in total, including 40 trials (80 s) and a rating (60 s) in each phase. Before the first trial, we carried out a practice cycle to make sure that participants understand the experimental requirements (**Figure 3**).

The real-time neurofeedback signal of each trial was updated every 2 s, including 1 s of real-time EEG acquisition and classification each. Online preprocessing (the same with offline processing mentioned above) was performed to remove noise. Processed EEG raw data were put into the classifier. Based on the SVM classifier, a probabilistic score (range, 0–1) was returned to characterize the similarity probability between the current brain activity and the brain activity pattern of smoking measured in smoking cue reactivity task. The probabilistic score was presented to participants in real time as a moving point in the feedback line at the bottom of the screen (**Figure 1B**). In order to prevent drastic changes of the line, the value of each point was obtained by averaging the value of the current point and the previous 2 points, and the first 2 points in the line were fixed 0.5 (no previous points to be averaged). At the same time, based on this value, the corresponding type of picture was displayed on the top of the screen according to adaptive closed-loop design. A higher probabilistic score corresponded to a picture with a higher craving level. This closed-loop neurofeedback program was written by Psychophysics Toolbox for MATLAB.

[1] http://psychtoolbox.org/

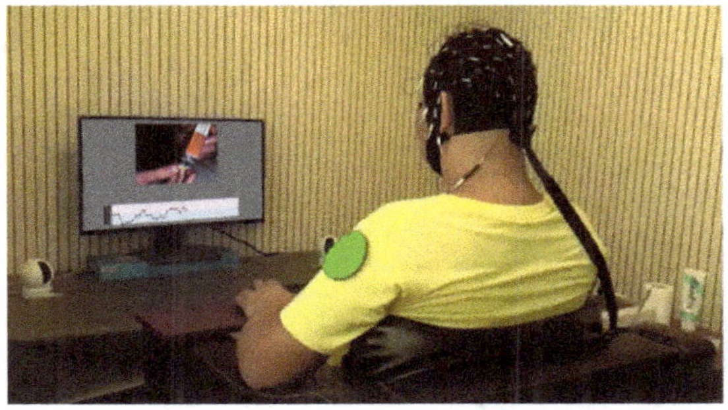

**FIGURE 3 |** One scene of a participant in the phase of neurofeedback regulation training. A participant is wearing EEG cap and watching neurofeedback display. A camera to monitor the status of the participant.

In this phase, participants were asked to downregulate the line repeatedly and continuously while fixating the picture. If one strategy failed to downgrade the line well, they needed to change the strategy until they found the most effective one. After finishing training and rating cycles (**Figure 1C**), participants were asked to record 10 mental strategies that may effectively downregulate the neurofeedback signals. To improve the initiative of participants, we informed them about the rewards they can get for completing the experiment in advance. Participants who completed eight cycles would receive a reward of up to 140 RMB according to their performance (proportional to mean probabilistic score). After completing a cycle, participants would have a rest for 1 min.

## Data Acquisition

EEG raw data were collected using a SynAmps RT amplifier (NeuroScan, Inc., Sterling, VA, United States), and an electrode cap was with 64 Ag/AgCl electrodes located according to international 10–20 system. Additionally, the left (M1) and right mastoids (M2) were also recorded. The impedance of all electrodes was kept under 5 k$\Omega$ based on the reference electrode attached to the tip of the nose. The EOG was recorded by VEOG (above and below the left eye) and HEOG (lateral to the outer canthi of both eyes) using four electrodes (VEOL, VEOU, HEOL, and HEOR). In order to reduce the influence of electromagnetic interference on EEG signals, we grounded the AFz electrode. The sampling rate of the EEG raw data was 250 Hz. In neurofeedback sessions, EEG raw signals were collected with the same parameters and sent to MATLAB program using NeuroScan Access SDK (NeuroScan, Inc., Sterling, VA, United States).

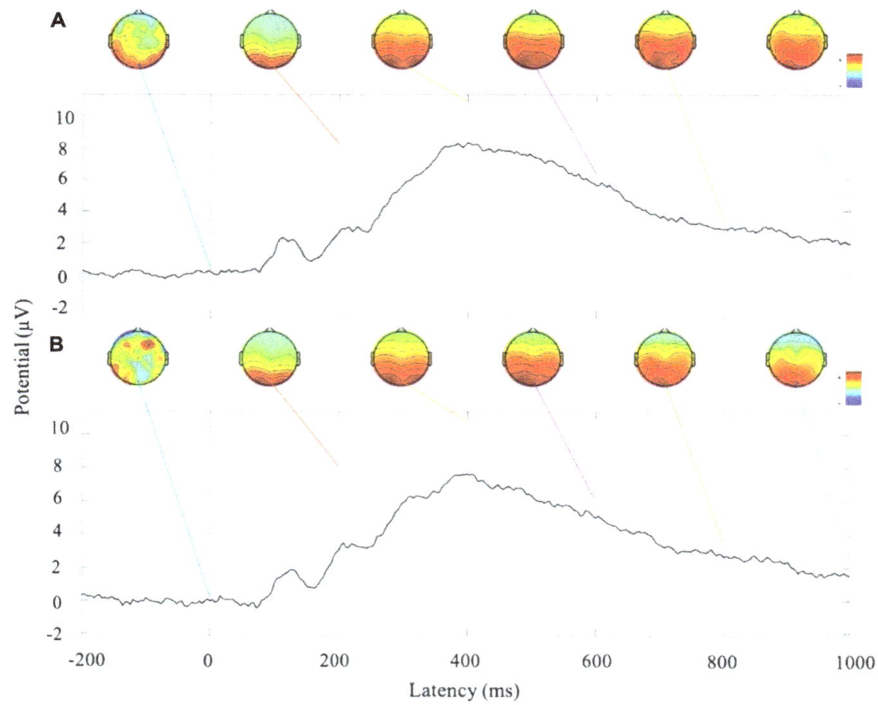


**FIGURE 4 |** Analysis of ERP amplitude and topographic map of cue reactivity task. **(A)** ERP waveform and topographic maps of the first visit of cue reactivity task phase. **(B)** ERP waveform and topographic maps of the second visit of cue reactivity task phase.

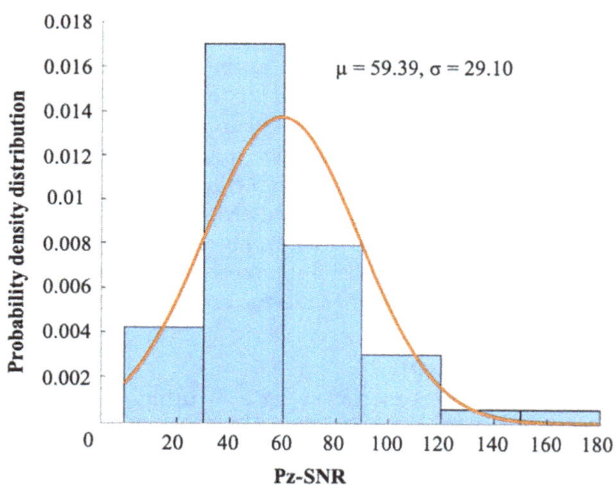


**FIGURE 5 |** The distribution of the SNR of Pz channel ($\mu$ = 59.39, $\sigma$ = 29.10). There were 55 runs of 28 subjects. There was no significant difference between the distribution and the normal distribution by KS test ($p$ = 0.29).

## Data Processing

The EEG raw data processing was conducted by EEGLAB toolbox (version 14_1_1b) for MATLAB. The preprocessing steps included high-pass filter (0.5 Hz), epoch (−200 to 1,000 ms, −200 to 0 ms as prestimulus interval to conduct baseline correction), and blink artifacts (using a conventional recursive least squares algorithm). ERP analysis was also conducted in EEGLAB. Epochs containing the amplitude changes exceeding ±100 mV were rejected. The ERPs were grand averaged based on different types of stimulus (smoking and neutral) across participants. The power characteristics of the time–frequency domain were mainly obtained based on the wavelet analysis algorithm. The frequency of the EEG data was divided into five ranges: alpha, low beta, high beta, low gamma, and high gamma waves.

## Data Evaluation

At the offline classifier construction phase of the cue reactivity task, EEG raw data were collected, and the signal-to-noise ratio (SNR) of Pz channel was calculated to verify the quality of the data (Hu et al., 2010). EEG epochs from −200 to 1,000 ms were preprocessed and averaged to calculate ERP waveforms separately for two visits. Besides, topographic maps were shown every 200 ms in the time window of 0–1,000 ms. Processed EEG data were imported to the classifier, and fivefold cross-validation accuracy was used to calculate its prediction accuracy.

In neurofeedback training phase, 1-s EEG data were preprocessed and shown at only channels located on the frontal midline. Topographic maps were shown every 200 ms in the time window of 0–1,000 ms. These 1-s EEG data were inputted to the personalized classifier model built in the offline phase, and a probabilistic score of smoking cue reactivity patterns was given. The score reflected the matching degree between the participant's current brain activity pattern and the pattern

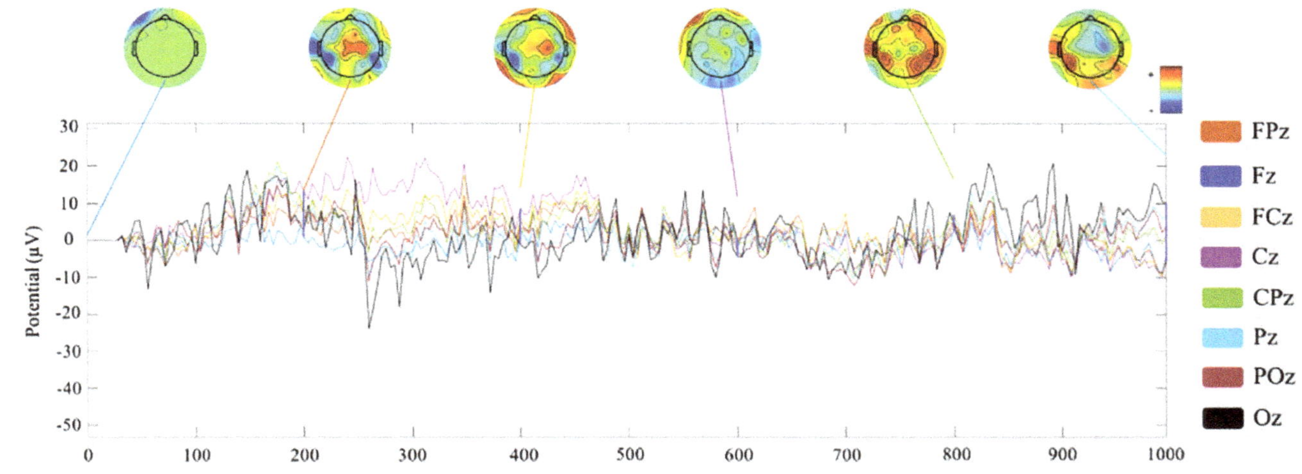


**FIGURE 6 |** Channel waveform and topographic map of real-time neurofeedback training phase.

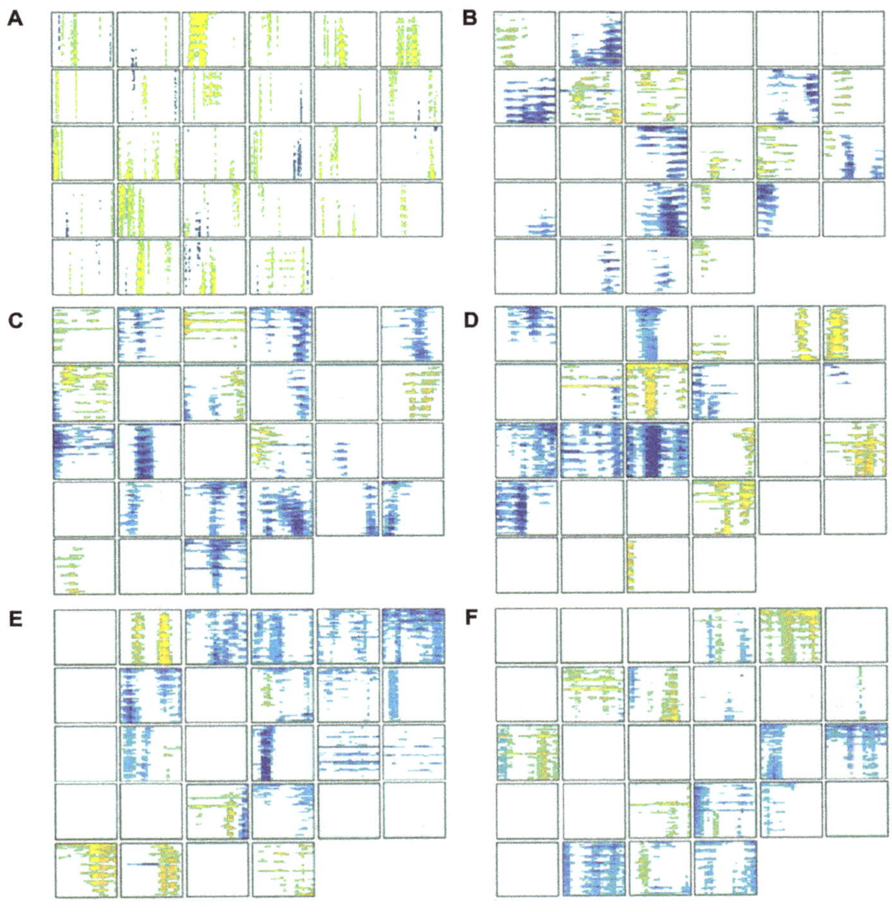


**FIGURE 7 |** The statistically significant features used to construct the classifier. **(A)** The features of each subject in the time domain; **(B)** the features in the alpha (8–13 Hz) frequency band; **(C)** the features in the low beta (14–20 Hz) frequency band; **(D)** the features in the high beta (21–30 Hz) frequency band; **(E)** the features in the low gamma (31–48 Hz) frequency band; **(F)** the features in the high-gamma (52–80 Hz) frequency band.

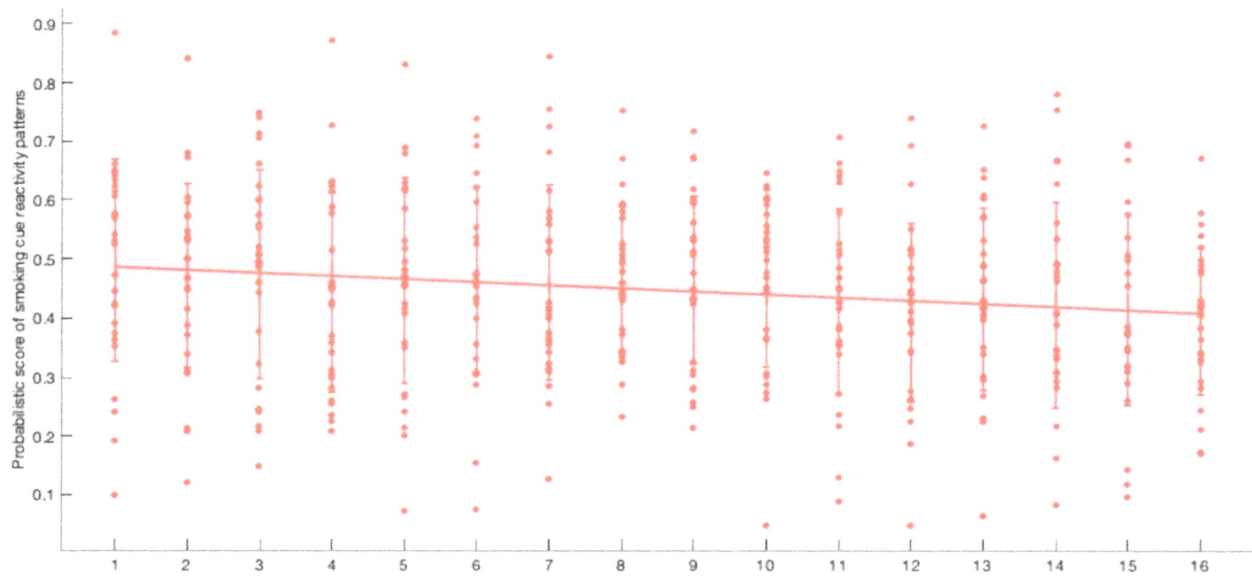


**FIGURE 8 |** Within two visit of neurofeedback learning, participants tried to reduce the probabilistic score ($r = -0.1545$, $p = 0.0010$). Error bar: SD; shaded area: 95% CI.

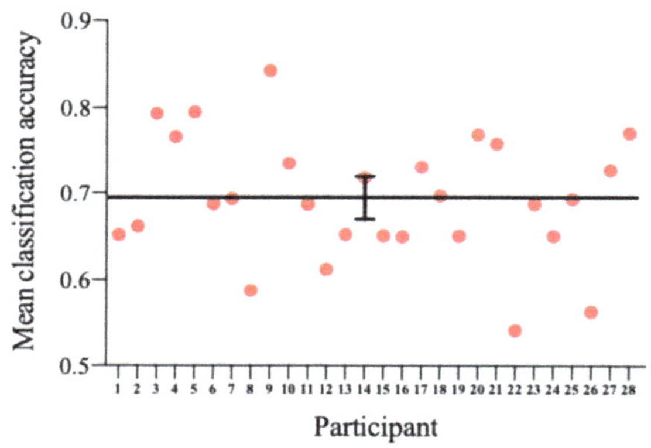


**FIGURE 9 |** The accuracy of the classifier for each participant. Horizontal line: average; error bar: SE.

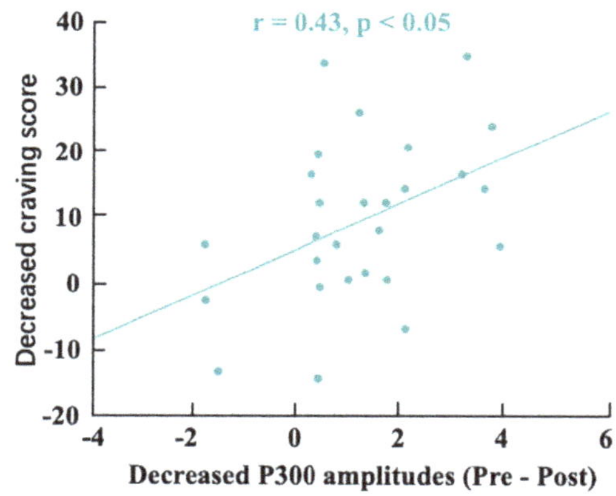


**FIGURE 10 |** The correlation between the mean decreased P300 amplitudes and decreased craving score ($r = 0.43$).

while viewing smoking cues in cue reactivity task. A high score indicated closely matched patterns. After training, the correlation between decreased P300 amplitudes (pre–post) and decreased craving score [score of tobacco craving questionnaire (TCQ), pre vs. post] was performed.

## Statistical Analysis

Statistical analysis was conducted in Statistics and machine learning toolbox in MATLAB. The comparison of features was performed with a non-parametric permutation test. The correlation of probabilistic score and training cycles was analyzed using Pearson's correlation. The comparison between the prediction accuracy and chance level used one-sample Student's $t$-test. The normality test was based on Kolmogorov–Smirnov (KS) test. Fivefold cross-validation was used to calculate the classification accuracy of the classifier. The reported $p$-values were all two-tailed. The significant threshold $\alpha$ is 0.05.

# RESULTS

## EEG Data Evaluation

The database is 3.96 GB, including 2.44 GB EEG data of cue reactivity task, 1.52 GB EEG data of neurofeedback, 16.8 kB demographic data, and 1.81 kB channel location file. Twenty-eight subjects were included in this database. The cue reactivity data were divided into two files: "cue reactivity_1.zip" and "cue reactivity_2.zip." Each subject had two runs, and each run contained six CNT files, which could be read in EEGLAB toolbox. The neurofeedback data were in "nf_eeg.zip." Each subject had two runs, and each run contained eight EEG MAT files (channel*time), which can be read in MATLAB. To facilitate subsequent data processing, electrode-position file and marker information were also provided. The channel location file named "chan62.zip," the baseline demographic and clinical characteristics named "baseline.mat," and trigger information file named "trigger.md" can be found in the root directory.

**Figures 4A,B** show the ERP amplitude and topographic map of cue reactivity task in the first and second visits. The data of the two visits have good consistency. The P300 component of ERP caused by addictive substance-related cues is usually a feature of substance use disorders, and the P300 amplitude is found to be related to the craving for smoking (Littel et al., 2012; Campanella et al., 2014). In our research, the P300 ERP component induced by smoking cues can be observed at approximately 300–550 ms. We evaluated the distribution of the Pz-SNR (**Figure 5**). KS test was performed to check the normality of distribution. There was no significant difference between the data distribution and the normal distribution ($p = 0.29$).

Channel waveform and topographic map of preprocessed 1-s real-time neurofeedback training data of eight channels (including FPz, Fz, FCz, Cz, CPz, Pz, POz, and Oz) are shown in different color to express brain electrical activity. We used the data of the 10th trial, the first cycle, the first visit (run1) of subject 1 (s1) as an example (**Figure 6**).

## Feature Extraction Evaluation

These time (**Figure 7A**) and frequency domain (**Figures 7B–F**) features from 28 participants were used to construct the classifier. For each block diagram, the abscissa represents the time information (ms), and the ordinate represents electrode channel information (60 channels) respectively. The yellow and blue areas in the figure represent the characteristic signals that were statistically significant with smoking > non-smoking conditions and the characteristic signal that was statistically significant with smoking < non-smoking conditions ($\alpha = 0.05$), respectively.

## Neurofeedback Performance Evaluation

Participants were trained for 16 cycles in two visits. In each trial of the neurofeedback cycle, the average score of 40 probabilistic scores was recorded as neurofeedback performance in the respective cycle. We performed a linear regression analysis on the probabilistic score and the training cycles. A significant negative correlation ($r = -0.1545$, $p = 0.0010$) was found, which showed that the match probability (the current brain activity patterns and the patterns when viewing smoking cues) decreased with training progressed (**Figure 8**). In other words, the difference in brain activity patterns between viewing the smoking cues and the neutral cue was smaller after neurofeedback training.

## Classifier Power Evaluation

Each point in **Figure 9** represents fivefold cross-validation accuracy of one participant. The accuracy of the classifier varies between 0.5409 and 0.8427, with a mean accuracy of 0.6935. One-sample $t$-test showed a significant difference between the prediction accuracy and the chance level ($p = 4.4176 \times 10^{-14}$).

# CONCLUSION AND DISCUSSION

In this paper, we developed a novel cognition-guided neurofeedback paradigm. Neurofeedback technology is an effective method to regulate brain signals and neuroplasticity, which involves brain networks of reward, control, and learning (Sitaram et al., 2017). Among them, dorsolateral prefrontal cortex (dlPFC) and posterior parietal cortex (PPC) in the control network will be activated during the execution of the strategy, and the learning network [mainly includes the dorsal striatum (DS)] is responsible for strategy learning in neurofeedback. The theoretical models of neurofeedback learning include operant (or instrumental) learning, motor learning, dual process theory, awareness theory, global workspace theory, and skill learning theory (Sitaram et al., 2017). These theoretical models are not mutually exclusive but compatible. Operant learning can be regarded as part of the dual process theory, which includes automatically process and controlled process (Enriquez-Geppert et al., 2017). Normally, approximately 15–30% of subjects do not respond to neurofeedback/BCI (Weber et al., 2011). Strategies are extremely important for neurofeedback. In the process of neurofeedback learning, strategies may promote or hinder neurofeedback learning, depending on the appropriate degree of scheduling cognitive resources in the process (Gaume et al., 2016; Davelaar, 2018).

In our implicit neurofeedback, the significant negative correlation ($r = -0.1545$, $p = 0.0010$) of the probabilistic score and training cycles demonstrates good neurofeedback learning effect. It also shows that the brain activity pattern in response to smoking stimuli represented by EEG signals can be successfully downregulated after two neurofeedback trainings. This is similar to previous rt-fMRI neurofeedback studies based on visual perception and attention brain activity patterns (deBettencourt et al., 2015; Amano et al., 2016). Our research also shows that the changes in brain patterns influenced addictive behaviors. The subjects' TCQ craving score and P300 amplitude decreased significantly after neurofeedback training (Bu et al., 2019), and there was a positive correlation between them (**Figure 10**). The results revealed the relationship between neural signals and behavioral indicators.

In particular, previous neurofeedback studies based on the regulation of brain activity patterns focused on training normal subjects to improve their cognitive abilities. The results of our study further extended these findings to patients with mental illness (smoking addicts), which also had the potential to regulate brain activity patterns. Our dataset provided important support for the extension of neurofeedback training of multivariable brain activity pattern regulation to clinical research in the future.

This dataset is of high quality and good integrity. In order to reduce artifacts as much as possible and improve the SNR, we added simple cognitive activities while performing the cue reactivity task to ensure that the collected data were brain electrical signals from the experiment rather than distractions. Additionally, in the cue reactivity task phase and the neurofeedback training phase, an intertrial interval (ITI) was used to eliminate the detention effect of the previous trial and gave participants a certain time to rest until they felt comfortable enough for the next trial. During the experiment, participants were instructed to blink and swallow as little as possible to obtain purer EEG raw data. As can be seen in **Figure 4**, ERP waveforms and topographic maps have strong consistency and repeatability between visits. In addition, we checked the strategies reported by the participants and the surveillance video during neurofeedback and found that no subjects used the strategies that were not allowed, such as not watching the screen. The decline in smoking cue reactivity patterns and the relatively high model prediction accuracy provided a guarantee for the intervention effect and method reliability of neurofeedback BCI. Nevertheless, the dataset also had some limitations. Considering that the prevalence among female smokers in China was very low (2.7%), we only recruited male participants. The dataset we present is the first cognition-guided neurofeedback BCI dataset on nicotine addiction to our knowledge. Participants completing two separate visits of training showed improvement in smoking cue reactivity patterns. High-quality EEG raw data are provided, and the classifier is evaluated and proven to have relatively high classification accuracy. Our two-visit, cognition-guided neurofeedback BCI can be compared with other neurofeedback paradigms to develop new neurofeedback systems.

Our previous research extracted the characteristics of the EEG signal in the time and frequency domains for SVM modeling. As far as we know, the cue reactivity task is commonly studied in substance addiction (Hardy et al., 2017). The dataset we provided contains the participants' brain electrical activity exposed to both smoking-related cues and neutral cues. There are other methods to analyze the dataset, such as the microstate (Michel, 2018) and source analysis (Zhou et al., 2019). These methods can be implemented on this dataset to discover mechanisms of nicotine addiction. The EEG data provided in this study can be used to verify other existing models or optimize parameters. In addition, the dataset can be used to development other ERP-based BCI algorithms.

In future research, BCI datasets can still be improved from the following aspects. First, a higher number of channels and sampling rate can be applied to obtain higher BCI bandwidth. Second, the extraction of feature can be improved. Different network connection of participants toward smoking and neutral cues can be incorporated into classification features to obtain a higher degree of discrimination (Ai et al., 2019). Third, SVM classifier was used in this study, and a relatively high classification accuracy rate was obtained. Subsequent studies can use other machine learning method to obtain higher model prediction rates, such as logistic regression and decision tree. For example, a feature extraction method was developed based on autoregression and used random forest classifiers to identify the EEG features of patients with epilepsy with a best accuracy of 97.352% (Zhang et al., 2017). Fourth, this study conducted two visits of neurofeedback training, which was mainly based on skill learning theory (Hinterberger et al., 2005; Koralek et al., 2012) and previous MRI research (Young et al., 2017a,b). In future BCI studies, longer training periods can be used to evaluate the impact of training time on neurofeedback effects. Finally, this study used a simple floating line as the visual form of neurofeedback. Nowadays, BCI is moving in the direction of gamification (de Castro-Cros et al., 2020), which is also the direction for future BCI datasets.

In conclusion, our novel neurofeedback BCI dataset has a significant contribution to this field. We offer the community access to our EEG data from our BCI experiment. The neurofeedback protocol that we developed and applied is based on the long-term research on nicotine addiction of our group and will act as a reference for subsequent neurofeedback BCI research.

## AUTHOR CONTRIBUTIONS

JB and XZ contributed to the experimental design. JB and GC contributed to the data collection. JB, CL, HGo, HGa, YC, ML, GQZ, and XZ contributed to the manuscript writing. CL, RN, and ZL contributed to the data processing. CL and HGo contributed to the data uploading. All listed authors made direct contributions to the article and approved it for publication.

## FUNDING

This work was supported by grants from the National Key Basic Research Program (2018YFC0831101). The National Natural Science Foundation of China (31771221, 71942003, 61773360, 31800927, 31900766, 32000750, and 71874170). Major Project of Philosophy and Social Science Research, Ministry of Education of China (19JZD010), CAS-VPST Silk Road Science Fund 2021 (GLHZ202128), Collaborative Innovation Program of Hefei Science Center, CAS (2020HSC-CIP001), Anhui Provincial Natural Science Foundation (2008085QH369), Major Project of Natural Science Foundation of the Anhui Higher Education Institutions (KJ2020ZD16), China Postdoctoral Science Foundation (2019TQ0312 and 2019M662203), Basic and Clinical Collaborative Research Improvement Project of Anhui Medical University (2020xkjT020), School Foundation of Anhui Medical University (2019xkj016), and Grants for Scientific Research of BSKY (XJ201907) from Anhui Medical University. A portion of the numerical calculations in this study was performed with the supercomputing system at the Supercomputing Centre of USTC.

## ACKNOWLEDGMENTS

We sincerely acknowledge Wei Hong (WH) for their assistance with subject assessment.

## REFERENCES


1. Ai, Q., Chen, A., Chen, K., Liu, Q., Zhou, T., Xin, S., et al. (2019). Feature extraction of four-class motor imagery EEG signals based on functional brain network. *J. Neural Eng.* 16:026032. doi: 10.1088/1741-2552/ab0328
2. Amano, K., Shibata, K., Kawato, M., Sasaki, Y., and Watanabe, T. (2016). Learning to associate orientation with color in early visual areas by associative decoded fMRI neurofeedback. *Curr. Biol.* 26, 1861–1866. doi: 10.1016/j.cub.2016.05.014 Bu, J., Young, K. D., Hong, W., Ma, R., Song, H., Wang, Y., et al. (2019). Effect of deactivation of activity patterns related to smoking cue reactivity on nicotine addiction. *Brain* 142, 1827–1841. doi: 10.1093/brain/awz114
3. Campanella, S., Pogarell, O., and Boutros, N. (2014). Event-related potentials in substance use disorders: a narrative review based on articles from 1984 to 2012. *Clin. EEG Neurosci.* 45, 67–76. doi: 10.1177/1550059413495533
4. Chiamulera, C. (2005). Cue reactivity in nicotine and tobacco dependence: a "multiple-action" model of nicotine as a primary reinforcement and as an enhancer of the effects of smoking-associated stimuli. *Brain Res. Rev.* 48, 74–97. doi: 10.1016/j.brainresrev.2004.08.005
5. Cui, X., Bray, S., Bryant, D. M., Glover, G. H., and Reiss, A. L. (2011). A quantitative comparison of NIRS and fMRI across multiple cognitive tasks. *NeuroImage* 54, 2808–2821. doi: 10.1016/j.neuroimage.2010.10.069
6. Cui, Y., Versace, F., Engelmann, J. M., Minnix, J. A., Robinson, J. D., Lam, C. Y., et al. (2013). Alpha oscillations in response to affective and cigarette-related stimuli in smokers. *Nicotine Tob. Res.* 15, 917–924. doi: 10.1093/ntr/nts209
7. Davelaar, E. J. (2018). Mechanisms of Neurofeedback: A Computation-theoretic Approach. *Neuroscience* 378:175-188.
8. de Castro-Cros, M., Sebastian-Romagosa, M., Rodríguez-Serrano, J., Opisso, E., Ochoa, M., Ortner, R., et al. (2020). Effects of gamification in BCI functional rehabilitation. *Front. Neurosci.* 14:882. doi: 10.3389/fnins.2020.00882
9. deBettencourt, M. T., Cohen, J. D., Lee, R. F., Norman, K. A., and Turk-Browne, N. B. (2015). Closed-loop training of attention with real-time brain imaging. *Nat. Neurosci.* 18, 470–475. doi: 10.1038/nn.3940
10. Enriquez-Geppert, S., Huster, R. J., and Herrmann, C. S. (2017). EEG-neurofeedback as a tool to modulate cognition and behavior: a review tutorial. *Front. Hum. Neurosci.* 11:51. doi: 10.3389/fnhum.2017.00051
11. Gadea, M., Aliño, M., Hidalgo, V., Espert, R., and Salvador, A. (2020). Effects of a single session of SMR neurofeedback training on anxiety and cortisol levels. *Neurophysiol. Clin.* 50, 167–173. doi: 10.1016/j.neucli.2020.03.001
12. Garavan, H., Pankiewicz, J., Bloom, A., Cho, J.-K., Sperry, L., Ross, T. J., et al. (2000). Cue-induced cocaine craving: neuroanatomical specificity for drug users and drug stimuli. *Am. J. Psychiatry* 157, 1789–1798. doi: 10.1176/appi.ajp. 157.11.1789
13. Gaume, A., Vialatte, A., Mora-Sánchez, A., Ramdani, C., and Vialatte, F. B. (2016). A psychoengineering paradigm for the neurocognitive mechanisms of biofeedback and neurofeedback. *Neurosci. Biobehav. Rev.* 68, 891–910. doi: 10.1016/j.neubiorev.2016.06.012
14. Gruzelier, J. H. (2014). EEG-neurofeedback for optimising performance. III: a review of methodological and theoretical considerations. *Neurosci. Biobehav. Rev.* 44, 159–182. doi: 10.1016/j.neubiorev.2014.03.015
15. Hardy, L., Mitchell, C., Seabrooke, T., and Hogarth, L. (2017). Drug cue reactivity involves hierarchical instrumental learning: evidence from a biconditional Pavlovian to instrumental transfer task. *Psychopharmacology (Berl.)* 234, 1977– 1984. doi: 10.1007/s00213-017-4605-x
16. Hinterberger, T., Veit, R., Wilhelm, B., Weiskopf, N., Vatine, J.-J., and Birbaumer, N. (2005). Neuronal mechanisms underlying control of a brain-computer interface. *Eur. J. Neurosci.* 21, 3169–3181. doi: 10.1111/j.1460-9568.2005. 04092.x
17. Hsueh, J.-J., Chen, T.-S., Chen, J.-J., and Shaw, F.-Z. (2016). Neurofeedback training of EEG alpha rhythm enhances episodic and working memory: alpha neurofeedback on Memory. *Hum. Brain Mapp.* 37, 2662–2675. doi: 10.1002/ hbm.23201
18. Hu, L., Mouraux, A., Hu, Y., and Iannetti, G. D. (2010). A novel approach for enhancing the signal-to-noise ratio and detecting automatically event-related potentials (ERPs) in single trials. *NeuroImage* 50, 99–111. doi: 10.1016/ j.neuroimage.2009.12.010
19. Ihssen, N., Sokunbi, M. O., Lawrence, A. D., Lawrence, N. S., and Linden, D. E. J. (2017). Neurofeedback of visual food cue reactivity: a potential avenue to alter incentive sensitization and craving. *Brain Imaging Behav.* 11, 915–924. doi: 10.1007/s11682-016-9558-x
20. Janapati, R., Dalal, V., Govardhan, N., and Gupta, R. S. (2020). Review on EEG- BCI classification techniques advancements. *IOP Conf. Ser. Mater. Sci. Eng.* 981:032019. doi: 10.1088/1757-899X/981/3/032019
21. Karelitz, J. L. (2020). Differences in magnitude of cue reactivity across durations of smoking history: a meta-analysis. *Nicotine Tob. Res.* 22, 1267–1276. doi: 10.1093/ntr/ntz071
22. Kirschner, M., Sladky, R., Haugg, A., Stämpfli, P., Jehli, E., Hodel, M., et al. (2018). Self-regulation of the dopaminergic reward circuit in cocaine users with mental imagery and neurofeedback. *EBioMedicine* 37, 489–498. doi: 10.1016/j.ebiom. 2018.10.052
23. Koralek, A. C., Jin, X., Long, J. D. II, Costa, R. M., and Carmena, J. M. (2012). Corticostriatal plasticity is necessary for learning intentional neuroprosthetic skills. *Nature* 483, 331–335. doi: 10.1038/nature10845
24. Korostenskaja, M., Kapeller, C., Prueckl, R., Ortner, R., Chen, P. C., Guger, C., et al. (2014). "Improving ecog-based P300 speller accuracy," in *Proceedings of the 6th International Brain-Computer Interface Conference (Verlag der Technischen Universität Graz)*, 1–4. doi: 10.3217/978-3-85125-378-8-88
25. Kwon, J., Shin, J., and Im, C.-H. (2020). Toward a compact hybrid brain-computer interface (BCI): performance evaluation of multi-class hybrid EEG-fNIRS BCIs with limited number of channels. *PLoS One* 15:e0230491. doi: 10.1371/journal. pone.0230491
26. Li, X., Hartwell, K. J., Borckardt, J., Prisciandaro, J. J., Saladin, M. E., Morgan, P. S., et al. (2013). Volitional reduction of anterior cingulate cortex activity produces decreased cue craving in smoking cessation: a preliminary real-time fMRI study: Nicotine and real-time fMRI. *Addict Biol.* 18, 739–748. doi: 10.1111/j.1369- 1600.2012.00449.x
27. Littel, M., Euser, A. S., Munafò, M. R., and Franken, I. H. A. (2012). Electrophysiological indices of biased cognitive processing of substance-related cues: a meta-analysis. *Neurosci. Biobehav. Rev.* 36, 1803–1816. doi: 10.1016/j. neubiorev.2012.05.001
28. Martz, M. E., Hart, T., Heitzeg, M. M., and Peltier, S. J. (2020). Neuromodulation of brain activation associated with addiction: a review of real-time fMRI neurofeedback studies. *NeuroImage Clin.* 27:102350. doi: 10.1016/j.nicl.2020. 102350
29. Michel, C. M. (2018). EEG microstates as a tool for studying the temporal dynamics of whole-brain neuronal networks: a review. *Neuroimage* 180(Pt. B), 577–593.
30. Posson, D. (2019). Automated neurofeedback brain-training as a primary addiction intervention. *Int. J. Educ. Soc. Sci.* 6, 21–27.
31. Rees, V. W., and Heather, N. (1995). "Individual differences and cue reactivity," in *Addictive Behaviour: Cue Exposure Theory and Practice. The Wiley Series in Clinical Psychology*, eds D. C. Drummond, S. T. Tiffany, S. Glautier, and B. Remington (Oxford: John Wiley & Sons), 99–118.
32. Sitaram, R., Ros, T., Stoeckel, L., Haller, S., Scharnowski, F., Lewis-Peacock, J., et al. (2017). Closed-loop brain training: the science of neurofeedback. *Nat. Rev. Neurosci.* 18, 86–100. doi: 10.1038/nrn.2016.164
33. Sokhadze, T. M., Cannon, R. L., and Trudeau, D. L. (2008). EEG Biofeedback as a Treatment for Substance Use Disorders: Review, Rating of Efficacy, and Recommendations for Further Research. *Appl. Psychophysiol. Biofeedback* 33, 1–28. doi: 10.1007/s10484-007-9047-5
34. Sokunbi, M. O. (2014). Real-time fMRI brain-computer interface: development of a "motivational feedback" subsystem for the regulation of visual cue reactivity. *Front. Behav. Neurosci.* 8:392.
35. Stam, C. J. (2010). Use of magnetoencephalography (MEG) to study functional brain networks in neurodegenerative disorders. *J. Neurol. Sci.* 289, 128–134. doi: 10.1016/j.jns.2009.08.028
36. Trambaiolli, L. R., Kohl, S. H., Linden, D. E. J., and Mehler, D. M. A. (2021). Neurofeedback training in major depressive disorder: a systematic review of clinical efficacy, study quality and reporting practices. *Neurosci. Biobehav. Rev.* 125, 33–56. doi: 10.1016/j.neubiorev.2021.02.015
37. Versace, F., Engelmann, J. M., Deweese, M. M., Robinson, J. D., Green, C. E., Lam, C. Y., et al. (2017). Beyond cue reactivity: non-drug-related motivationally relevant stimuli are necessary to understand reactivity to drug-related cues. *Nicotine Tob. Res.* 19, 663–669. doi: 10.1093/ntr/ntx002
38. Weber, E., Köberl, A., Frank, S., and Doppelmayr, M. (2011). Predicting successful learning of SMR neurofeedback in healthy participants: methodological considerations. *Appl. Psychophysiol. Biofeedback* 36, 37–45. doi: 10.1007/ s10484-010-9142-x
39. Young, K. D., Misaki, M., Harmer, C. J., Victor, T., Zotev, V., Phillips, R., et al. (2017a). Real-time functional magnetic resonance imaging amygdala neurofeedback changes positive information processing

in major depressive disorder. *Biol. Psychiatry* 82, 578–586. doi: 10.1016/j.biopsych.2017. 03.013

40. Young, K. D., Siegle, G. J., Zotev, V., Phillips, R., Misaki, M., Yuan, H., et al. (2017b). Randomized clinical trial of real-time fMRI amygdala neurofeedback for major depressive disorder: effects on symptoms and autobiographical memory recall. *Am. J. Psychiatry* 174, 748–755. doi: 10.1176/appi.ajp.2017.16060637
41. Zafar, R., Dass, S. C., and Malik, A. S. (2017). Electroencephalogram-based decoding cognitive states using convolutional neural network and likelihood ratio based score fusion. *PLoS One* 12:e0178410. doi: 10.1371/journal.pone. 0178410
42. Zhang, T., Chen, W., and Li, M. (2017). AR based quadratic feature extraction in the VMD domain for the automated seizure detection of EEG using random forest classifier. *Biomed. Signal Process. Control* 31, 550–559. doi: 10.1016/j.bspc. 2016.10.001
43. Zhang, X. (2011). Anatomical differences and network characteristics underlying smoking cue reactivity. *Neuroimage* 54, 131–141.
44. Zhou, L., Wang, G., Nan, C., Wang, H., Liu, Z., and Bai, H. (2019). Abnormalities in P300 components in depression: an ERP-sLORETA study. *Nord. J. Psychiatry* 73, 1–8. doi: 10.1080/08039488.2018.1478991
45. Zotev, V., Phillips, R., Yuan, H., Misaki, M., and Bodurka, J. (2014). Self- regulation of human brain activity using simultaneous real-time fMRI and EEG neurofeedback. *NeuroImage* 85, 985–995. doi: 10.1016/j.neuroimage.2013.04.126

# 16

# The Relation between College Students' Social Anxiety and Mobile Phone Addiction: The Mediating Role of Regulatory Emotional Self-Efficacy and Subjective Well-Being

*Zhenlei Xiao[1] and Jianhao Huang[2]**

[1] Hengshui University, Hengshui, China, [2] Dhurakij Pundit University, Bangkok, Thailand

***Correspondence:**
Jianhao Huang
rollancekimo@gmail.com

The present study explores the underlying mechanism of the relationship between college students' social anxiety and mobile phone addiction. Adopting college students' social anxiety scale, regulatory emotional self-efficacy scale, subjective well-being scale and mobile phone addiction scale, this research tested valid samples of 680 Chinese college students. The results indicated that social anxiety exerted a significant and positive impact on mobile phone addiction. Regulatory emotional self-efficacy played a partial mediating role between social anxiety and mobile phone addiction. Subjective well-being also played a partial mediating role between social anxiety and mobile phone addiction. Moreover, both regulatory emotional self-efficacy and subjective well-being were found to play a chain mediating role between social anxiety and mobile phone addiction. The study provides valuable insights into the impact of college students' social anxiety on mobile phone addiction.

**Keywords: social anxiety, regulatory emotional self-efficacy, subjective well-being, mobile phone addiction, college students**

## INTRODUCTION

The advent of smartphones has remarkably changed people's living standards and made our life convenient; however, the simultaneously aroused problem of mobile phone addiction cannot be ignored. Addiction to mobile phones, particularly among teenagers, has become a vital social issue (Caprara et al., 2002; Lian, 2017; Elhai et al., 2018; Zsido et al., 2021). This newly emerged addiction behavior is associated with a series of mental and behavioral problems among individuals because of their excessive dependence on and usage of mobile phones (Lapierre et al., 2019). College students are open-minded, display good social adaptability, and are flexible at embracing new technology. However, they have more free time, and thus, they treat mobile phones as their personal friends. Consequently, college students are addicted to various mobile phone functions, and their addiction behavior is particularly serious (Kim and Koh, 2018; Yu et al., 2021).

Davis (2001) asserted that the individual susceptible qualities such as depression, social anxiety, and material dependence are the root causes of Internet addiction. Numerous studies conducted on the possible factors for mobile phone addiction suggest that social anxiety is one of the most direct factors leading to mobile phone addiction (Kong et al., 2020). According to social psychology, the long-term use of mobile phones to communicate with people significantly increases the probability of personal sociability decline, and the lack of normal social communication can increase the probability of loneliness and emptiness; thus, mobile phone addiction possibly contributes to the development of negative emotions (Maya and Nazir, 2016; Liu et al., 2017; Zhang et al., 2018). Social anxiety is a psychosocial problem, and people with social anxiety prefer other forms of communication, rather than face-to-face communication, particularly through mobile technology devices because this mode of communication can reduce anxiety (Darcin et al., 2016).

Individuals with social anxiety exhibit emotional instability, impatience, and impulsivity; express their emotions through repression and concealing (Wu and Liu, 2006); and display poor emotion regulation ability and low self-efficacy (Kashdan et al., 2011). Regulatory emotional self-efficacy, a type of self-efficacy, not only has a direct impact on behaviors but also can indirectly affect behaviors by influencing cognition, motivations, decisions and emotions, thereby playing a pivotal role in regulating individual personality and behavior and further maintaining the mental health state of individuals (Tang et al., 2010). The impact of emotions on health and behavior is mediated by regulatory emotional self-efficacy. Furthermore, it enables individuals to effectively cope with stress, improve their subjective well-being, and also plays a crucial role in addiction behavior (Bandura et al., 2003). Individuals with high regulatory emotional self-efficacy can actively change their environment to better deal with various problems under adverse situations, which may improve their subjective well-being (Huang et al., 2016). Teenagers who are dissatisfied with their well-being in real life achieve satisfaction by indulging in the Internet. According to a study, the individual Internet addiction and subjective well-being are significantly correlated (Akin, 2012). Given the aforementioned facts, the present research aims to explore the effect of social anxiety on college students' mobile phone addiction behavior, as well as the mediating role of regulatory emotional self-efficacy and subjective well-being. Knowledge of the underlying mechanism behind the correlation between social anxiety and college students' mobile phone addiction behavior may be useful in reducing the impact of social anxiety on college students' mobile phone addiction. Therefore, reinforcing the educational management of college students holds great practical significance.

## Social Anxiety and Mobile Phone Addiction

Social anxiety refers to the individuals' experience of negative emotions such as worry, fear, and nervousness under social situations (Li et al., 2003). It is a psychosocial problem, and people with social anxiety prefer other forms of communication to face-to-face communication, especially through mobile technology devices, because a communication method not involving face-to-face communication can reduce anxiety (Darcin et al., 2016). Generally, social anxiety tends to persist from childhood to adolescence. A study reported that the social anxiety of college students is as high as 45.7% (Li et al., 2019). People with social anxiety are extremely afraid of real social situations and tend to be shy, nervous, embarrassed, afraid, and produce other negative emotions while communicating with others (Ashbaugh et al., 2010). Online communication can help people with social anxiety avoid the negative emotions and pressure produced during real communication, and these individuals feel more comfortable in online communication than in real communication (Prizant-Passal et al., 2016). According to the cognitive model of problematic Internet use, individuals experience interpersonal control in online communication, which is conducive to the alleviation of their negative emotions. Moreover, their Internet use behavior is strengthened by negative reinforcement, and they are prone to develop abstinence syndromes (Caplan, 2002). Lee et al. (2013) verified that the use of mobile media for social communication to escape social anxiety in real life is one of the reasons for the excessive use of social networks. Kim et al. (2006) demonstrated that people with a high social anxiety level are more likely to exhibit Internet addiction. Therefore, we hypothesize that college students' social anxiety has a significant predictive effect on mobile phone addiction (H1).

## Social Anxiety, Regulatory Emotional Self-Efficacy, and Mobile Phone Addiction

Regulatory emotional efficacy represents a confidence level through which individuals can regulate their emotional state, and self-confidence is a manifestation of high self-efficacy (Bandura et al., 2003). It involves the perceived self-efficacy in expressing the positive affect, managing anger and irritation, and managing despondency and distress (Caprara et al., 2008). Kashdan and McKnight (2010) found that some individuals with social anxiety have poor emotion regulation ability, face difficulty in adapting to environmental changes, and experience varied negative emotions and strong hostile impulses. Individuals with social anxiety are emotionally instable, impatient, and impulsive; they express their emotions through repression and concealing and exhibit poor emotion regulation ability (Kashdan et al., 2011). In addition, the self-negative belief held by socially anxious individuals has an influence on their meta-evaluation of mood; therefore, their regulatory emotional self-efficacy is lower than that of other individuals (Mennin et al., 2005; Bassi et al., 2018). Kashdan and Roberts (2004) found a negative correlation between social anxiety and self-efficacy. Individuals with a high social anxiety level experience stronger negative effects and worse self-efficacy than those with a low social anxiety level. Previous studies have shown that regulatory emotional self-efficacy exerts an impact on individuals' psychosocial adaptation and that it can effectively regulate externalized problems (such as aggression and crime) and internalized problems (such as depression and shyness) (Caprara et al., 2010). Furthermore, studies have demonstrated that regulatory emotional self-efficacy has not only a short-term influence on depression and aggression but also a long-term effect (Caprara et al., 2002, 2010). Therefore, college students' social anxiety possibly exerts an influence on regulatory emotional self-efficacy and then leads to mobile phone addiction. Based on this assumption, we hypothesize that regulatory emotional self-efficacy plays a role in mediating the impact of college students' social anxiety on their mobile phone addiction behavior (H2).

## Social Anxiety, Subjective Well-Being, and Mobile Phone

Subjective well-being represents an individual's subjective evaluation and experience of life quality, and it serves as a significant psychological indicator that reflects the quality of life of an individual under a particular social situation (Diener et al., 1999). It is assessed according to the health condition, life, work, and interpersonal relationships (Diener and Ryan, 2009). Social anxiety is a crucial factor that affects individuals' subjective well-being. It can substantially reduce individuals' social motivations and the sense of pleasure generated by social communication, thereby reducing their perception of happiness (Li et al., 2017). People with social anxiety generally resort to negative means such as self-comfort, relying on others, fantasy, and exhibiting forgetfulness to avoid problems and relieve anxiety and tension (Li et al., 2003). However, social relations can exert a strong impact on subjective well-being. Individuals' life satisfaction is increased once their social needs are met (Leung et al., 2011). Ye et al. (2021) observed a significant negative correlation between social anxiety and subjective well-being of college students. The authors attached great importance to the social skills and interpersonal relationships among college students, whereas the emergence of social anxiety was reported to reduce the students' overall well-being. Another study on college students with different anxiety levels showed that the higher the level of social anxiety, the lower is the subjective well-being, and the lower the social anxiety level, the higher is the subjective well-being (Öztürk and Mutlu, 2010). Social anxiety is a key factor that influences individuals' subjective well-being, which in turn can significantly reduce the motivation of individual social behavior and the sense of pleasure derived from social communication, thereby reducing the individual perception of happiness.

Previous studies have found that subjective well-being has a significant impact on both physical and mental health of individuals and their Internet addiction behavior (Li et al., 2017). According to the compensation theory of network satisfaction, the unmet psychological needs in realities strongly influence the college students' Internet addiction behavior through network satisfaction compensation (Parker and Plank, 2000). Empirical research has demonstrated a significant negative correlation between subjective well-being and dependence on mobile phone; the higher the subjective well-being, the lower is the mobile phone addiction (Deng et al., 2015). A high level of subjective well-being serves as a protective factor for Internet addiction (Durak, 2011; Bozoglan et al., 2013). Therefore, social anxiety has an impact on subjective well-being, which in turn has an influence on addiction behavior. Thus, it is reasonable to predict that subjective well-being plays a mediating role in the relation between social anxiety and mobile phone addiction among college students. Based on this assumption, we propose the third hypothesis that subjective well-being plays a mediating role in the impact of social anxiety on mobile phone addiction among college students (H3).

## Social Anxiety, Regulatory Emotional Self-Efficacy, Subjective Well-Being, and Mobile Phone Addiction

Although social anxiety, as a type of negative emotion, has a negative impact on subjective well-being, Tsapelas et al. (2010) described regulatory emotional self-efficacy as a significant predictor of subjective well-being. Emotion regulation theory has been put forward to identify factors that affect the relation between emotions and behaviors; among these, self-efficacy is a key regulating factor (Heuven et al., 2006). Caprara et al. (2002) found that the differences in emotion regulation among individuals depend on the belief in their own emotion regulation ability, whereas such belief has an impact on the actual effect of individuals' emotion regulation. As a type of self-efficacy, regulatory emotional self-efficacy not only has a direct impact on behaviors but also can indirectly affect behaviors by influencing cognition, motivations, decisions, and emotions, thereby playing a vital role in regulating individual personality and behavior and maintaining the individual mental health level (Tang et al., 2010). Research suggests that regulatory emotional self-efficacy has an impact on the individuals' evaluation of life quality, that is, their subjective well-being. It is mainly reflected in the fact that the individuals having a high level of regulatory emotional self-efficacy are capable of effectively dealing with their emotions and timely adjust and control their negative emotions, thus maintaining a positive attitude toward things and exhibiting higher subjective well-being (Caprara and Steca, 2006). Moreover, the level of negative indicators such as depressive symptoms that reflect well-being from the negative aspect will be lower (Au et al., 2009). Other studies have found that individuals with a high self-efficacy exhibit stronger well-being experience (Cohen and Cairns, 2012). A study on the three fields of self-efficacy (academic, social, and emotional) demonstrated that regulatory emotional self-efficacy is a key factor for the well-being of adolescents (Andretta and McKay, 2020). The aforementioned findings suggest that social anxiety may lead to the reduction of regulatory emotional self-efficacy, and subjective well-being is conducive to the reduction of mobile phone addiction among college students. Therefore, it is reasonable to predict that the decrease in social anxiety among college students may be associated with better regulatory emotional self-efficacy, which in turn exert a positive impact on subjective well-being, and the improved subjective well-being may help in reducing mobile phone addiction among college students. Based on this assumption, we put forward the fourth hypothesis that both regulatory emotional self-efficacy and subjective well-being play a chain mediating role in the influence of social anxiety on mobile phone addiction of college students (H4).

# MATERIALS AND METHODS

## Participants

Using the convenient sampling method, we conducted a questionnaire survey on students at a university in Hebei Province, China, on an online questionnaire platform. In September 2021, teachers at the administration office sent the questionnaires in electronic forms to the students at our request. It took a university student approximately 30 min to fill in the questionnaire. We distributed 735 questionnaires and received 680 valid ones after eliminating invalid ones, with a 92.5% response rate. Among the students who returned the valid questionnaires, 450 were female and 230 were male; 216 were freshmen, 188 were sophomores, 174 were juniors, and 100 were seniors (see **Table 1** for details). According to the formula provided by Israel (1992) for calculating the sample size, that is, sample size = $z^2 \times p(1-p)/e^2/1 + (z^2 \times p(1-p)/e^2N)$, $z = 2.58$, $p = 0.5$, $N = 3{,}000$, and $e^2 = 0.0025$, the formal sample size should be no less than 545. The size of our study met the sampling criteria. The study was conducted in accordance with the Declaration of Helsinki and all subjects were willing to cooperate and had signed informed consent forms. We gave due consideration to their privacy and wishes and informed them that they could refuse to participate or withdraw from the study at any time (Goodyear et al., 2007). The study was also approved by the Ethics Committee of Hengshui College, China.

## Measurement

### Social Anxiety

The social anxiety scale of college students compiled by Qian et al. (2005) was used to assess the social anxiety level; the scale comprises 22 items from three dimensions, namely tension and anxiety, social sensitivity, and social confidence; among these, the third dimension involves a reverse scoring question pattern. The five-point scoring system, from 1 = "Completely do not conform" to 5 = "Completely conform," was adopted. The higher the score, the higher is the individual social anxiety level. The Cronbach α value of the scale in the present study was 0.946. The result of confirmatory factor analysis indicated that the $\chi^2$/df ratio was 5.990. This ratio is susceptible to the sample size; thus, when it is greater than 3, other fitness indicators should be determined (Wheaton, 1987). Regarding other fitness indicators, RMSEA = 0.08 (lower than the standard value of 0.1); SRMR = 0.051 (lower than the standard value of 0.8) (MacCallum et al., 1992); CFI = 0.898; NFI = 0.880; GFI = 0.859; and TLI = 0.884, and the fitting indices of the four variables were greater than 0.8, which indicated that the model fitted well (Bollen, 1989; Gefen et al., 2000; Schumacker et al., 2004).

### Regulatory Emotional Self-Efficacy

The regulatory emotional self-efficacy scale compiled by Caprara et al. (2010) was adopted. The scale was first translated into Chinese language by Wen et al. (2009) to conduct tests in college students; the results proved the reliability and validity of the scale. The scale comprises 12 items from three dimensions, namely the perceived self-efficacy in expressing positive affect, the perceived self-efficacy in regulating despondency and distress, and the perceived self-efficacy in regulating anger and irritation. The five-point scoring system, from 1 = "Completely do not conform" to 5 = "Completely conform" was adopted. The total score of each item was summed up to obtain the total score for regulatory emotional self-efficacy. A high score denoted the high individual regulatory emotional self-efficacy. The Cronbach α value of the scale in the present study was 0.869. The results of confirmatory factor analysis are as follows: $\chi^2$/df = 4.008, RMSEA = 0.067, SRMR = 0.064, CFI = 0.961, NFI = 0.949, GFI = 0.953, and TLI = 0.950, indicating that the model fitted well.

**TABLE 1** | Background variable characteristics.

| Variables | Grouping | Percentages |
|---|---|---|
| Gender | Male | 33.8% |
| | Female | 66.2% |
| College grade | Freshman | 31.8% |
| | Sophomore | 27.6% |
| | Junior | 25.6% |
| | Senior | 14.7% |

### Subjective Well-Being

The subjective well-being scale compiled by Pontin et al. (2013) was adopted. The scale comprises 24 items from three dimensions, namely psychological well-being, physical well-being, and interpersonal relationship well-being. An item "Are you satisfied with your sexual life?" was deemed unsuitable for college students and hence excluded. Altun et al. (2014) proved the reliability and validity of the scale for college students. The five-point scoring system, from 1 = "Never have" to 5 = "Always have," was used. The Cronbach α value of the scale in the present study was 0.950. The results of confirmatory factor analysis are as follows: $\chi^2$/df = 5.430, RMSEA = 0.081, SRMR = 0.039, CFI = 0.929, NFI = 0.914, GFI = 0.888, and TLI = 0.917, indicating that the model fitted well.

### Mobile Phone Addiction

The mobile phone addiction scale compiled by Leung (2008) was adopted. The scale comprises 17 items from four dimensions, namely uncontrolled addiction, abstinent addiction, avoidant addiction, and inefficient addiction. The five-point scoring system, from 1 = "Never have" to 5 = "Always have," was adopted. The total score of each item was summed up to obtain the total score for mobile phone addiction. The higher the score, the more severe is the mobile phone addiction. The scale has displayed good reliability and validity in previous studies (Lian et al., 2016). The Cronbach α value of the scale in the present study was 0.945. The results of confirmatory factor analysis are as follows: $\chi^2$/df = 8.887, RMSEA = 0.108, SRMR = 0.046, CFI = 0.937, NFI = 0.929, GFI = 0.883, and TLI = 0.916, indicating that the model fitted well.

### Data Analysis

SPSS and AMOS were used to manage and analyze the data; SPSS was used mainly for preliminary data processing, descriptive statistics, reliability and validity tests, and correlation analysis, whereas AMOS was used for confirmatory factor analysis and mediating effect analysis through the structural equation model of latent variables. Harman single-factor test was performed in SPSS to determine the influence of common method variance on the study results. Furthermore, we conducted a test on the analysis result of non-rotating factor by including the social anxiety level, regulatory emotional self-efficacy, subjective well-being, and mobile phone addiction in the exploratory

**TABLE 2** | Descriptive statistics and correlation between observed variables.

| Variables | M | SD | TA | SIC | SIS | POS | DES | ANG | PSY | PHY | INT | UNC | ABS | AVO | INE |
|---|---|---|---|---|---|---|---|---|---|---|---|---|---|---|---|
| TA | 2.59 | 0.86 | – | | | | | | | | | | | | |
| SIC | 2.62 | 0.70 | 0.65 | – | | | | | | | | | | | |
| SIS | 2.57 | 0.83 | 0.75 | 0.60 | – | | | | | | | | | | |
| POS | 4.02 | 0.68 | −0.26 | −0.40 | −0.25 | – | | | | | | | | | |
| DES | 3.46 | 0.75 | −0.51 | −0.54 | −0.53 | 0.32 | – | | | | | | | | |
| ANG | 3.35 | 0.78 | −0.41 | −0.45 | −0.49 | 0.21 | 0.68 | – | | | | | | | |
| PSY | 3.63 | 0.80 | −0.52 | −0.55 | −0.56 | 0.43 | 0.60 | 0.52 | – | | | | | | |
| PHY | 3.71 | 0.82 | −0.45 | −0.47 | −0.50 | 0.27 | 0.54 | 0.49 | 0.75 | – | | | | | |
| INT | 3.79 | 0.83 | −0.46 | −0.48 | −0.47 | 0.33 | 0.45 | 0.37 | 0.68 | 0.67 | – | | | | |
| UNC | 2.12 | 0.97 | 0.53 | 0.56 | 0.56 | −0.35 | −0.52 | −0.50 | −0.63 | −0.59 | −0.57 | – | | | |
| ABS | 2.27 | 1.12 | 0.56 | 0.57 | 0.57 | −0.30 | −0.54 | −0.48 | −0.57 | −0.55 | −0.52 | 0.74 | – | | |
| AVO | 2.76 | 1.17 | 0.44 | 0.49 | 0.49 | −0.22 | −0.45 | −0.45 | −0.44 | −0.42 | −0.37 | 0.59 | 0.63 | – | |
| INE | 2.60 | 1.10 | 0.56 | 0.54 | 0.51 | −0.27 | −0.52 | −0.50 | −0.50 | −0.53 | −0.50 | 0.73 | 0.68 | 0.58 | – |

*The correlation coefficients all reached significant levels ($p < 0.001$). M, mean; SD, standard deviation; TA, tension and anxiety; SIC, social interaction confidence; SIS, social interaction sensitivity; POS, positive affect; DES, despondency and distress; ANG, anger and irritation; PSY, psychological well-being; PHY, physical well-being; INT, interpersonal relationship well-being; UNC, uncontrolled addiction; ABS, abstinent addiction; AVO, avoidant addiction; INE, inefficient addiction.*

factor analysis. The results showed that a total of 11 factors exhibited characteristic roots greater than 1, with the variance interpretation rate of the first factor being 38.6% (less than 50%) (Harris et al., 2009), which indicated that the common method variance has a slight impact on the present study results.

## RESULTS

### Descriptive Statistics and the Correlation Among the Studied Variables

**Table 2** shows the descriptive statistics of each studied variable including the mean value, standard deviation, and correlation strength among the variables. The correlation coefficients between the studies variables ranged from 0.21 to 0.75, all of which exhibited a significance level of $p < 0.001$. Therefore, no collinearity problem was evident.

In this questionnaire, the skewness absolute values for the 74 items were between 0.028 and 0.875, and the kurtosis absolute values for the 74 items were between 0.01 and 1.156 (see **Supplementary Appendix** for details). The results satisfied the standards of the absolute value for skewness < 2 and kurtosis < 7 (Curran et al., 1996). The research data met normal distribution.

### Structural Model

In this research, *t*-test and ANOVA analysis result show that gender ($t = -0.761$, $p > 0.050$) and college grade ($F = 1.109$, $p > 0.050$) have no significant difference in college students' mobile phone addiction. Therefore, this research does not control the impact on college students' mobile phone addiction of gender and college grade.

A structural model was used to examine the relationship among social anxiety, regulatory emotional self-efficacy, subjective well-being, and mobile phone addiction, which showed that $\chi^2/df = 5.201$, RMSEA = 0.079, SRMR = 0.040, CFI = 0.956, NFI = 0.946, GFI = 0.935, and TLI = 0.942, indicating that the model fitted well. The results are shown in **Figure 1**. First, social anxiety was found to have a significant positive impact on mobile phone addiction ($\beta = 0.391$, $p < 0.01$), thus verifying H1. Second, social anxiety was found to have a significant negative impact on regulatory emotional self-efficacy ($\beta = -0.726$, $p < 0.001$), whereas regulatory emotional self-efficacy was found to have a significant negative influence on mobile phone addiction ($\beta = -0.202$, $p < 0.01$). This finding indicated that social anxiety may indirectly affect mobile phone addiction by virtue of regulatory emotional self-efficacy. In addition, social anxiety was found to have a significant negative impact on subjective well-being ($\beta = -0.354$, $p < 0.001$), whereas subjective well-being was found to have a significant negative impact on mobile phone addiction ($\beta = -0.336$, $p < 0.001$). The finding suggested that social anxiety affects mobile phone addiction possibly by affecting subjective well-being. Finally, regulatory emotional self-efficacy was found to significantly and positively affect subjective well-being ($\beta = 0.497$, $p < 0.01$), indicating that social anxiety influences subjective well-being possibly by affecting regulatory emotional self-efficacy and finally affects mobile phone addiction.

In the present study, the deviation correction percentile Bootstrap method (repeated the sampling for 500 times) was used to determine the mediating effect, and the confidence interval was set at 95%. Exclusion of 0 in the confidence interval indicates a significant mediating effect (Hayes, 2013). The results are shown in **Table 3**. Regulatory emotional self-efficacy was found to play a significant mediating role in the relation between social anxiety and mobile phone addiction, indicating that H2 is tenable. Furthermore, subjective well-being had a significant mediating impact on the relation between social anxiety and mobile phone addiction, indicating that H3 is tenable. In addition, both regulatory emotional self-efficacy and subjective well-being were found to play a significant chain mediating role in the relation between social anxiety and mobile phone addiction, thereby verifying H4.

## DISCUSSION

Based on the previous studies, we developed a chain mediating effect model, with social anxiety as the predictive variable,

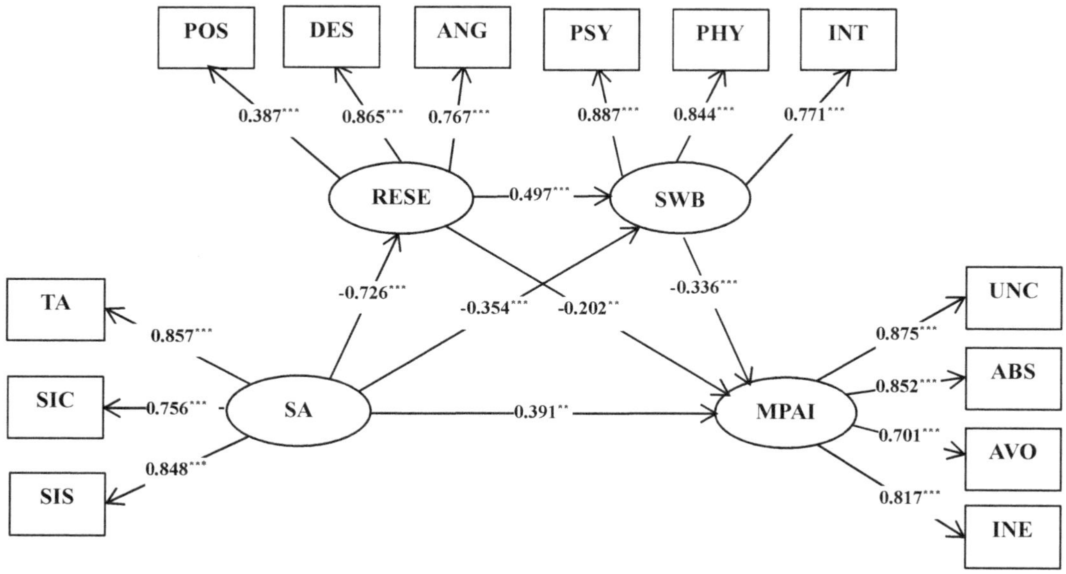


**FIGURE 1 |** Final standardized parameter values of the mode. SA, social anxiety; RESE, regulatory emotional self-efficacy; SWB, subjective well-being; MPAI, mobile phone addiction; TA, tension and anxiety; *SIC*, social interaction confidence; SIS, social interaction sensitivity; POS, positive affect; DES, despondency and distress; ANG, anger and irritation; PSY, psychological well-being; PHY, physical well-being; INT, interpersonal relationship well-being; UNC, uncontrolled addiction; ABS, abstinent addiction; AVO, avoidant addiction; INE, inefficient addiction. ***$p < 0.001$, **$p < 0.01$.

**TABLE 3 |** Mediation effect with bootstrapping.

| Path | Effect value | Proportion | 95% confidence interval | |
|---|---|---|---|---|
| | | | Lower limit | Upper limit |
| SA → RESE → MPAI | (−0.726) × (−0.202) = 0.147** | 0.147/0.778 = 0.189 | −0. 009 | −0. 308 |
| SA → SWB → MPAI | (−0.354) × (−0.336) = 0.119*** | 0.119/0.778 = 0.153 | −0. 039 | −0. 232 |
| SA → RESE → SWB → MPAI | (−0.726)×0.497 × (−0.336) = 0.121*** | 0.121/0.778 = 0.156 | −0. 049 | −0. 234 |
| Direct effect (SA → MPAI) | 0.391** | 0.391/0.778 = 0.503 | – | – |
| Total mediation | 0.387 | 0.387/0.778 = 0.497 | – | – |
| Total effect | 0.778 | – | – | – |

*The effect values in the table are standardized parameter values.* **$p < 0.01$, ***$p < 0.001$. *SA, social anxiety; RESE, regulatory emotional self-efficacy; SWB, subjective well-being; MPAI, mobile phone addiction.*

regulatory emotional self-efficacy and subjective well-being as the mediating variables, and mobile phone addiction as the outcome variable. The results of our study supported the self-efficacy theory, which suggests that regulatory emotional self-efficacy, as a type of self-efficacy, both directly and indirectly influences behaviors by influencing cognition, motivations, decisions, and emotions (Caprara and Steca, 2006; Caprara et al., 2008).

The present study indicated that college students' social anxiety has a significant positive impact on their mobile phone addiction; the finding is consistent with those of previous studies (Kim and Koh, 2018; Kong et al., 2020). Kardefelt-Winther (2014) proposed the compensatory Internet use theory, while considering the fact that various needs of adolescents are driven by individual development needs, and if the needs are hindered by interference factors, a "psychological compensation" process will occur. If the needs of adolescents cannot be met, a "pathological compensation" will occur, and they are likely to seek compensation through a way that is easy to produce a sense of achievement, such as playing games on the Internet. Social anxiety is characterized mainly by the fear of evaluation from other people, with individuals believing that other people will provide negative feedback, resulting in fear while communicating (Haxby et al., 2000). In the new social communication mode, college students can avoid face-to-face communication, thus reducing the possibility of cognitive processing deviation due to the negative expression of other people (Yoon et al., 2007). Therefore, students can communicate more comfortably using mobile phones and the Internet (Lee and Stapinski, 2012). People with high social anxiety tend to choose mobile phones or the Internet as substitutes for real social communication, eventually exhibiting high dependence on mobile phones and the Internet.

The present study results suggest that the regulatory emotional self-efficacy mediates the relation between social anxiety and mobile phone addiction of college students, consistent with the finding of previous studies indicating that regulatory emotional self-efficacy has a significant impact on mobile phone addiction (Mesurado and Malonda, 2018). Regulatory emotional self-efficacy plays a crucial role in maintaining mental health (Fredrickson et al., 2008). As a negative emotion, social anxiety influences the individual regulatory emotional self-efficacy (Sommers and Vodanovich, 2000). Individuals having a low regulatory emotional self-efficacy level tend to experience negative emotions for a long time, eventually exhibiting uncontrolled and aggressive or addictive behaviors (Liu et al., 2021). On the one hand, college students with a high social anxiety level lack social skills and use inappropriate coping strategies in social activities, leading to unfavorable social outcomes (Li et al., 2003) and thus addiction behaviors. On the other hand, college students with a high social anxiety level have poor emotion regulation ability and cognition, which render them incapable of adjusting their emotional state well (Kashdan et al., 2011), leading to the low regulatory emotional self-efficacy and thus mobile phone addiction.

Subjective well-being has a partial mediation effect on the relation between social anxiety and mobile phone addiction of college students, which is consistent with a study indicating that subjective well-being can significantly and negatively predict mobile phone addiction (Bozoglan et al., 2013). College students generally face problems in learning, interpersonal relationship, and emotions. In the face of learning pressure, coping with the pressure through positive means can improve individual subjective well-being, whereas the use of negative means can deteriorate individual subjective well-being (Karlsen et al., 2006). Individuals with strong subjective well-being exhibit better mental health, self-esteem, and self-control (Bozoglan et al., 2013), less negative emotional experience such as depression and anxiety, and strong adaptability (Klug and Maier, 2015). Such individuals can flexibly adjust to the interaction between themselves and surrounding environment; they not only achieve satisfaction in playing online games without becoming addicted but also display sufficient ability to deal with setbacks in life and achieve satisfaction in real life (Mascia et al., 2020).

College students' social anxiety exerts an impact on mobile phone addiction possibly through the mediation of regulatory emotional self-efficacy and subjective well-being, which is an important means by which social anxiety affects mobile phone addiction in college students. This finding is consistent with those of previous studies suggesting that regulatory emotional self-efficacy can significantly and positively affect subjective well-being (Caprara and Steca, 2006; Tsapelas et al., 2010). High regulatory emotional self-efficacy is conducive to the improvement in interpersonal relationship efficacy, which in turn can facilitate the formation of satisfactory and harmonious interpersonal relationships, improve subjective well-being, and enable individuals to effectively cope with addiction behaviors (Tang et al., 2010). College students with social anxiety generally tend to lose control of their emotions and lack confidence in effectively regulating their emotions, leading to more negative emotional experience, decreased well-being, and mobile phone addiction (Bozoglan et al., 2013). College students with high regulatory emotional self-efficacy can effectively communicate with others. In the presence of a negative stimulus, these individuals take effective measures, for example, by changing view of events to eliminate inside depression, and display strong confidence in effectively regulating their emotions. Therefore, they experience fewer negative emotions and reduced risk of developing mobile phone addiction (Caprara et al., 2002; Durak, 2011).

### Practical Significance

The present study provides ideas for the prevention of mobile phone addiction among college students. First, social anxiety can directly and significantly predict mobile phone addiction. Therefore, colleges should pay more attention to the social anxiety of students, and reduce their social anxiety by organizing various activities and encouraging students to actively participate in those activities. Second, social anxiety can affect mobile phone addiction through chain mediation between regulatory emotional self-efficacy and subjective well-being, indicating that both these variables are the key factors influencing college students' mobile phone addiction. Thus, colleges should attach importance to the cultivation of regulatory emotional self-efficacy and subjective well-being of students. In practical college education, emotion education courses or activities should be considered as the carrier to transfer emotion regulation knowledge and skills to college students and guide them to effectively regulate their emotions to gradually improve their regulatory emotional self-efficacy. The improvement of regulatory emotional self-efficacy is not only conducive to the improvement of students' emotional state but also essential for students to gain a sense of control in daily emotional experience and thus enhance their self-confidence.

### Limitations and Future Research Directions

The present study has some limitations. First, the study design was cross-sectional. Although previous studies have provided the basis for such studies, establishing a precise causal relationship using this method is challenging. Therefore, longitudinal studies are warranted to ascertain the causal relationship between social anxiety and mobile phone addiction. Second, the study adopted the questionnaire method; thus, future studies should adopt a qualitative or quasi-experimental design to further explore the possible causes of mobile phone addiction.

## AUTHOR CONTRIBUTIONS

ZX designed the study, analyzed the data, and drafted the manuscript. JH assisted in analyzing and interpreting the data and participated in the revision of the manuscript. Both authors contributed to the study and approved the submitted version.

## REFERENCES

1. Akin, A. (2012). The relationships between internet addiction. Subjective vitality, and subjective happiness. *Cyberpsychol. Behav. Soc. Netw.* 15, 404–410. doi: 10.1089/cyber.2011.0609

2. Altun, I., Zba, G. K., and Arli, E. (2014). Subjective well-being in university students. *Iran. J. Public Health* 43, 1585–1586.
3. Andretta, J. R., and McKay, M. T. (2020). Self-efficacy and well-being in adolescents: a comparative study using variable and person-centered analyses. *Child. Youth Serv. Rev.* 118:105374. doi: 10.1016/j.childyouth.2020.105374
4. Ashbaugh, A., Antony, M. M., Liss, A., Summerfeldt, L. J., Mccabe, R. E., and Swinson, R. P. (2010). Changes in perfectionism following cognitive-behavioral treatment for social phobia. *Depress. Anxiety* 24, 169–177. doi: 10.1002/da. 20219
5. Au, A., Lai, M. K., Lau, K. M., Pan, P. C., Lam, L., Thompson, L., et al. (2009). Social support and well-being in dementia family caregivers: the mediating role of self-efficacy. *Aging Ment. Health* 13, 761–768. doi: 10.1080/13607860902918223
6. Bandura, A., Caprara, G. V., Barbaranelli, C., Gerbino, M., and Pastorelli, C. (2003). Role of affective self-regulatory efficacy in diverse spheres of psychosocial functioning. *Child Dev.* 74, 769–782. doi: 10.1111/1467-8624.00567
7. Bassi, M., Fave, A. D., Steca, P., and Caprara, G. V. (2018). Adolescents' regulatory emotional self-efficacy beliefs and daily affect intensity. *Motiv. Emot.* 42, 287– 298. doi: 10.1007/s11031-018-9669-3
8. Bollen, K. A. (1989). *Structural Equations with Latent Variables.* (New York, NY: John Wiley & Sons), 289–308. doi: 10.1037/028856
9. Bozoglan, B., Demirer, V., and Sahin, I. (2013). Loneliness, self-esteem, and life satisfaction as predictors of Internet addiction: a cross-sectional study among Turkish university students. *Scand. J. Psychol.* 54, 313–319. doi: 10.1111/sjop. 12049
10. Caplan, S. E. (2002). Problematic Internet use and psychosocial well-being: development of a theory-based cognitive–behavioral measurement instrument. *Comput. Hum. Behav.* 18, 553–575. doi: 10.1016/S0747-5632(02)00004-3
11. Caprara, G. V., Gerbino, M., Paciello, M., Giunta, L. D., and Pastorelli, C. (2010). Counteracting Depression and delinquency in late adolescence: the role of regulatory emotional and interpersonal self-efficacy beliefs. *Eur. Psychol.* 15, 34–48. doi: 10.1027/1016-9040/a000004
12. Caprara, G. V., Giunta, L. D., Eisenberg, N., Gerbino, M., Pastorelli, C., and Tramontano, C. (2008). Assessing regulatory emotional self-efficacy in three countries. *Psychol. Assess.* 20, 227–237. doi: 10.1037/1040-3590.20.3.227
13. Caprara, G. V., Regalia, C., and Bandura, A. (2002). Longitudinal impact of perceived self-regulatory efficacy on violent conduct. *Eur. Psychol.* 7, 63–69. doi: 10.1027//1016-9040.7.1.63
14. Caprara, G. V., and Steca, P. (2006). The contribution of self-regulatory efficacy beliefs in managing affect and family relationships to positive thinking and hedonic balance. *J. Soc. Clin. Psychol.* 25, 603–627. doi: 10.1521/jscp.2006.25. 6.603
15. Cohen, K., and Cairns, D. (2012). Is searching for meaning in life associated with reduced subjective well-being? Confirmation and Possible Moderators. *J. Happiness Stud.* 13, 313–331. doi: 10.1007/s10902-011-9265-7
16. Curran, P. J., West, S. G.,, Finch, J. F. and John, F. (1996). The robustness of test statistics to nonnormality and specification error in confirmatory factor analysis. *Psychol. Methods* 1, 16–29. doi: 10.1037/1082-989X.1.1.16
17. Darcin, A. E., Kose, S., Noyan, C. O., Nurmedov, S., Yılmaz, O., and Dilbaz, N. (2016). Smartphone addiction and its relationship with social anxiety and loneliness. *Behav. Inf. Technol.* 35, 1–6. doi: 10.1080/0144929x.2016.1158319
18. Davis, R. A. (2001). A cognitive-behavioral model of pathological Internet use. *Comput. Hum. Behav.* 17, 187–195. doi: 10.1016/S0747-5632(00)00041-8
19. Deng, Z. J., Huang, H., Gui, Y. F., Niu, L. Y., and Zhou, C. Y. (2015). Mobile phone dependence,parenting style and subjective well-being in college students. *Chin. Ment. Health J.* 29, 68–73.
20. Diener, E., and Ryan, K. (2009). Subjective well-being: a general overview. *S. Afr. J. Psychol.* 39, 391–406. doi: 10.1177/008124630903900402
21. Diener, E., Suh, E. M., Lucas, R. E., and Smith, H. L. (1999). Subjective well-being: three decades of progress. *Psychol. Bull.* 125, 276–302. doi: 10.1037/0033-2909. 125.2.276
22. Durak, S. D. (2011). The mediator roles of life satisfaction and self-esteem between the affective components of psychological well-being and the cognitive symptoms of problematic internet use. *Soc. Indic. Res.* 103, 23–32. doi: 10.1007/s11205-010-9694-4
23. Elhai, J. D., Tiamiyu, M. F., Weeks, J. W., Levine, J. C., Picard, K. J., and Hall, B. J. (2018). Depression and emotion regulation predict objective smartphone use measured over one week. *Pers. Individ. Dif.* 133, 21–28. doi: 10.1016/j.paid. 2017.04.051
24. Fredrickson, B. L., Cohn, M. A., Coffey, K. A., Pek, J., and Finkel, S. M. (2008). Open hearts build lives: positive emotions, induced through loving-kindness meditation, build consequential personal resources. *J. Pers. Soc. Psychol.* 95, 1045–1062. doi: 10.1037/a0013262
25. Gefen, D., Straub, D. W., and Boudreau, M. (2000). Structural equation modeling and regression: guidelines for research practice. *Commun. Assoc. Inf. Syst.* 4:7. doi: 10.17705/1cais.00407
26. Goodyear, M. D., Krleza-Jeric, K., and Lemmens, T. (2007). The declaration of Helsinki. *BMJ* 335, 624–625. doi: 10.1136/bmj.39339.610000
27. Harris, K. J., Wheeler, A. R., and Kacmar, K. M. (2009). Leader–member exchange and empowerment: direct and interactive effects on job satisfaction, turnover intentions, and performance. *Leadersh. Q.* 20, 371–382. doi: 10.1016/j.leaqua. 2009.03.006
28. Haxby, J. V., Hoffman, E., and Gobbini, M. I. (2000). The distributed human neural system for face perception. *Trends Cogn. Sci.* 4, 223–233. doi: 10.1016/S1364- 6613(00)01482-0
29. Hayes, A. (2013). Introduction to mediation, moderation, and conditional process analysis. *J. Educ. Meas.* 51, 335–337. doi: 10.1111/jedm.12050
30. Heuven, E., Bakker, A. B., Schaufeli, W. B., and Huisman, N. (2006). The role of self-efficacy in performing emotion work. *J. Vocat. Behav.* 69, 222–235. doi: 10.1016/j.jvb.2006.03.002
31. Huang, S. H., Wen, Z. M., Zeng, Y. F., Li, Y. J., and Yang, Y. D. (2016). The Mediating role of Mental Toughness and social support in the relationship between emotional self-efficacy and subjective well-being of College Students. *Chin. J. Sch. Health* 37, 1559–1561. doi: 10.16835/j.cnki.1000-9817.2016.10.037
32. Israel, G. D. (1992). *Determining Sample Size.* Gainesville, FL: University of Florida.
33. Karlsen, E., Dybdahl, R., and Vitters, J. (2006). The possible benefits of difficulty: how stress can increase and decrease subjective well-being. *Scand. J. Psychol.* 47, 411–417. doi: 10.1111/j.1467-9450.2006.00549.x
34. Kashdan, T. B., and McKnight, P. E. (2010). The darker side of social anxiety. *Curr. Dir. Psychol. Sci.* 19, 47–50. doi: 10.1177/0963721409359280
35. Kashdan, T. B., and Roberts, J. E. (2004). Social Anxiety's impact on affect, curiosity, and social self-efficacy during a high self-focus social threat situation. *Cogn. Ther. Res.* 28, 119–141. doi: 10.1023/B:COTR.0000016934.20981.68
36. Kashdan, T. B., Weeks, J. W., and Savostyanova, A. A. (2011). Whether, how, and when social anxiety shapes positive experiences and events: a self-regulatory framework and treatment implications. *Clin. Psychol. Rev.* 31, 786–799. doi: 10.1016/j.cpr.2011.03.012
37. Kim, E., and Koh, E. (2018). Avoidant attachment and smartphone addiction in college students: the mediating effects of anxiety and self-esteem. *Comput. Hum. Behav.* 84, 264–271. doi: 10.1016/j.chb.2018.02.037
38. Kim, K., Ryu, E., Chon, M. Y., Yeun, E. J., Choi, S. Y., Seo, J. S., et al. (2006). Internet addiction in Korean adolescents and its relation to depression and suicidal ideation: a questionnaire survey. *Int. J. Nurs. Stud.* 43, 185–192. doi: 10.1016/j.ijnurstu.2005.02.005
39. Klug, H., and Maier, G. W. (2015). Linking goal progress and subjective well-being: a meta-analysis. *J. Happiness Stud.* 16, 37–65. doi: 10.1007/s10902-013-9493-0
40. Kong, F. C., Qin, J. K., Huang, B., Zhang, H. B., and Lei, L. (2020). The effect of social anxiety on mobile phone dependence among Chinese adolescents: a moderated mediation model. *Child. Youth Serv. Rev.* 108:104517. doi: 10.1016/j.childyouth.2019.104517


40. Kong, F. C., Qin, J. K., Huang, B., Zhang, H. B., and Lei, L. (2020). The effect of social anxiety on mobile phone dependence among Chinese adolescents: a moderated mediation model. *Child. Youth Serv. Rev.* 108:104517. doi: 10.1016/j.childyouth.2019.104517


41. Lapierre, M. A., Zhao, P., and Custer, B. E. (2019). Short-term longitudinal relationships between smartphone use/dependency and psychological well-being among late adolescents. *J. Adolesc. Health* 65, 607–612. doi: 10.1016/j.jadohealth.2019.06.001
42. Lee, B. W., and Stapinski, L. A. (2012). Seeking safety on the internet: relationship between social anxiety and problematic internet use. *J. Anxiety Disord.* 26, 197–205. doi: 10.1016/j.janxdis.2011.11.001
43. Lee, S., Tam, C. L., and Chie, Q. T. (2013). Mobile phone usage preferences: the contributing factors of personality, social anxiety and loneliness. *Soc. Indic. Res.* 118, 1205–1228. doi: 10.1007/s11205-013-0460-2
44. Leung, A., Yu, H. C., and Liu, X. Y. (2011). The relations between life domain satisfaction and subjective well-being. *J. Manag. Psychol.* 26, 155–169. doi: 10. 1108/02683941111102182
45. Leung, L. (2008). Linking psychological attributes to addiction and improper use of the mobile phone among adolescents in Hong Kong. *J. Child. Media* 2, 93–113. doi: 10.1080/17482790802078565
46. Li, B., Zhong, J., and Qian, M. Y. (2003). Regression analysis on social anxiety proneness among college students. *Chin. Ment. Health J.* 17, 109–112. doi: 10.3321/j.issn:1000-6729.2003.02.014

47. Li, C., Xu, K. Y., Huang, X. Y., Chen, N. N., Li, J. Q., Wang, J., et al. (2019). The Mediating role of negative body self in emotion regulation strategies and social anxiety. *China J. Health Psychol.* 27, 1564–1567. doi: 10.13342/j.cnki.cjhp.2019. 10.030
48. Li, Wang, T. T., Yin, L., and Wang, M. H. (2017). The relationship between mobile phone addiction and subjective well-being in college students: the mediating effect of social anxiety. *Stud. Psychol. Behav.* 15, 562–568. doi: 10.3969/j.issn. 1672-0628.2017.04.018
49. Lian, L., You, X. Q., Huang, J., and Yang, R. J. (2016). Who overuses Smartphones? Roles of virtues and parenting style in Smartphone addiction among Chinese college students. *Comput. Hum. Behav.* 65, 92–99. doi: 10.1016/j.chb.2016.08.027
50. Lian, L. (2017). Alienation as mediator and moderator of the relationship between virtues and smartphone addiction among Chinese University Students. *Int. J. Ment. Health Addict.* 16, 1208–1218. doi: 10.1007/s11469-017-9842-z
51. Liu, H. Y., Dou, K., Yu, C. F., Nie, Y. G., and Zheng, X. (2021). The relationship between peer attachment and aggressive behavior among Chinese adolescents: the mediating effect of regulatory emotional self-efficacy. *Int. J. Environ. Res. Public Health* 18:7123. doi: 10.3390/ijerph18137123
52. Liu, Q. Q., Zhou, Z. K., Niu, G. F., and Fan, C. Y. (2017). Mobile phone addiction and sleep quality in adolescents: mediation and moderation analyses. *Acta Psychol. Sin.* 49, 1524–1536. doi: 10.3724/SP.J.1041.2017.01524
53. MacCallum, R. C., Roznowski, M., and Necowitz, L. B. (1992). Model modifications in covariance structure analysis: the problem of capitalization on chance. *Psychol. Bull.* 111, 490–504. doi: 10.1037//0033-2909.111.3.490
54. Mascia, M. L., Agus, M., and Penna, M. P. (2020). Emotional intelligence, self- regulation, smartphone addiction: Which relationship with student well-being and quality of life? *Front. Psychol.* 11:375. doi: 10.3389/fpsyg.2020.00375
55. Maya, S., and Nazir, S. H. (2016). Relationships among smartphone addiction, stress, academic performance, and satisfaction with life. *Comput. Hum. Behav.* 57, 321–325. doi: 10.1016/j.chb.2015.12.045
56. Mennin, D. S., Heimberg, R. G., Turk, C. L., and Fresco, D. M. (2005). Preliminary evidence for an emotion dysregulation model of generalized anxiety disorder. *Behav. Res. Ther.* 43, 1281–1310. doi: 10.1016/j.brat.2004.08.008
57. Mesurado, B., and Malonda, E. (2018). Negative emotions and behaviour: the role of regulatory emotional self-efficacy. *J. Adolesc.* 64, 62–71. doi: 10.1016/j. adolescence.2018.01.007
58. Öztürk, A., and Mutlu, T. (2010). The relationship between attachment style, subjective well-being, happiness and social anxiety among university students'. *Procedia Soc. Behav. Sci.* 9, 1772–1776. doi: 10.1016/j.sbspro.2010.12.398
59. Parker, B. J., and Plank, R. E. (2000). A uses and gratifications perspective on the Internet as a new information source. *Latin Am. Bus. Rev.* 18, 43–49.
60. Pontin, E., Schwannaue, M., Tai, S., and Kinderman, P. (2013). A UK validation of a general measure of subjective well-being: the modified BBC subjective well- being scale (BBC-SWB). *Health Qual. Life Outcomes* 11:150. doi: 10.1186/1477- 7525-11-150
61. Prizant-Passal, S., Shechner, T., and Aderka, I. M. (2016). Social anxiety and internet use - A meta-analysis: What do we know? What are we missing? *Comput. Hum. Behav.* 62, 221–229. doi: 10.1556/2006.2021.00083
62. Qian, M. Y., Zhong, J., Xu, K. Y., Li, B., and Jiang, X. (2005). The development of social anxiety inventory for Chinese College Students. *Chin. Ment. Health J.* 19, 53–56. doi: 10.3321/j.issn:1000-6729.2005.01.016
63. Schumacker, R. E., Lomax, R., and Routledge. (2004). A Beginner's guide to structural equation modeling. *Technometrics* 47, 522–522. doi: 10.1198/tech. 2005.s328
64. Sommers, J., and Vodanovich, S. J. (2000). Boredom proneness: its relationship to psychological- and physical-health symptoms. *J Clin. Psychol.* 56, 149–155. doi: 10.1002/(sici)1097-4679(200001)56:1<149::aid-jclp14>3.0.co;2-y
65. Tang, D. L., Dong, Y., Yu, G. L., and Wen, S. F. (2010). The regulatory emotional self-efficacy: a new research topic. *Adv. Psychol. Sci.* 18, 598–604.
66. Tsapelas, I., Aron, A., and Orbuch, T. (2010). Marital boredom now predicts less satisfaction 9 years later. *Psychol. Sci.* 20, 543–545. doi: 10.1111/j.1467-9280. 2009.02332.x
67. Wen, S. F., Tang, D. L., and Yu, G. L. (2009). The characteristics of regulatory emotional self-efficacy in Chinese graduate students. *Psychol. Sci.* 32, 666–668. doi: 10.16719/j.cnki.1671-6981.2009.03.025
68. Wheaton, B. (1987). Assessment of Fit in Overidentified Models with Latent Variables. *Sociol. Methods Res.* 16, 118–154. doi: 10.1177/0049124187016001005 Kardefelt-Winther D. (2014). A conceptual and methodological critique of internet addiction research: towards a model of compensatory internet use. *Comput. Hum. Behav.* 31, 351–354. doi: 10.1016/j.chb.2013.10.059
69. Wu, L. L., and Liu, X. H. (2006). The relationship between adult attachment style and personality characteristics of social anxiety disorder patients. *Chin. J. Tissue Eng. Res.* 10, 18–22. doi: 10.3321/j.issn:1673-8225.2006.14.011
70. Ye, B., Li, L., Wang, P., Wang, R., and Yang, Q. (2021). Social anxiety and subjective well-being among Chinese college students: a moderated mediation model. *Pers. Individ. Dif.* 175:110934. doi: 10.1016/j.paid.2021.110680
71. Yoon, K. L., Fitzgerald, D. A., Angstadt, M., Mccarron, R. A., and Phan, K. L. (2007). Amygdala reactivity to emotional faces at high and low intensity in generalized social phobia: a 4-Tesla functional MRI study. *Psychiatry Res.* 154, 93–98. doi: 10.1016/j.pscychresns.2006.05.004
72. Yu, P. A., Hz, B., Bz, A., Hm, A., Rh, A., and Hj, C. (2021). Perceived stress and Mobile phone addiction among college students during the 2019 coronavirus disease: the mediating roles of rumination and the moderating role of self- control. *Pers. Individ. Dif.* 185:111222. doi: 10.1016/j.paid.2021.111222
73. Zhang, L., Bian, Y. W., Wang, Y. L., and You, Z. L. (2018). The effect of social anxiety on mobile phone addiction: the mediating effect of the belief in a just world. *Chin. J. Spec. Educ.* 1, 92–96.
74. Zsido, A. N., Arato, N., Lang, A., Labadi, B., and Bandi, S. A. (2021). The role of maladaptive cognitive emotion regulation strategies and social anxiety in problematic smartphone and social media use. *Pers. Individ. Dif.* 173:110647. doi: 10.1016/j.paid.2021.110647

# 17

# The Mediating Roles of Emotional Regulation on Negative Emotion and Internet Addiction among Chinese Adolescents from a Development Perspective

*Lijuan Liang*[1], *Mingrui Zhu*[2], *Jiali Dai*[3], *Min Li*[4] *and Ya Zheng*[5]*

[1] *Department of Psychology, The First Affiliated Hospital, Hainan Medical University, Haikou, China,* [2] *Department of Neurology, The People's Hospital of Liaoning Province, Shenyang, China,* [3] *Daqing No.3 Hospital, Daqing, China,* [4] *HeBei Institute of International Business and Economics, Qinghuangdao, China,* [5] *Department of Psychology, Dalian Medical University, Dalian, China*

***Correspondence:***
*Ya Zheng*
*zhengya@dmu.edu.cn*

Previous researches indicated that emotional regulation can be associated with depression and anxiety, which may be an important mediating factor between emotional regulation and internet addiction. However, the mechanism between these associations has received little attention and it is still unclear. This study has examined 716 Chinese adolescents, 341 were males (47.6%), aged 13 to 18(Mean = 14.58, SD = 1.50), using a cross-sectional survey involving Young's Diagnostic Questionnaire for Internet Addiction, the nine-item Patient Health Questionnaire (PHQ-9), the seven-item Generalized Anxiety (GAD-7) scale, and the Emotion Regulation Questionnaire (ERQ). Correlation analysis, multiple-group analysis and structural equation modeling were carried out in SPSS Statistics version 23 (IBM, Armonk, NY) and AMOS version 21. Cognitive reappraisal had a significantly negative direct effect on Internet addiction ($\beta = -0.118$, $p < 0.05$). Furthermore, negative emotions mediated the relationships between expression suppression and Internet addiction [$\beta = 0.149$, 95% CI = (0.099, 0.212)] and the relationship between cognitive reappraisal and Internet addiction [$\beta = -0.101$, 95% CI = (−0.147, −0.065)]. The differences in the structure path coefficients for different development stages demonstrated that recognitive reappraisal showed more protective roles for negative emotion ($p < 0.01$), and negative emotion also predict Internet addiction more effectively in high school students ($p < 0.001$). However, cognitive reappraisal directly predicted negative Internet addiction in junior high school students. Therefore, the intervention on adolescents for internet addiction should not only focus on emotional regulation and negative emotion, but also development stages of adolescents.

**Keywords: depression, anxiety, stress, internet addiction, expressive suppression, cognitive reappraisal**

## INTRODUCTION

With the development of society and information technology, the internet has brought convenience, but also some problems, especially for adolescents. Physical and psychological characteristics show that adolescents have relatively poor self-control and immature psychology and behavior. Adolescents may be prone to internet addiction (IA), which can affect their physical

(1) and mental health (2) and academic performance (3), even generating suicidal ideation (4). Internet addiction is characterized by psychological dependence, tolerance, and withdrawal symptoms and is included in the "Internet Addiction" chapter of the Diagnostic and Statistical Manual of Mental Disorders, Fifth Edition (DSM-V; American Psychiatric Association, 2013) (5). The prevalence of internet addiction among Chinese adolescents was found to be 10.4% (6). Many adolescents with internet addiction show more problematic internet usage, which may be associated with significantly more negative emotion and greater deficits in emotional regulation (7). There are obvious differences between boys and girls in Internet addiction. For example, adolescents with masculine temperament prefer competitive games, while adolescents with feminine temperament show low preference for competitive games. However, due to the virtuality of cyberspace, there may be cross gender behavior in adolescents' online behavior (8). Meanwhile, adolescents experience more negative emotions, which may be related to the contradiction between the demand for emotional autonomy and immature emotion regulation in adolescence (9). However, fewer studies simultaneously focused on the mediating roles of cognitive reappraisal and expressive suppression in internet addiction and the model invariance across gender and age.

## Depression, Anxiety and Internet Addiction

Owing to factors that pertain to academic performance (10), interpersonal problems (11), and family (12), many adolescents suffered from emotion problems, especially negative emotion of depression and anxiety (13). Many studies have considered that depression and anxiety may be the main risk factors for internet addiction among adolescents (14, 15). Internet addiction should be a negative coping style of avoiding problems. Therefore, the behavior of internet addiction may further aggravate the symptoms of negative emotions. The internal mechanism between emotion problems and internet addiction has played an important role in intervention and the treatment of internet addiction (16, 17). A possible explanation for these associations is that individuals with depression and anxiety may try to self-regulate emotional states through internet addictive behaviors (18). Positive emotional regulation strategies may be mediating roles between emotion problems and internet addiction.

According to Cognitive Behavior Theory (CBT), anxiety and depression of adolescents may be the mediator variables between emotional regulation and problem behavior (19). The problem behaviors of adolescents mainly include internalization and externalization. Internalization problems include all kinds of over-inhibited or inward-directed behavior, such as anxiety and depression, while externalization problems include all kinds of uninhibited or outward-focused behavior, such as internet addiction and aggression. Therefore, internet addiction as an externalized behavior may also be influenced by emotion regulation, but few researches have explored the relationship and psychological mechanism between emotion regulation and internet addiction.

## The Mediating Role of Expressive Suppression and Cognitive Reappraisal

Emotional regulation deficits have been theoretically and empirically associated with affective disorders and addiction. Some studies have tried to intervene in internet addiction in adolescents with cognitive behavioral therapy (CBT) (20). Cognitive factors may be key factors in internet addiction. Some studies have supported the notion that the ability to regulate emotions may predict internet addiction, and therefore producing changes in cognition may be an effective intervention method (21, 22). Cognitive reappraisal, as an adaptive strategy, is defined as cognitively transforming a situation in order to modify its impact on one's emotions (23). Cognitive reappraisal may help individuals to re-evaluate a situation of maladjustment and improve the ability of self-control. However, expressive suppression is a maladaptive strategy defined as inhibiting emotion expressive behavior (24). Some studies have shown that adolescents with internet addiction had greater difficulty in emotional regulation, manifested by excessive expressive suppression and too little cognitive reappraisal (25, 26). Owing to excessive suppression of negative emotional experiences, the correlation between negative and internet addiction may be enhance. Therefore, a deficit of emotional regulation may further strengthen the association between negative emotions and internet addiction.

According to previous studies, depression (27) and anxiety (28) are positively associated with internet addiction, and emotional regulation may have a mediating role between negative emotion and internet addiction.

## The Effect of Age and Gender

Many related studies have shown that internet addiction and emotional features of adolescents vary with age and sex (29). Although the related research supports the fact that negative emotion, such as depression and anxiety, play important roles in the severity of internet addiction, gender also plays an important role in the structural equation model (30). In addition, compared with boys, girls were found to be at a higher risk of mood symptoms only and of comorbid IA and mood symptoms (13). However, few studies have referred to the invariance of the structural model relating negative emotion and internet addiction, and some research shows that the path relating emotion and internet addiction shows no difference, which assumed negative emotion as mediator between school climate problematic internet use and ignore the comparison of progressive equivalence models (31). According to the different psychological mechanisms of age and gender, the treatment of internet addiction should consider the variables of age (32) and gender (33, 34).

## The Present Study

Emotion problems, such as depression (35) and anxiety (36) have been associated with internet addiction, so emotion problems may be risk factors for internet addiction. Expressive suppression may be a risk mediating factor between emotion problems and internet addiction. Internet addiction is affected directly by depression and anxiety, and indirectly by expressive suppression and cognitive reappraisal. Given the mediating effects of gender and age, we also considered the roles of gender and age in this model to determine whether the model developed for all participants was suitable for all adolescents regardless of age and gender.

# MATERIALS AND METHODS

## Participants

A total of 716 adolescents participated in the study. The valid data set comprised 690 participants after deleting invalid data, and the data efficiency was 96.37%. All adolescents gave informed consent before starting to fill out the form by choosing whether agree to participate in this study or not.

## Procedure

The participants in this study were students who completed a self-reported questionnaire from the provinces of Sichuan and Hainan. They were first asked to read an informed consent declaration and entered the survey only if they agreed by QR (quick response) code or web page. They could opt to remain anonymous or use their real name when filling in the questionnaire.

## Ethics Statement

Ethical approval for this study was obtained from the Hainan Medical University Ethics Committee (HYLL2020005). Parents and schools were informed to obtain the consent prior to the study. All participants were volunteered to participate in the study and receive individual psychometric results at the end of the measurement.

## Measurement

### Depression

The nine-item Patient Health Questionnaire (PHQ-9) has been widely utilized to assess symptoms of depression (37). The nine items of the PHQ correspond to the diagnostic criteria of depressive symptoms in DSM-V. The PHQ-9requiresparticipants to self-report the frequency of related symptoms over the past 2 weeks. As a severity measure, the PHQ-9 score can range from 0 to 27, because each of the nine items is scored from 0 (not at all) to 3 (nearly every day). Cronbach's alpha for the PHQ-9 was 0.911 in the current sample.

### Anxiety

The seven-item Generalized Anxiety Disorder (GAD) scale is generally utilized to measure anxiety symptoms among adolescents (38). The GAD asks participants to self-report on the status and frequency of symptoms during the last 2 weeks (39). The score for the GAD can range from 0 to 21, and the Cronbach's alpha was 0.924 among all participants in this study.

### Expressive Suppression and Cognitive Reappraisal

The Chinese version of the Emotion Regulation Questionnaire (ERQ) consists of 10 items that measure two factors: expressive suppression (four items) and cognitive reappraisal (six items). Each item of the ERQ is scored one (completely disagree) to seven (completely agree). Scores of for all four expressive suppression items were summed to generate a single expressive suppression score, while scores for all six cognitive reappraisal items were added up to yield a single cognitive reappraisal scores (40, 41). The Chinese version of the ERQ shows good internal consistency, adequate validity in Chinese individuals. In the present study, the Cronbach's alpha coefficients for the expressive suppression and the cognitive reappraisal were 0.752 and 0.857, respectively.

### Internet Addiction

Young's Diagnostic Questionnaire for Internet Addiction (YDQ) was applied to assess Internet addiction (42). The YDQ was modified according to the DSM-IV criteria for pathological gambling and consists of eight "yes" or "no" questions. The total score of the eight items ranged from 0 to 8, which also showed good reliability and validity in Chinese adolescents. Cronbach's alpha was 0.771 in this study.

## Data Analysis

First, we conducted descriptive statistics, Student's *t*-test, correlation analyses using SPSS Statistics version 23 (IBM, Armonk, NY). Next, Amos 21.0 was adopted to examine the hypothesized models. Structural equation modeling (SEM) was performed to test the mediating role of negative emotions in the relationships among expressive suppression, cognitive reappraisal and Internet addiction. Specially, The SEM analysis was conducted in two steps. Firstly, we tested the measurement model to examine whether the observed variables were properly chosen for the indicators of the latent variables. Secondly, we tested the structural model to examine the proposed associations among the latent variables. Indirect effects were also calculated using bias-corrected bootstrapping (5,000 bootstrap samples) with 95% confidence intervals (CIs) (43). The 95% CIs not including zero shows a significant effect. Furthermore, to assess the structural equivalence across gender and developmental stages, two multi-group (by adolescent gender or developmental stages of adolescents) SEMs were performed.

In the present study, several goodness-of-fit indices were adopted to assess the model-data fit. The first one was the Chi-square statistic and its associated $p$ value. If the $p$ value is not significant, it may show good model-data fit. However, the Chi-square statistic is sensitive to sample size (44). Therefore, we adopted the Chi-square to degrees of freedom ratio ($\chi^2$/df) to assess the model fit. A $\chi^2$/df ratio of $<3$ indicated a good model fit. Other substitutive indices were also used in the current study, including the Tucker-Lewis Index (TLI) (45), the comparative fit index (CFI) (46), the standardized root mean square residual (SRMR) (47), and the root mean square error of approximation (RMSEA) (48). A TLI and CFI larger than 0.95 and a SRMR and RMSEA $<0.08$ show good model fit (48). For the comparison of the nested models, differences in the $\chi^2$ ($\Delta\chi^2$) and the degree of freedom ($\Delta$df) were employed to compare the models with the goodness of fit to test the model that best fit the data (49, 50). Specifically, the standard of comparison between the two nested models is as follows: when the degrees of freedom increase with a significant increase in the corresponding Chi-square value (that is, $\Delta\chi^2/\Delta$df is significant), the better model is the one with a smaller degrees of freedom. Otherwise, the larger degrees of freedom model are better. The predictive and explanatory powers of the model were assessed using path coefficients and $R^2$.

## RESULTS

### Descriptive Statistics and *t*-Tests

The characteristics of the participants and the distribution of Interent addiction are shown in **Table 1**. The average age of the adolescents in the current study was 14.59 (SD = 1.50) years, and the age range was 12 to 18 years; the study included 332 boys (48.1%) and 358 girls (51.9%). According to the standard definition of Interent addiction, the prevalence of Interent addiction was 10.72% ($n$ = 74) among the adolescent internet users in this study. There were no gender differences in expressive suppression, cognitive reappraisal, Internet addiction, while depression and anxiety yielded significant gender differences. Compared with boys, girls had higher scores on the depression and anxiety scales. Forthermore, there were no developmental stages differences in expressive suppression, cognitive reappraisal, and Internet addiction, while depression and anxiety yielded significant developmental stages differences. High school students showed higher level of depression and anxiety than the junior high school students (**Table 1**).

### Correlation Analysis

For all participants, expressive suppression was significantly positively related to depression, anxiety and Interent addiction ($r = 0.298$, $p < 0.001$, $r = 0.309$, $p < 0.001$, $r = 0.08$, $p <$ 0.05, respectively), while cognitive reappraisal was significantly negatively associated with depression, anxiety and Internet addiction ($r = -0.243$, $p < 0.001$ and $r = -0.219$, $p < 0.001$, $r = -0.180$, $p < 0.001$, respectively). In addition, depression and anxiety were significantly correlated to Internet addiction ($r = 0.332$, $p < 0.001$ and $r = 0.323$, $p < 0.001$, respectively) (**Table 2**).

### Mediational Model Analysis

Firstly, the hypothesized measurement model contained 20 observed variables and five latent variables: expression suppression, cognitive reappraisal, depression, anxiety and Internet addiction (**Figure 1**). Depression and anxiety were loaded on the latent variable of negative emotion, while other all items were loaded on their corresponding latent variables in the measurement model. For example, the total eight items in the YDQ were loaded on the latent variable of Internet addiction. The measurement model was a good fit to the data, ($\chi^2 = 275.551$, $\chi^2/df = 1.680$, TLI = 0.969, CFI = 0.974, SRMR = 0.038, RMSEA = 0.032). The indicators loaded well-onto each latent variable with standardized factor loadings ranging from 0.470 to 0.903. When evaluating the structural model, we analyzed the significance of the entire model as well as the significance of the relationship and variances among the multiple factors in the model. According to the fit standards, our model fits well with the empirical data ($\chi^2 = 275.551$, $\chi^2/df = 1.680$, TLI = 0.969, CFI = 0.974, SRMR = 0.038, RMSEA = 0.032). Expression suppression had no significant direct effect on Internet addiction ($\beta = -0.071$, $p > 0.05$), while cognitive reappraisal had a significantly negative direct effect on Internet addiction ($\beta = -0.118$, $p < 0.05$). Furthermore, negative emotions mediated the relationships between expression suppression and Internet addiction [$\beta = 0.149$, 95% CI = (0.099, 0.212)]. In addition, negative emotions also mediated the associations between cognitive reappraisal and Internet addiction [$\beta = -0.101$, 95% CI = (−0.147, −0.065)]. Finally, we found that 17.2% variance of Internet addiction could be explained by this model.

### Structural Invariance of the Mediated Model Analysis

To assess the structural invariance of the mediated model across gender and developmental stages of adolescents, two nested models were estimated, respectively. The first model allowed the structure coefficient of the two models to be estimated freely according to gender, while the second model was conducted for the structure path coefficients to be equal. The results found that these two models were not significantly different, $\Delta\chi^2[(5), N = 676] = 7.012$, $p = 0.220$, indicating that they were not differed according to gender. In addition, the first model allowed the structure coefficient of the two models to be estimated freely according to the developmental stages of adolescents, while the second model was conducted for the structure path coefficients to be equal. The results found that these two models were also not significantly different, $\Delta\chi^2[(5), N = 676] = 18.058$, $p = 0.003$, indicating that they differed according to the developmental stages of adolescents. In addition, we utilized critical ratios of differences (CRDs) as an index to examine the differences in the structure path coefficients between junior high school students and high school students. If the CRD was larger than 1.96, then the associations between these two variables would demonstrate a significant developmental stages difference as $p < 0.05$. First, the results showed that the structure path from cognitive reappraisal to negative emotions revealed a significant developmental stages difference (CRD = −2.065, $P < 0.05$). More specifically, first, the path coefficient for junior high school students was $\beta = -0.23$, $p < 0.01$, while the path coefficient for high school students was $\beta = -0.35$, $p < 0.01$. Therefore, cognitive reappraisal had a far greater protective role against the negative emotions among high school students than junior high school students. Second, the results showed that the structure path from negative emotions to Internet addiction revealed a significant developmental stages difference (CRD = 3.057, $P < 0.001$). More specifically, the path coefficient for junior high school students was $\beta = 0.28$, $p < 0.01$, while the path coefficient for high school students was $\beta = 0.70$, $p < 0.001$. Therefore, negative emotions had a far greater prediction to Internet addiction among high school students than junior high school students. Finally, the results showed that the structure path from cognitive reappraisal to Internet addiction revealed a significant developmental stages difference (CRD = 2.711, $p < 0.01$). More specifically, the path coefficient for junior high school students was $\beta = -0.19$, $p < 0.01$, while the path coefficient for high school students was $\beta = 0.11$, $p > 0.05$. Therefore, cognitive reappraisal had a far greater direct prediction to Internet addiction among junior high school students than high school students. Thus, there were the

**TABLE 1** | Descriptive statistics among the variables.

| Variables | Gender | | | | | Developmental stage of adolescents | | | | |
|---|---|---|---|---|---|---|---|---|---|---|
| | Girls ($N$ = 358) | | Boys ($N$ = 332) | | $t$ | Junior high school students ($N$ = 504) | | High school students ($N$ = 186) | | $t$ |
| | Mean | SD | Mean | SD | | Mean | SD | Mean | SD | |
| Expressive suppression | 15.20 | 4.77 | 14.97 | 4.73 | 0.65 | 14.99 | 4.94 | 15.35 | 4.20 | −0.95 |
| Cognitive reappraisal | 29.08 | 5.92 | 28.71 | 6.74 | 0.77 | 29.00 | 6.47 | 28.63 | 5.93 | 0.69 |
| Depression | 6.36 | 6.13 | 4.69 | 5.16 | 3.87** | 5.09 | 5.57 | 6.83 | 6.02 | −3.58** |
| Anxiety | 6.19 | 5.11 | 4.92 | 4.56 | 3.43** | 5.29 | 4.80 | 6.34 | 5.06 | −2.51* |
| Internet addiction | 1.65 | 2.38 | 1.72 | 2.71 | −0.40 | 1.65 | 2.58 | 1.77 | 2.45 | −0.54 |

*$p < 0.05$; **$p < 0.01$.

**TABLE 2** | Correlation among the main variables for all sample.

| | Range | Mean + SD | 1 | 2 | 3 | 4 | 5 |
|---|---|---|---|---|---|---|---|
| 1. Expressive suppression | 4–28 | 15.09 ± 4.75 | – | | | | |
| 2. Cognitive reappraisal | 6–42 | 28.91 ± 6.32 | −0.003 | – | | | |
| 3. Depression | 0–27 | 5.56 ± 5.74 | 0.298*** | −0.243*** | – | | |
| 4. Anxiety | 0–21 | 5.58 ± 4.89 | 0.309*** | −.219*** | 0.804*** | – | |
| Internet addiction | 0–8 | 1.85 ± 2.01 | 0.080* | −0.180*** | 0.332*** | 0.323*** | – |

*$p < 0.05$; ***$p < 0.001$.

structural invariance of the mediated model across gender, while the developmental stages of adolescents played the moderating effects in the structural paths in the mediated model.

# DISCUSSION

## Gender and Age Differences

Our study showed that symptoms of depression and anxiety were significantly more common in girls than in boys. This result is consistent with most previous studies that female sex may be a risk factor for depression and anxiety (51). Among adolescents, the high school students showed significantly higher levels of depression and anxiety symptoms than junior school students, which may be related to more academic pressure, as well as emotional problems linked with physical and mental development.

## Correlation Among Main Variables

Expressive suppression showed significant positive correlation with depression, anxiety and Internet addiction. Depression and anxiety are highly comorbid, which is broadly characterized by an overreliance on expressive suppression. Previous researched also supported that expressive suppression was associated with negative emotion consequences (52). Negative emotion of depression and anxiety is also characterized by ineffective utilization of cognitive reappraisal, which inhibits the potential positive emotion. Similar with previous researches, cognitive reappraisal showed negative correlation to depression and anxiety (53, 54). The high school students may suffer from stressful or uncontrollable situations, due to underutilization of cognitive reappraisal. For negative emotion, treatment intervention may appear to increase cognitive reappraisal but decrease expressive suppression. In addition, expressive suppression was negative correlated with Internet addiction, but cognitive reappraisal was positively correlated with Internet addiction. The results were consistent with related research that emotion dysregulation may be a potential risk factor for Internet addiction (55). Because of the outbreak of COVID-19, adolescence may also have troubles, for example, lack of social communication, lack of peer communication and academic pressure. However, there are some difficulties in emotion regulation among some adolescents, which may enhance the negative emotion. Negative emotions may lead to externalized behaviors, such as Internet addiction. Therefore, dysregulated negative emotions in adolescents may be a risk factor for psychopathology, but appropriate emotion regulation strategy may be a protective factor for psychopathology (56).

## Mediating Effect of Negative Emotion

This study demonstrated that expressive suppression couldn't predict Interent addiction directly, cognitive reappraisal could predict Internet addiction directly. Negative emotion of depression and anxiety conducted mediating variables between emotional regulation and Interent addiction. On the one hand, similar to previous research, negative emotion was the partial mediating factor between cognitive reappraisal and Interent addiction (57–59). Negative emotion are important mechanisms in the relationship between emotional regulation and Interent addiction. The higher the score of cognitive reappraisal corresponded to the lower the negative emotion and the less the Interent addiction. On the other hand, depression and anxiety were also completely mediating factor between expressive

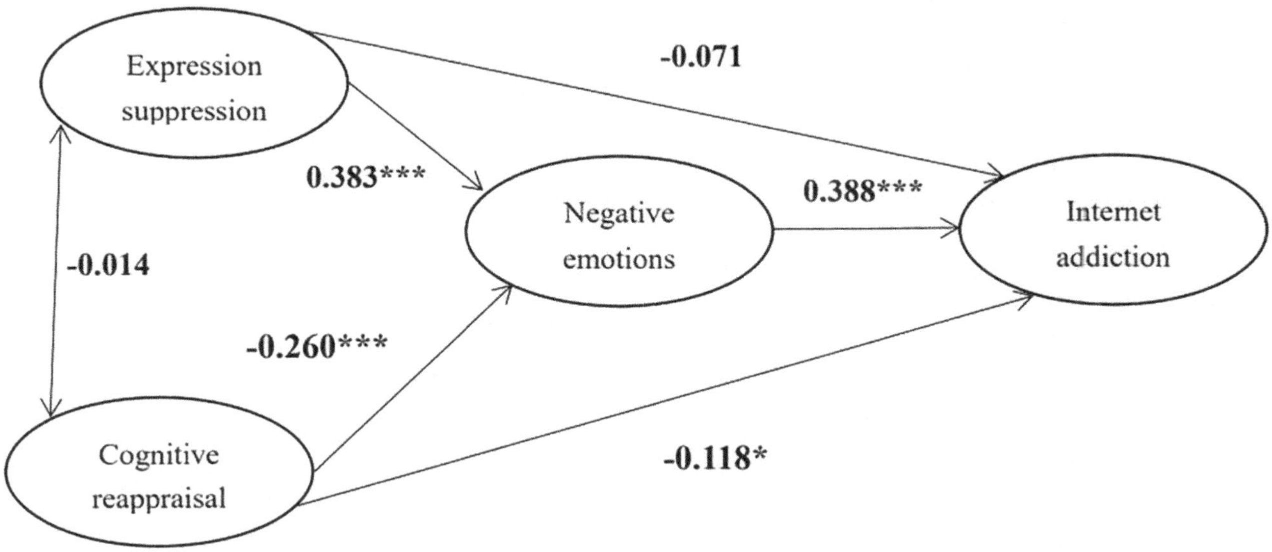


**FIGURE 1** | Standardized estimates of the mediated model. $^{*}p < 0.05$; $^{***}p < 0.001$.

suppression and Interent addiction. The higher the score of expressive suppression predicted the higher the negative emotion and the more the Interent addiction. Cognitive reappraisal allows individuals to reframe negative emotional situations and reassess emotional events, which enables them to have better adaptability to negative situations, and to gain more control (23). Expressive suppression is a negative coping style, which may enhance negative emotional experience, leading to deterioration of self-control, cognitive bias, and maladaptive behavior problems (24). At the same time, expressive suppression may also be harmful for an individual's social functioning and reduce the acquisition of social support (60, 61). For younger adolescents, there are a lot of social support from parents, teachers, friends and so on. Compared with older adolescents, they also confront with less academy stress. This study demonstrated that expressive suppression may be not the important mediating role between negative emotions and internet. Adolescents may still be more inclined to express their emotions rather than over restrain them. Cognitive reappraisal could be beneficial in enabling individuals to distinguish negative emotions, experience lower emotional intensity, and adopt more and various emotional regulation strategies. Research has shown that cognitive reappraisal reduced not only emotional experience but also bilateral amygdala activation (62).

## Invariance of the Model

To determine whether both different genders and different development stages of adolescents are applicable in the models, an invariance study of the structural models was conducted. The results showed that structural invariance across gender was accepted, but the invariance across different development stages of adolescents was not established. The structure models could be suitable for both boys and girls. Previous studies revealed that over-suppression of negative emotion may be harmful to the relief of negative emotions and lead to more behavioral problems and physical diseases, especially in females (63, 64). In our study, almost of adolescents are in the early stage of adolescents, psychological and behavioral differences between boys and girls haven't appeared particularly significance. With the development of adolescents, the differences may be more and more significant. As a result of social expectations, males are less likely to express themselves when they are faced with depression and anxiety, but are more willing to take on negative emotions and deal with bad situations by themselves.

According to invariance across different development stage of adolescents, the structure models couldn't also suitable for different stages of adolescents. Compared with junior high school students, cognitive reappraisal could be more protective factors for negative emotion of depression and anxiety among high school students. With the development of adolescents, cognitive function gradually improved, high school students could be better at cognitive reappraisal than junior high school students (65). The cognitive-affective process suggested that the improvement of cognitive level may be beneficial to the improvement of negative emotional experience. Similar with previous studies, anxiety and depression positively predicted Internet addiction of adolescents (15). However, negative emotion of high school students could be more effectively predicting roles in Internet addiction than junior high school students. Compared with junior high school students, high school students have more academic pressure, which is associated with more negative emotions. Finally, cognitive reappraisal is more effective in predicting Internet addiction of junior high school students. Related studies have demonstrated that emotion dysregulation is risk factors for Internet addiction. More students. Related studies have demonstrated that emotion dysregulation is risk factors for Internet addiction. More cognitive reappraisal predicted greater reduction in negative emotion (66).

## Conclusion

According to cognitive behavior theory, emotional regulation plays important roles in Internet addiction. The way of emotion regulation affects emotional experience, which directly positively predicts Internet addiction. In this study, expressive suppression was a risk factor of negative emotion and Internet addiction, while expressive reappraisal was a protective factor of negative emotion and Internet addiction. Expressive suppression affects Internet addiction through negative emotions, while cognitive reappraisal affects Internet addiction directly. At the same time, there are some differences in the path coefficient of the model among the different development stages of high school students. This found reminds that psychological intervention should consider emotional regulation and negative emotion, but also development stages of adolescents.

## LIMITATIONS AND IMPLICATIONS

Longitudinal study may be more beneficial to explore the psychological development mechanism between negative emotions and Interent addiction. Insufficient of older adolescents may affect this invariance of age, we should increase the sample of older adolescents in the future. According to the result, relief of depression and anxiety could be main intervention strategies to decrease Interent addiction for adolescent. In addition, cognitive reappraisal should be benefit for reducing of Interent addiction, which played a positive mediating role between depression, anxiety and Interent addiction.

## AUTHOR CONTRIBUTIONS

LL carried out experiments, conducted the statistical analysis, and wrote the manuscript. MZ, JD, and ML conducted data collection work and revised the manuscript. YZ designed experiments and critically reviewed the manuscript. All authors contributed to the article and approved the submitted version.

## REFERENCES


1. Alaca N. The impact of internet addiction on depression, physical activity level and trigger point sensitivity in Turkish university students. *J Back Musculoskelet Rehabil.* (2020) 33:623–30. doi: 10.3233/BMR-171045
2. Lam LT. The roles of parent-and-child mental health and parental internet addiction in adolescent internet addiction: does a parent-and-child gender match matter? *Front Public Health.* (2020) 8:142. doi: 10.3389/fpubh.2020.00142
3. Fossion P, Antonetti S, Lays C. Internet: abuse, addiction and benefits. *Rev Med Brux.* (2018) 39:250–4.
4. Lu L, Jian SY, Dong M, Gao J, Zhang TT., Chen XQ, et al. Childhood trauma and suicidal ideation among chinese university students: the mediating effect of internet addiction and school bullying victimisation. *Epidemiol Psychiatr Sci.* (2020) 29:108. doi: 10.1017/S2045796020000682
5. Block JJ. Issues for DSM-V: internet addiction. *Am J Psychiat.* (2008) 165:306–7. doi: 10.1176/appi.ajp.2007.07101556
6. Dong B, Zhao F, Wu XS, Wang WJ, Li YF, Zhang ZH, et al. Social anxiety may modify the relationship between internet addiction and its determining factors in chinese adolescents. *Int J Mental Health Addict.* (2019) 17:1508–20. doi: 10.1007/s11469-018-9912-x
7. Drach RD, Orloff NC, Hormes JM. The emotion regulatory function of online social networking: preliminary experimental evidence. *Addict Behav.* (2020) 112:106559. doi: 10.1016/j.addbeh.2020.106559
8. Yeh YC, Ko HC, Wu JY, Cheng CP. Gender differences in relationships of actual and virtual social support to internet addiction mediated through depressive symptoms among college students in Taiwan. *Cyberpsychol Behav.* (2008) 11:485–7. doi: 10.1089/cpb.2007.0134
9. Marusak HA, Thomason ME, Sala-Hamrick K, Crespo L, Rabinak CA. What's parenting got to do with it: emotional autonomy and brain and behavioral responses to emotional conflict in children and adolescents. *Dev Sci.* (2018) 21:e12605. doi: 10.1111/desc.12605
10. Cardenas SD, Vergara KA, Simancas-Pallares M. Internet addiction and academic performance in dental students. *Rev Colomb Psiquiatr.* (2019) 48:198–207. doi: 10.1016/j.rcpeng.2018.03.009
11. Simcharoen S, Pinyopornpanish M, Haoprom P, Kuntawong P, Wongpakaran N, Wongpakaran T. Prevalence, associated factors and impact of loneliness and interpersonal problems on internet addiction: a study in chiang mai medical students. *Asian J Psychiatr.* (2018) 31:2–7. doi: 10.1016/j.ajp.2017.12.017
12. Copello A, Templeton L, Orford J, Velleman R, Patel A, Moore L, et al. The relative efficacy of two levels of a primary care intervention for family members affected by the addiction problem of a close relative: a randomized trial. *Addiction.* (2009) 104:49–58. doi: 10.1111/j.1360-0443.2008.02417.x
13. Gao T, Li M, Hu Y, Qin Z, Cao R, Mei S, et al. When adolescents face both internet addiction and mood symptoms: a crosssectional study of comorbidity and its predictors. *Psychiatr Res.* (2020) 284. doi: 10.1016/j.psychres.2020.112795. [Epub ahead of print].
14. Seki T, Hamazaki K, Natori T, Inadera H. Relationship between internet addiction and depression among Japanese university students. *J Affect Disord.* (2019) 256:668–72. doi: 10.1016/j.jad.2019.06.055
15. Li G, Hou G, Yang D, Jian H, Wang W. Relationship between anxiety, depression, sex, obesity, and internet addiction in chinese adolescents: a short-term longitudinal study. *Addict Behav.* (2019) 90:421–7. doi: 10.1016/j.addbeh.2018.12.009
16. Santos VA, Freire R, Zugliani M, Cirillo P, Santos HH, Nardi AE, et al. Treatment of internet addiction with anxiety disorders: treatment protocol and preliminary before-after results involving pharmacotherapy and modified cognitive behavioral therapy. *JMIR Res Protoc.* (2016) 5:e46. doi: 10.2196/resprot.5278
17. Zhang YY, Chen JJ, Ye H, Volantin L. Psychological effects of cognitive behavioral therapy on internet addiction in adolescents: a systematic review protocol. *Medicine.* (2020) 99:e18456. doi: 10.1097/MD.0000000000018456
18. Scimeca G, Bruno A, Cava L, Pandolfo G, Muscatello MR, Zoccali R. The relationship between alexithymia, anxiety, depression, and internet addiction severity in a sample of Italian high school students. *Sci World J.* (2014) 2014:504376. doi: 10.1155/2014/504376
19. Herbert JD, Gaudiano BA, Forman EM. The importance of theory in cognitive behavior therapy: a perspective of contextual behavioral science. *Behav Ther.* (2013) 44:580–91. doi: 10.1016/j.beth.2013.03.001
20. Kim S, Noh D. The current status of psychological intervention research for internet addiction and internet gaming disorder. *Issues Ment Health Nurs.* (2019) 40:335–41. doi: 10.1080/01612840.2018.1534910
21. King DL, Delfabbro PH, Griffiths MD, Gradisar M. Cognitive-behavioral approaches to outpatient treatment of internet addiction in children and adolescents. *J Clin Psychol.* (2012) 68:1185–95. doi: 10.1002/jclp.21918
22. Tsai JK, Lu WH, Hsiao RC, Hu HF, Yen CF. Relationship between difficulty in emotion regulation and internet addiction in college students: a one-year prospective study. *Int J Environ Res Public Health.* (2020) 17:1–11. doi: 10.3390/ijerph17134766

23. Gross JJ, John OP. Individual differences in two emotion regulation processes: implications for affect, relationships, and well-being. *J Pers Soc Psychol.* (2003) 85:348–62. doi: 10.1037/0022-3514.85.2.348
24. Gross JJ, Levenson RW. Emotional suppression: physiology, self-report, and expressive behavior. *J Pers Soc Psychol.* (1993) 64:970–86. doi: 10.1037/0022-3514.64.6.970
25. Karaer Y, Akdemir D. Parenting styles, perceived social support and emotion regulation in adolescents with internet addiction. *Compr Psychiatry.* (2019) 92:22–7. doi: 10.1016/j.comppsych.2019.03.003
26. Hormes JM, Kearns B, Timko CA. Craving facebook? Behavioral addiction to online social networking and its association with emotion regulation deficits. *Addiction.* (2014) 109:2079–88. doi: 10.1111/add.12713
27. Senormanci O, Saracli O, Atasoy N, Senormanci G, Kokturk F, Atik L. Relationship of internet addiction with cognitive style, personality, and depression in university students. *Compr Psychiatry.* (2014) 55:1385–90. doi: 10.1016/j.comppsych.2014.04.025
28. Yucens B, Uzer A. The relationship between internet addiction, social anxiety, impulsivity, self-esteem, and depression in a sample of Turkish undergraduate medical students. *Psychiatry Res.* (2018) 267:313–8. doi: 10.1016/j.psychres.2018.06.033
29. Duan L, Shao X, Wang Y, Huang Y, Miao J, Yang X, et al. An investigation of mental health status of children and adolescents in china during the outbreak of COVID-19. *J Affect Disord.* (2020) 275:112–8. doi: 10.1016/j.jad.2020.06.029
30. Jeonga B, Lee JY, Kim BM, Park E, Kwon JG, Kim DJ, et al. Associations of personality and clinical characteristics with excessive internet and smartphone use in adolescents: a structural equation modeling approach. *Addict Behav.* (2020) 110. doi: 10.1016/j.addbeh.2020.106485. [Epub ahead of print].
31. Zhai B, Li D, Li X, Liu Y, Zhang J, Sun W, et al. Perceived school climate and problematic internet use among adolescents: mediating roles of school belonging and depressive symptoms. *Addict Behav.* (2020) 110. doi: 10.1016/j.addbeh.2020.106501. [Epub ahead of print].
32. Hsieh KY, Hsiao RC, Yang YH, Liu TL, Yen CF. Predictive effects of sex, age, depression, and problematic behaviors on the incidence and remission of internet addiction in college students: a prospective study. *Int J Environ Res Public Health.* (2018) 15: 1–10. doi: 10.3390/ijerph15122861
33. Jang MH, Ji ES. Gender differences in associations between parental problem drinking and early adolescents' internet addiction. *J Spec Pediatr Nurs.* (2012) 17:288–300. doi: 10.1111/j.1744-6155.2012.00344.x
34. Li Q, Dai W, Zhong Y, Wang L, Dai B, Liu X. The mediating role of coping styles on impulsivity, behavioral inhibition/approach system, and internet addiction in adolescents from a gender perspective. *Front Psychol.* (2019) 10:2402. doi: 10.3389/fpsyg.2019.02402
35. Chi X, Liu X, Guo T, Wu M, Chen X. Internet addiction and depression in chinese adolescents: a moderated mediation model. *Front Psychiatry.* (2019) 10:816. doi: 10.3389/fpsyt.2019.00816
36. Kim K, Ryu E, Chon MY, Yeun EJ, Choi SY, Seo JS, et al. Internet addiction in Korean adolescents and its relation to depression and suicidal ideation: a questionnaire survey. *Int J Nurs Stud.* (2006) 43:185–92. doi: 10.1016/j.ijnurstu.2005.02.005
37. Lai J, Ma S, Wang Y, Cai Z, Hu J, Wei N, et al. Factors associated with mental health outcomes among health care workers exposed to coronavirus disease 2019. *JAMA Netw Open.* (2020) 3:e203976. doi: 10.1001/jamanetworkopen.2020.3976
38. Bartolo A, Monteiro S, Pereira A. Factor structure and construct validity of the generalized anxiety disorder 7-item (GAD-7) among portuguese college students. *Cad Saude Publica.* (2017) 33:e00212716. doi: 10.1590/0102-311x00212716
39. Tiirikainen K, Haravuori H, Ranta K, Kaltiala-Heino R, Marttunen M. Psychometric properties of the 7-item generalized anxiety disorder scale (GAD-7) in a large representative sample of Finnish adolescents. *Psychiatry Res.* (2019) 272:30–5. doi: 10.1016/j.psychres.2018.12.004
40. Hutchison AN, Yeung DY, Gerstein LH, Wettersten KB. Psychometric comparison of chinese and english versions of the emotion regulation questionnaire with bilingual Hong Kong chinese students. *Int J Psychol.* (2021) 56:296–303. doi: 10.1002/ijop.12699
41. Liu W, Chen L, Tu X. Chinese adaptation of emotion regulation questionnaire for children and adolescents (ERQ-CCA): a psychometric evaluation in chinese children. *Int J Psychol.* (2017) 52:398–405. doi: 10.1002/ijop.12233
42. Young KS. Internet addiction: the emergence of a new clinical disorder. *Cyberpsychol Behav.* (1998) 1:237–44. doi: 10.1089/cpb.1998.1.237
43. Hayes AF. *Introduction to Mediation, Moderation, and Conditional Process Analysis: A Regression-Based Approach.* New York, NY: Guilford Press (2013).
44. Bollen KA. A new incremental fit index for general structural equation models. *Sociol Meth Res.* (1989) 17:303–16. doi: 10.1177/0049124189017003004
45. Tucker LR, Lewis C. A reliability coefficient for maximum likelihood factor analysis. *Psychometrika.* (1973) 38:1–10. doi: 10.1007/BF02291170
46. Rigdon EE. CFI versus RMSEA: a comparison of two fit indexes for structural equation modeling. *Struct Equ Model A Multidis J.* (1996) 3:369–79. doi: 10.1080/10705519609540052
47. Browne MW, Cudeck R. Alternative ways of assessing model fit. In: Bollen KA, Long JS, editors. *Testing Structural Equation Models.* SAGE Focus Editions ed. Newbury Park; Sage Publication (1993). p. 136–62.
48. Hooper D, Coughlan J, Mullen MR. Structural equation modelling: guidelines for determining model fit. *Electron J Bus Res Methods.* (2008) 6:53–60.
49. Heijmans RDH, Pollock DSG, Satorra A. *Scaled and Adjusted Restricted tests in Multi-sample Analysis of Moment Structures. Innovations in Multivariate Statistical Analysis: A Festschrift for Heinz Neudecker.* Boston, MA: Springer US (2000). p. 233–47.
50. Byrne BM, Stewart SM. Teacher's corner: the MACS approach to testing for multigroup invariance of a second-order structure: a walk through the process. structural equation modeling: a multidisciplinary journal. *Struct Equ Model A Multidis J.* (2006) 13:287–321. doi: 10.1207/s15328007sem1302_7
51. Pospos S, Tal I, Iglewicz A, Newton IG, Tai-Seale M, Downs N, et al. Gender differences among medical students, house staff, and faculty physicians at high risk for suicide: a HEAR report. *Dep Anxiety.* (2019) 36:902–20. doi: 10.1002/da.22909
52. Dryman MT, Heimberg RG. Emotion regulation in social anxiety and depression: a systematic review of expressive suppression and cognitive reappraisal. *Clin Psychol Rev.* (2018) 65:17–42. doi: 10.1016/j.cpr.2018.07.004
53. Goldin PR, Ziv M, Jazaieri H, Hahn K, Heimberg R, Gross JJ. Impact of cognitive behavioral therapy for social anxiety disorder on the neural dynamics of cognitive reappraisal of negative self-beliefs: randomized clinical trial. *JAMA Psychiatry.* (2013) 70:1048–56. doi: 10.1001/jamapsychiatry.2013.234
54. Andreotti C, Thigpen JE, Dunn MJ, Watson K, Potts J, Reising MM, et al. Cognitive reappraisal and secondary control coping: associations with working memory, positive and negative affect, and symptoms of anxiety/depression. *Anxiety Stress Coping.* (2013) 26:20–35. doi: 10.1080/10615806.2011.631526
55. Mo PKH, Chan VWY, Chan SW, Lau JTF. The role of social support on emotion dysregulation and internet addiction among chinese adolescents: a structural equation model. *Addict Behav.* (2018) 82:86–93. doi: 10.1016/j.addbeh.2018.01.027
56. Gilbert KE. The neglected role of positive emotion in adolescent psychopathology. *Clin Psychol Rev.* (2012) 32:467–81. doi: 10.1016/j.cpr.2012.05.005
57. Chung MC, Di X, Wan KH. Exploring the interrelationship between alexithymia, defense style, emotional suppression, homicide-related posttraumatic stress disorder and psychiatric co-morbidity. *Psychiatry Res.* (2016) 243:373–81. doi: 10.1016/j.psychres.2016.05.057
58. Ottonello M, Fiabane E, Pistarini C, Spigno P, Torselli E. Difficulties in emotion regulation during rehabilitation for alcohol addiction: correlations with metacognitive beliefs about alcohol use and relapse risk. *Neuropsychiatr Dis Treat.* (2019) 15:2917–25. doi: 10.2147/NDT.S214268
59. Gullone E, Taffe J. The emotion regulation questionnaire for children and adolescents (ERQ-CA): a psychometric evaluation. *Psychol Assess.* (2012) 24:409–17. doi: 10.1037/a0025777
60. Cundiff JM, Jennings JR, Matthews KA. Social stratification and risk for cardiovascular disease: examination of emotional suppression as a pathway to risk. *Pers Soc Psychol Bull.* (2019) 45:1202–15. doi: 10.1177/0146167218808504
61. Chung MC, Symons C, Gilliam J, Kaminski ER. Posttraumatic stress disorder, emotional suppression and psychiatric co-morbidity in patients with chronic idiopathic urticaria: a moderated mediation analysis. *J Ment Health.* (2018) 27:442–9. doi: 10.1080/09638237.2018.1437601
62. Chen S, Chen C, Yang J, Yuan J. Trait self-consciousness predicts amygdala activation and its functional brain connectivity during emotional suppression:

an fMRI analysis. *Sci Rep.* (2017) 7:117. doi: 10.1038/s41598-017-00073-3
63. Brandao T, Schulz MS, Gross JJ, Matos PM. The emotion regulation questionnaire in women with cancer: a psychometric evaluation and an item response theory analysis. *Psychooncology.* (2017) 26:1647–53. doi: 10.1002/pon.4356
64. Baziliansky S, Cohen M. Emotion regulation and psychological distress in cancer survivors: a systematic review and meta-analysis. *Stress Health.* (2021) 37:3–18. doi: 10.1002/smi.2972
65. Li Y, Wang Y, Ren Z, Gao M, Liu Q, Qiu C, et al. The influence of environmental pressure on internet use disorder in adolescents: the potential mediating role of cognitive function. *Addict Behav.* (2020) 101:105976. doi: 10.1016/j.addbeh.2019.04.034
66. Pettorruso M, Valle S, Cavic E, Martinotti G, di Giannantonio M, Grant JE. Problematic internet use (PIU), personality profiles and emotion dysregulation in a cohort of young adults: trajectories from risky behaviors to addiction. *Psychiatry Res.* (2020) 289:113036. doi: 10.1016/j.psychres.2020.113036

# Permissions

All chapters in this book were first published by Frontiers; hereby published with permission under the Creative Commons Attribution License or equivalent. Every chapter published in this book has been scrutinized by our experts. Their significance has been extensively debated. The topics covered herein carry significant findings which will fuel the growth of the discipline. They may even be implemented as practical applications or may be referred to as a beginning point for another development.

The contributors of this book come from diverse backgrounds, making this book a truly international effort. This book will bring forth new frontiers with its revolutionizing research information and detailed analysis of the nascent developments around the world.

We would like to thank all the contributing authors for lending their expertise to make the book truly unique. They have played a crucial role in the development of this book. Without their invaluable contributions this book wouldn't have been possible. They have made vital efforts to compile up to date information on the varied aspects of this subject to make this book a valuable addition to the collection of many professionals and students.

This book was conceptualized with the vision of imparting up-to-date information and advanced data in this field. To ensure the same, a matchless editorial board was set up. Every individual on the board went through rigorous rounds of assessment to prove their worth. After which they invested a large part of their time researching and compiling the most relevant data for our readers.

The editorial board has been involved in producing this book since its inception. They have spent rigorous hours researching and exploring the diverse topics which have resulted in the successful publishing of this book. They have passed on their knowledge of decades through this book. To expedite this challenging task, the publisher supported the team at every step. A small team of assistant editors was also appointed to further simplify the editing procedure and attain best results for the readers.

Apart from the editorial board, the designing team has also invested a significant amount of their time in understanding the subject and creating the most relevant covers. They scrutinized every image to scout for the most suitable representation of the subject and create an appropriate cover for the book.

The publishing team has been an ardent support to the editorial, designing and production team. Their endless efforts to recruit the best for this project, has resulted in the accomplishment of this book. They are a veteran in the field of academics and their pool of knowledge is as vast as their experience in printing. Their expertise and guidance has proved useful at every step. Their uncompromising quality standards have made this book an exceptional effort. Their encouragement from time to time has been an inspiration for everyone.

The publisher and the editorial board hope that this book will prove to be a valuable piece of knowledge for researchers, students, practitioners and scholars across the globe.

# List of Contributors

**Elisa Schroder, Clémence Dousset, Xavier Noel, Charles Kornreich and Salvatore Campanella**
Laboratoire de Psychologie Médicale et d'Addictologie, ULB Neuroscience Institute (UNI), CHU Brugmann-Université Libre de Bruxelles (U.L.B.), Brussels, Belgium

**Samantha V. Abram**
Department of Psychology, University of Minnesota Twin Cities, Minneapolis, MN, United States
Sierra Pacific Mental Illness Research Education and Clinical Centers, San Francisco VA Medical Center, and the University of California, San Francisco, San Francisco, CA, United States

**A. David Redish**
Department of Neuroscience, University of Minnesota Twin Cities, Minneapolis, MN, United States

**Angus W. MacDonald III**
Department of Psychology, University of Minnesota Twin Cities, Minneapolis, MN, United States
Department of Psychiatry, University of Minnesota Twin Cities, Minneapolis, MN, United States

**Kell Grandjean Costa, Daniel Aranha Cabral and Eduardo Bodnariuc Fontes**
NEUROex: Research Group in Physical Activity, Cognition and Behavior, Center of Health Sciences, Federal University of Rio Grande do Norte, Natal, Brazil

**Rodrigo Hohl**
Department of Physiology, Federal University of Juiz de Fora, Juiz de Fora, Brazil

**Serenella Tolomeo**
Department of Psychology, National University of Singapore, Singapore, Singapore
Centre for Family and Population Research, National University of Singapore, Singapore, Singapore

**Fleur Davey**
NHS Fife, Queen Margaret Hospital, Dunfermline, United Kingdom

**J. Douglas Steele**
School of Medicine, University of Dundee, Ninewells Hospital and Medical School, Dundee, United Kingdom

**Alexander Mario Baldacchino**
School of Medicine, University of Dundee, Ninewells Hospital and Medical School, Dundee, United Kingdom
Division of Population and Behavioural Science, Medical School, University of St Andrews, St Andrews, United Kingdom

**Limin Chen, Shuai Wang, Jun Wang, Lin Tian, Hongmei Zhu and Zhenhe Zhou**
Wuxi Mental Health Center, Wuxi, China

**Hongliang Zhou**
Nanjing Brain Hospital Affiliated to Nanjing Medical University, Wuxi, China

**Yue Gu**
Basic Medicine College of Nanjing Medical University, Nanjing, China

**Tonisha E. Kearney-Ramos**
Division on Substance Use Disorders, Columbia University Irving Medical Center, New York, NY, United States

**Oliver J. Mithoefer and William Devries**
Department of Psychiatry, Medical University of South Carolina, Charleston, SC, United States

**Logan T. Dowdle**
Department of Psychiatry, Medical University of South Carolina, Charleston, SC, United States
Department of Neurosciences, Medical University of South Carolina, Charleston, SC, United States

**Colleen A. Hanlon**
Department of Psychiatry, Medical University of South Carolina, Charleston, SC, United States
Department of Neurosciences, Medical University of South Carolina, Charleston, SC, United States
Center for Biomedical Imaging, Medical University of South Carolina, Charleston, SC, United States

**Mark S. George**
Department of Psychiatry, Medical University of South Carolina, Charleston, SC, United States
Department of Neurosciences, Medical University of South Carolina, Charleston, SC, United States
Center for Biomedical Imaging, Medical University of South Carolina, Charleston, SC, United States
Ralph S. Johnson VA Medical Center, Charleston, SC, United States

**Manoranjan S. D'Souza**
Department of Pharmaceutical and Biomedical Sciences, The Raabe College of Pharmacy, Ohio Northern University, Ada, OH, United States

**Meredith Halcomb**
Department of Radiology and Imaging Sciences, Indiana University School of Medicine Indianapolis, Indianapolis, IN, United States

**Evangelia Argyriou and Melissa A. Cyders**
Department of Psychology, Indiana University–Purdue University, Indianapolis, IN, United States

**Marsha E. Bates and Jennifer F. Buckman**
Cardiac Neuroscience Laboratory, Department of Kinesiology and Health, Rutgers University-New Brunswick, Piscataway, NJ, United States
Center of Alcohol Studies, Rutgers University-New Brunswick, Piscataway, NJ, United States

**Laura M. Lesnewich and Sarah Grace Uhouse**
Center of Alcohol Studies, Rutgers University-New Brunswick, Piscataway, NJ, United States
Cardiac Neuroscience Laboratory, Department of Psychology, Rutgers University-New Brunswick, Piscataway, NJ, United States

**Suril Gohel**
Department of Health Informatics, School of Health Professions, Rutgers University-Newark, Newark, NJ, United States

**Kevin Butler**
Translational Addiction Research Laboratory, Centre for Addiction and Mental Health, University of Toronto, Toronto, ON, Canada

**Bernard Le Foll**
Translational Addiction Research Laboratory, Centre for Addiction and Mental Health, University of Toronto, Toronto, ON, Canada
Alcohol Research and Treatment Clinic, Acute Care Program, Centre for Addiction and Mental Health, Toronto, ON, Canada
Campbell Family Mental Health Research Institute, Centre for Addiction and Mental Health, Toronto, ON, Canada
Department of Family and Community Medicine, University of Toronto, Toronto, ON, Canada
Department of Pharmacology and Toxicology, University of Toronto, Toronto, ON, Canada
Division of Brain and Therapeutics, Department of Psychiatry, University of Toronto, Toronto, ON, Canada
Institute of Medical Sciences, University of Toronto, Toronto, ON, Canada

**Nicole J. Roberts, Briana N. Sprague and Charles F. Geier**
Department of Human Development and Family Studies, The Pennsylvania State University, University Park, PA, United States

**Zita Oravecz**
Department of Human Development and Family Studies, The Pennsylvania State University, University Park, PA, United States
Institute for CyberScience, The Pennsylvania State University, University Park, PA, United States

**Jamie A. Burns, Danielle S. Kroll, Dana E. Feldman, Christopher Kure Liu, Peter Manza, Corinde E. Wiers and Gene-Jack Wang**
National Institute on Alcohol Abuse and Alcoholism, Bethesda, MD, United States

**Nora D. Volkow**
National Institute on Alcohol Abuse and Alcoholism, Bethesda, MD, United States
National Institute on Drug Abuse, Bethesda, MD, United States

**Matthias Vonmoos, Katrin H. Preller and Lea M. Hulka**
Experimental and Clinical Pharmacopsychology, Department of Psychiatry, Psychotherapy and Psychosomatics, Psychiatric Hospital of the University of Zurich, Zurich, Switzerland

**Christoph Eisenegger**
Neuropsychopharmacology and Biopsychology Unit, Department of Basic Psychological Research and Research Methods, Faculty of Psychology, University of Vienna, Vienna, Austria

**Oliver G. Bosch**
Experimental and Clinical Pharmacopsychology, Department of Psychiatry, Psychotherapy and Psychosomatics, Psychiatric Hospital of the University of Zurich, Zurich, Switzerland
Department of Psychiatry, Psychotherapy and Psychosomatics, Psychiatric Hospital of the University of Zurich, Zurich, Switzerland

**Erich Seifritz**
Department of Psychiatry, Psychotherapy and Psychosomatics, Psychiatric Hospital of the University of Zurich, Zurich, Switzerland
Neuroscience Center Zurich, University and ETH Zurich, Zurich, Switzerland

**Markus Baumgartner**
Center of Forensic Hairanalytics, Institute of Forensic Medicine, University of Zurich, Zurich, Switzerland

**Boris B. Quednow**
Experimental and Clinical Pharmacopsychology, Department of Psychiatry, Psychotherapy and Psychosomatics, Psychiatric Hospital of the University of Zurich, Zurich, Switzerland
Neuroscience Center Zurich, University and ETH Zurich, Zurich, Switzerland

**Christos Kouimtsidis, Emily Palmer and Anne Lingford-Hughes**
Centre for Psychiatry, Imperial College London, London, United Kingdom

**Theodora Duka**
Sussex Addiction Research and Intervention Centre (SARIC), School of Psychology, University of Sussex, Brighton, United Kingdom

**Junjie Bu**
Department of Radiology, The First Affiliated Hospital of USTC, Hefei National Laboratory for Physical Sciences at the Microscale and School of Life Science, Division of Life Science and Medicine, University of Science and Technology of China, Hefei, China
Department of Intelligent Medical Engineering, School of Biomedical Engineering, Anhui Medical University, Hefei, China

**Chang Liu, Huixing Gou, Ginger Qinghong Zeng and Hefan Gan**
Department of Radiology, The First Affiliated Hospital of USTC, Hefei National Laboratory for Physical Sciences at the Microscale and School of Life Science, Division of Life Science and Medicine, University of Science and Technology of China, Hefei, China

**Zhen Liang**
Department of Intelligent Medical Engineering, School of Biomedical Engineering, Anhui Medical University, Hefei, China

**Zhenlei Xiao**
Hengshui University, Hengshui, China

**Jianhao Huang**
Dhurakij Pundit University, Bangkok, Thailand

**Yan Cheng and Mengyuan Liu**
Department of Psychology, School of Humanities and Social Science, University of Science and Technology of China, Hefei, China

**Rui Ni**
Department of Life Sciences, Imperial College London, London, United Kingdom

**Guanbao Cui**
Institute of Advanced Technology, University of Science and Technology of China, Hefei, China

**Xiaochu Zhang**
Department of Radiology, The First Affiliated Hospital of USTC, Hefei National Laboratory for Physical Sciences at the Microscale and School of Life Science, Division of Life Science and Medicine, University of Science and Technology of China, Hefei, China
Department of Psychology, School of Humanities and Social Science, University of Science and Technology of China, Hefei, China
Institute of Advanced Technology, University of Science and Technology of China, Hefei, China
Hefei Medical Research Center on Alcohol Addiction, Anhui Mental Health Center, Hefei, China
Academy of Psychology and Behavior, Tianjin Normal University, Tianjin, China

**Lijuan Liang**
Department of Psychology, The First Affiliated Hospital, Hainan Medical University, Haikou, China

**Mingrui Zhu**
Department of Neurology, The People's Hospital of Liaoning Province, Shenyang, China

**Jiali Dai**
Daqing No.3 Hospital, Daqing, China

**Min Li**
HeBei Institute of International Business and Economics, Qinghuangdao, China

**Ya Zheng**
Department of Psychology, Dalian Medical University, Dalian, China

# Index

## P



## R



## S



## T



## V



## W